**FOURTH EDITION**

# Handbook of
# Obstetric and
# Gynecologic
# Emergencies

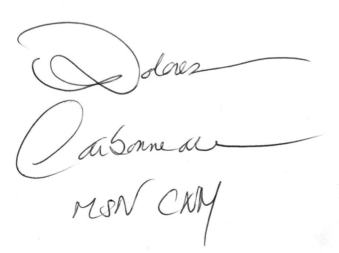

**FOURTH EDITION**

# Handbook of Obstetric and Gynecologic Emergencies

Edited by

## Guy I. Benrubi, MD

Senior Associate Dean for Clinical Affairs
Robert J. Thompson Professor and Chair
Department of Obstetrics and Gynecology
University of Florida College of Medicine-Jacksonville
Jacksonville, Florida

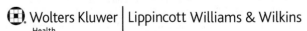
Wolters Kluwer | Lippincott Williams & Wilkins
Health

Philadelphia · Baltimore · New York · London
Buenos Aires · Hong Kong · Sydney · Tokyo

*Acquisitions Editor*: Sonya Seigafuse
*Product Manager*: Nicole Walz
*Senior Manufacturing Manager*: Ben Rivera
*Marketing Manager*: Kimberly Schonberger
*Vendor Manager*: Bridgett Dougherty
*Design Coordinator*: Terry Mallon
*Cover Designer*: Karen Quigley
*Production Services*: SPi Technologies

© 2010 by LIPPINCOTT WILLIAMS & WILKINS, a WOLTERS KLUWER business
© 2005, 2001 by Lippincott Williams & Wilkins
© 1994 by J.B. Lippincott

530 Walnut Street
Philadelphia, PA 19106 USA
LWW.com

Printed in China

**Library of Congress Cataloging-in-Publication Data**
Handbook of obstetric and gynecologic emergencies / edited by Guy I. Benrubi. —4th ed.
   p. ; cm.
   Includes bibliographical references and index.
   ISBN-13: 978-1-60547-666-7 (alk. paper)
   ISBN-10: 1-60547-666-8
   1. Obstetrical emergencies—Handbooks, manuals, etc. 2. Gynecologic emergencies—Handbooks, manuals, etc. I. Benrubi, Guy I.
   [DNLM: 1. Pregnancy Complications—diagnosis. 2. Pregnancy Complications—therapy. 3. Emergencies. 4. Emergency Treatment—methods. 5. Genital Diseases, Female—diagnosis. 6. Genital Diseases, Female—therapy. WQ 240 H2362 2010]

   RG571.O245    2010
   618'.0425—dc22

                                                                                    2009046290

To purchase additional copies of this book, call our customer service department at (800) 638-3030 or fax orders to (301) 223-2320. International customers should call (301) 223-2300.

Visit Lippincott Williams & Wilkins on the Internet: at LWW.com. Lippincott Williams & Wilkins customer service representatives are available from 8:30 am to 6 pm, EST.

CCS0110

*To the memory of*
Michael "Bam Bam" D'Agostino

*"Hi doctor…"*
*"Give me half…"*

*"… Don't put off things till it's too late.*
*You are the DJ of your fate."*

—Vikram Seth
(*The Golden Gate*, 1986)

*después de Purim, platicos*
(loose translation: pointless after the fact)
—Old European Proverb

Physicians are faced, increasingly, with diagnosis and management decisions in obstetric and gynecologic emergency settings. Whether the setting is the emergency department of a busy inner-city hospital or the office of a gynecologist or other primary care provider, an understanding of the pathophysiology and management considerations is critical to good patient care. During the last decade, it has become apparent that a large portion of the young women and children at greatest risk for obstetric and gynecologic emergencies increasingly fall out of the health care system. In several areas of the country, up to 25% of women receive no prenatal care. In other areas, close to 50% of young women have no primary care providers to handle emergencies. Currently, an estimated 50 million US citizens are not medically insured. The increasing demands on the health care dollar and the increasing percentage of care delivered under managed systems create a premium on either no hospitalization or early discharge. Consequently, complications of delivery, as well as of gynecologic surgery, are not recognized until after the patient has left the hospital. To this must be added the effects of the Great Recession, which became evident on health care in mid-2008. Unemployment, underemployment, and loss of health benefits have had a severe impact on preventative care. Even if employed women still have benefits, their deductibles and co-pays have significantly increased. All of these factors result in management being provided in emergent care settings, whether in the hospital or in the office.

This book intends to address the need for a continuing up-to-date understanding of these obstetric and gynecologic emergencies. It seeks its audience among obstetricians, gynecologists, emergency department physicians, family practitioners, and other primary health care providers. The book is organized in two main sections: obstetric emergencies and gynecologic emergencies. Although the organization is along the lines of the traditional major emergencies that occur in these two disciplines, several problems are addressed by multiple authors from different perspectives. It is the editor's belief that additional understanding of the management of these conditions can be gained from divergent points of view. Finally, it must be recognized that obstetric and gynecologic emergencies change over time. What are frequent problems today may become relatively infrequent tomorrow. New challenges face the physician. For example, approximately 80% of women in this country do not have legal abortion services available to them. It is, therefore, probable that physicians will see emergency situations arising from illegal abortions. Additionally, violence has become a pervasive disease in our society; physicians who treat women must be conversant with both clinical and psychological problems that arise from rape and other traumas to the reproductive organs. Tragically, in the 21st century, emergent conditions due to terrorist acts also need to be addressed.

I thank all of the contributors for their excellent work and their diligent, careful, and astute analysis of the issues raised. Thanks are also due to Louise Bierig for her efficiency and editing skills. Special thanks are due to Ms. Georgette Andreason whose technical and organizational expertise cannot be matched and without whom this project would not have been undertaken nor completed.

**Guy I. Benrubi, MD**

**A. Ben Abdu, MD**
Obstetrics and Gynecology
University of Tennessee
  College of Medicine
Chattanooga, Tennessee

**C. David Adair, MD**
Professor and Vice Chair
Department of Obstetrics
  and Gynecology
Section on Maternal Fetal Medicine
University of Tennessee
  College of Medicine
Chattanooga, Tennessee

**Pam Adams, RN, EMT-P**
Registered Nurse/Paramedic
President
OB STAT, Inc.
Arden, North Carolina

**Sarah Adams, MD**
Assistant Professor
Division of Gynecologic Oncology
University of Pennsylvania Hospitals
Philadelphia, Pennsylvania

**Kurt Barnhart, MD, MSCE**
Associate Professor of Obstetrics
  and Gynecology
Director, Women's Health Clinical
  Research Center
Assistant Dean for Clinical
  Research Operations
University of Pennsylvania School
  of Medicine
Philadelphia, Pennsylvania

**Paula H. Bednarek, MD, MPH**
Assistant Professor
Department of Obstetrics
  and Gynecology
Oregon Health & Science
  University
Portland, Oregon

**Guy I. Benrubi, MD**
Senior Associate Dean
  for Clinical Affairs
Robert J. Thompson Professor
  and Chair
Department of Obstetrics
  and Gynecology
University of Florida College
  of Medicine-Jacksonville
Jacksonville, Florida

**Kelly A. Best, MD**
Assistant Professor
Associate Residency Program
  Director
Department of Obstetrics
  and Gynecology
University of Florida College
  of Medicine-Jacksonville
Jacksonville, Florida

**Rosanne L. Botha, MD**
Family Planning Fellow
Oregon Health & Science
  University
Portland, Oregon

**David Caro, MD**
Associate Professor
Residency Program Director
Department of Emergency
    Medicine
University of Florida College
    of Medicine-Jacksonville
Jacksonville, Florida

**Joseph G. Cernigliaro, MD**
Assistant Professor of Radiology
Mayo Clinic College of Medicine
Rochester, Minnesota
Consultant, Department
    of Radiology
Mayo Clinic
Jacksonville, Florida

**Stephen A. Contag, MD**
Clinical Instructor Maternal Fetal
    Medicine
Wake Forest University
Winston-Salem, North Carolina

**Isaac Delke, MD**
Professor
Department of Obstetrics
    and Gynecology
University of Florida College
    of Medicine-Jacksonville
Chief, Division of Maternal-Fetal
    Medicine
Director, Obstetrics
Director, HIV in Pregnancy
    Program
Shands Jacksonville Medical
    Center
Jacksonville, Florida

**Charles J. Dunton, MD**
Professor of Obstetrics
    and Gynecology
Jefferson Medical College
Active Staff Physician
Main Line Gynecology
Oncology, Lankenau Hospital
Wynnewood, Pennsylvania

**Alison B. Edelman, MD, MPH**
Associate Professor
Assistant Director, Family
    Planning Fellowship
Department of Obstetrics
    and Gynecology
Oregon Health & Science University
Portland, Oregon

**Gwyn Grabner, RDMS**
Registered Diagnostic Medical
    Sonographer
University of Florida College
    of Medicine-Jacksonville
Jacksonville, Florida

**Victor J. Hassid, MD**
Fellow, Division of Plastic Surgery
University of Illinois College of
    Medicine
Chicago, Illinois

**Linda Hastings, PharmD**
Pediatric Practitioner
Department of Pharmacy
Shands Jacksonville
    Medical Center
Clinical Assistant Professor
University of Florida College
    of Pharmacy
Jacksonville, Florida

**Thanh T. Hogan, PharmD**
Clinical Associate Professor
University of Florida College
    of Pharmacy
Director of Pharmacy
Shands Jacksonville Medical Center
Jacksonville, Florida

**Cheryl B. Iglesia, MD, FACOG**
Director, Section of Female Pelvic
    Medicine and Reconstructive
    Surgery
Washington Hospital Center
Associate Professor,
Georgetown University School
    of Medicine
Washington, District of Columbia

**David C. Jones, MD**
Director, Fetal Diagnostic Center
Fletcher Allen Health Care
Associate Professor of Obstetrics,
Gynecology & Reproductive
Sciences
University of Vermont College
of Medicine
Burlington, Vermont

**James L. Jones, MD, PhD**
Assistant Professor
Department of Obstetrics
and Gynecology
University of Florida College
of Medicine-Jacksonville
Jacksonville, Florida

**Jason Joseph, MD**
Obstetrics and Gynecology
University of Tennessee
College of Medicine
Chattanooga, Tennessee

**Saju D. Joy, MD, MS**
Assistant Professor
Wake Forest University
Baptist Medical Center
Winston-Salem, North Carolina

**Andrew M. Kaunitz, MD**
Professor and Associate
Chairman
Department of Obstetrics
and Gynecology
University of Florida College
of Medicine-Jacksonville
Jacksonville, Florida

**Joseph H. Kipikasa, MD**
Associate Professor, Section
on Maternal-Fetal Medicine
Department of Obstetrics
and Gynecology
University of Tennessee College
of Medicine
Chattanooga, Tennessee

**Bela I. Kudish, MD, MS**
Fellow in Female Pelvic
Medicine and Reconstructive
Surgery
Washington Hospital Center
Georgetown University
Washington, District of Columbia

**Allison H. Luper, MSN, CNM**
Certified Nurse Midwife
Winston-Salem Womancare
Winston-Salem, North Carolina

**Deborah S. Lyon, MD**
Associate Professor
Director, Gynecology Division
Director, Residency Program
Department of Obstetrics
and Gynecology
University of Florida College
of Medicine-Jacksonville
Jacksonville, Florida

**Marcia E. Murakami, MD**
Assistant Professor of Radiology
Mayo Clinic College of Medicine
Rochester, Minnesota
Consultant, Department
of Radiology
Mayo Clinic
Jacksonville, Florida

**Tracey Maurer, MD**
Assistant Clinical Professor
University of Vermont College
of Medicine
Attending, Fletcher Allen
Health Care
Burlington, Vermont

**Andrea L. McKeever, PharmD, BCPS**
Assistant Professor, Department
of Pharmacy Practice
Director, Drug Information Service
South University School
of Pharmacy
Savannah, Georgia

**Mehdi Parva, MD**
Resident Physician
Department of Obstetrics
  and Gynecology
Lankenau Hospital
Wynnewood, Pennsylvania

**Mary E. Rausch, MD**
Fellow, Reproductive
  Endocrinology and Infertility
University of Pennsylvania School
  of Medicine
Philadelphia, Pennsylvania

**Marghani M. Reever, PhD**
Courtesy Faculty
Department of Obstetrics
  and Gynecology
University of Florida College
  of Medicine-Jacksonville
Jacksonville, Florida

**William Renfro, PharmD**
Neonatology Practitioner,
  Department of Pharmacy
Shands Jacksonville Medical Center
Clinical Associate Professor
University of Florida College
  of Pharmacy
Jacksonville, Florida

**Stephen C. Rubin, MD**
Franklin Payne Professor and Chief
Division of Gynecologic Oncology
University of Pennsylvania Health
  System
Philadelphia, Pennsylvania

**Luis Sanchez-Ramos, MD**
Professor
Division of Maternal-Fetal
  Medicine
Department of Obstetrics
  and Gynecology
University of Florida College
  of Medicine-Jacksonville
Jacksonville, Florida

**Miren A. Schinco, MD**
Associate Professor of Surgery
Chief, Acute Care Surgery
University of Florida College
  of Medicine-Jacksonville
Jacksonville, Florida

**Brent E. Seibel, MD**
Assistant Professor
Associate Clerkship Director
Department of Obstetrics
  and Gynecology
University of Florida College
  of Medicine-Jacksonville
Jacksonville, Florida

**Shireen Madani Sims, MD**
Clinical Assistant Professor
Department of Obstetrics
  and Gynecology
University of Florida College
  of Medicine
Gainesville, Florida

**Karl H.S. Smith, MD**
Assistant Professor
Chief, Division of Gynecologic
  Oncology
Department of Obstetrics
  and Gynecology
University of Florida College
  of Medicine-Jacksonville
Jacksonville, Florida

**Shawn P. Stallings, MD**
Assistant Professor and Residency
  Director
Section on Maternal-Fetal
  Medicine
Department of Obstetrics
  and Gynecology
University of Tennessee College
  of Medicine
Chattanooga, Tennessee

**Lama L. Tolaymat, MD, MPH**
Assistant Professor
Director of Ultrasound
    and Prenatal Diagnosis
Division of Maternal-Fetal Medicine
Department of Obstetrics
    and Gynecology
University of Florida College
    of Medicine-Jacksonville
Jacksonville, Florida

**Stephen Topp, MD**
Department of Emergency
    Medicine
University of Florida College
    of Medicine-Jacksonville
Jacksonville, Florida

**Carlos Torres, MD, FACOG**
Associate Professor, Section on
    Maternal-Fetal Medicine
Department of Obstetrics and
    Gynecology
University of Tennessee College
    of Medicine
Chattanooga, Tennessee

**Kristina E. Ward, PharmD, BCPS**
Clinical Assistant Professor
Director, Drug Information
    Services
University of Rhode Island,
    College of Pharmacy
Kingston, Rhode Island

# CONTENTS

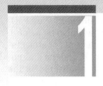

# Medical Emergencies in the Pregnant Patient

## Saju D. Joy and Stephen A. Contag

This chapter highlights five serious medical complications during pregnancy. These conditions affect two patients, the pregnant woman and her fetus. The clinician's goal is to treat the acute condition and concurrently address the possibility of pregnancy in women of childbearing age. Determining the gestational age and viability of the pregnancy is extremely important. The clinician must expeditiously evaluate and treat each of the following medical complications: pulmonary embolism (PE), asthma, diabetic ketoacidosis, thyroid storm, and seizures.

## PULMONARY EMBOLISM

Venous thromboembolism is five times more likely in the pregnant patient than in the nonpregnant patient due to the increase in venous stasis, changes in coagulation factors, and tissue trauma (1). Symptomatic venous thromboembolism has been shown to complicate 0.5 to 3 in 1,000 pregnancies (1,2), while PE complicates 1.3 per 10,000 pregnancies (3) and has been the leading cause of pregnancy-related deaths. During the period between 1991 and 1999, it was responsible for nearly 20% of all pregnancy-related maternal deaths in the United States (4). Recent data suggest that the frequency has decreased to approximately 10% of all pregnancy-related deaths (5). Deep venous thrombosis (DVT) occurs with equal frequency in all three trimesters; however, PE is more common during the postpartum period (1,2). The likelihood of developing a pulmonary embolus is greatly affected by the adequate treatment of DVT. If left untreated, 24% of patients with a DVT will suffer a pulmonary embolus, with a mortality rate of 15%. In patients who receive adequate therapy with anticoagulants, the risk for PE declines to approximately 5% and the mortality rate decreases to <1% (6).

### Patient Presentation

Thromboembolism in the pregnant patient may be difficult to diagnose since many symptoms such as lower extremity edema, dyspnea, and tachycardia are common during normal pregnancy. Signs and symptoms of PE include tachypnea, dyspnea, pleuritic chest pain, apprehension, cough, tachycardia, hemoptysis, and fever. The most common presenting sign is tachypnea, which was present in 89% of patients with proven PE (7) in one study. Dyspnea was the second most common finding, followed by pleuritic pain. Ten percent of symptomatic PE cases are fatal within the first hour following the onset of symptoms. Five to ten percent of patients will present with cardiovascular shock (7). Approximately 50% of patients with PE will have echocardiographic findings suggestive of cor pulmonale or intracardiac emboli that are associated with an increased risk of short-term mortality (7,8). A high level of suspicion must be maintained and rapid evaluation performed in pregnant patients presenting with signs or symptoms of PE.

## Diagnostic Tests

Any pregnant patient who presents with signs or symptoms of PE should be fully evaluated. Initial evaluation should include auscultation and arterial blood gas analysis. A normal $PaO_2$ in room air is reassuring; however, a pulmonary embolus may still be present. Up to 14% of patients with a pulmonary embolus have a $PaO_2$ of >85 mm Hg. Chest radiography and electrocardiography may also be helpful. A chest radiograph may reveal an infiltrate suggestive of pneumonia or atelectasis. These findings, however, do not rule out the possibility of PE, and the diagnosis should be pursued whenever one has a high suspicion of embolism (8,9). The most common ECG abnormality during a pulmonary embolus is tachycardia; however, findings suggestive of acute right-heart failure may be seen including S1, Q3, T3 patterns, right bundle-branch block, P-wave pulmonale, or right axis deviation. These are more common with massive embolism than with smaller emboli, but these findings are also nonspecific (10,11).

D-dimer test measures plasma levels of cross-linked fibrin formed after fibrin lysis by plasmin. This test is a nonspecific indicator of venous thrombosis, and PE is a possible diagnosis. It may be positive in patients with pregnancy, surgery, infection, cancer, trauma, and other inflammatory states and cannot guide decisions about treatment (11,12). Highly sensitive enzyme-linked immunosorbent assay (ELISA)–based D-dimer tests have sensitivity for the diagnosis of PE and DVT of 96% to 98% and a negative likelihood ratio of 0.12 that yield a high certainty for excluding DVT or PE. The sensitivity and positive likelihood values that are between 1.5 and 2.5 do not greatly increase the certainty of diagnosis because of the high frequency of false-positive results. These highly sensitive D-dimer tests can be used to rule out pulmonary embolus. The negative predictive value for these tests when used alone is not high enough to rule out PE, but they may be useful when used in conjunction with another test for PE (13,14). Troponin and brain natriuretic peptide have also been used as indirect markers of PE secondary to the development of myocardial ischemia or right ventricular overload (7).

Evidence of DVT can be used as a surrogate method for diagnosis of PE. In patients who present with acute PE, bilateral venography and compression ultrasonography detect DVT in approximately 75% and 50% of patients, respectively. Additional methods include CT venography and magnetic resonance imaging (MRI) of the lower extremities (7). When there is a high clinical suspicion of PE, and a DVT has been detected, anticoagulation therapy should be started. A negative imaging study for DVT reduces the likelihood of PE; however, the diagnosis cannot be excluded (14).

Ventilation–perfusion (V/Q) lung scanning can be used to evaluate for PE. A normal scan rules out PE but is obtained in only 25% of patients in whom the diagnosis is suspected (15). A high-probability V/Q scan is associated with a prevalence of PE of >80%, but only 45% of patients with suspected pulmonary embolus will have a high-probability scan. Patients with intermediate- or low-probability scans will require further evaluation (14).

Spiral computed tomography (CT) is becoming more widely used for detection of PE. Intraluminal filling defects in lobar or main pulmonary arteries have a positive predictive value for PE of 85%. The sensitivity for subsegmental emboli is only 30%; therefore, intraluminal defects in segmental or subsegmental pulmonary vessels require further evaluation. The combination of CT venography with CT of the pulmonary arteries increases the sensitivity for the diagnosis of PE from 85% to 90% (7). A normal spiral CT significantly reduces the likelihood of PE but does not exclude the diagnosis. Contrast-enhanced CT arteriography has advantages over V/Q scanning, including speed, characterization of nonvascular structures, and detection of venous thrombosis (7).

Pulmonary angiography is the gold standard for diagnosis of PE. Maternal morbidity is associated with catheterization and injection of the contrast solution at a rate of 4% to 5%. The procedure-related maternal mortality rate is 0.2% to 0.3%. Pulmonary angiography is used only when a high suspicion of PE is present, but the other less invasive diagnostic tests are inconclusive (9,10).

The fetal radiation dose with chest radiography (<100 mrad), V/Q scan (<64 mrad), spiral CT (<200 mrad), or pulmonary angiography (<2,000 mrad) is low. Even when chest radiography, V/Q scan, and pulmonary angiography are used in combination, the total radiation dose to the fetus is significantly below the generally accepted dose associated with adverse fetal and neonatal outcomes (5 rad) (10,16). The radiation dose may also be decreased by using abdominal shielding.

MRI has not been used as extensively for detection of PE but seems to have an accuracy similar to that of spiral CT. MRI has the added benefit of avoiding radiation exposure to the fetus (14). The limitations of MRI include availability at the health care facility, time, and cost.

### Therapy

Bed rest is not recommended for DVT unless there is substantial pain and swelling. The data for PE are not conclusive. When PE is diagnosed, inpatient therapy with initial bed rest for 24 to 48 hours is often recommended (7,17,18). Inpatient parenteral anticoagulation with low molecular weight heparin (LMWH) or unfractionated heparin should be initiated unless contraindicated (18). Anticoagulation improves survival among patients with symptomatic PE, but the risk of recurrent, nonfatal venous thromboembolism is estimated at 5% to 10% during the 1st year after diagnosis (18). If the suspicion of PE is high, parenteral anticoagulation should be considered even before imaging, as long as the risk of bleeding does not appear to be excessive. Among pregnant patients, parenteral anticoagulation with subcutaneous unfractionated heparin or LMWH should be maintained throughout pregnancy. Heparin is the drug of choice for acute PE in pregnancy. It has a high molecular weight, is negatively charged, and does not cross the placenta. A heparin bolus of 5,000 units (80 IU/kg) should be given, followed by an hourly infusion of 1,000 units. The dose should be adjusted to keep the activated partial thromboplastin time (aPTT) at 1.5 to 2.5 times normal levels. After 5 to 10 days of intravenous anticoagulation, subcutaneous heparin injections may be started at doses of 7,500 to 10,000 units every 8 to 12 hours to keep the aPTT at 1.5 to 2.5 times normal. Monitoring LMWH by measuring the level of activity against activated factor X (anti–factor Xa) is common practice in patients who are morbidly obese (weighing >150 kg) or very small (<40 kg), in patients with either very severe renal insufficiency or rapidly changing renal function or in patients who are pregnant (19). Full anticoagulation should be continued for 3 to 6 months or longer depending on the presence of risk factors (20). After that time, there is controversy regarding whether to continue full-dose or low-dose prophylactic heparin for the remainder of the pregnancy and for 6 to 12 weeks postpartum (21). Among postpartum patients diagnosed with PE, coumadin can be initiated simultaneously on the 1st day of therapy with subcutaneous LMWH, fondaparinux, or weight-based intravenous unfractionated heparin administered for at least 5 days, preferably until the international normalized ratio (INR) is in the therapeutic range (2.0 to 3.0) for 2 consecutive days (18).

The main complication associated with heparin therapy is hemorrhage. The incidence is 4% in nonsurgical patients receiving intravenous heparin (21). Heparin is associated with two types of heparin-induced thrombocytopenia. The more common form of thrombocytopenia is benign and self-limiting. The more severe form is due to heparin-dependent IgG antiplatelet antibodies and occurs 5 to 14 days after starting full-dose heparin in 3% of patients. Platelet levels should be checked for the first 2 to 3 weeks after instituting heparin therapy, and the medication should be discontinued if severe thrombocytopenia is detected (21). If a patient develops heparin-induced thrombocytopenia, the heparin therapy should be discontinued. Subsequent management options should include consultation with a maternal-fetal medicine specialist and/or hematologist/ oncologist or an internist with an expanded knowledge in hematology. Options for treatment with a direct thrombin inhibitor (e.g., argatroban or lepirudin) may be considered. Similarly, newer alternatives include oral direct thrombin inhibitors (dabigatran), oral anti–factor Xa inhibitors (rivaroxaban and apixaban that are in phase 3 trials), and reversible parenteral anti–factor Xa inhibitor requiring dosing only once a week (biotinylated idraparinux) (22). Heparin can lead to significant bone loss, especially in pregnant women. This effect can be decreased, and we recommend supplementing vitamin D and calcium (21).

LMWH may be superior to unfractionated heparin for the treatment of DVT, and it is at least as effective as unfractionated heparin in reducing the risk of death and the risk of major bleeding during initial therapy for PE (23). Initial dosing should be according to maternal weight, and anti-Xa levels should be checked 4 hours after the morning dose every week. The dose should be adjusted to keep the anti-Xa level between 0.7 and 1.2 U/mL. LMWHs present less risk for the severe form of heparin-induced thrombocytopenia and for osteoporosis than unfractionated heparin; however, they are much more costly (21,24).

Coumarin derivatives cross the placenta and can lead to embryopathy in the first trimester, which consists of nasal and limb hypoplasia. Midtrimester exposure can lead to optic atrophy, microcephaly, and mental retardation. Bleeding within the fetoplacental unit may result in a high fetal loss rate. Coumarin derivatives are relatively contraindicated in pregnancy and should be used with extreme caution. There is an exception of the mechanical heart valve patient whose extreme risk for thrombosis even with anticoagulation with heparin may exceed the risk for embryopathy with coumarin, and she may be an appropriate candidate for coumarin during pregnancy. These medications may be used after delivery if full anticoagulation is still required (21,24).

The primary indications for placement of an inferior vena cava filter include contraindications to anticoagulation, major bleeding complications during anticoagulation, and recurrent embolism while the patient is receiving adequate therapy (18).

## ASTHMA

Asthma is the most common obstructive pulmonary disease in pregnancy and complicates 4% to 8% of pregnancies nationwide (25). In 2005, approximately 4,000 deaths in the United States were attributable to asthma (26). Asthma mortality is threefold higher in African American women than in Caucasian women (26). In approximately one third of women, asthma worsens during pregnancy (27,28). The most important predictor for worsening of a disease during pregnancy is poor control of moderate or severe asthma. Better controlled mild to moderate asthma during pregnancy is associated with excellent maternal and perinatal outcomes. Exacerbations during pregnancy among severe asthmatic patients occur in up to 52% of patients, and the hospitalization rate has been reported as 27% (28,29).

Asthma is characterized by inflammation and reversible airway obstruction owing to hyperresponsive bronchi following exposure to stimuli. Stimuli include known allergens, psychological stressors, and physical exertion. In some patients, the obstruction cannot be completely reversed despite treatment (30).

Asthma may increase the risk for maternal and fetal pregnancy complications among those with poorly controlled or severe disease. The result of previous studies is contradictory (28,29). Two large cohort studies evaluating the risk of maternal asthma on perinatal outcomes have examined the risk for gestational diabetes mellitus, preeclampsia, preterm delivery, and intrauterine growth restriction (31,32). One of the largest prospective trials evaluating pregnancy complications associated with asthma found no association of the disease with preterm delivery. The only significant association found was an increased risk for cesarean delivery (32). Most studies suggest that patients receiving chronic medications for asthma, especially oral corticosteroids, have the highest risk for preterm delivery and small-for-gestational-age infants (31,33). An increased risk for preeclampsia has been noted among patients with daily symptoms or requiring theophylline (34). A lower forced expiratory volume at 1 second ($FEV_1$) has been associated with an increased risk for low birth weight and prematurity (35). It remains unclear whether the pregnancy complications are due to the chronic medications, the severity of the disease, or both factors combined.

## Pharmacologic Agents

The treatment goal for the pregnant asthmatic is to obtain optimal therapy by maintaining control of her asthma thus ensuring improved maternal health and normal fetal maturation (36). The components of caring for a patient with asthma include assessment and monitoring of asthma, including objective measures of pulmonary function; control of factors contributing to asthma severity; patient education; and pharmacologic therapy using a stepwise approach (36).

Most asthma medications are safe and better than the alternative of asthma symptoms and exacerbations that may impair fetal oxygenation during pregnancy (36). Prevention of inflammation, airway hyperresponsiveness, and symptoms is the cornerstone of therapy. Stepwise therapy requires additional medications and dosages adjusted to the symptom severity. A patient not responding to any given treatment should be stepped up to the next level of therapy. Medications are categorized in two general classes: (a) long-term control medications to achieve and maintain control of persistent asthma—especially important is daily medication to suppress the inflammation that is considered an early and persistent component in the pathogenesis of asthma—and (b) quick-relief medications that are taken as needed to treat symptoms and exacerbations (36).

Inhaled $\beta_2$-agonists are recommended for the acute asthma exacerbation by relieving acute bronchospasm of any severity. They are also the first-line medication for mild intermittent and exercise-induced asthma. They are not very effective in preventing airway hyperresponsiveness among patients with persistent asthma (37). To date, no congenital anomalies have been associated with these medications in animals or humans (38). Subcutaneous injection of selective $\beta_2$-agonists, such as terbutaline, may be used in patients with severe exacerbation who are unconscious, cannot use an inhaler, or is moving air very poorly (39). Exclusive use of short-acting $\beta_2$-agonists for management of persistent asthma is associated with an increased mortality (40). Long-acting $\beta_2$-agonists have been shown to significantly decrease the number and severity of exacerbations when used in combination with inhaled corticosteroids; however, their safety in pregnancy has not been proven (30,38).

Inhaled corticosteroids are the mainstay of long-term control of persistent asthma of any severity. These medications decrease airway inflammation, thereby decreasing the number and severity of exacerbations as well as the need for additional inhaled $\beta_2$-agonist therapy. The majority of inhaled corticosteroids are pregnancy category C, with the exception of budesonide, which is now pregnancy category B. Several large studies have shown no increased risk for congenital anomalies when budesonide was used during pregnancy (36,41,42). Oral corticosteroids have been associated with orofacial clefting and intrauterine growth restriction in some trials; however, poor asthma control may lead to worse maternal and fetal complications (28,38,42,43). The main indication for oral steroids is patients not responsive to short-acting bronchodilators and inhaled corticosteroids regardless of the severity of the disease. Quick-relief medication $\beta_2$-agonists should be available to all patients with persistent asthma being treated with inhaled corticosteroids or other long-term anti-inflammatory medications (36).

Theophylline is rarely used for asthma management during pregnancy because of its side effects. Drug levels may change dramatically during the course of pregnancy due to pregnancy-related changes in pharmacokinetics and interactions with other drugs. Serum levels must be checked regularly since theophylline has a narrow therapeutic window, and supratherapeutic drug levels can cause death (38,42). The recommended serum concentration is 5 to 12 $\mu$g/mL. It is used as an alternative treatment for mild persistent asthma or adjunctive treatment to be used with inhaled corticosteroids in moderate to severe persistent asthma (36).

Cromolyn and nedocromil are mast cell stabilizers dispensed as inhalers. They are used as an alternative to inhaled corticosteroids for therapy in mild persistent asthma. Leukotriene receptor antagonists, including zafirlukast and montelukast, may also be considered as an alternative for mild persistent asthma and as an adjunctive therapy for long-term control in moderate persistent asthma (36).

Ipratropium bromide is an inhaled anticholinergic agent and is pregnancy category B. A recent metaanalysis revealed significantly improved pulmonary function following administration of anticholinergic inhalers in combination with inhaled $\beta_2$-agonists for patients with a severe exacerbation (44).

## Emergency Therapy

Treatment of an acute asthma exacerbation during pregnancy is very similar to treatment for nonpregnant patients (Fig. 1.1). Treatment of an acute exacerbation begins at home. Patients should have individualized treatment plans. Treatment begins with inhaled albuterol 2 to 4 puffs every 20 minutes for up to 1 hour (36). This is followed by inhaled or oral corticosteroids for long-term management and suppression of inflammation and hyperreactivity. For the patient that has a severe exacerbation not responsive to home therapy, rapid evaluation upon presentation is critical. Initially, airway patency should be established. The physical examination should include auscultation, heart rate and respiratory rate evaluation, and, in addition, observing if the patient is using accessory muscles. Pulse oximetry should be obtained. In the pregnant patient, supplemental oxygen should be administered to maintain the pulse oximetry value at ≥95% to assure adequate fetal oxygenation. In patients at ≥24 weeks of gestation, external fetal heart rate (FHR) monitoring should be continued until significant maternal improvement. Pulmonary function should be determined using both spirometry and $FEV_1$ or a peak expiratory flow meter (45). Peak expiratory flow rate (PEFR) appears to be equivalent to $FEV_1$ for determining airway constriction. Arterial blood gas testing should be considered for any patient with pulse oximetry values <95%, severe distress, or a PEFR ≤30% of the predicted value after initial therapy (45).

If the initial PEFR is >50% of that predicted, an inhaled $\beta_2$-agonist should be administered every 20 minutes for 1 hour. Oral systemic corticosteroids should be added if there is no response or if the patient recently took inhaled corticosteroids. If the initial PEFR is <50% of the predicted value, it is considered a severe exacerbation, and inhaled ipratropium bromide should be given in conjunction with the $\beta_2$-agonist every 20 minutes for 1 hour (36). Metered dose inhalers used with inhaler spacer devices provide doses of medications equivalent to those

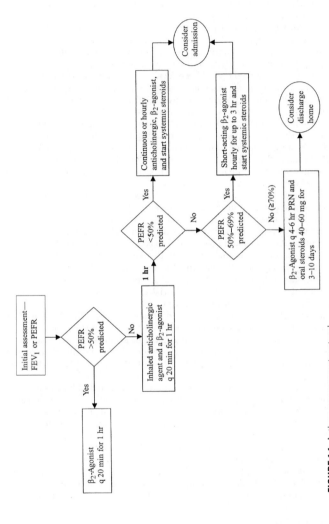

**FIGURE 1.1** Asthma management protocol.

with nebulizer therapy (45). Subcutaneous terbutaline may be administered in patients who cannot comply with the administration of inhaled medications (39). In cases of severe exacerbation, patients should be started on oral systemic corticosteroids. Patients with impending or actual respiratory arrest should continue with dual inhaled therapy and intravenous systemic corticosteroids.

After 1 hour, the patient must be reassessed. A PEFR of 50% to 70% of the predicted value suggests a moderate exacerbation, and the patient should receive a short-acting inhaled $\beta_2$-agonist every 60 minutes. Systemic steroids should be initiated in all patients with a suboptimal response. The patient may continue this regimen for up to 3 hours as long as there is continued clinical improvement. A PEFR of <50% of the predicted value or evidence of severe obstruction, such as accessory muscle usage and retractions, suggests a severe exacerbation. The patient should be given an inhaled $\beta_2$-agonist with an inhaled anticholinergic agent hourly or continuously, and systemic corticosteroids should be started (36,45).

A patient with an incomplete response to initial management, a PEFR 50% to 70% of the predicted value, and persistent dyspnea/wheezing should be considered for hospital admission and intravenous steroids. Any patient at high risk for asthma-related mortality or with recent steroid use, comorbidities, or a recent admission should be hospitalized (45). Generally, any pregnant patient with a viable pregnancy and an incomplete response should be admitted and fetal well-being assured. Patients who are discharged should continue inhaled medications and oral steroids as described above (45).

A patient with a good response to initial therapy, a PEFR ≥70% of the predicted value, and no symptoms 60 minutes after the last inhaler treatment may be discharged home. Patients should be advised to continue $\beta_2$-agonist therapy every 4 to 6 hours as needed for dyspnea. A 3- to 10-day course of oral steroids at a dosage of 40 to 60 mg per day should be continued without a taper (45). A steroid course of <2 weeks' duration should not lead to adrenal suppression, and tapering the medication has not been shown to decrease the risk of relapse (30). The patient should be followed up closely by her primary care provider.

Any patient with a poor response to initial therapy, a PEFR <50% of the predicted value, or severe dyspnea should be admitted for intravenous corticosteroids. $\beta_2$-Agonists and anticholinergics should be given hourly or continuously until significant clinical improvement is seen. The bioavailability of oral corticosteroids appears to be equivalent to that of intravenous steroids; however, the onset of action may be quicker via the intravenous route (45).

All asthmatic patients with an acute exacerbation should be closely monitored for signs of impending respiratory distress. Decreasing level of consciousness, absence of wheezing despite clinically severe symptoms, and hypercapnia ($PCO_2$ > 45 mm Hg) are all ominous findings suggestive of impending respiratory arrest. Intubation should not be delayed once it is deemed necessary, given the difficulty of reversing respiratory failure once it has begun in the asthmatic patient (45,46).

Patients may be discharged when the PEFR is ≥70% of the predicted value. The patient should be advised to continue short-acting inhaled medications as needed and to complete a 3- to 10-day course of oral steroids at a dose of 40 to 60 mg per day. A single daily dose may be used or the dose may be divided twice daily (45).

## THYROID STORM

The prevalence of overt thyroid disease in the pregnant population is 1%. The prevalence of subclinical hypothyroidism is 2% to 3% and antibody positivity 10% to 15% (47). Hyperthyroidism occurs in 0.2% of pregnancies, and Graves disease is the diagnosis in 95% of these cases (48,49). Thyroid hormone is secreted from the thyroid gland as thyroxine ($T_4$) and converted peripherally mostly in the liver and the kidneys to the active form triiodothyronine ($T_3$). $T_3$ then interacts with nuclear hormone binding sites that regulate the transcription of gene products. These gene products are critical to the regulation of calorigenesis, cardiovascular function, oxygen consumption, and other metabolic processes (49). Abnormal thyroid function in pregnancy has been associated with significant maternal and neonatal morbidity including IUGR, preeclampsia, placental abruption, preterm delivery, and perinatal death.

Thyroid storm occurs in 1% of pregnant patients with hyperthyroidism (50). It is characterized by an extreme hypermetabolic state with symptoms including fever, neurologic changes from irritability to coma, cardiac arrhythmias and decompensation, gastrointestinal distress, leukocytosis, and elevated liver function tests (49). The onset is generally abrupt, and the disease is usually fatal if left untreated. Maternal morbidity has been reported in up to 25%, but with recognition and early, aggressive management, it can be significantly less (51,52). It is also seen occasionally in patients with toxic multinodular goiter and rarely with trophoblastic tumors (53). A precipitating event can be identified in 50% to 75% of cases (54). Thyroid function test findings and the most common precipitating events for thyroid storm are listed in Tables 1.1 and 1.2, respectively.

### Diagnostic Criteria

Fever in excess of 37.8 °C (100 °F) is present and may be as high as 41.1 °C (106 °F), with or without concurrent infection. Especially important for the emergency physician, sudden puerperal fever, even without a history of hyperthyroidism, can be the presentation of thyroid storm, especially in the patient who has not received prenatal care (55). Exaggerated peripheral manifestations of thyrotoxicosis may be present including cardiovascular, gastrointestinal, and central nervous system dysfunctions.

Cardiovascular abnormalities are seen in up to 50% of patients (56). In addition to *arrhythmias* such as atrial fibrillation and premature ventricular contractions, complete heart block may occur. Patients may also complain of palpitations with tachycardia out of proportion to the maternal fever. A *widened*

 **TABLE 1.1** Thyroid Function Tests in Pregnancy and Hyperthyroidism

| Thyroid Test | Change in Pregnancy | Change in Hyperthyroidism |
|---|---|---|
| Total thyroxine ($TT_4$) | Increased | Increased |
| Free $T_4$ ($FT_4$) | Unchanged | Increased |
| Total triiodothyronine ($TT_3$) | Increased | Increased or unchanged |
| Free $T_3$ ($FT_3$) | Unchanged | Increased or unchanged |
| Thyroid-stimulating hormone (TSH) | Unchanged | Decreased |
| Free thyroxine index (FTI) | Unchanged | Increased |
| Resin $T_3$ uptake ($RT_3U$) | Decreased | Increased |
| Thyroid-binding globulin (TBG) | Increased | Unchanged |

**TABLE 1.2**     Events That May Precipitate Thyroid Storm

Infection, especially pulmonary

Surgery

Trauma

Labor

Delivery

Induction of anesthesia

Complications of pregnancy (preeclampsia, DKA)

Gestational trophoblastic disease (up to 2% of cases)

Myocardial infarction

Vascular accident

Pulmonary embolus

*pulse pressure* is generally present, because of increased stroke volume, cardiac output, peripheral vasodilation, and myocardial oxygen consumption. Congestive heart failure is also common and may be the presenting symptom in patients with thyroid storm. Progressive cardiac dysfunction often leads to pulmonary edema and, subsequently, cardiogenic shock may occur.

Central nervous system dysfunction is seen in up to 90% of patients with thyroid storm (56). Manifestations vary from change in mental status, restlessness, anxiety, confusion, and agitation to the extremes of delirium, disorientation, and psychosis. Tremor and proximal muscle weakness are common. Without expedient treatment, severe consequences of thyroid storm include emotional lability, seizures, obtundation, and coma (52). Gastrointestinal manifestations may result in the patient experiencing weight loss, despite an increased appetite (54). Other symptoms include diarrhea, anorexia, nausea, vomiting, and crampy abdominal pain, a constellation that mimics an acute abdomen. Occasionally, jaundice and/or tender hepatomegaly are noted.

### Differential Diagnosis

Thyroid storm may be confused with other hyperkinetic states but should be suspected in any thyrotoxic patient with fever (54). A careful medication history should be obtained. The review of systems should be focused to include the above-mentioned cardiac, central nervous system, and gastrointestinal manifestations. During the physical examination, the clinician should examine the patient for a palpable goiter or eye signs suggestive of Graves' ophthalmopathy. The differential diagnosis includes anxiety states, psychosis, drug abuse (cocaine toxicity), pheochromocytoma, heat stroke, malignant neuroleptic syndrome, acute abdomen, alcoholic complications, and sepsis.

### Laboratory Evaluation

Thyroid function tests do not distinguish storm from uncomplicated thyrotoxicosis, because the values overlap (57). However, serum-free thyroxine ($FT_4$), free triiodothyronine ($FT_3$), and thyroid-stimulating hormone levels need to be

| TABLE 1.3 | Management of Thyroid Storm |
|---|---|

I. Inhibit thyroid hormone synthesis

  a. **Thionamide**

    • ***Propylthiouracil (PTU):***—first-line agent: 600–800 mg PO, then 150–200 mg q 4–6 hr

    • ***Methimazole***: 40 mg rectally t.i.d or 15–25 mg PO q 6 hr

II. Inhibit thyroid hormone release

  a. **Thionamide**

  b. **Sodium iodide:** 1–2 hr post thionamide administration

    • ***Saturated solution of potassium iodide (SSKI)***: 2–5 drops PO q 8 hr

    • ***Sodium iodide***: 0.5–1 g IV q 8 hr

    • ***Lugol's solution*** (5% KI, 10% $KI_2$): 8 drops q 6 hr

  c. **Iodide allergy:** 1–2 hr post thionamide administration

    • ***Lithium carbonate***: 300 mg PO q 6 hr

III. Block peripheral effects/conversion to active hormone

  a. **Thionamide**

  b. **Dexamethasone:** 2 mg IV or IM q 6 hr for four doses

IV. Identify and treat precipitating factor(s)

  Treat underlying hypertension, infection, or bleeding

V. General supportive/symptomatic care

  a. **Tachycardia**

    • $\beta$-Blocker: ***Propranolol***—20–80 mg PO q 4–6 hr ***or*** 1–2 mg IV q 5 min to total of 6 mg, then 1–10 mg IV q 4 hr

    • Bronchospasm history: ***Diltiazem***—60 mg PO q 6–8 hr

  b. **Hyperthermia:** Acetaminophen ± cooling blanket

  c. **Dehydration:** Fluid replacement; caution for heart failure; consider central hemodynamic monitoring

  d. **Restlessness:** ***Phenobarbital***—30–60 mg PO q 6–8 hr as needed

    • Electrolyte replacement

    • Consider plasma exchange

obtained. If thyroid storm is suspected, the clinician should not await the results of these laboratory tests but proceed with empiric management.

## Management

The key to successful management of thyroid storm requires supportive care, prompt identification of etiology, and quadruple therapy (thionamide, iodide, glucocorticoids, and $\beta$-blockers). These efforts to resuscitate and treat should occur in an intensive care unit. Quadruple therapy is used in (a) preventing the synthesis and the release of $T_4$, (b) preventing the conversion of $T_4 \rightarrow T_3$, and (c) blocking the actions of thyroid hormone on the cardiovascular system (24). A management protocol for thyroid storm with suggested medications is outlined in Table 1.3 (52,55).

Supportive care includes hydration with intravenous fluids and electrolytes to replace gastrointestinal and insensible losses. Supplemental oxygen with continuous cardiac monitoring should be employed. Congestive heart failure should be treated the same as in the nonpregnant individual, but patients may be refractory to digoxin and require higher doses (57). Control of tachycardia with $\beta$-blockade may pose problems in the face of recalcitrant congestive heart failure. Alternatives to $\beta$-blockade include IM reserpine, guanethidine, and diltiazem. Fever should be controlled with antipyretics (acetaminophen) and, if necessary, a cooling blanket. Phenobarbital is used to reduce extreme agitation and can increase the catabolism of thyroid hormone. Aspirin is contraindicated in thyrotoxic crisis because it displaces $T_3$ and $T_4$ from binding proteins.

Identifying and treating precipitating factors are critical in the management of thyroid storm. A thorough search as to the cause, such as infection, trauma, labor, or pulmonary embolus, should be conducted. Broad-spectrum antibiotic coverage should be initiated early and continued until final cultures are negative, unless another precipitating cause is identified.

In pregnancy, the drug of choice for medical treatment of hyperthyroidism is propylthiouracil (PTU), rather than methimazole. PTU will block thyroid hormone synthesis by inhibiting both the organification of tyrosine residues and the peripheral conversion of $T_4$ to $T_3$ (58). A loading dose of 600 to 800 mg orally should be given, followed by 150 to 200 mg orally every 4 to 6 hours (52). PTU is only available orally but can be administered via nasogastric tube. Although PTU begins to act in the 1st hour after administration, the full therapeutic effect is not achieved for 3 to 6 weeks (56). Newborns of treated mothers generally have small goiters, if one is present at all, and mild hypothyroidism, which resolves shortly after birth. Although the evidence linking methimazole to aplasia cutis in the newborn is debated, practitioners in the United States still hesitate to use the drug unless the patient cannot tolerate PTU (54) or oral administration is not possible. Methimazole does not inhibit the peripheral conversion of $T_4$ to $T_3$. Methimazole is administered 40 mg rectally three times a day.

Iodide treatment blocks the release of thyroid hormone and thus it is included as part of the quadruple therapy. Options include (a) a saturated solution of potassium iodide, 2 to 5 drops orally or by nasogastric tube every 8 hours; (b) sodium iodide, 0.5 to 1.0 g every 8 hours by slow intravenous infusion; (c) Lugol's solution, 8 drops every 6 hours; and (d) lithium carbonate, 300 mg orally every 6 hours (especially for patients allergic to iodine) (52). Iodide administration should not be initiated until 1 to 2 hours after PTU or methimazole therapy has begun, so that there is no further buildup of hormone stores (57).

Glucocorticoids decrease thyroid hormone release and inhibit peripheral tissue conversion of $T_4$ to $T_3$, decreasing the peripheral manifestations of thyrotoxicosis. Dexamethasone can be used at 2 mg intravenously or intramuscularly every 6 hours for four doses.

Propranolol can be used to control tachycardia, tremor, and restlessness. The intravenous protocol recommends 1 to 2 mg intravenously per 5 minutes for a total of 6 mg, then 1 to 10 mg intravenously every 4 hours, versus the oral protocol of 20 to 80 mg orally every 4 to 6 hours. If the patient has a history of severe bronchospasm, reserpine (1 to 5 mg intramuscularly every 4 to 6 hours), guanethidine (1 mg/kg orally every 12 hours), or diltiazem (60 mg orally every 6 to 8 hours) may be administered (52). Plasmapheresis and peritoneal dialysis are reserved for patients for whom conservative therapy fails.

After initial clinical improvement, iodine and glucocorticoid therapy can be discontinued. Antithyroid medications should be continued until the patient is euthyroid. In general, the therapeutic goal is to maintain high to normal maternal thyroid hormone levels to minimize the potential for suppression of the fetal gland.

If storm occurs early in pregnancy, a subtotal thyroidectomy can be performed in the second trimester. Use of the preceding management protocol has resulted in a decrease in mortality to the range of 10% to 20% (57). Death, however, is usually the result of cardiac failure or intercurrent infection (56).

## DIABETIC KETOACIDOSIS

Diabetic ketoacidosis (DKA) complicates about 1% to 3% of all diabetic pregnancies (58–62). In one study, 30% of cases of DKA occurred in women who did not have known diabetes (63). Despite improved supportive care, DKA is still a significant cause of mortality. Although maternal mortality in DKA has been reduced from 50% in the pre-insulin era to <1% today, some authorities quote maternal mortality rates of 5% to 15% (62,64). Similarly, fetal loss rates have historically ranged from 9% to 90% and continue to remain high, at 22% to 35% (60,63,65). Women with brittle diabetes and recurrent DKA are of greater concern, with fetal loss resulting in nearly one half of their pregnancies (63,66).

### Pathophysiology

DKA is a state of inadequate insulin action with hypoglycemia perceived at the level of the target cell (67). A relative or an absolute insulin deficiency results in decreased peripheral usage of glucose and subsequent hyperglycemia with production of counterregulatory hormones to increase glucose production and availability. Glucagon appears to enhance the uptake and conversion of amino acids to glucose in the liver. Glucagon can also augment hepatic ketone production and induce gluconeogenesis and glycolysis (62). Deficient amounts and impaired function of insulin result in decreased glucose uptake by the liver, fat, and muscle as well as reduced stimulation of adipocytes to store free fatty acids. DKA results when there is a metabolic imbalance in levels of insulin and glucagon disturbing the euglycemic state.

The hyperglycemia causes an osmotic diuresis, which leads to volume depletion and electrolyte loss. Water is excreted in proportion to the increase in osmotic pressure and electrolytes are lost with the free water. Intracellular glucose unavailability leads to lipolysis with free fatty acid breakdown by oxidation, and the resulting ketogenesis leads to metabolic (keto) acidosis. There is usually a concurrent stressor, such as an infection, that can cause release of glucagon, catecholamines, growth hormone, and cortisol. These glucose counterregulatory hormones cause increased glycogenolysis, which increases circulating glucose levels, and gluconeogenesis, which both increases glucose levels and depletes hepatic amino acid stores (68).

The natural progression of osmotic diuresis results in a decreased cardiac output with low blood pressure, and, ultimately will lead to vascular collapse with shock. Metabolic acidosis is a result of decreased peripheral perfusion with production of lactic acid as well as ketone production secondary to free fatty acid oxidation and formation of acetoacetic acid and $3\beta$-hydroxybutyric acid. Pregnancy is normally a state of compensated respiratory alkalosis which is compensated through renal bicarbonate excretion. This leaves fewer buffers available to neutralize ketones despite an increase in the respiratory rate, in an attempt to compensate for the rising levels of ketones. The increased respiratory rate results in even further (insensible) fluid loss.

Although DKA is more frequently seen in insulin-dependent diabetics, cases have been documented in gestational diabetics (69,70). DKA is observed in conjunction with $\beta$-mimetic therapy, whereby the breakdown of glycogen to glucose and increases in cellular metabolism may result in lactic acidosis (71). DKA has also been documented in a woman with no history of glucose intolerance being treated with terbutaline and betamethasone (72).

The fetal status can be compromised by decreased uteroplacental perfusion secondary to hypovolemia and maternal acidosis. Additional factors affecting the fetus include fetal hyperglycemia and osmotic diuresis which can lead to fetal hypovolemia and lactic acidosis, relative hypoxia secondary to increased oxygen requirements induced by fetal hyperinsulinemia, and decreased oxygen transfer caused by a leftward shift of the maternal oxygen dissociation curve secondary to decreased 2,3 diphosphoglycerol concentrations. This leads to increased affinity of maternal hemoglobin for oxygen.

### Diagnosis

The diagnosis of DKA is made by clinical findings and confirmed by laboratory studies which include hyperglycemia, acidosis, and ketonemia. The patient with DKA may present with malaise, headache, nausea, vomiting, thirst, weight loss, and a change in mental status. Other frequent complaints include polydipsia, polyuria, and shortness of breath. The patient may also have a characteristic "fruity" breath resulting from increased acetone production (68). The differential diagnosis for high–anion gap metabolic acidosis in pregnancy includes lactic acidosis, chronic renal failure, salicylate overdose, and ingestion of ethylene glycol (73).

Diagnostic criteria are listed in Table 1.4. In general, hyperglycemia with high–anion gap metabolic acidosis plus ketonemia or ketonuria confirms DKA. Pregnant patients can present with DKA at lower serum glucose concentrations (<200 mg/dL or 11.1 mmol/L) as seen in up to 36% of cases in one series (74). This is due to a decreased buffer reserve. The increased anion gap ($Na^+ - [Cl^- + HCO_3^-]$) of >12 mEq/L is indicative of a decreased serum bicarbonate concentration. Large fluid shifts result in peripheral vascular depletion. As a result, the patient may suffer from dehydration and hypotension, and secondary to reduced uterine blood flow, the fetal cardiac tracing may indicate uteroplacental insufficiency. Consequent prerenal azotemia may also be evident.

The clinician should be acutely aware of the potential rapid onset of DKA during pregnancy; DKA may develop within hours in a severely dehydrated pregnant patient that may have occurred over several days in the nonpregnant patient. This may be precipitated by the hyperemesis commonly found during the first trimester of pregnancy. The hyperglycemia in DKA can lead to profound diuresis with decreased cardiac output, a fall in blood pressure, and shifts in the concentration of serum sodium and potassium. Potassium is usually increased as a result of protein breakdown secondary to gluconeogenesis as well as decreased potassium entry into cells secondary to insulin resistance. Low serum potassium levels reflect severe potassium depletion. Although sodium concentrations can vary, they may decrease secondary to osmotic diuresis that subsequently leads to shock (75).

| TABLE 1.4 | Diagnostic Criteria for Diabetic Ketoacidosis |
|---|---|

Maternal arterial pH, <7.30

$HCO_3^-$, <15

Serum ketones, present

Blood glucose, ≥300 mg/dL[a]

[a]DKA may develop in pregnant patients with serum glucose <200 mg/dL.

## Management

The ABCs of resuscitation apply to the pregnant patient with DKA. If she has extreme malaise or is obtunded, an indwelling bladder catheter should be used and a nasogastric tube placed to keep the stomach empty, thereby decreasing the risk of aspirating gastric contents (68). Prompt and aggressive treatment of hypovolemia and insulin resistance is essential as well as the identification and treatment of precipitating factors.

The total body water deficit may be as high as 100 to 150 mL/kg or up to 10 L. This deficit should initially be corrected with 1 L of saline (0.9% sodium chloride) administered over the first hour. An additional 2 L of saline (if no hypernatremia) or half-normal saline (0.45% sodium chloride) may be administered 1 L per hour during the 2nd and 3rd hours. Then, 250 to 500 mL of half-normal saline per hour should be given until approximately 75% of the deficit is corrected. When the serum glucose falls below 250 mg/dL, the intravenous fluids can be changed to a 5% dextrose solution (62). Six to eight liters of fluids should be replaced over the first 24 hours of treatment to compensate for approximately 75% of the estimated fluid loss. Solutions containing lactate should be avoided. Urine output must be monitored closely, continuously checking for glucose and ketones.

After initial blood studies have been done and hydration begun, insulin therapy should be started. There are many regimens for insulin replacement; one option is as follows: initially, 0.1 U/kg body weight should be given as an intravenous push; then, an intravenous drip of regular insulin is given, at 0.1 U/kg body weight per hour (equivalent to 8 to 10 units per hour). Serum glucose should be checked every 1 to 2 hours, and if a decrease of 25% or more (50 to 75 mg) is not achieved within the first 2 hours, the insulin infusion rate should be doubled (62). As mentioned previously, when the serum glucose falls below 250 mg/dL, the intravenous solution should include 5% dextrose with half-normal saline, and the insulin infusion rate should be decreased by half. When the blood glucose drops below 150 mg/dL, a basal rate of 1 to 2 U of insulin per hour should be adequate to maintain homeostasis, with the patient able to eat and return to split-dosing of subcutaneous insulin (62). The insulin drip may then be tapered over 4 to 6 hours and discontinued.

Potassium loss due to vomiting and massive osmotic diuresis is usually in the range of 5 to 10 mEq/kg body weight. Acidosis causes displacement of intracellular potassium to the extracellular space, giving the clinician spurious reassurance that potassium stores are adequate. Correcting the acidosis drives potassium back into the cell, rapidly decreasing the serum potassium level. Potassium can also be bound by ketones that are being removed by increasing diuresis. The calculated potassium deficit is 5 to 10 mEq/kg of body weight. Potassium repletion does not need to be initiated until serum concentrations are below 5.3 mEq/L. Potassium chloride, up to 40 mEq/L, should be added to the intravenous solution (half-normal saline), and the serum electrolytes should be checked every 2 to 4 hours (68). If phosphorus is low, 10 to 20 mEq/L of potassium phosphate can replace 10 to 20 mEq/L of potassium chloride as long as renal function is adequate (62).

Bicarbonate replacement is somewhat controversial and should be considered only if the pH is <7.10. One ampule (44 mEq $NaHCO_3$) may be administered in a liter of half-normal saline. Administration of bicarbonate does not affect the recovery of outcome variables (rates of decrease in glucose and ketone levels and rates of increase in pH or bicarbonate) in the mother (70). Bicarbonate is broken down to hydrogen ions and $CO_2$ by carbonic anhydrase. Free hydrogen ions may theoretically cross the placenta and thereby exacerbate the hypoxic effects of DKA on the fetus.

Identifying and treating the precipitating cause of the acidosis are paramount. A thorough search for infection should be undertaken after initial resuscitation has begun, including obtaining blood, urine, and sputum cultures. A thorough physical examination of the integumentary, respiratory, genitourinary, and gastrointestinal systems should be performed. Chorioamnionitis should be considered as a possible source. Broad-spectrum antibiotics should be administered empirically, pending culture results (68).

If the gestation is sufficiently advanced that the fetus is potentially capable of extrauterine survival, the FHR should be electronically monitored. Late decelerations and decreased FHR variability (both signs of fetal distress) may be seen because of the maternal acidosis. However, the mother should be stabilized before any intervention to delivery. The FHR abnormalities will usually resolve as the maternal status normalizes, and thus delivery can often be delayed (68).

A common error is to discontinue or decrease volume therapy after glucose levels normalize. Acidemia may still be present despite correction of hyperglycemia, and restoration of circulating volume is critical to its resolution. Without continued and adequate fluid replacement, the possibility for recurrence of DKA exists (67).

## SEIZURE DISORDERS

A seizure in pregnancy should be treated as any emergency resuscitation protocol, with the ABCs. First, the airway is secured and then patient breathing efforts are supported. Then, attention should focus on evaluating the cause of the seizure episode. Although the majority of seizures during pregnancy are due to previously diagnosed epilepsy, denovo seizures in the absence of signs of preeclampsia require the exclusion of metabolic alterations such as hyponatremia, hypoglycemia, hyperglycemia, or acute hepatic failure from fatty liver of pregnancy, viral hepatitis, or structural lesions such as intracranial hemorrhage, venous sinus thrombosis, or ischemic stroke (76). When evaluating a patient for a seizure, the first question is whether this incident is related to the patient's pregnancy (e.g., eclampsia) or does she have a history of a seizure disorder? Could drug overdose, head trauma, infection, or any metabolic abnormalities have been the trigger for this episode? Can the patient or witness provide any information regarding provoking factors, including preictal and postictal symptoms, headaches, and sleep deprivation?

Eclampsia is the most common cause of new onset seizures in pregnancy (76). Tonic–clonic seizures in pregnancy must include an evaluation for eclampsia. Preeclampsia is a condition that complicates approximately 7% of all pregnancies, with findings of high blood pressure, proteinuria, and multiple laboratory and clinical manifestations suggesting end-organ damage. Severe preeclampsia can include neurologic symptoms of visual disturbances, scotomata, or headaches and, with the inclusion of seizures, can be categorized as eclampsia. Although most cases of preeclampsia occur in the third trimester of pregnancy, cases of second-trimester (>20 weeks' gestation) and postpartum eclampsia are noted to be more frequent occurrences.

Essential in the diagnosis of eclampsia is the presence of a seizure concurrent with the diagnosis of preeclampsia (hypertension and proteinuria). The progression of preeclampsia leads to end-organ damage. Associated laboratory abnormalities include an elevation of the serum uric acid level, serum creatinine >1 mg/dL, blood urea nitrogen >10 mg/dL, and sometimes an elevation of the serum transaminases or depression of the platelet count. The serum alkaline phosphatase level cannot be used to assess liver function, as the placenta produces alkaline phosphatase, and this will give a misleading, elevated result. It is important to note, however, that these blood tests are not always uniformly abnormal in the eclamptic patient and that an elevated blood pressure may be the only objective sign seen in these patients. Prodromal complaints indicating severe preeclampsia include excessive weight gain in the preceding few weeks, right upper quadrant pain, visual disturbances consisting of scotomata or blurry vision, and a headache unresponsive to acetaminophen.

Idiopathic epilepsy affects 0.5% to 1.0% of the population of North America. It complicates approximately 0.3% to 0.6% of pregnancies (77). These seizures can be categorized as generalized tonic–clonic seizures, partial complex seizures that may or may not generalize, and absence seizures. While 17% to 33% of epileptic women report an increase in seizure frequency (78) during pregnancy, up to 25% report a decrease and up to 50% report no change in frequency (79). In part, the increased seizure risk is due to the pharmacokinetic changes during pregnancy (decreased protein binding, increased volume of distribution, increased renal clearance, with impaired intestinal absorption, and increased hepatic metabolism), which combine to lower the free circulatory levels of antiepileptic drugs (AED). However, patient noncompliance with anticonvulsant therapy is a more frequent reason for low circulatory levels of AED. Often, as soon as the pregnancy test is positive, gravidas stop taking their anticonvulsant medications, because of the perceived teratogenicity. Although one would expect an increase in seizure activity during the first trimester, there persists an increased risk throughout gestation with the highest incidence in the peripartum period because of the combination of noncompliance and pharmacokinetic changes (80).

## Pregnancy Effects on Epilepsy

As mentioned previously, low serum concentrations of AED can accompany the increased seizure frequency seen in some pregnancies. This finding may be because of our present ability to measure levels of anticonvulsant drugs in epileptic patients. Table 1.5 lists the first- and second-generation antiepileptic medications. Pregnancy is known to change the disposition of anticonvulsant medications (81). The increase in plasma volume, the presence of fetal and placental compartments, and the increase in extracellular fluid all increase the volume of distribution of anticonvulsant medications and can lower the total serum concentration of these medicines. Free serum drug levels best represent the drug available to the central nervous system for anticonvulsant activity, therefore, only the free, unbound drug that is pharmacologically active is measured. Bardy et al. (82) measured serum phenytoin levels during pregnancy in 111 patients and concluded that they are lowest at the time of delivery. During the late third trimester and in labor, free levels of carbamazepine have been noted to fall 11%, phenytoin 31%, and phenobarbital 50% (78). Furthermore, many patients experience nausea and vomiting in the first trimester of pregnancy, which reduces the absorption of anticonvulsant drugs from the gastrointestinal tract (83). Barbiturates and phenytoin induce hepatic microsomal enzymes, which hasten their own metabolism. In addition, pregnancy increases the liver's ability to hydroxylate these medications (81). This

| TABLE 1.5 | First- and Second-Generation AED | |
|---|---|---|
| **Generation** | **Category** | **Antiepileptic drug** |
| First | C | Carbamazepine |
| | D | Phenytoin, phenobarbital, valproic acid, primidone |
| Second | C | Felbamate, gabapentin, lamotrigine, levetiracetam, oxacarbazepine, tiagabine, topiramate, zonisamide |

is only a brief example of the many ways in which serum anticonvulsant levels can change during a normal pregnancy and why it is important to measure these drug levels in epileptic patients who are seen after a seizure. Some authors recommend checking levels each trimester and after delivery (76).

### Fetal Effects of Anticonvulsant Medications

Many pregnant women become noncompliant because they are concerned about the teratogenicity associated with AED. Major malformations occur in 2% to 4% of the general population. Whereas the incidence is approximately twice as high among women with epilepsy not using any AEDs, among epileptics on monotherapy, it is 4% to 6% (84). Major congenital malformations associated with AEDs include heart defects, neural tube defects including anencephaly, and cleft lip and palate. Certain abnormalities have been associated with the specific medications. Barbiturate use is associated with facial clefts and congenital heart disease. Carbamazepine and valproic acid use in the first trimester is associated with neural tube defects of <1% and 1% to 2%, respectively. Other abnormalities associated with antiepileptic medications include ocular hypertelorism, epicanthal folds, nasal growth deficiency, abnormal ears, distal digital hypoplasia, and nail hypoplasia.

The teratogenic potentials of phenobarbital and primidone (which is metabolized to phenobarbital) are debatable. Generally, carbamazepine and phenobarbital are considered to have the least teratogenic potential, but even phenobarbital has been implicated as a pathogen (85). Second-generation antiepileptic medications may be less teratogenic (Table 1.6), but there are very few data from clinical studies and registries available via the Internet. Patients should not change anticonvulsants without first consulting a physician once they confirm pregnancy. When physicians and patients attempt to change medications at this time, seizure activity usually increases, jeopardizing both the mother and the fetus. The emerging concept appears to be that there is a teratogenic pattern for all of the older AEDs that are metabolized through the liver. This lends support to the concept of the AED drug syndrome. The basic tenet in pharmacotherapy for epilepsy is to simplify drug regimens. It is preferable to avoid polytherapy particularly that which involves valproic acid which alone or in combination is associated with a two- to three-fold increased risk for teratogenicity (86).

Teratogenesis mostly occurs in the first 2 months of pregnancy during the critical organogenesis period, and any negative effects of anticonvulsants have often occurred by the time the patient realizes that she is pregnant. Therefore, preconceptional and prenatal counseling is highly recommended.

### Management of an Acute Seizure

Status epilepticus occurs in 1% of the population that develops seizures (76). In the general population, status epilepticus has been associated with a 22% to 35% mortality rate. Generalized convulsive status epilepticus at any time during pregnancy is similarly life-threatening to the woman and her fetus. Recent improvements in care have improved outcomes for the pregnant patient and her fetus (80). Although a single seizure is generally well tolerated by a healthy fetus, there are reports of intracranial hemorrhage, miscarriages, transient fetal hypoxia, and prolonged bradycardia (78,87). A more frequent concern is trauma sustained during a seizure.

Patients may present with nonconvulsive status epilepticus (NCSE), in which there is a prolonged impairment of consciousness or a change in behavioral function including confusion, agitation, staring, aphasia, and lethargy without obvious epileptic motor features. NCSE accounts for approximately 20% of all status epilepticus. Prompt diagnosis is again essential since the complex partial status epilepticus form can result in cognitive or memory loss, motor and sensory dysfunction, and even death.

| TABLE 1.6 | Second-Generation AED in Pregnancy | | |

| Drug | Starting dose | Malformations | Findings |
|---|---|---|---|
| Gabapentin (Neurontin) | 300 mg t.i.d | 4.5% (51 pregnancies) | |
| Lamotrigine (Lamictal) | Multiple regimens depending on concomitant therapy | 1.8%–10% (334 pregnancies) | MonoTx (1.8%), polyTx w/o (4.3%), or w/valproic acid (10%). Crosses placenta |
| Oxcarbazepine (Trileptal) | 300 mg b.i.d | 62 cases total w/prospective 42 pregnancies | Spina bifida (polyTx), cleft palates, facial dysmorphisms. *MonoTx* cases—no malformations. *PolyTx*—one with ventricular septal defect (polyTx w/phenobarbital). Crosses placenta |
| Topiramate (Topamax) | 50 mg q.d. | 167 cases | Clinical trial, 28 pts: one malformation, two anomalies, postmarket surveillance—five cases of hypospadias. Crosses placenta |
| Zonisamide (Zonegran) | 100 mg q.d. | 7.7% (26 cases) | PolyTx w/phenytoin, one malformation; w/phenytoin and valproic acid, one malformation. Crosses placenta |

*Note*: MonoTx, monotherapy; polyTx, polytherapy

In a patient experiencing a tonic–clonic convulsion, it is frequently impossible to distinguish between idiopathic epilepsy and eclampsia without further history or laboratory investigation. However, in a pregnant patient with the uterine fundus extending to or above the level of the umbilicus, the clinician would suspect a pregnancy of >20 weeks' gestation. In this situation, the clinician should have a high suspicion of eclampsia in the presence of hypertension and proteinuria. These patients should be treated as if they are eclamptic until further studies and history can be obtained.

There are several steps in managing a pregnant patient with a seizure. The ABCs for resuscitation should be followed. First, an adequate airway must be maintained to allow oxygenation after the patient's respirations resume, following the convulsion. Breathing and circulation need to be assessed after the convulsion ceases. During the seizure, it is necessary to prevent self-injury and uterine (fetal) trauma. After the seizure, the airway should be cleared and the patient should be suctioned to reduce the risk of aspiration of secretions or vomitus. She should also be watched carefully to prevent bodily injury, lacerations, and fractures (85,88). If seizures persist, the airway must be protected, possibly requiring intubation.

If an eclamptic seizure is the working diagnosis, the patient should be treated with intravenous magnesium sulfate, if possible. The usual initial dose is 6 g, administered intravenously and slowly, over 1 to 2 minutes. If intravenous access is not available, 10 g may be administered intramuscularly. Overdoses of magnesium can lead to respiratory depression, and inadequate doses can result in continued seizures. If seizures continue, another 2 g of magnesium sulfate may be given intravenously. After controlling the eclamptic seizure, a maintenance dose of 2 g per hour should be administered. Renal function should be evaluated (magnesium is cleared renally) and a Foley catheter placed. Magnesium toxicity progresses from loss of deep tendon reflexes to ECG variations to apnea and cardiac arrest, because of electrical–mechanical disassociation. Calcium gluconate 1 g IV (1 ampule) may be administered to reverse magnesium toxicity.

If the patient has a history of epilepsy, she should be treated with the parenteral form of the medication she has been taking. If the etiology of the seizures is uncertain, phenytoin may be used for acute treatment. The usual loading dose is 10 to 15 mg/kg prepregnancy weight, given intravenously over an hour. The infusion is started at a rate of up to 50 mg per minute to a total dose of 20 mg/kg. Phosphenytoin may also be administered, in place of phenytoin, at a rate of 150 mg per minute in cases of status epilepticus. The patient should be placed on a cardiac monitor while phenytoin or phosphenytoin is being administered. Subsequently, the patient should be given 200 mg either orally or intravenously, beginning 12 hours after the bolus. This dosage regimen also has been used successfully to treat eclampsia (88).

Diazepam and the other benzodiazepines are *considered first-line treatments* for status epilepticus. They can be used to treat seizures acutely until the patient can be transported to a labor floor and treated appropriately for eclampsia. Lorazepam at a dose of 4 mg IV can be given slowly over 2 to 5 minutes, which may be repeated in 10 to 15 minutes; usual maximum dose is 8 mg. Alternatively, diazepam can be administered at 0.1 to 0.3 mg/kg intravenously, with termination of seizures within 20 seconds of administration. However, because of subsequent redistribution of the drug into adipose tissue, the duration of diazepam's acute anticonvulsant effect is typically <20 minutes. A rectal gel formulation of diazepam may be used when intravenous access is problematic (75). Diazepam, at high doses, can lead to maternal and neonatal respiratory depression and loss of FHR variability on the monitor tracing. In status epilepticus, prompt recognition and therapy are critical given that prolonged status epilepticus is associated with a loss of $\gamma$-aminobutyric acid receptors. The principal anti–status epilepticus medications are aimed at activating $\gamma$-aminobutyric acid receptors. Therefore, any delay in recognition has a direct impact on treatment.

Fetal well-being must be assessed during the seizure and the postictal state. Determining the fetal gestational age is critical, since often during a tonic–clonic seizure, the fetus will experience an episode of bradycardia. This bradycardia may represent the hypoxic maternal state or, worse yet, fetal compromise due to a placental abruption. If it is the former, the fetus will often regain a normal FHR within 15 minutes after the seizure. If it is an abruption, palpating the uterus will confirm tetanic contractions, and some women may experience vaginal bleeding. The gestational age will determine whether the surgeon needs to proceed with an emergency cesarean delivery or whether it is unnecessary to perform a major surgery and administer anesthetics to an unstable mother.

## References

1. Heit JA, Kobbervig CE, James AH, Petterson TM, Bailey KR, Melton LJ III. Trends in the incidence of venous thromboembolism during pregnancy or postpartum: a 30-year population-based study. *Ann Intern Med*. 2005;143(10):697–706. Summary for patients in: *Ann Intern Med*. 2005;143(10):I12.

2. ACOG. *Thromboembolism in Pregnancy*. ACOG Practice Bulletin 19. Washington, DC: American College of Obstetricians and Gynecologists; 2000.

3. Knight M; UKOSS. Antenatal pulmonary embolism: risk factors, management and outcomes. *BJOG*. 2008;115(4):453–461.

4. Centers for Disease Control and Prevention. Surveillance Summaries, February 21, 2003. *MMWR*. 2003:52(No. SS-2):3–5.

5. Clark SL, Belfort MA, Dildy GA, Herbst MA, Meyers JA, Hankins GD. Maternal death in the 21st century: causes, prevention, and relationship to cesarean delivery. *Am J Obstet Gynecol*. 2008;199(1):36.e1–36.e5.

6. Villasanta U. Thromboembolic disease in pregnancy. *Am J Obstet Gynecol*. 1965;93:142–160.

7. Tapson VF. Acute pulmonary embolism. *N Engl J Med*. 2008;358(10):1037–1052.

8. Grifoni S, Olivotto I, Cecchini P, et al. Short-term outcome of patients with acute pulmonary embolism, normal blood pressure, and echocardiographic right ventricular dysfunction. *Circulation*. 2000;101(24):2817–2822.

9. Nolan TE, Hankins GDV. Acute pulmonary dysfunction and distress. *Obstet Gynecol Clin North Am*. 1995;22(1):39–54.

10. Whitty J, Dombrowski M. Respiratory diseases in pregnancy. In: Gabbe SG, Niebyl JR, Simpson JL, eds. *Obstetrics: Normal and Problem Pregnancies*. 4th Ed. Philadelphia, PA: Churchill Livingstone; 2002:1046–1053.

11. Stein PD, Terrin ML, Hales CA, et al. Clinical, laboratory, roentgenographic, and electrocardiographic findings in patients with acute pulmonary embolism and no pre-existing cardiac or pulmonary disease. *Chest*. 1991;100:598–603.

12. Di Nisio M, Squizzato A, Rutjes AW, Büller HR, Zwinderman AH, Bossuyt PM. Diagnostic accuracy of D-dimer test for exclusion of venous thromboembolism: a systematic review. *J Thromb Haemost*. 2007;5:296–304.

13. Stein PD, Hull RD, Patel KC, et al. D-dimer for the exclusion of acute venous thrombosis and pulmonary embolism: a systematic review. *Ann Intern Med*. 2004; 140:589–602.

14. Kearon C. Diagnosis of pulmonary embolism. *CMAJ*. 2003;168(2):183–194.

15. Miniati M, Pistolesi M, Marini C, et al. Value of perfusion lung scan in the diagnosis of pulmonary embolism: results of the Prospective Investigative Study of Acute Pulmonary Embolism Diagnosis (PISA-PED). *Am J Respir Crit Care Med*. 1996;154(5):1387–1393.

16. Gei AF, Vadhera RB, Hankins GDV. Embolism during pregnancy: thrombus, air, and amniotic fluid. *Anesthesiol Clin North Am*. 2003;21(1):165–182.

17. Partsch H, Blättler W. Compression and walking versus bed rest in the treatment of proximal deep venous thrombosis with low molecular weight heparin. *J Vasc Surg*. 2000;32:861–869.

18. Büller HR, Agnelli G, Hull RD, Hyers TM, Prins MH, Raskob GE. Antithrombotic therapy for venous thromboembolic disease: the Seventh ACCP Conference on Antithrombotic and Thrombolytic Therapy. *Chest*. 2004;126(Suppl.):401S–428S.

19. Harenberg J. Is laboratory monitoring of low-molecular-weight heparin therapy necessary? Yes. *J Thromb Haemost*. 2004;2:547–550.

20. Campbell IA, Bentley DP, Prescott RJ, Routledge PA, Shetty HG, Williamson IJ. Anticoagulation for three versus six months in patients with deep vein thrombosis or pulmonary embolism, or both: randomised trial. *Br Med J*. 2007;334:674.

21. Laros R. Thromboembolic disease. In: Creasy RK, Resnik R, Iams JD, eds. *Maternal Fetal Medicine Principles and Practice*. 5th Ed. Philadelphia, PA: Elsevier; 2004: 845–857.

22. Bauer K. New anticoagulants. *Hematology Am Soc Hematol Educ Program*. 2006: 450–456.

23. Segal JB, Streiff MB, Hofmann LV, Thornton K, Bass EB. Management of venous thromboembolism: a systematic review for a practice guideline. *Ann Intern Med*. 2007;146:211–222.

24. Ginsberg JS, Greer I, Hirsh J. Use of antithrombotic agents during pregnancy. *Chest*. 2001;119:122S–131S.

25. Kwon HL, Belanger K, Bracken MB. Asthma prevalence among pregnant and child-bearing-aged women in the United States: estimates from National Health Surveys. *Ann Epidemiol.* 2003;13(5):317–324.

26. Kung HC, Hoyert DL, Xu JQ, Murphy SL. *Deaths: Final Data for 2005. National Vital Statistics Reports*; Vol 56, No 10. Hyattsville, MD: National Center for Health Statistics, 2008.

27. Schatz M, Harden K, Forsythe A, et al. The course of asthma during pregnancy, post-partum, and with successive pregnancies: a prospective analysis. *J Allergy Clin Immunol.* 1998;81(3):509–517.

28. Dombrowski MP. Asthma and pregnancy. *Obstet Gynecol.* 2006;108(3, pt 1):667–681.

29. Schatz M, Dombrowski MP, Wise R, et al. Asthma morbidity during pregnancy can be predicted by severity classification. *J Allergy Clin Immunol.* 2003;112(2):283–288.

30. National Asthma Education and Prevention Program. Expert panel report: guidelines for the diagnosis and management of asthma update on selected topics. *J Allergy Clin Immunol.* 2002;110(5 Suppl.):13–29.

31. Bracken MB, Triche EW, Belanger K, et al. Asthma symptoms, severity, and drug therapy: a prospective study of effects on 2205 pregnancies. *Obstet Gynecol.* 2003;102(4):739–752.

32. Dombrowski MP, Schatz M, Wise R, et al. Asthma during pregnancy. *Obstet Gynecol.* 2004;103(1):5–12.

33. Schatz M, Dombrowski MP, Wise R, et al. The relationship of asthma medication use to perinatal outcomes. *J Allergy Clin Immunol.* 2004;113:1040–1045.

34. Triche EW, Saftlas AF, Belanger K, Leaderer BP, Bracken MB. Association of asthma diagnosis, severity, symptoms, and treatment with risk of preeclampsia. *Obstet Gynecol.* 2004;104: 585–593.

35. Schatz M, Dombrowski MP, Wise R, et al. Spirometry is related to perinatal outcomes in pregnant women with asthma. *Am J Obstet Gynecol.* 2006;194:120–126.

36. U.S. Department of Health and Human Services. National Institutes of Health National Heart, Lung, and Blood Institute, National Asthma Education and Prevention Program. *Working Group Report on Managing Asthma during Pregnancy: Recommendations for Pharmacologic Treatment, Update 2004.* NIH Publication No. 05–5236, March 2005. Available at: http://www.nhlbi.nih.gov/ health/prof/lung/asthma/astpreg.htm. Retrieved November 20, 2008.

37. Cockcroft DW, Murdock KY. Comparative effects of inhaled salbutamol, sodium cromoglycate, and beclomethasone dipropionate on allergen-induced early asthmatic responses, late asthmatic responses, and increased bronchial responsiveness to histamine. *J Allergy Clin Immunol.* 1987;79:734–740.

38. Demoly P, Piette V, Daures J-P. Asthma therapy during pregnancy. *Expert Opin Pharmacother.* 2003;4(7):1019–1023.

39. Papiris S, Kotanidou A, Katerina M, Rousos C. Clinical review: severe asthma. *Crit Care.* 2002;6(1):30–44.

40. Spitzer WO, Suissa S, Ernst P, et al. The use of beta-agonists and the risk of death and near death from asthma. *N Engl J Med.* 1992;326:501–506.

41. Kallen B, Rydhstroem H, Aberg A. Congenital malformations after the use of inhaled budesonide in early pregnancy. *Obstet Gynecol.* 1999;93:392–395.

42. Liccardi G, Cazzola M, Canonica GW, et al. General strategy for the management of bronchial asthma in pregnancy. *Respir Med.* 2003;97(7):778–789.

43. Park-Wyllie L, Mazzotta P, Pastuszak A, et al. Birth defects after maternal exposure to corticosteroids: prospective cohort study and meta-analysis of epidemiological studies. *Teratology.* 2000;62:385–392.

44. Rodrigo G, Rodrigo C, Burschtin O. A meta-analysis of the effects of ipratropium bromide in adults with acute asthma. *Am J Med.* 1999;107(4):363–370.

45. National Asthma Education and Prevention Program. *Practical Guide for the Diagnosis and Management of Asthma.* Publication 97–4053. Bethesda, MD: National Heart, Lung, and Blood Institute of the National Institutes of Health; 1997.

46. Adams BK, Cydulka RK. Asthma evaluation and management. *Emerg Med Clin North Am.* 2003;21(2):315–330.

47. Allan WC, Haddow JE, Palomaki GE, et al. Maternal thyroid deficiency and pregnancy complications: implications for population screening. *J Med Screen.* 2000;7:127–130.

48. Fernández-Soto ML, Jovanovic LG, González-Jiménez A, et al. Thyroid function during pregnancy and the postpartum period: iodine metabolism and disease states. *Endocr Pract.* 1998;4(2):97–105.
49. Ecker JL, Musci TJ. Treatment of thyroid disease in pregnancy. *Obstet Gynecol Clin North Am.* 1997;24(3):575–589.
50. Davis LE, Lucas MJ, Hankins GD, Roark ML, Cunningham FG. Thyrotoxicosis complicating pregnancy. *Am J Obstet Gynecol.* 1989;160(1):63–70.
51. Tietgens ST, Leinung MC. Thyroid storm. *Med Clin North Am.* 1995;79(1):169–184.
52. ACOG. *Thyroid Disease in Pregnancy.* ACOG Technical Bulletin 37. Washington, DC: American College of Obstetricians and Gynecologists, 2002.
53. Hershman JM. Human chorionic gonadotropin and the thyroid: hyperemesis gravidarum and trophoblastic tumors. *Thyroid.* 1999;9(7):653–657.
54. Mestman JH. Diagnosis and management of maternal and fetal thyroid disorders. *Curr Opin Obstet Gynecol.* 1999;11:167–175.
55. Calhoun BC, Brost B. Emergency management of sudden puerperal fever. *Obstet Gynecol Clin North Am.* 1995;22:357–367.
56. Mestman JH. Hyperthyroidism in pregnancy. *Clin Obstet Gynecol.* 1997;40:45–64.
57. Mestman J. Severe hyperthyroidism in pregnancy. In: Clark SL, Phelan JP, Cotton DB, eds. *Critical Care Obstetrics.* Oradell, NJ: Medical Economics Books; 1987:262.
58. Gittoes NJ, Franklyn JA. Hyperthyroidism: current treatment guidelines. *Drugs.* 1998;55:543–553.
59. Kilvert J, Nicholson HO, Wright AD. Ketoacidosis in diabetic pregnancy. *Diabet Med.* 1993;10:278–281.
60. Cullen MT, Reece EA, Homko CJ, et al. The changing presentations of diabetic ketoacidosis during pregnancy. *Am J Perinatol.* 1996;13:449–451.
61. Schneider M, Umpierrez GE, Ramsey RD, et al. Pregnancy complicated by diabetic ketoacidosis: maternal and fetal outcomes. *Diabetes Care.* 2003;26:958–959.
62. Ramin KD. Diabetic ketoacidosis in pregnancy. *Obstet Gynecol Clin North Am.* 1999;26:481–488.
63. Montoro MN, Myers VP, Mestman JH, et al. Outcome of pregnancy in diabetic ketoacidosis. *Am J Perinatol.* 1993;10:17–20.
64. Gabbe SG, Mestman JH, Hibbard LT. Maternal mortality in diabetes mellitus: a 1-year survey. *Obstet Gynecol.* 1976;48(5):549–551.
65. Schneider MB, Umpierrez GE, Ramsey RD, Mabie WC, Bennett KA. Pregnancy complicated by diabetic ketoacidosis. *Diabetes Care.* 2003;26(3):958–959.
66. Kent LA, Gill GV, Williams G. Mortality and outcome of patients with brittle diabetes and recurrent acidosis. *Lancet.* 1994;344:778–781.
67. Parker JA, Conway DL. Diabetic ketoacidosis in pregnancy. *Obstet Gynecol Clin North Am.* 2007;34(3):533–543.
68. Brumfield CG, Huddleston JF. The management of diabetic ketoacidosis in pregnancy. *Clin Obstet Gynecol.* 1984;27:50–59.
69. Pitteloud N, Binz K, Caulfield A, et al. Ketoacidosis during gestational diabetes: case report. *Diabetes Care.* 1998;21:1031–1032.
70. Metzgar BE, Coustan DR. Summary and recommendations of the Fourth International Workshop-Conference on Gestational Diabetes. *Diabetes Care.* 1998;21:B161–B167.
71. Tibaldi JM, Lorber DL, Nerenberger A. Diabetic ketoacidosis and insulin resistance with subcutaneous terbutaline infusion: a case report. *Am J Obstet Gynecol.* 1990;163:509–510.
72. Bernstein IM, Catalano PM. Ketoacidosis in pregnancy associated with the parenteral administration of terbutaline and betamethasone: a case report. *J Reprod Med.* 1990;35:818–820.
73. Hollingsworth DR. Medical and obstetric complications of diabetic pregnancies: IDDM, NIDDM, and GDM. In: Brown C-L, Mitchell C, eds. *Pregnancy, Diabetes and Birth: A Management Guide.* 2nd Ed. Baltimore, MD: Williams & Wilkins; 1992.
74. Cullen MT, Reece EA, Homko CJ, Sivan E. The changing presentations of diabetic ketoacidosis during pregnancy. *Am J Perinatol.* 1996;13:449–451.
75. Stecker MM. Management of status epilepticus. *UpToDate* (electronic journal), October 24, 2002.

76. Beach RL, Kaplan PW. Seizures in pregnancy: diagnosis and management. *Int Rev Neurobiol*. 2008;83:259–271.
77. ACOG. *Seizure Disorders in Pregnancy*. ACOG Educational Bulletin 231. Washington, DC: American College of Obstetricians and Gynecologists; 1996.
78. Shuster EA. Seizures in pregnancy. *Emerg Med Clin North Am*. 1994;12(4):1013–1025.
79. Treiman DM. Current treatment strategies in selected situations in epilepsy. *Epilepsia*. 1993;34(Suppl. 5):s17–s23.
80. EURAP Study Group. Seizure control and treatment in pregnancy: observations from the EURAP epilepsy pregnancy registry. *Neurology*. 2006;66(3):354–360.
81. Nulman I, Laslo D, Koren G. Treatment of epilepsy in pregnancy. *Drugs*. 1999;57:535–544.
82. Bardy AH, Hiilesmaa VII, Teramo KA. Serum phenytoin during pregnancy, labor and puerperium. *Acta Neurol Scand*. 1987;75:374–375.
83. Ramsay RE, Strauss RG, Wilder J, Wilmore U. Status epilepticus in pregnancy: effect of phenytoin malabsorption on seizure control. *Neurology*. 1978;28:85–89.
84. McAuley JW, Anderson GD. Treatment of epilepsy in women of reproductive age. *Clin Pharmacokinet*. 2002;41(8):559–579.
85. Gedekoh RH, Hayashi TF, McDonald HM. Eclampsia at Magee-Womens Hospital, 1970–1980. *Am J Obstet Gynecol*. 1981;140(8):860–866.
86. Harden CL. Antiepileptic drug teratogenesis: what are the risks for congenital malformations and adverse cognitive outcomes? *Int Rev Neurobiol*. 2008;83:205–213.
87. Pennell PB. Antiepileptic drug pharmacokinetics during pregnancy and lactation. *Neurology*. 2003;61(6 Suppl. 2):S35–S42.
88. Morrell MJ. Guidelines for the care of women with epilepsy. *Neurology*. 1998;51(Suppl. 4):S21–S27.

# 2 Acute Abdominal Pain in Pregnancy

### Kelly A. Best

Acute abdominal pain in pregnancy poses a unique challenge for both the clinician and the patient. The physiologic and physical changes associated with pregnancy must be considered when conducting a history, performing a physical examination, and interpreting diagnostic and other laboratory results in the pregnant patient with acute abdominal pain. Surgical interventions for nonobstetric reasons during pregnancy are reported to occur in 0.2% to 2.2% of all gestations (1). The most common etiologies for these surgical interventions include adnexal masses, acute appendicitis, and gallstone disease (2). Therefore, it is of critical importance to involve the expertise of the obstetrician, the general surgeon, and the radiologist in the evaluation of the pregnant patient who presents with acute abdominal pain.

This chapter reviews common causes of acute abdominal pain in pregnancy and facilitates interpretation of laboratory and diagnostic tests in pregnant women. The diagnostic approach to pregnant as well as nonpregnant patients should be similar. Clinicians should resist the temptation to uniformly attribute the patient's symptoms to her pregnancy. In addition, clinicians should have a high index of suspicion as classical findings may not be present for certain disease states. Delay in diagnosis resulting in complications associated with the underlying condition may lead to premature labor and delivery (3).

## PHYSIOLOGIC CHANGES IN PREGNANCY

Expansion of the plasma volume and an increase in red blood cell mass begin as early as the 4th week of pregnancy, peak at 28 to 34 weeks of gestation, and then plateau until parturition (4,5). Plasma volume expansion is accompanied by a lesser increase in red cell volume (6). As a result, there is a modest reduction in hematocrit, with peak hemodilution occurring at 24 to 26 weeks. The blood volume in pregnant women at term is about 100 mL/kg (7). The cardiac output rises 30% to 50% (1.8 L per minute) above baseline during normal pregnancy in part from changes in three important factors that determine cardiac output: preload is increased due to the associated rise in blood volume, afterload is reduced due to the decline in systemic vascular resistance, and maternal heart rate rises by 15 to 20 beats per minute (8).

During pregnancy, white cell volume increases from 5,000 to 6,000 cells/$mm^3$ to 16,000 cells/$mm^3$ in the second and third trimesters and to 20,000 to 30,000 cells/$mm^3$ in early labor (9). The glomerular filtration rate (GFR) and renal blood flow rise markedly during pregnancy. The increase in GFR can be demonstrated within 1 month of conception and reaches a peak approximately 40% to 50% above baseline levels by the end of the first trimester, resulting in a decrease in blood urea nitrogen and serum creatinine as well as glucosuria despite normal plasma glucose levels (10). Both kidneys increase in size by 1 to 1.5 cm during pregnancy primarily due to an increase in renal vascular and interstitial volumes (10). Ureteral dilatation during pregnancy results from hormonal effects, external compression, and intrinsic changes in the ureteral wall (11). Physiologic hydronephrosis typically occurs and is more common on the right than the left side (90% versus 10%).

In the respiratory system, the diaphragm rises by up to 4 cm, and the chest diameter can increase by 2 cm or more (12). Diaphragmatic excursion is not limited by the uterus and actually increases by up to 2 cm. Pregnancy is a state of relative hyperventilation, which may be centrally mediated through progesterone. The respiratory rate does not change while the tidal volume increases, resulting in an approximately 50% increase in minute ventilation. The normal $PaO_2$ in pregnant women ranges from 100 to 110 mm Hg (13–16). In addition, there is a decrease in arterial carbon dioxide levels ($PCO_2$ and $PaCO_2$) from the nonpregnant average of 40 mm Hg to a plateau of 27 to 32 mm Hg during pregnancy (14,15). This respiratory alkalosis is followed by compensatory renal excretion of bicarbonate, so that the resultant arterial pH is normal to slightly alkalotic (usually 7.40 to 7.45) (16). The decrease in $PaCO_2$ probably helps the fetus to eliminate carbon dioxide across the placenta.

## PHYSICAL EXAMINATION CHANGES IN PREGNANCY

Pain perceived from the abdomen is caused by peritoneal irritation, mechanical stretching, or ischemia (17). Physical exam findings in pregnancy may be blunted compared with those of nonpregnant patients with the same disease or process. Peritoneal signs may be absent due to the lifting and stretching of the anterior abdominal wall in pregnancy, preventing contact with the parietal peritoneum and eliminating rebound tenderness or guarding (18). In addition, the gravid uterus may distort the clinical picture by obstructing the movement of the omentum to an area of inflammation. Performing an examination with a pregnant patient in the left or right decubitus position, displacing the uterus to one side, may be of some benefit in certain clinical situations.

## IMAGING TECHNIQUES

Diagnostic imaging is often necessary during pregnancy. Sonographic examination is a common occurrence in pregnant women, but other types of radiological evaluation may also be required. Although the safety of radiation exposure during pregnancy is a common concern, a missed or delayed diagnosis can pose a greater risk to the woman and her pregnancy than any hazard associated with ionizing radiation (19). In many cases, the perception of fetal risk is higher than the actual risk (20,21). Table 2.1 provides an overview of the total fetal exposure of ionizing radiation in some commonly performed radiologic studies. Ionizing radiation can result in the following three harmful effects: (a) cell death and teratogenic effects, (b) carcinogenesis, and (c) genetic effects or mutations in germ cells (22). The threshold at which an increased risk of congenital malformations is observed in radiation-exposed embryos/fetuses has not been definitively determined. The best evidence suggests that the risk of malformations is increased at doses above 0.10 Gy, whereas the risk between 0.05 and 0.10 Gy is less clear (23). The American College of Obstetricians and Gynecologists makes the following recommendations for the use of diagnostic imaging techniques in pregnancy (24):

> Women should be counseled that X-ray exposure from a single diagnostic procedure does not result in harmful fetal effects. Specifically, exposure to less than 5 rad has not been associated with an increase in fetal anomalies or pregnancy loss.
>
> Concern about possible effects of high-dose ionizing radiation exposure should not prevent medically indicated diagnostic X-ray procedures from being performed on a pregnant woman. During pregnancy, other imaging procedures not associated with ionizing radiation (ultrasonography, MRI) should be considered instead of X-rays when appropriate.

| TABLE 2.1 | Estimated Fetal Exposure from Common Radiologic Procedures |
|---|---|

| Procedure | Fetal Exposure |
|---|---|
| Chest x-ray (two views) | 0.02–0.07 mrad |
| Abdominal film (single view) | 100 mrad |
| Intravenous pyelogram | ≥1 rad |
| Mammography | 7–20 mrad |
| Barium enema or small bowel series | 2–4 rad |
| CT scan (head or chest) | <1 rad |
| CT scan (abdomen) | 3.5 rad |
| CT pelvimetry | 250 mrad |

*Note*: 1 rad = 0.01 gray (Gy).
*Source*: Adapted from Ref. 24; Data from Cunningham FG, Gant NF, Leveno KJ, Gilstrap LC III, Hauth JC, Wenstrom KD (eds). General considerations and maternal evaluation. In: *Williams Obstetrics*. 21st Ed. New York, NY: McGraw-Hill; 2001:1143–1158.

## COMMON CAUSES OF ACUTE ABDOMINAL PAIN IN PREGNANCY

The differential diagnosis of acute abdominal pain in pregnancy includes etiologies similar to those in the nonpregnant patient as well as causes specific to the pregnancy (Table 2.2). The following sections review common causes of acute abdominal pain in pregnancy and detail safe diagnostic strategies for both the mother and the fetus.

### Appendicitis
Acute appendicitis is the most common nonobstetric surgical diagnosis during pregnancy (25). The incidence ranges from 0.06% to 0.1%, or 1 in 1,500 deliveries (26–28). Appendicitis is more frequently seen in the second trimester when compared with the first and third trimesters or during the postpartum period (29). An infected appendix appears to be more likely to rupture during pregnancy, possibly because of delay in diagnosis and intervention (30,31).

Right lower quadrant pain is the most common symptom of appendicitis. Although older studies suggested that the location of the appendix migrates upward with the enlarging uterus, this theory has been refuted by subsequent studies which have found that the most common symptom of appendicitis, that is, right lower quadrant pain, occurs within a few centimeters of McBurney's point in the vast majority of pregnant women, regardless of the stage of pregnancy (31,32).

The physiologic changes of pregnancy can confound the diagnosis of appendicitis. Leukocytosis can be a normal finding in pregnant women. Indigestion, bowel irregularity, nausea/vomiting, as well as a sense of not feeling well are also common symptoms of both appendicitis and normal pregnancy. The temporal relationship of these symptoms is essential in differentiating early appendicitis from the nausea and vomiting of pregnancy. In appendicitis, nausea and vomiting, if present, typically follow the onset of pain, whereas nausea and vomiting associated with pregnancy are not usually associated with pain. Microscopic hematuria and pyuria are found in up to one third of patients with acute

| TABLE 2.2 | Common Causes of Abdominal Pain | | | |
|---|---|---|---|---|
| **Upper Quadrants** | **Lower Quadrants** | **Epigastrium** | **Periumbilical** | **Pelvic (Female)** |
| Hepatitis | Appendicitis | GERD | Appendicitis | Ectopic pregnancy |
| Cholecystitis | Irritable bowel syndrome | Peptic ulcer disease | Gastroenteritis | Salpingitis |
| Pancreatitis | Nephrolithiasis | Gastritis | Bowel obstruction | PID/TOA |
| Pneumonia | Inguinal hernia | Pancreatitis | | Adnexal pathology |
| Gastritis/ ulcer | Diverticular disease | Myocardial infarction | | Endometritis |
| Splenic abscess | | | | Leiomyomata (torsion/ degeneration) |
| | | | | Placental abruption Uterine rupture Dysmenorrhea Labor |

appendicitis, and a decrease in the direct contact between the area of inflammation and the parietal peritoneum results in less muscle response or guarding.

The gold standard for diagnostic imaging of the appendix in pregnancy is graded compression ultrasonography. Appendicitis is diagnosed if a noncompressible blind-ended tubular structure is visualized in the right lower quadrant with a maximal diameter >6 mm (33,34). Magnetic resonance imaging (MRI) can be useful for the next step in cases with diagnostic uncertainty and provides an attractive alternative to CT because it avoids exposure to ionizing radiation.

Consultation with a general surgeon should be obtained in women whose imaging studies or physical examination suggest appendicitis. The decision to proceed to laparotomy should be based upon the clinical findings, the diagnostic imaging results, and the clinical judgment. Given the diagnostic difficulties and the significant risk of fetal morbidity or mortality with perforation (36% versus 1.5%) (26) or with peritonitis or abscess (fetal loss: 6% versus 2%; early delivery: 11% versus 4%), a higher negative laparotomy rate (20% to 35%) compared with nonpregnant women has generally been considered to be acceptable (35,36).

A transverse incision at McBurney's point, or more commonly over the point of maximal tenderness, can be utilized in pregnancy (37). When the diagnosis is less certain, a lower midline vertical incision can be utilized since it permits adequate exposure of the abdomen for diagnosis and treatment of surgical conditions that mimic appendicitis. A vertical incision can also be used for a cesarean delivery, if subsequently required for obstetric indications. Case reports and small case series regarding laparoscopic appendectomy in pregnancy suggest that such procedures can be performed successfully during all trimesters and with few complications (38–41). The decision to proceed with such an approach should take into consideration the skill and experience of the surgeon, as well as clinical factors such as the size of the gravid uterus. Modifications of the technique during pregnancy should include the following: a slight left lateral positioning of the patient, avoiding the use of any cervical instruments; use of open entry techniques or placement of trocars under direct visualization; and limiting the intra-abdominal pressure to <12 mm Hg (42).

## Cholecystitis

The incidence of biliary disease requiring surgery in pregnancy is 0.2 to 0.5 cases per 1,000 pregnancies (43). Hormonal changes associated with pregnancy predispose to the development of gallstones (44,45). Cholelithiasis is the main cause of cholecystitis in pregnancy, accounting for over 90% of cases (46).

Patients with acute cholecystitis typically complain of abdominal pain, most commonly in the right upper quadrant or epigastrium. The pain may radiate to the right shoulder or back. Characteristically, acute cholecystitis pain is steady and severe. Associated complaints may include nausea, vomiting, and anorexia. Elicitation of "Murphy's sign" may be a useful diagnostic maneuver. While palpating the area of the gallbladder fossa, the patient is asked to inspire deeply, causing the gallbladder to descend toward the examining fingers. Patients with acute cholecystitis commonly experience increased discomfort and may have an associated inspiratory arrest. Patients with acute cholecystitis are usually ill appearing, febrile, and tachycardic and lie still on the examining table because cholecystitis is associated with true local parietal peritoneal inflammation that is aggravated by movement. Abdominal examination usually demonstrates voluntary and involuntary guarding but may be blunted in pregnancy. Liver enzymes may be difficult to interpret in pregnancy as alkaline phosphatase may be elevated in normal pregnancy. Bilirubin and transaminases, however, will not be elevated in normal pregnancy and may provide evidence of biliary obstruction.

Ultrasonography represents an appropriate first choice when imaging pregnant women with suspected cholecystitis and can often establish the diagnosis. The sensitivity and specificity of ultrasonography for the detection of gallstones are in the range of 84% (95% CI 0.76 to 0.92) and 99% (95% CI 0.97 to 1.00), respectively (45,46).

As a general rule, surgery is safest to perform during the second trimester, when the risk of premature labor is lowest and uterine obstruction of the gallbladder is not present. Laparoscopic cholecystectomy has been performed during pregnancy but its safety is uncertain. In one small series, the laparoscopic approach was associated with adverse fetal outcomes (47). In other reports, however, laparoscopic cholecystectomy was safe if performed by a skilled laparoscopic surgeon and was not associated with fetal mortality, although tocolytic therapy was required in some patients (48,49).

## Adnexal Masses

Increasing use of ultrasound during pregnancy suggests that clinically significant adnexal masses complicate 0.2% to 2% of pregnancies (50). The ultrasound appearance of the mass suggests whether it is benign or malignant. In a large series, about 1% of ovarian masses in pregnant women were malignant, with germ cell tumors and epithelial tumors being the most common subgroups (50). Complications include torsion, rupture, hemorrhage, and suspicion of malignancy. In the majority of cases, adnexal masses can be managed expectantly throughout pregnancy, while surgical management of complicated adnexal masses is necessary in approximately 1 in 1,300 pregnancies (51,52).

Adnexal torsion is more common in pregnancy than in the nonpregnant state (26) and has been reported in up to 7% of pregnant patients with adnexal masses (53). Pain associated with torsion is often intermittent, crampy and may radiate to the ipsilateral thigh or flank. Nausea and vomiting may also develop. Examination findings may include a palpable fullness in the pelvis or lower quadrant and, in the presence of rupture, peritoneal signs may be present. While the patient may remain afebrile with a normal or slightly elevated white count, hemoglobin may be decreased when rupture results in hemoperitoneum (and in severe cases, hypovolemic shock). Transvaginal and transabdominal ultrasound examinations are the imaging modalities of choice when evaluating an adnexal mass.

While laparotomy (with a vertical midline incision to facilitate exposure and allow for extension if indicated) should be regarded as the preferred approach for the surgical management of ovarian torsion in pregnancy, several reports have suggested that laparoscopy by a surgeon skilled in this approach may be acceptable (53–55). In some circumstances, adnexal cyst rupture may be treated expectantly if the clinical condition remains stable.

A persistent adnexal cyst larger than 5 cm in a pregnant woman should be removed electively during the early second trimester of pregnancy because torsion, rupture, or hemorrhage often requires emergency surgery and can lead to preterm delivery (51). On occasion, a simple cyst that is 5 to 10 cm in size can be managed expectantly if the patient is asymptomatic and serial ultrasound examinations show no increase in size. If the cyst persists, excision can be performed at cesarean delivery or postpartum. It is important to consider that a large adnexal cyst in the posterior cul-de-sac has the potential to produce obstructed labor and delivery. Surgical intervention is indicated for an adnexal mass of any size suspicious for malignancy or if torsion, rupture, or hemorrhage is suspected. An adnexal mass identified incidentally at the time of cesarean delivery should be removed (56). Complete surgical removal is preferred to aspiration since malignancy could be missed even with simple, smooth-walled cysts (57).

Postoperative progesterone is recommended when the corpus luteum is removed prior to 8 to 10 weeks of gestation.

## Pyelonephritis and Nephrolithiasis

Acute pyelonephritis is a common complication of pregnancy as the physiologic changes in pregnancy often predispose women to this condition. Ascending infection from the urinary bladder is the likely etiology in the majority of cases. As the gravid uterus enlarges, increased pressure on the ureters at the pelvic brim, as well as the relaxant effect of circulating progesterone on the ureters, predisposes the pregnant patient to urinary stasis (58).

Patients with acute pyelonephritis often appear acutely ill and may complain of flank pain, dysuria, frequency, fever, and shaking chills. Costovertebral angle tenderness may be present on the affected side while abdominal pain is less common. The white count will likely be elevated with a concomitant left shift. Urinalysis typically reveals both pyuria and bacteriuria. Urine culture with sensitivity will guide treatment; however, initiation of intravenous antibiotics directed at Gram-negative enteric bacteria should be initiated as soon as possible while urinary cultures are pending.

The development of symptomatic nephrolithiasis during pregnancy is a rare event, occurring in about 1 in every 1,500 to 3,000 pregnancies (59). Affected patients usually present in the second or third trimester (~20% in the first trimester) with acute flank pain (90%), which often radiates to the groin or lower abdomen. Nausea, vomiting, urinary frequency, and urgency are also typical. Microscopic hematuria is present in 75% to 95% of patients, one third of whom have gross hematuria (59).

Renal and pelvic ultrasound should be performed when an obstructing calculus is suspected. This modality avoids exposure to radiation and is useful for detecting secondary signs of obstruction, such as hydronephrosis or hydroureter (60). Physiologic hydronephrosis of pregnancy must be distinguished from pathological hydronephrosis from obstruction. When the ultrasound examination is negative and the patient has continued discomfort suggestive of nephrolithiasis, two options are available for diagnosis: a limited intravenous pyelogram (IVP) in which a single abdominal radiograph is taken approximately 5 minutes after intravenous administration of contrast material (60) or, if available, ureteroscopy (61). The single-shot IVP, which delivers about 50 mrad to the fetus, is positive in most pregnant women with a symptomatic stone (60). MRI can also be a useful adjunct in assessing stones during pregnancy. $T_2$-weighted MRI can offer differing urographic appearances in physiologic and calculus obstruction (62).

Most (75% to 85%) stones pass spontaneously, due in part to the normally dilated urinary tract in pregnant women (58,59). Cystoscopy with insertion of a ureteral stent or ureteroscopy to remove or fragment the stone may be required in the patient who is septic, has persistent severe pain, or has obstruction in a solitary functioning kidney (61,63). Ureteral stenting or placement of a nephrostomy tube to relieve obstruction or pain is a valid option for managing pregnant patients. However, pregnancy significantly increases the risk of stent encrustation, necessitating the need for frequent ureteral stent exchange (64). If conservative management fails, ureteroscopy with lithotripsy may be an option. Although shock wave lithotripsy has been inadvertently performed in a few pregnant women, its use during pregnancy is currently contraindicated (65,66).

## Bowel Obstruction

Bowel obstruction complicates 1 in 1,500 to 3,500 deliveries (67). Risk factors for bowel obstruction in pregnancy are related to adhesions from pelvic infection and previous surgery, complications of Crohn's disease, intussusception, and more rarely neoplasm.

Symptoms of intestinal obstruction are similar to those in the nonpregnant population and include abdominal distention, vomiting, abdominal pain, and an inability to pass flatus. Pain is generally periumbilical, paroxysmal, and crampy. On physical examination, the large, gravid abdomen may pose a diagnostic challenge as it may mask the usual findings during auscultation, percussion, and palpation. In general, abdominal tenderness, abnormal bowel sounds (high pitched or hypoactive), tachycardia, and hypotension may be present.

While laboratory studies are not helpful in establishing the diagnosis of bowel obstruction, they may be utilized to monitor the white blood cell count (a sharp rise over a short period of time may indicate strangulation) and to assess the degree of dehydration. The diagnosis of small bowel obstruction can be made by a history and a physical examination in the majority of patients. Plain abdominal radiography is used to confirm the diagnosis of bowel obstruction. Ordering an upright chest film to rule out the presence of free air, as well as supine and upright abdominal films, is appropriate in this setting. Of note, plain films can be equivocal in 20% to 30% of patients and are "normal, nonspecific, or misleading" in 10% to 20% (68,69). Multiple air-fluid levels with distended loops of small bowel are seen in small bowel obstruction, although occasionally they can be seen in the setting of a paralytic ileus. Abdominal ultrasonography can also be useful, especially as a bedside test for the critically ill (70,71).

Treatment of small bowel obstruction in pregnancy is similar to that in nonpregnant individuals. Aggressive intervention is warranted because delay in treatment increases maternal and fetal morbidity and mortality. Fluid and electrolyte replacement, bowel decompression, and prompt surgical intervention in cases resistant to decompression are suggested.

## LAPAROSCOPIC SURGERY IN PREGNANCY

Laparotomy has generally been accepted as the approach of choice for surgical exploration in pregnancy. Recent case reports and case series of successful laparoscopy in pregnancy have called into question this long-held belief (55,72,73). Theoretical areas of concern have included the potential decrease in uteroplacental blood flow resulting in fetal hypoxia due to the rise in intra-abdominal pressure during pneumoperitoneum, fetal acidosis from absorption of carbon dioxide, and direct or indirect fetal injury if the uterus is perforated by a trocar or a Veress needle.

Although prospective studies are lacking, multiple case series evaluating the safety of laparoscopy in pregnancy have reported laparoscopic procedures in all trimesters with minimal morbidity to the fetus with regard to fetal weight, gestational duration, intrauterine growth restriction, congenital malformations, stillbirths, or neonatal deaths (73).

The benefits of laparoscopy for pregnant and nonpregnant women include less postoperative pain, less postoperative ileus, reduction in adhesion formation, shorter hospital stay, less narcotic use, improved respiratory efforts, and faster return to usual activities (74). In addition, there may be less uterine manipulation and improved visualization in the gravid population when compared with laparotomy (73–75). The following are considerations when laparoscopy is performed in pregnancy:

1. Laparoscopy can be performed in any trimester; however, the optimal time for nonemergent indications is the early second trimester.
2. Use of an oral or nasogastric tube for gastric decompression.
3. Use of prophylactic pneumatic compression devices (with the need for pharmacologic thromboprophylaxis determined on a case-by-case basis) to prevent thrombosis.
4. Avoidance of uterine/cervical manipulators.
5. Supine or low lithotomy position with a leftward tilt.
6. Establishment of pneumoperitoneum is dependent on the surgeon's experience and comfort.
7. Intra-abdominal pressure should be maintained between 8 and 12 mm Hg and should not exceed 15 mm Hg.
8. Fetal heart rate should be confirmed and documented before and after the procedure. If fetal monitoring is necessary during the procedure, consideration for transabdominal or transvaginal ultrasound assessment should be made.
9. Fetal heart rate and uterine activity should be monitored in the recovery room by protocols appropriate for gestational age.
10. Nonsteroidal antiinflammatory drugs should be avoided, especially after 32 weeks of gestation, while opioids and antiemetics can be used as needed.

## SUMMARY

The presence of the fetus should not delay the decision to perform the indicated diagnostic testing or to initiate treatment, as delays in this setting often result in significant morbidity and mortality for both the mother and the fetus. A multidisciplinary approach with early consultation from obstetric, surgical, laboratory, and radiologic services is warranted. Because obstetric causes for abdominal pain exist in many patients, however, consultation with an obstetric provider will help to define the subset of patients who warrant further investigation into nonobstetric sources for acute abdominal pain.

## References

1. Hunt MG, Martin JN Jr, Martin RW, Meeks GR, Wiser WL, Morrison JC. Perinatal aspects of abdominal surgery for nonobstetric disease. *Am J Perinatol.* 1989;6(4):412–417.
2. Semin, GS. Anesthesia for nonobstetric surgery in the pregnant patient. *Perinatology.* 2002;26(2):136–145.
3. Kilpatrick CC, Orejuela FJ. Management of the acute abdomen in pregnancy: a review. *Curr Opin Obstet Gynecol.* 2008;20(6):534–539.
4. Assali NS, Brinkman CR III. *Pathophysiology of Gestation, Vol 1: Maternal Disorders.* New York, NY: Academic Press; 1972:278.
5. Ueland K. Cardiorespiratory physiology of pregnancy. In Vanassa A Barss, MD (ed): *Gynecology and Obstetrics.* Vol. 3. Baltimore, MD: Harper & Row; 1979.
6. Pritchard JA. Changes in the blood volume during pregnancy and delivery. *Anesthesiology.* 1965;26:393.
7. Metcalfe J, Ueland K. Maternal cardiovascular adjustments to pregnancy. *Prog Cardiovasc Dis.* 1974;16:363.
8. Robson SC, Hunter S, Boys RJ, Dunlop W. Serial study of factors influencing changes in cardiac output during human pregnancy. *Am J Physiol.* 1989;256:H1060.
9. Pritchard JA, Baldwin RM, Dickey JC, et al. Blood volume changes in pregnancy and the puerperium. *Am J Obstet Gynecol.* 1962;84:1271.
10. Davison JM, Dunlop W. Renal haemodynamics and tubular function in normal human pregnancy. *Kidney Int.* 1980;18:152.
11. Beydoun SN. Morphologic changes in the renal tract in pregnancy. *Clin Obstet Gynecol.* 1985;28:249.
12. Weinberger SE, Weiss ST, Cohen WR, et al. Pregnancy and the lung. *Am Rev Respir Dis.* 1980;121:559.
13. Gilroy RJ, Mangura BT, Lavietes MH. Rib cage and abdominal volume displacements during breathing in pregnancy. *Am Rev Respir Dis.* 1988;137:668.
14. Liberatore SM, Pistelli R, Patalano F, et al. Respiratory function during pregnancy. *Respiration.* 1984;46:145.
15. Pernoll ML, Metcalfe J, Kovach PA, et al. Ventilation during rest and exercise in pregnancy and postpartum. *Respir Physiol.* 1975;25:295.
16. Artal R, Wiswell R, Romem Y, Dorey F. Pulmonary responses to exercise in pregnancy. *Am J Obstet Gynecol.* 1986;154:378.
17. Mayen IE, Hussain H. Abdominal pain during pregnancy. *Gastroenterol Clin North Am.* 1998;27:1.
18. Sivanesaratnam V. The acute abdomen and the obstetrician. *Clin Obstet Gynaecol.* 2000;14(1):89–102.
19. McCollough CH, Schueler BA, Atwell TD, et al. Radiation exposure and pregnancy: when should we be concerned? *Radiographics.* 2007;27:909.
20. Ratnapalan S, Bona N, Chandra K, Koren G. Physicians'perceptions of teratogenic risk associated with radiography and CT during early pregnancy. *Am J Roentgenol.* 2004;182:1107.
21. Bentur Y, Horlatsch N, Koren G. Exposure to ionizing radiation during pregnancy: perception of teratogenic risk and outcome. *Teratology.* 1991;43:109.
22. Hall EJ. Scientific view of low-level radiation risks. *Radiographics.* 1991;11:509–518.
23. www.icrp.org
24. ACOG Committee Opinion No. 299. Guidelines for diagnostic imaging during pregnancy. *Obstet Gynecol.* 2004;104:647.
25. Tamir IL, Bongard FS, Klein SR. Acute appendicitis in the pregnant patient. *Am J Surg.* 1990;160:571.
26. Sharp HT. Gastrointestinal surgical conditions during pregnancy. *Clin Obstet Gynecol.* 1994;37:306.
27. Andersen B, Nielsen TF. Appendicitis in pregnancy: diagnosis, management and complications. *Acta Obstet Gynecol Scand.* 1999;78:758.
28. Mourad J, Elliott JP, Erickson L, Lisboa L. Appendicitis in pregnancy: new information that contradicts long-held clinical beliefs. *Am J Obstet Gynecol.* 2000;182:1027.
29. Andersson B, Lambe M. Incidence of appendicitis during pregnancy. *Int J Epidemiol.* 2001;30:1281.

30. Bickell NA, Aufses AH Jr, Rojas M, Bodian C. How time affects the risk of rupture in appendicitis. *J Am Coll Surg.* 2006;202:401.

31. Weingold AB. Appendicitis in pregnancy. *Clin Obstet Gynecol.* 1983;26:801.

32. Hodjati, H, Kazerooni, T. Location of the appendix in the gravid patient: a re-evaluation of the established concept. *Int J Gynaecol Obstet.* 2003;81:245.

33. Barloon TJ, Brown BP, Abu-Yousef MM, et al. Sonography of acute appendicitis in pregnancy. *Abdom Imaging.* 1995;20:149.

34. Lim HK, Bae SH, Seo GS. Diagnosis of acute appendicitis in pregnant women: value of sonography. *Am J Roentgenol.* 1992;159:539.

35. Babaknia A, Parsa H, Woodruff JD. Appendicitis during pregnancy. *Obstet Gynecol.* 1977;50:40.

36. McGory ML, Zingmond DS, Tillou A, et al. Negative appendectomy in pregnant women is associated with a substantial risk of fetal loss. *J Am Coll Surg.* 2007;205:534.

37. Popkin CA, Lopez PP, Cohn SM, et al. The incision of choice for pregnant women with appendicitis is through McBurney's point. *Am J Surg.* 2002;183:20.

38. Curet MJ, Allen, D, Josloff, RK, Pitcher, DE. Laparoscopy during pregnancy. *Arch Surg.* 1996;131:546.

39. Gurbuz AT, Peetz ME. The acute abdomen in the pregnant patient. Is there a role for laparoscopy? *Surg Endosc.* 1997;11:98.

40. Affleck DG, Handrahan DL, Egger MJ, Price RR. The laparoscopic management of appendicitis and cholelithiasis during pregnancy. *Am J Surg.* 1999;178:523.

41. Wu JM, Chen KH, Lin HF, et al. Laparoscopic appendectomy in pregnancy. *J Laparoendosc Adv Surg Tech.* 2005;15:447.

42. Al-Fozan H, Tulandi T. Safety and risks of laparoscopy in pregnancy. *Curr Opin Obstet Gynecol.* 2002;14:375.

43. Landers D, Carmona R, Crombleholme W, Lim R. Acute cholecystitis in pregnancy. *Obstet Gynecol.* 1987;69:131.

44. Mazze RI, Kallen B. Reproductive outcome after anesthesia and operation during pregnancy: a registry study of 5405 cases. *Am J Obstet Gynecol.* 1989;161:1178.

45. Stauffer RA, Adams A, Wygal J, Lavery JP. Gallbladder disease in pregnancy. *Am J Obstet Gynecol.* 1982;144:661.

46. Shea JA, Berlin JA, Escarce JJ, et al. Revised estimates of diagnostic test sensitivity and specificity in suspected biliary tract disease. *Arch Intern Med.* 1994;154:2573.

47. Amos JD, Schorr SJ, Norman PF, et al. Laparoscopic surgery during pregnancy. *Am J Surg.* 1996;171:435.

48. Lanzafame RJ. Laparoscopic cholecystectomy during pregnancy. *Surgery.* 1995;118:627.

49. Lachman E, Schienfeld A, Voss E, et al. Pregnancy and laparoscopic surgery. *J Am Assoc Gynecol Laparosc.* 1999;6:347.

50. Hoffman MS, Sayer RA. Adnexal masses in pregnancy. *OBG Management.* 2007;19:27.

51. Hess LW, Peaceman A, O'Brien WF, Winkel CA. Adnexal mass occurring with intra-uterine pregnancy: report of fifty-four patients requiring laparotomy for definitive management. *Am J Obstet Gynecol.* 1988;158:1029.

52. Whitecar MP, Turner S, Higby MK. Adnexal masses in pregnancy: a review of 130 cases undergoing surgical management. *Am J Obstet Gynecol.* 1999;181:19.

53. Shalev E, Peleg D. Laparoscopic treatment of adnexal torsion. *Surg Gynecol Obstet.* 1993;176:448.

54. Cohen SB, Oelsner G, Seidman DS, Admon D, Mashiach S, Goldenberg M. Laparoscopic detorsion allows sparing of the twisted ischemic adnexa. *J Am Assoc Gynecol Laparosc.* 1999;6:139.

55. Soriano D, Yefet Y, Seidman DS, Goldenberg M, Mashiach S, Oelsner G. Laparoscopy versus laparotomy in the management of adnexal masses during pregnancy. *Fertil Steril.* 1999;71:955.

56. Koonings PP, Platt LD, Wallace R. Incidental adnexal neoplasms at cesarean section. *Obstet Gynecol.* 1988;72:767.

57. Rodin A, Coltart TM, Chapman MG. Needle aspiration of simple ovarian cysts in pregnancy. Case reports. *Br J Obstet Gynaecol.* 1989;96:994.

58. Gilstrap LC, Ramin SM. Urinary tract infections during pregnancy. *Obstet Gynecol Clin North Am.* 2001;28(3):581–591.
59. Butler EL, Cox SM, Eberts EG, Cunningham FG. Symptomatic nephrolithiasis complicating pregnancy. *Obstet Gynecol.* 2000;96:753.
60. Boridy IC, Maklad N, Sandler CM. Suspected urolithiasis in pregnant women: imaging algorithm and literature review. *AJR Am J Roentgenol.* 1996;167:869.
61. Scarpa RM, De Lisa A, Usai E. Diagnosis and treatment of ureteral calculi during pregnancy with rigid ureteroscopes. *J Urol.* 1996;155:875.
62. Spencer JA, Chahal R, Kelly A, et al. Evaluation of painful hydronephrosis in pregnancy: magnetic resonance urographic patterns in physiological dilatation versus calculous obstruction. *J Urol.* 2004;171:256.
63. McAleer SJ, Loughlin KR. Nephrolithiasis and pregnancy. *Curr Opin Urol.* 2004;14:123.
64. Parulkar BG, Hopkins TB, Wollin MR, et al. Renal colic during pregnancy: a case for conservative treatment. *J Urol.* 1998;159:365.
65. Asgari MA, Safarinejad MR, Hosseini SY, Dadkhah F. Extracorporeal shock wave lithotripsy of renal calculi during early pregnancy. *BJU Int.* 1999;84:615.
66. Deliveliotis CH, Argyropoulos B, Chrisofos M, Dimopoulos CA. Shockwave lithotripsy in unrecognized pregnancy: interruption or continuation? *J Endourol.* 2001;15:787.
67. Coleman MT, Trianfo VA, Rund DA. Nonobstetric emergencies in pregnancy: trauma and surgical conditions. *Am J Obstet Gynecol.* 1997;177:497.
68. Megibow AJ, Balthazar EJ, Cho KC, et al. Bowel obstruction: evaluation with CT. *Radiology.* 1991;180:313.
69. Balthazar EJ. George W. Holmes Lecture. CT of small-bowel obstruction. *AJR Am J Roentgenol.* 1994;162:255.
70. Suri S, Gupta S, Sudhakar PJ, et al. Comparative evaluation of plain films, ultrasound and CT in the diagnosis of intestinal obstruction. *Acta Radiol.* 1999;40:422.
71. Ogata M, Imai S, Hosotani R, et al. Abdominal ultrasonography for the diagnosis of strangulation in small bowel obstruction. *Br J Surg.* 1994;81:421.
72. Reedy MB, Kallen B, Kuehl TJ. Laparoscopy during pregnancy: a study of five fetal outcome parameters with use of the Swedish Health Registry. *Am J Obstet Gynecol.* 1997;177:673.
73. Yumi H. Guidelines for diagnosis, treatment, and use of laparoscopy for surgical problems during pregnancy: this statement was reviewed and approved by the Board of Governors of the Society of American Gastrointestinal and Endoscopic Surgeons (SAGES), September 2007. *Surg Endosc.* 2008;22:849.
74. Andreoli M, Servakov M, Meyers P, Mann WJ Jr. Laparoscopic surgery during pregnancy. *J Am Assoc Gynecol Laparosc.* 1999;6:229.
75. Stepp K, Falcone T. Laparoscopy in the second trimester of pregnancy. *Obstet Gynecol Clin North Am.* 2004;31:485.

# 3 Ectopic Pregnancy

### Mary E. Rausch, Andrew M. Kaunitz, and Kurt Barnhart

The term "ectopic pregnancy" (EP) refers to any pregnancy resulting from the implantation of a fertilized ovum outside of the uterine cavity, most commonly in the fallopian tube. Although EPs account for approximately 2% of pregnancies, the true incidence is difficult to ascertain given the underreporting of EPs treated in outpatient units (1). The most concerning acute danger of an EP is tubal rupture with massive intra-abdominal hemorrhage, and this is a leading cause of first trimester morbidity and mortality (2). EP resulted in 7% of all pregnancy-related deaths between 1991 and 1997, with 85% to 92% of fatalities secondary to hemorrhage (3).

Pregnancy-related deaths associated with an EP are on the decline, likely because of earlier detection and treatment (3). One half of deaths could have been prevented by more prompt diagnosis and treatment of EP by health professionals, and one third of deaths could have been prevented by more prompt notification of a physician by the patient (4). Although the average age of women with an EP is 28 years, the mortality rate is highest for teenagers (4). Misdiagnosis of a gastrointestinal disorder, intrauterine pregnancy (IUP), or pelvic inflammatory disease (PID) is common in this setting.

## ETIOLOGY

Of the 96% of EPs found in the fallopian tube, 70% are ampullary, 12% isthmic, 11% fimbrial, and 2% interstitial, with extratubal sites being rare (5) (Fig. 3.1). The tube serves a complex function in the process of fertilization and transport of the oocyte from the ovary to the uterus, where the blastocyst implants. At ovulation, the fimbriated end of the fallopian tube picks up the expelled oocyte with its cumulus mass of follicular cells. Conduction of the egg toward the uterus is thought to be effected primarily by the negative tubal intraluminal pressure generated by muscular contractions, with a secondary contribution from ciliary beating. Impaired muscular contractions, loss of ciliary action, or physical blockade could therefore prevent the embryo from reaching its normal location in the uterus. Tubal transport takes approximately 3 days, with fertilization occurring in the ampullary portion of the tube. Damage to the tube from prior infection, surgery, or tubal pregnancy can therefore subsequently increase one's risk of future EP (6–8) (Table 3.1). A woman who experiences one EP has an increased risk of a second; women with an EP are 2.4 to 25 times as likely to have had a prior EP (8).

Although any form of contraception decreases the overall risk of pregnancy including EP, when contraceptive failure occurs in women using an intrauterine device (IUD) or following tubal sterilization, the risk of EP is elevated (7,9). With the copper T, approximately 6% of failures represent ectopic implantations (10). With the levonorgestrel IUD, this percentage is approximately 50 (11). Other factors in the history which may be associated with risk of EP include a history of salpingitis, tubal infertility, and DES exposure (6,7).

Among patients presenting to the emergency room with an early symptomatic pregnancy, the incidence of EP was lower for adolescents than adults (9.7% versus 21.7%) (12) and younger women (<25 years old) (8). However,

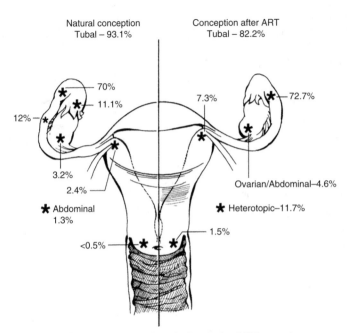

Natural conception
Tubal – 93.1%

Conception after ART
Tubal – 82.2%

70%

11.1%

12%

7.3%

72.7%

3.2%

2.4%

Ovarian/Abdominal–4.6%

✱ Abdominal
1.3%

✱ Heterotopic–11.7%

1.5%

<0.5%

**FIGURE 3.1** Locations of ectopic implantation in natural and ART conceptions.

adolescents with EP present more often than adults with pain and a positive chlamydia and/or gonorrhea culture and less often with the classic risk factors of prior EP and prior pelvic surgery (12).

## CLINICAL PRESENTATION

Although the classic signs and symptoms of EP are pain, amenorrhea, and vaginal bleeding, this diagnosis should be suspected in any reproductive-age woman presenting with pain or abnormal bleeding, as well as in women with symptoms of shock. The character of the pain is often nonspecific and may be diffuse, unilateral, bilateral, or even contralateral to the side involved. In tubal pregnancies, the pain may begin as vague lower abdominal discomfort that later becomes sharp and colicky as periodic tubal distention occurs. By contrast, the pain associated with the spontaneous abortion of an IUP is usually central and is likened to that of labor or menstrual cramps. Tubal rupture may be accompanied by a significant hemoperitoneum, resulting in poorly localized abdominal pain. Shoulder pain is possible secondary to phrenic nerve irritation when blood contacts diaphragmatic surfaces.

Although a history of recent amenorrhea is common in women with EPs, it is not unusual for a patient initially to deny having missed any menstrual periods. On a careful review, however, the most recent period may be described as lighter or abnormally timed, perhaps representing pathologic bleeding from decidualized endometrium. The abnormal vaginal bleeding reported by women with EPs is usually mild. Heavy bleeding or passage of clots is distinctly atypical and is more characteristic of inevitable or incomplete abortion of an IUP.

| **TABLE 3.1** | Risk Factors for EP |
|---|---|

Tubal infection (salpingitis; PID)

Previous EP

Tubal sterilization

Tubal surgery

Infertility

Increasing age

Endometriosis

Prior spontaneous abortion

Ovulation induction

ARTs

IUD

Smoking

Abdominal surgery

Pelvic tuberculosis

Pelvic schistosomiasis

Factors in the patient's history may increase the physician's suspicion for EP. Questions regarding prior tubal surgery, pelvic infections, history of infertility, and type of birth control are appropriate. Current data indicate an ectopic rate for conceptions after the use of assisted reproductive technologies (ARTs) comparable to the estimated incidence of EP in the United States of 2% (13), but one third of conceptions resulting from sterilization are EPs (14). A history of induced or spontaneous abortion does not eliminate the possibility of an EP.

It should be stressed that history and physical findings, although necessary and important for assessing the patient and planning the appropriate follow-up and treatment, are not sufficient for exclusion or confirmation of an EP diagnosis (7). It should also be noted that whereas certain elements of the history may be more suggestive of a spontaneous abortion, such as heavy bleeding, passing of tissue, or midline cramping, they can also be found in some patients ultimately found to have an EP (7). Ultrasound in conjunction with human chorionic gonadotropin (hCG) levels may provide a definite diagnosis, and in stable patients in whom the diagnosis is uncertain, close follow-up is warranted.

## DIFFERENTIAL DIAGNOSIS

The clinical presentation of a patient with an EP can mimic a number of other gynecologic and nongynecologic disorders (Table 3.2). Because most of these disorders are not immediately life threatening, it is important that the clinician excludes EP when considering these and other conditions in a woman of reproductive age with abdominal pain or abnormal bleeding. In addition, EP must be immediately suspected in a woman of reproductive age who presents with signs of hemorrhagic shock. The list of differential diagnoses can be easily separated

**TABLE 3.2** Differential Diagnosis of EP

| **Pregnancy Test** | |
| --- | --- |
| **Positive Urine**[a] | **Negative Urine** |
| Normal IUP | Salpingitis, PID |
| Threatened abortion | Functional ovarian cyst ± rupture or torsion |
| Inevitable abortion | Ovarian neoplasm |
| Incomplete abortion | Appendicitis |
| Completed abortion | Endometriosis |
| Corpus luteum cyst ± rupture or torsion | Pelvic adhesions |
| | Fibroids |
| | Polycystic ovary disease |
| | Gastroenteritis |
| | Urinary tract infection |
| | Renal stone |

[a]A positive pregnancy test does not preclude the possibility of other conditions occurring with pregnancy, either intrauterine or ectopic.

into those associated with pregnancy and those that usually are not. Of course, a positive pregnancy test does not eliminate the possibility that the patient could have another process occurring in addition to pregnancy.

Functional ovarian cysts are common in reproductive-age women. Rupture or torsion of an ovarian cyst can cause lateral pelvic pain, mimicking EP. A ruptured, hemorrhagic corpus luteum cyst can occur with both IUP and EP. It may be extremely difficult to differentiate an EP from a ruptured corpus luteum of pregnancy because pain and bleeding can occur with both, as well as evidence of hemoperitoneum. Although pelvic sonography may be able to demonstrate an intrauterine gestation, the presence of a substantial hemoperitoneum may mandate surgical intervention (15).

Nonviable IUPs are readily confused with ectopic gestation. Vaginal bleeding with threatened, inevitable, or incomplete abortion is usually described as being much heavier than a menstrual period, and the pain is often reported to be midline, similar to menstrual cramps or labor. If the abortion is indeed inevitable or incomplete, the cervical os may be noticeably dilated, with extruding tissue or clot. A decidual cast may be shed in patients with an EP and may be confused with products of conception associated with an incomplete abortion. If possible, all tissue passed by the patient should be examined. While an experienced observer may be able to identify the presence of chorionic villi without microscopy, false-positive results have potential life-threatening consequences. The histological presence of chorionic villi obtained from the uterus/cervix, or passed vaginally by the patient virtually excludes the diagnosis of EP. The use of serial quantitative serum hCG titers and transvaginal sonography to distinguish viable IUP from nonviable IUP and EP is discussed below.

Pelvic pain and abnormal vaginal bleeding may also occur with salpingitis (PID). Usually, the pregnancy test will be negative, and fever and leukocytosis will be present. In rare cases, PID can occur in the presence of a very early pregnancy. Gastrointestinal disorders including appendicitis are also included in the differential diagnosis of EP.

## AMBULATORY EVALUATION

Diagnostic modalities available in ambulatory settings can expedite the diagnosis of EP, minimizing this condition's morbidity, mortality, and cost. The initial evaluation of any woman of reproductive age complaining of abdominal pain or abnormal vaginal bleeding should include a directed gynecologic history, a physical evaluation, and a sensitive and rapid urine pregnancy test. An algorithm for the evaluation and management of suspected EPs is presented in Fig. 3.2.

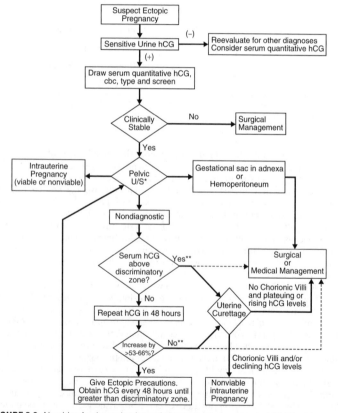

**FIGURE 3.2** Algorithm for the evaluation and management of a suspected EP. *If pelvic ultrasound is not readily available, consider culdocentesis. **Recommend uterine curettage to rule out an abnormal IUP; however, this may be bypassed depending on the clinical scenario.

## History

An appropriate interview in this setting focuses not only on the nature of the pain but also on menstrual history, sexual activity, contraceptive use, prior pregnancies, and gynecologic disease. Pain is a common symptom with EP, and it varies considerably in clinical presentation, owing to the duration of the gestation, the site of implantation, and the existence of rupture and a hemoperitoneum. A history of amenorrhea or abnormal vaginal bleeding may be difficult to elicit in some patients. It is imperative that the timing and character of the last two or three menstrual periods be investigated through direct questioning. Finally, attention must be paid to the obstetric and gynecologic history, particularly with regard to known risk factors for EP.

## Physical Examination

The physical examination of the patient with an EP varies, depending on the gestational age and the presence of rupture with a resulting hemoperitoneum. The physical exam should include vital signs, with attention to orthostatic changes in pulse and blood pressure, as well as abdominal and pelvic examinations. Tachycardia or hypotension can indicate hypovolemia due to intra-abdominal bleeding, but this can also occur in patients with spontaneous abortions due to vaginal bleeding as well as in patients with IUP who have a ruptured corpus luteum cyst or hyperemesis (7). Orthostatic changes and narrowed pulse pressure are unusual except in the case of massive intra-abdominal bleeding.

On abdominal exam, tenderness is the most common physical finding. The tenderness is classically unilateral and in the lower quadrant, but it can be bilateral. Rebound tenderness, guarding, and rigidity are not usually present except in cases with significant hemoperitoneum. Peritoneal signs are not commonly found in patients with EP but, when present, are predictive of EP (7,16).

A speculum exam of the vagina should be performed, looking closely at the source of any bleeding, the amount of blood present, and the presence of tissue at the cervical os. A bimanual pelvic exam will allow estimation of uterine size, determination of cervical dilation, and evaluation of the presence and tenderness of adnexal masses. A pelvic mass is found in the minority of patients with EP and is not predictive of EP—in fact, most of the patients with a palpable mass have an IUP, with the mass likely representing a corpus luteum cyst (7). Given the potential risk for tubal rupture and subsequent hemoperitoneum with a digital vaginal exam, some authors have suggested that the limited additional diagnostic information obtained may not warrant the hazards of performing the exam in patients with suspected EPs, especially in light of the diagnostic capability of ultrasound and serum hCG levels (17).

A minority of EPs result from implantation in the interstitial portion of the oviduct or in the uterine cornu. These cases characteristically present at a more advanced gestational age. On examination, the uterus is enlarged to a degree consistent with an uncomplicated IUP, and fetal heart motion may be detected. These patients may have only vague pain and an unimpressive examination until rupture occurs, at which time they often present with hypovolemic shock.

## Pregnancy Tests

Given that the differential diagnosis for abnormal vaginal bleeding with or without pain in a woman of reproductive age is dependent on knowing her pregnancy status, a screening urine pregnancy test should be done as part of the initial evaluation. This will facilitate more timely diagnosis and minimize the risk of misdiagnosis. Using currently available urine pregnancy tests, 54% of tests are positive 11 days from the LH surge, and 98% are positive 14 days from the LH surge (18). However, these data are from normal pregnancies and may vary for abnormal pregnancies. Some women with EPs will have hCG titers below that detectable by even the sensitive urine screening tests. To exclude this remote possibility, a serum hCG should be obtained in a woman with a presentation consistent with EP despite a negative urine pregnancy test.

## Ultrasonography

Once a symptomatic patient is known to be pregnant, vaginal ultrasound plays a key role in differentiating first trimester pregnancy pathology. Hardware for performing vaginal ultrasound is becoming more accessible in emergency departments and physician's offices, and the finding of an IUP on ultrasound virtually eliminates the possibility of an EP as heterotopic pregnancies are rare. Caution should be exercised in patients whose pregnancies are the result of ART, however, as the rate of heterotopics in these patients may be as high as 1% (19), although more recent data estimate the heterotopic pregnancy rate in the United States to be 0.15% for patients undergoing ART (20).

Accurate gestational age is the best determinant of when an IUP should be seen within the uterus, and a gestational sac or sacs should be visible by approximately 5 weeks on transvaginal ultrasound (21). In the absence of proper gestational dating, a discriminatory zone, or level above which a normal IUP should be visible, can guide management. Transvaginal ultrasound is more accurate and diagnostic of both IUPs and EPs than is transabdominal ultrasound (22) and is therefore the modality of choice. A commonly accepted cutoff for visualization of IUP via transvaginal ultrasound is 1,500 to 2,500 IU/L (23), although this may vary between institutions depending on the hCG assay as well as the equipment and experience of the sonographer. In the situation of multiple pregnancies, the hCG values are higher than singletons for any given gestational age and may reach well above 2,000 IU/L before ultrasound recognition of the pregnancy. Accordingly, the hCG level should be interpreted with caution in situations where multiples may be expected, as with the use of infertility treatment.

Although an IUP should be identified when the hCG level is above the discriminatory zone, ultrasound may provide useful information in symptomatic women whose hCG levels are below this level. In two studies of women ultimately found to have EPs, 39% with hCG <1,000 mIU/mL (24) and 42% with hCG <1,500 mIU/mL (25) were diagnosed on initial ultrasound. Free fluid can give insight into the presence and degree of hemoperitoneum, and alternative sources of pain, such as adnexal pathology, can be found. However, looking at all women who present with symptomatic pregnancies below the discriminatory zone, only 14% of women were diagnosed accurately and definitively with initial ultrasound. To avoid interrupting a desired viable pregnancy or subjecting the women to unnecessary surgery, caution must be exercised when correlating ultrasound findings with hCG values when the latter are found to be below the discriminatory zone (25).

When performing a transvaginal ultrasound, the bladder should be empty. First, the clinician should evaluate the uterus for the presence of a gestational sac. A gestational sac is defined as a central sonolucency surrounded by an echogenic ring, which can be detected when it reaches the dimensions of 2 to 3 mm (Table 3.3). Gestational sacs 5 mm or greater in dimensions can consistently be imaged using vaginal ultrasound (21). This "double decidual sac sign," thought to represent a distinct decidua vera and decidua capsularis, must be differentiated from a "pseudogestational sac," an intrauterine collection of fluid which can mimic a gestational sac. Generally, IUPs are *eccentrically* located within the uterus, while pseudogestational sacs are *central*. The double sac sign is far less reliable than a gestational sac with a yolk sac, which should be seen when the

| | | |
|---|---|---|
| **TABLE 3.3** | Correlation of hCG, Gestational Age, and Expected Transvaginal Ultrasound Findings in Normal Intrauterine Pregnancies | |

| $\beta$-hCG Level (mIU/mL) | Gestational Age (Days from LMP) | TVUS Finding |
|---|---|---|
| 1,000–2,000 | 35–38 | 2- to 3-mm gestational sac |
| 2,500 | 37–40 | Yolk sac |
| 5,000 | 39–42 | Fetal pole |
| 17,000 | 42–49 | Fetal pole with cardiac activity |

hCG, human chorionic gonadotropin; LMP, last menstrual period; TVUS, transvaginal ultrasound.

mean sac diameter is 8 mm, during the 5th week (21). Fetal heart motion should be noted by 6 to 6.5 weeks, at an embryo length of 4 to 5 mm, and the absence of cardiac activity at a fetal length >5 mm indicates an embryonic demise (21).

After evaluating the uterine cavity, the clinician should examine the adnexa bilaterally, evaluating for the presence of masses. Any suspicious masses should be measured for use in determining management pathways. A corpus luteum may be confused with an ovarian pregnancy. Ultrasound is diagnostic for EP if a gestational sac, possibly with a yolk sac or fetal pole, can be identified and localized outside the uterus. Other findings on transvaginal ultrasound can also be predictive of EP. These include a thick-walled cyst or complex mass separate from the ovary and/or a large amount of free fluid in the posterior cul-de-sac.

Both the cul-de-sac of Douglas and the abdominal cavity should be evaluated by ultrasound to assess for masses and free fluid. Although the presence of blood in the cul-de-sac in the appropriate clinical setting suggests EP, hemoperitoneum may also be encountered in women with a ruptured corpus luteum, spleen/liver, or hepatic adenoma. Blood in the cul-de-sac may also be found during menses, with threatened or incomplete abortion, or after uterine curettage.

Special ultrasound studies have been researched in patients at increased risk for EP. The thickness of the endometrial stripe on transvaginal imaging is one example. A stripe of >8 mm has been associated with the increased likelihood of an intrauterine IUP, while a stripe of <8 mm has been associated with EP; however, there is an overlap between the two groups (26). Doppler imaging has also been studied. High-velocity flow by Doppler ultrasound was found to detect EP with a sensitivity of 73% (27). Care must be taken not to confuse a corpus luteum with an EP, as the corpus luteum has increased blood flow but is always located within the ovary. To further confuse the evaluation, 90% of ectopic implantations will be found on the same side as the corpus luteum. Using Doppler techniques, blood flow to the side of an EP has been shown to increase by as much as 20% over that to the unaffected side (28). Characteristic blood flow patterns of the endometrium give Doppler evaluation an 84% sensitivity and a 100% specificity for detecting an abnormal IUP versus a pseudogestational sac (29).

## Culdocentesis

As time and technology have progressed, the painful and invasive procedure of culdocentesis has become less important in evaluating women felt to have an EP. At sites where a sensitive hCG assay and transvaginal ultrasound cannot be obtained in a timely fashion, however, culdocentesis may expedite the evaluation of women suspected of having an EP. Culdocentesis entails puncturing the cul-de-sac of Douglas with a needle and aspirating its contents. The aspiration results are usually classified into three categories: (i) positive—nonclotting blood or blood with a hematocrit of >12%; (ii) negative—clear (serous) cul-de-sac fluid or blood-tinged fluid with a hematocrit of <5%; and (iii) nondiagnostic—no fluid or clotting blood. Unfortunately, since intra-abdominal bleeding from a corpus luteum cyst in women with an IUP is common, culdocentesis may also be positive in women who prove not to have an ectopic gestation. A nondiagnostic culdocentesis should neither raise nor lower a clinician's suspicion of EP.

## Serial hCG Evaluation

If the initial hCG is below the discriminatory zone and the transvaginal ultrasound cannot definitively diagnose either an intrauterine or an extrauterine pregnancy in a hemodynamically stable woman without evidence of hemoperitoneum, then the patient must be followed up closely with serial hCG levels. If the hCG is rising, this most likely indicates either an early viable IUP or EP. The minimum rise for a viable pregnancy in a woman presenting with symptoms is 53% in 2 days (30), and a vaginal ultrasound should be performed to document an IUP once the discriminatory zone is reached. Falling hCG levels may indicate a miscarriage or EP. There is no one predictable single rate of decline associated with miscarriage. With this diagnosis, the rate of decline assessed over 48 hours is dependent on the initial hCG value and ranges from 21% to 35% for hCG values up to 5,000 mIU/mL (31). When initial hCG levels are low (50 to 500 mIU/mL), the slowest decline range in 2 days is 12% to 24% (32). Among women with EPs, 60% will have an initial rise and 40% will have an initial decline, and the hCG trend in an EP can mimic the pattern of a viable IUP or miscarriage in 29% of cases (33). Therefore, careful monitoring of these patients is crucial until a definitive diagnosis is made, with prompt intervention required if a woman develops symptoms of an evolving EP or if her hCG trend fails to indicate an evolving miscarriage or viable pregnancy.

## Suction Curettage and Endometrial Biopsy

Once an EP is suspected in a stable woman with a nonviable gestation determined by an abnormal hCG trend below the discriminatory zone or lack of evidence of an intrauterine gestation on transvaginal ultrasound above the discriminatory zone, a dilation and curettage can be used to look for histological evidence of a failed IUP. Of patients with an hCG >2,000 mIU/mL and no evidence of an intrauterine gestation on ultrasound, 54% will ultimately have a failed IUP (miscarriage) (34). In the situation where serial hCG assessment has detected an abnormal pattern (below 2,000 mIU/mL), 31% will actually have a miscarriage and not an EP (34). Presumptive treatment with medical management would therefore incorrectly treat a large number of patients if a definitive diagnosis is not made (34). Although dilation and curettage may yield a more accurate diagnosis, one must weigh the risks of a surgical procedure (rare, but potentially serious) against the risks of incorrectly treating some women with nonviable IUPs with methotrexate (MTX) (whose side effects are more common, but typically mild and resolve quickly). A cost-effectiveness study of presumptive MTX treatment versus dilation and curettage prior to MTX found no difference in side effects or treatment success, with a minimal cost difference of $200 between the two strategies (35). Clinicians, however, should keep in mind that a definitive diagnosis is necessary to provide a prognosis regarding a woman's future reproductive potential and the need for a workup of recurrent miscarriage or tubal factor infertility.

In patients with an uncertain diagnosis, curettage can be performed in an ambulatory setting under local anesthesia. In many institutions, however, this may only be accomplished in an operating room with anesthesia, and not in the office or emergency room. Although it may be preferable in terms of cost and convenience to detect the presence of chorionic villi with an endometrial biopsy, multiple studies have shown the 3-mm plastic piston-type endometrial biopsy devices (e.g., Pipelle) to be inferior to curettage for this purpose, with sensitivities of 30% to 63% (36,37), and as low as 13.3% for frozen endometrial biopsies (38).

Since the pathology results of the curettage are typically not available until at least the following day, frozen section has been proposed as a way to gain more rapid information to guide management. The sensitivity of frozen section is reported as 62% to 88% with a specificity of 98% to 100% (37,39–41). Although frozen section can guide initial management, given that false-negative results can occur on frozen section, following hCG levels for dropping levels the next morning and final pathology can help ensure the correct diagnosis is made.

### Serum Markers

Serum progesterone levels have been proposed to help distinguish normal from abnormal pregnancies. Proposed algorithms use a progesterone level over the cutoff of 25 ng/mL to exclude EP, <5 ng/mL to indicate an abnormal pregnancy, and any value between as indeterminate, which must be followed further with ultrasound and serial hCG levels (42). A meta-analysis looking at the predictive value of a single progesterone level to diagnose EP found that it was able to discriminate a first trimester pregnancy failure from a viable IUP, but it could not differentiate an EP from a failed IUP (43). Therefore, a low progesterone level (≤5 ng/mL) may be useful for identifying patients at risk of EP who need to be closely followed up, but it cannot definitely diagnose them.

There are a number of other serum markers reported in the literature (interleukin-6, interleukin-8, vascular endothelial growth factor, tumor necrosis factor-$\alpha$, activin A, creatine kinase, and cancer antigen-125, among others). However, at present, the results are not conclusive and none can be recommended for clinical use without further study.

## MANAGEMENT

The presentation of patients with EP ranges from minimal symptoms to irreversible shock preceding death. If the patient appears to have a surgical abdomen, a complete blood count and blood type and cross-match should be obtained, and intravenous access should be ensured with two large-bore cannulas. If needed, fluid resuscitation should be commenced, followed by appropriate blood-component therapy. Although hemodynamic stability is desirable before subjecting a patient to surgical anesthesia, it must be remembered that often the surgical intervention itself will be required to achieve stability through control of active hemorrhage. Transfer to another facility is appropriate in the clinically stable patient if it will facilitate performance of diagnostic studies not available in the referring ambulatory setting. It may also be necessary for patients with a ruptured EP and/or hemoperitoneum if immediate surgery cannot be performed at the referring site. In this case, the most expeditious mode of transportation is indicated, with appropriate intravenous infusions, advanced cardiac life support, and even consideration of the use of military antishock trousers. For the patient presenting in shock, an emergency consultation should be obtained from any readily available physician with the surgical expertise to perform a laparotomy.

More frequently, however, the patient suspected of having an EP will be hemodynamically stable. The earlier the diagnosis of EP is made, the more likely it is that fallopian tube conserving measures can be employed. This is of particular importance for the younger patient. Regardless of the treatment for EP, Rh immunoglobulin (Rhogam) should be given to all unsensitized Rh-negative women (44).

## Surgical Management

Surgical management is required in patients with an EP who are hemodynamically unstable as well as those that fail medical therapy. Primary surgical therapy is also indicated for patients without tubal rupture who decline or are poor candidates for medical therapy. (See "Medical Management" below.)

The surgical options for a tubal pregnancy include salpingostomy and salpingectomy. Salpingostomy preserves the tube but bears the risk for persistent trophoblast and repeat ipsilateral EP. Salpingectomy avoids this risk but leaves a reproductive-age woman with one less potentially functional tube. Pooled data from nonrandomized studies have reported comparable pregnancy rates after either salpingectomy or salpingostomy, but with an increased 15% subsequent ectopic rate following salpingostomy compared with 10% subsequent to salpingectomy (45,46). More recent studies have suggested improved fertility rates with conservative surgery (47–49), though definitive studies are lacking. Concern has also been raised about ovarian function following salpingectomy for EP. In a comparison of the ovaries in the same patient postsalpingectomy, the operated side had lower antral follicle counts and 3D power Doppler indices than the nonsurgical side (50). In a study directly comparing postsalpingectomy versus postsalpingostomy patients undergoing IVF, fewer follicles developed and fewer oocytes were retrieved from the operated side in women who had undergone salpingectomy, but this had no effect on the overall number of follicles, oocytes, cycle characteristics, or pregnancy rates when these cycles were compared with those from postsalpingostomy patients (51). Of note, similar concerns about ovarian function have also been raised following MTX therapy, although decreased oocyte production with ovarian stimulation appears to be temporary (52). Overall, definitive data regarding long-term fertility outcomes comparing the various treatments are lacking.

As laparoscopic techniques and experience continue to improve, even EPs with a large degree of hemoperitoneum may be treated without laparotomy in some settings. Two recent meta-analyses examined the differences between laparoscopic and open salpingostomies. They found that laparoscopic salpingostomy is superior to laparotomy in terms of decreased cost, shorter operating time, shorter hospital stay, less blood loss, and shorter convalescence time (53,54). In stable patients with small, unruptured EPs, the open approach was more successful in eliminating the pregnancy, with a higher persistent trophoblast rate in the laparoscopic group (53,54), although it is of note that these pooled studies were from the 1980s and 1990s, when laparoscopy was a newer technique. Long-term follow-up of treated patients demonstrates no evidence of difference in subsequent IUPs, but a nonsignificant trend toward lower repeat EP in the laparoscopy versus the laparotomy groups (53,54). The addition of a single prophylactic dose of MTX within 24 hours of salpingostomy significantly decreases the risk of persistent trophoblast (53,54) and can be considered for patients undergoing conservative surgery.

## Medical Management

MTX, a folic acid antagonist originally used as a chemotherapeutic agent, inhibits dihydrofolic acid reductase. MTX affects proliferating cells by interfering with DNA synthesis and repair and with cellular replication. All replicating cells are affected, including intestinal and buccal mucosa, respiratory epithelium, bone marrow, bladder, and fetal cells. Patients considered for this medical management must be hemodynamically stable, be reliable and able to comply with follow-up, and have no medical contraindications to the use of MTX (see Table 3.4). Given its toxicity to rapidly dividing tissues, it should not be given to women with blood dyscrasias, active gastrointestinal (peptic ulcer) disease, or respiratory disease. As it is renally excreted and may have a toxic effect on hepatocytes, renal and liver diseases (including alcoholism and alcoholic liver disease) are also contraindications. For these reasons, normal serum creatinine, liver transaminases, and complete blood count to check for leukopenia, thrombocytopenia, and anemia should be checked prior to administration, and these are rechecked 1 week after administration prior to further doses to ensure that the results of these tests remain normal. Other absolute contraindications include IUP, breastfeeding, and known sensitivity to MTX (23,55).

Success with MTX depends on both the baseline characteristics of the patient's pregnancy as well as the protocol utilized. Studies have reported increased failure with elevated hCG levels as well as fetal cardiac activity (56–58). A systematic review demonstrated a 3.7% failure rate with hCG levels <5,000 mIU/ mL, but a 14.3% failure rate with hCG levels >5,000 mIU/mL when a single-dose MTX regimen was used (59). Relative contraindications endorsed by both the American College of Obstetricians and Gynecologists (ACOG) as well as the American Society for Reproductive Medicine (ASRM) include embryonic cardiac motion and an ectopic mass size cutoff of 3.5 cm (ACOG) or 4 cm (ASRM) (23,55). ASRM also includes high initial hCG concentration (>5,000 mIU/mL) and refusal to accept blood transfusion as relative contraindications to MTX use (23).

MTX can be administered as a single-dose, a two-dose, or a multidose regimen. These regimens are outlined below according to the ACOG guidelines (55). Prior to administration, a normal complete blood count, liver, and renal tests should be documented as detailed above. Screening for blood type and Rh status should also be completed to assess the need for rhogam.

> ***Single-dose regimen***: MTX (50 mg/m$^2$) is administered intramuscularly on day 1. hCG levels are checked on post treatment days 4 and 7, with an expected 15% drop. If the drop is as expected, hCG levels are measured

| TABLE 3.4 | Medical Contraindications to MTX Use |
|---|---|

Hemodynamically unstable patient

Alcoholism

Liver disease

Immunodeficiency

Blood dyscrasias

Breastfeeding

Unreliable patient

Peptic ulcer disease

Renal dysfunction

Hematologic dysfunction

Active pulmonary disease

weekly until they are negative, and an additional dose of MTX ($50\,mg/m^2$) may be considered for a plateau or increase in hCG during this time. If the drop is <15% on day 7, another $50\,mg/m^2$ dose is administered, the hCG levels are repeated again on days 4 and 7, and the patient followed up as detailed above.

**Two-dose regimen**: MTX ($50\,mg/m^2$) is administered intramuscularly on day 0 and repeated on day 4. hCG levels are checked on days 4 and 7. If the drop is 15% or greater between days 4 and 7, levels are repeated weekly until negative. If the drop is <15%, MTX is again given on days 7 and 11. If there is a 15% drop, hCG levels should be monitored weekly until negative.

**Multidose regimen**: MTX ($1\,mg/kg$) is administered intramuscularly alternating with Leucovorin (LEU, folinic acid $0.1\,mg/kg$) intramuscularly 1 day later. These alternating injections are continued until there is a 15% decline in serum hCG levels. A patient may need 1, 2, 3, or 4 courses of both MTX and LEU. Once hCG levels decline, they are followed up weekly until negative. If the hCG level plateaus or increases, one can consider repeating the regimen.

The single-dose regimen is the most simple and convenient regimen, and both single- and two-dose regimens avoid the need for folinic acid rescue. A meta-analysis incorporating 1,327 patients, albeit with no controlled trials, reported significantly improved success with the multidose regimen (88% versus 93%) (56). Recent meta-analyses incorporating two newer randomized controlled trials, though with much lower aggregate numbers of women ($N = 159$), did not demonstrate a statistically significant difference (53). A randomized controlled trial with 108 patients demonstrated the same magnitude of decreased efficacy of single dose (89% for single dose and 93% for multidose; the mean number of doses was 2.3 in this group) but was also underpowered; accordingly, the comparison of the success rates did not achieve statistical significance (60). In a prospective study of a newer two-dose protocol, which is a hybrid of the single-dose and multidose regimens (see protocols above), this regimen had an 87% success rate and was shown to be a safe and efficacious regimen (61), though comparative studies have yet to be published.

Candidates with suspected EPs who are contemplating MTX treatment should be counseled regarding the side effects of MTX. A randomized controlled trial reported complication rates of 28% for a single-dose regimen and 37% complication rate for a multidose regimen (60). Abdominal pain was the most frequent complication, reported by 20% of patients in the single-dose regimen and 22% in the multidose regimen (60). Other complications including diarrhea, elevated liver enzymes, stomatitis, dermatitis, and pruritis were found in 7% of the single-dose patients and 17% of the multidose patients (60). Abdominal pain, in particular, is not unusual 2 to 3 days after administration and is thought to result from the drugs' cytotoxic effect on the trophoblast, causing a tubal abortion (55). In general, the symptoms are usually mild and resolve over 1 to 2 weeks. Patients should be instructed to contact a physician for onset of severe abdominal pain or signs of hemodynamic instability, including syncope, dizziness, and tachycardia. Patients with these symptoms may require surgical therapy or admission to the hospital for observation, with ultrasound evaluation and monitoring of hemoglobin levels. Given that MTX is a folic acid antagonist, patients should be counseled to avoid vitamins with folic acid, and as gastrointestinal symptoms are more common side effects, avoidance of alcohol and nonsteroidal antiinflammatory agents is also prudent. Avoidance of sunlight and pelvic rest (including no sexual intercourse) are appropriate until the EP has resolved. Mean time to resolution of hCG after single-dose MTX is 4 weeks (62).

Compared with laparoscopic salpingostomy, there is a nonsignificant trend toward increased treatment success with a multidose MTX regimen, but with 61% complications compared with 22% in the salpingostomy group (most of these were associated with repeat MTX administration for persistent trophoblast) (63). Comparing laparoscopic salpingostomy with a single-dose regimen, a meta-analysis (which included 265 EP patients overall) found that MTX was significantly less successful than surgery (OR 0.82), but associated with better physical functioning and significant savings in direct costs, although savings in indirect costs were lost with an hCG >1,500 IU/L (53,54). The meta-analysis found that the likelihood of future IUPs was similar with surgical and medical treatment, but a trend toward a lower risk of future EP was noted with MTX therapy (53,54). Of the 27 women who failed medical therapy, 7 ultimately had surgery and 20 were treated with additional doses of MTX (from two to four doses) (54).

Local administration of MTX has also been used in treatment of EP. Using this modality, the drug is injected directly into the mass, and it requires the expertise of a clinician skilled in ultrasound-guided procedures. In pooled data, local administration of MTX showed a nonsignificant trend toward primary treatment success over intramuscular MTX therapy, with no difference in future likelihood of conceiving an IUP or a repeat EP (54). Systemic MTX administration is easier and requires no anesthesia or specialized clinical skills. Therefore, local MTX administration has limited applicability. Reports, however, have suggested that in women with interstitial or cervical pregnancies, direct injection of MTX or potassium chloride into the EP may be employed as adjunctive or definitive treatment (64,65).

### Expectant Management

Prior to the advent of sensitive pregnancy tests and ultrasound, many EPs were unknowingly managed expectantly. Today, with the increased and earlier recognition of EP, it can be difficult to differentiate women whose EPs will resolve safely with no intervention from those whose EPs are actively proliferating and will require treatment. Lund, in 1955 (66), was the first to describe expectant management of EP, with a success rate of 70%; 22% of patients in this report required emergent surgery. More recently, investigators have noted better results. Expectant management of a known EP may be considered in the setting of a low and falling hCG level occurring in a highly reliable patient without evidence of substantial bleeding. In carefully selected patients, success rates for expectant management have ranged from 69% to 82% (67–69). Independent predictors of successful expectant management include low initial hCG titer and the trend in hCG levels between the first and the second assessments (70). Clinicians, however, should recognize that tubal rupture can occur in women with low or declining hCG levels (71); accordingly, such patients should be followed up closely until resolution of the EP. The American College of Obstetrics and Gynecology defines candidates for expectant management as those who are asymptomatic, who have objective evidence of resolution, such as decreasing hCG levels, and who are willing to accept the potential risks of tubal rupture and hemorrhage (55). Expectant management should cease in the case of rupture, increased or intractable pain, or failure of hCG to decline (55).

## SUMMARY AND CONCLUSION

Because EP is a common and potentially life-threatening condition, physicians must remain alert to this entity. Initial evaluation, including directed history, examination, and laboratory and sonographic assessments as described in this chapter, usually allows a definitive diagnosis before catastrophic hemorrhage or rupture occurs. In stable patients, medical management with MTX offers a successful nonoperative treatment strategy for a substantial portion of women presenting with an EP.

## References

1. Zane SB, Kieke BA Jr, Kendrick JS, Bruce C. Surveillance in a time of changing health care practices: estimating ectopic pregnancy incidence in the United States. *Matern Child Health J*. 2002 Dec;6(4):227–236.
2. Goldner TE, Lawson HW, Xia Z, Atrash HK. Surveillance for ectopic pregnancy—United States, 1970–1989. *MMWR CDC Surveill Summ*. 1993 Dec;42(6):73–85.
3. Berg CJ, Chang J, Callaghan WM, Whitehead SJ. Pregnancy-related mortality in the United States, 1991–1997. *Obstet Gynecol*. 2003 Feb;101(2):289–296.
4. Dorfman SF, Grimes DA, Cates W Jr, Binkin NJ, Kafrissen ME, O'Reilly KR. Ectopic pregnancy mortality, United States, 1979 to 1980: clinical aspects. *Obstet Gynecol*. 1984 Sep;64(3):386–390.
5. Bouyer J, Coste J, Fernandez H, Pouly JL, Job-Spira N. Sites of ectopic pregnancy: a 10 year population-based study of 1800 cases. *Hum Reprod*. 2002 Dec;17(12):3224–3230.
6. Ankum WM, Mol BW, Van der Veen F, Bossuyt PM. Risk factors for ectopic pregnancy: a meta-analysis. *Fertil Steril*. 1996 Jun;65(6):1093–1099.
7. Dart RG, Kaplan B, Varaklis K. Predictive value of history and physical examination in patients with suspected ectopic pregnancy. *Ann Emerg Med*. 1999 Mar;33(3):283–290.
8. Barnhart KT, Sammel MD, Gracia CR, Chittams J, Hummel AC, Shaunik A. Risk factors for ectopic pregnancy in women with symptomatic first-trimester pregnancies. *Fertil Steril*. 2006 Jul;86(1):36–43.
9. Mol BW, Ankum WM, Bossuyt PM, Van der Veen F. Contraception and the risk of ectopic pregnancy: a meta-analysis. *Contraception*. 1995 Dec;52(6):337–341.
10. Mishell DR Jr. Intrauterine devices: mechanisms of action, safety, and efficacy. *Contraception*. 1998 Sep;58(3 Suppl.):45S–53S; quiz 70S.
11. Backman T, Rauramo I, Huhtala S, Koskenvuo M. Pregnancy during the use of levonorgestrel intrauterine system. *Am J Obstet Gynecol*. 2004 Jan;190(1):50–54.
12. Menon S, Sammel MD, Vichnin M, Barnhart KT. Risk factors for ectopic pregnancy: a comparison between adults and adolescent women. *J Pediatr Adolesc Gynecol*. 2007 Jun;20(3):181–185.
13. Assisted reproductive technology in the United States: 2001 results generated from the American Society for Reproductive Medicine/Society for Assisted Reproductive Technology registry. *Fertil Steril*. 2007 Jun;87(6):1253–1266.
14. Peterson HB, Xia Z, Hughes JM, Wilcox LS, Tylor LR, Trussell J. The risk of ectopic pregnancy after tubal sterilization. U.S. Collaborative Review of Sterilization Working Group. *N Engl J Med*. 1997 Mar;336(11):762–767.
15. Hallatt JG, Steele CH Jr, Snyder M. Ruptured corpus luteum with hemoperitoneum: a study of 173 surgical cases. *Am J Obstet Gynecol*. 1984 May;149(1):5–9.
16. Buckley RG, King KJ, Disney JD, Gorman JD, Klausen JH. History and physical examination to estimate the risk of ectopic pregnancy: validation of a clinical prediction model. *Ann Emerg Med*. 1999 Nov;34(5):589–594.
17. Mol BW, Hajenius PJ, Engelsbel S, et al. Should patients who are suspected of having an ectopic pregnancy undergo physical examination? *Fertil Steril*. 1999 Jan;71(1):155–157.
18. Johnson SR, Miro F, Barrett S, Ellis JE. Levels of urinary human chorionic gonadotrophin (hCG) following conception and variability of menstrual cycle length in a cohort of women attempting to conceive. *Curr Med Res Opin*. 2009 Mar;25(3):741–748.
19. Svare J, Norup P, Grove Thomsen S, et al. Heterotopic pregnancies after in-vitro fertilization and embryo transfer—a Danish survey. *Hum Reprod*. 1993 Jan;8(1):116–118.
20. Clayton HB, Schieve LA, Peterson HB, Jamieson DJ, Reynolds MA, Wright VC. Ectopic pregnancy risk with assisted reproductive technology procedures. *Obstet Gynecol*. 2006 Mar;107(3):595–604.
21. Albayram F, Hamper UM. First-trimester obstetric emergencies: spectrum of sonographic findings. *J Clin Ultrasound*. 2002 Mar–Apr;30(3):161–177.

22. Cacciatore B, Stenman UH, Ylostalo P. Comparison of abdominal and vaginal sonography in suspected ectopic pregnancy. *Obstet Gynecol.* 1989 May;73(5, pt 1): 770–774.
23. Medical treatment of ectopic pregnancy. *Fertil Steril.* 2008 Nov;90(5 Suppl.): S206–S212.
24. Dart RG, Kaplan B, Cox C. Transvaginal ultrasound in patients with low beta-human chorionic gonadotropin values: how often is the study diagnostic? *Ann Emerg Med.* 1997 Aug;30(2):135–140.
25. Barnhart KT, Simhan H, Kamelle SA. Diagnostic accuracy of ultrasound above and below the beta-hCG discriminatory zone. *Obstet Gynecol.* 1999 Oct;94(4):583–587.
26. Spandorfer SD, Barnhart KT. Endometrial stripe thickness as a predictor of ectopic pregnancy. *Fertil Steril.* 1996 Sep;66(3):474–477.
27. Taylor KJ, Ramos IM, Feyock AL, et al. Ectopic pregnancy: duplex Doppler evaluation. *Radiology.* 1989 Oct;173(1):93–97.
28. Kirchler HC, Seebacher S, Alge AA, Muller-Holzner E, Fessler S, Kolle D. Early diagnosis of tubal pregnancy: changes in tubal blood flow evaluated by endovaginal color Doppler sonography. *Obstet Gynecol.* 1993 Oct;82(4, pt 1):561–565.
29. Dillon EH, Feyock AL, Taylor KJ. Pseudogestational sacs: Doppler US differentiation from normal or abnormal intrauterine pregnancies. *Radiology.* 1990 Aug;176(2): 359–364.
30. Barnhart KT, Sammel MD, Rinaudo PF, Zhou L, Hummel AC, Guo W. Symptomatic patients with an early viable intrauterine pregnancy: HCG curves redefined. *Obstet Gynecol.* 2004 Jul;104(1):50–55.
31. Barnhart K, Sammel MD, Chung K, Zhou L, Hummel AC, Guo W. Decline of serum human chorionic gonadotropin and spontaneous complete abortion: defining the normal curve. *Obstet Gynecol.* 2004 Nov;104(5, pt 1):975–981.
32. Chung K, Sammel M, Zhou L, Hummel A, Guo W, Barnhart K. Defining the curve when initial levels of human chorionic gonadotropin in patients with spontaneous abortions are low. *Fertil Steril.* 2006 Feb;85(2):508–510.
33. Silva C, Sammel MD, Zhou L, Gracia C, Hummel AC, Barnhart K. Human chorionic gonadotropin profile for women with ectopic pregnancy. *Obstet Gynecol.* 2006 Mar;107(3):605–610.
34. Barnhart KT, Katz I, Hummel A, Gracia CR. Presumed diagnosis of ectopic pregnancy. *Obstet Gynecol.* 2002 Sep;100(3):505–510.
35. Ailawadi M, Lorch SA, Barnhart KT. Cost-effectiveness of presumptively medically treating women at risk for ectopic pregnancy compared with first performing a dilatation and curettage. *Fertil Steril.* 2005 Feb;83(2):376–382.
36. Ries A, Singson P, Bidus M, Barnes JG. Use of the endometrial pipelle in the diagnosis of early abnormal gestations. *Fertil Steril.* 2000 Sep;74(3):593–595.
37. Barnhart KT, Gracia CR, Reindl B, Wheeler JE. Usefulness of pipelle endometrial biopsy in the diagnosis of women at risk for ectopic pregnancy. *Am J Obstet Gynecol.* 2003 Apr;188(4):906–909.
38. Al-Ramahi M, Nimri C, Bata M, Saleh S. The value of frozen section Pipelle endometrial biopsy as an outpatient procedure in the diagnosis of ectopic pregnancy. *J Obstet Gynecol.* 2006 Jan;26(1):63–65.
39. Spandorfer SD, Menzin AW, Barnhart KT, LiVolsi VA, Pfeifer SM. Efficacy of frozen-section evaluation of uterine curettings in the diagnosis of ectopic pregnancy. *Am J Obstet Gynecol.* 1996 Sep;175(3, pt 1):603–605.
40. Heller DS, Hessami S, Cracchiolo B, Skurnick JH. Reliability of frozen section of uterine curettings in evaluation of possible ectopic pregnancy. *J Am Assoc Gynecol Laparosc.* 2000 Nov;7(4):519–522.
41. Barak S, Oettinger M, Perri A, Cohen HI, Barenboym R, Ophir E. Frozen section examination of endometrial curettings in the diagnosis of ectopic pregnancy. *Acta Obstet Gynecol Scand.* 2005 Jan;84(1):43–47.
42. Carson SA, Buster JE. Ectopic pregnancy. *N Engl J Med.* 1993 Oct;329(16):1174–1181.
43. Mol BW, Lijmer JG, Ankum WM, Van der Veen F, Bossuyt PM. The accuracy of single serum progesterone measurement in the diagnosis of ectopic pregnancy: a meta-analysis. *Hum Reprod.* 1998 Nov;13(11):3220–3227.
44. Jabara S, Barnhart KT. Is Rh immune globulin needed in early first-trimester abortion? A review. *Am J Obstet Gynecol.* 2003 Mar;188(3):623–627.

45. Yao M, Tulandi T. Current status of surgical and nonsurgical management of ectopic pregnancy. *Fertil Steril*. 1997 Mar;67(3):421–433.
46. Clausen I. Conservative versus radical surgery for tubal pregnancy. A review. *Acta Obstet Gynecol Scand*. 1996 Jan;75(1):8–12.
47. Mol BW, Matthijsse HC, Tinga DJ, et al. Fertility after conservative and radical surgery for tubal pregnancy. *Hum Reprod*. 1998 Jul;13(7):1804–1809.
48. Bouyer J, Job-Spira N, Pouly JL, Coste J, Germain E, Fernandez H. Fertility following radical, conservative-surgical or medical treatment for tubal pregnancy: a population-based study. *BJOG*. 2000 Jun;107(6):714–721.
49. Bangsgaard N, Lund CO, Ottesen B, Nilas L. Improved fertility following conservative surgical treatment of ectopic pregnancy. *BJOG*. 2003 Aug;110(8):765–770.
50. Chan CC, Ng EH, Li CF, et al. Impaired ovarian blood flow and reduced antral follicle count following laparoscopic salpingectomy for ectopic pregnancy. *Hum Reprod*. 2003 Oct;18(10):2175–2180.
51. Lass A, Ellenbogen A, Croucher C, et al. Effect of salpingectomy on ovarian response to superovulation in an in vitro fertilization-embryo transfer program. *Fertil Steril*. 1998 Dec;70(6):1035–1038.
52. McLaren JF, Burney RO, Milki AA, Westphal LM, Dahan MH, Lathi RB. Effect of methotrexate exposure on subsequent fertility in women undergoing controlled ovarian stimulation. *Fertil Steril*. 2009 Aug;92(2):512–519.
53. Mol F, Mol BW, Ankum WM, Van der Veen F, Hajenius PJ. Current evidence on surgery, systemic methotrexate and expectant management in the treatment of tubal ectopic pregnancy: a systematic review and meta-analysis. *Hum Reprod Update*. 2008 Jul–Aug;14(4):309–319.
54. Hajenius PJ, Mol F, Mol BW, Bossuyt PM, Ankum WM, Van der Veen F. Interventions for tubal ectopic pregnancy. *Cochrane Database Syst Rev*. 2007(1):CD000324.
55. ACOG Practice Bulletin No. 94: Medical management of ectopic pregnancy. *Obstet Gynecol*. 2008 Jun;111(6):1479–1485.
56. Barnhart KT, Gosman G, Ashby R, Sammel M. The medical management of ectopic pregnancy: a meta-analysis comparing "single dose" and "multidose" regimens. *Obstet Gynecol*. 2003 Apr;101(4):778–784.
57. Lipscomb GH, McCord ML, Stovall TG, Huff G, Portera SG, Ling FW. Predictors of success of methotrexate treatment in women with tubal ectopic pregnancies. *N Engl J Med*. 1999 Dec;341(26):1974–1978.
58. Elito J Jr, Reichmann AP, Uchiyama MN, Camano L. Predictive score for the systemic treatment of unruptured ectopic pregnancy with a single dose of methotrexate. *Int J Gynaecol Obstet*. 1999 Nov;67(2):75–79.
59. Menon S, Colins J, Barnhart KT. Establishing a human chorionic gonadotropin cutoff to guide methotrexate treatment of ectopic pregnancy: a systematic review. *Fertil Steril*. 2007 Mar;87(3):481–484.
60. Alleyassin A, Khademi A, Aghahosseini M, Safdarian L, Badenoosh B, Hamed EA. Comparison of success rates in the medical management of ectopic pregnancy with single-dose and multiple-dose administration of methotrexate: a prospective, randomized clinical trial. *Fertil Steril*. 2006 Jun;85(6):1661–1666.
61. Barnhart K, Hummel AC, Sammel MD, Menon S, Jain J, Chakhtoura N. Use of "2-dose" regimen of methotrexate to treat ectopic pregnancy. *Fertil Steril*. 2007 Feb;87(2):250–256.
62. Saraj AJ, Wilcox JG, Najmabadi S, Stein SM, Johnson MB, Paulson RJ. Resolution of hormonal markers of ectopic gestation: a randomized trial comparing single-dose intramuscular methotrexate with salpingostomy. *Obstet Gynecol*. 1998 Dec;92(6):989–994.
63. Hajenius PJ, Engelsbel S, Mol BW, et al. Randomised trial of systemic methotrexate versus laparoscopic salpingostomy in tubal pregnancy. *Lancet*. 1997 Sep;350(9080):774–779.
64. Tulandi T, Al-Jaroudi D. Interstitial pregnancy: results generated from the Society of Reproductive Surgeons Registry. *Obstet Gynecol*. 2004 Jan;103(1):47–50.
65. Kung FT, Chang SY. Efficacy of methotrexate treatment in viable and nonviable cervical pregnancies. *Am J Obstet Gynecol*. 1999 Dec;181(6):1438–1444.
66. Lund J. Early ectopic pregnancy; comments on conservative treatment. *J Obstet Gynaecol Br Emp*. 1955 Feb;62(1):70–76.

67. Carp HJ, Oelsner G, Serr DM, Mashiach S. Fertility after nonsurgical treatment of ectopic pregnancy. *J Reprod Med.* 1986 Feb;31(2):119–122.
68. Makinen JI, Kivijarvi AK, Irjala KM. Success of non-surgical management of ectopic pregnancy. *Lancet.* 1990 May;335(8697):1099.
69. Ylostalo P, Cacciatore B, Sjoberg J, Kaariainen M, Tenhunen A, Stenman UH. Expectant management of ectopic pregnancy. *Obstet Gynecol.* 1992 Sep;80(3, pt 1):345–348.
70. Trio D, Strobelt N, Picciolo C, Lapinski RH, Ghidini A. Prognostic factors for successful expectant management of ectopic pregnancy. *Fertil Steril.* 1995 Mar;63(3): 469–472.
71. Tulandi T, Hemmings R, Khalifa F. Rupture of ectopic pregnancy in women with low and declining serum beta-human chorionic gonadotropin concentrations. *Fertil Steril.* 1991 Oct;56(4):786–787.

# Trauma in Pregnancy

## Victor J. Hassid and Miren A. Schinco

Trauma is the primary cause of death in women of reproductive age and is the leading nonobstetric cause of both fetal and maternal death during pregnancy (1–4). The potential for pregnancy must be considered in any girl or woman between the ages of 10 and 50 years. Accidental injury is estimated to occur in 6% to 7% of all pregnancies, and its incidence increases as pregnancy progresses until, by the end of the third trimester, minor trauma occurs more frequently than at any other time during female adulthood (1,2,5–8).

The majority of blunt trauma during pregnancy results from motor vehicle crashes, with the remainder being relatively evenly distributed between falls and assaults (3,4,9–13). Some authors report that up to 11% of women are victims of physical abuse during pregnancy (14–17) and up to 31.5% of pregnant women admitted following trauma are victims of intentional injury (11). During the third trimester, an altered center of gravity (caused by the enlarged uterus) combined with pelvic ligamentous laxity produces a degree of gait instability that makes the pregnant woman particularly susceptible to injury by falls (1,9). This represents the second most common mechanism of injury during pregnancy (13).

In a recent review of over 77,000 women of childbearing age in the American College of Surgeon's National Trauma Data Bank, pregnant patients were significantly younger, more likely to be underinsured, and of African American or Hispanic descent than their nonpregnant counterparts. While they were less likely to have used alcohol or illicit drugs, still 13% had been drinking and 20% had used drugs prior to their trauma. Although pregnant trauma patients were more likely to use seat belts, still only two thirds were restrained. After admission for a trauma, 5.1% of patients went on to delivery, three quarters within 24 hours and by cesarean section.

The foundation of trauma management in pregnancy is that "the best chance for fetal survival is to assure maternal survival" (5). The physician caring for a pregnant trauma patient should always remember that there are two patients. Initial treatment priorities for an injured pregnant patient remain the same as for the nonpregnant patient. The use of imaging studies should not be withheld because of pregnancy. Because the anatomic and physiologic alterations of pregnancy can alter the gravid woman's response to injury, an understanding of these changes is critical when approaching trauma management. Early communication between the trauma surgeon and the obstetrician is very important in order to optimize the management of the pregnant trauma patient.

## OUTCOMES

Regardless of severity, trauma during pregnancy has been associated with spontaneous abortion, premature labor, uterine injury, placental abruption, maternal death, and low birth weight fetal loss. When comparing traumatized gravid women with nontrauma controls, for any injury, both maternal and fetal outcomes are worse, with progressively worse outcomes with higher injury severity score (ISS). Injuries associated with the highest maternal mortality are thoracoabdominal and pelvic followed by brain injuries. Women who sustain trauma, but do not deliver at that time, continue with significant risk of increased morbidity and mortality throughout their pregnancy and therefore require close monitoring (13).

Maternal predictors of fetal death consist of maternal factors (ISS >15, severe head injury, pelvic fractures, shock, hypoxemia, and absent fetal heart tones) and mechanisms of injury (auto-pedestrian collisions, maternal ejection, motorcycle collision, and lack of restraints) (18–21). Infants under 28 weeks' gestational age appear to have the highest potential for complications, possibly due to their intolerance of maternal stress (13).

## ANATOMIC AND PHYSIOLOGIC ALTERATIONS OF PREGNANCY

### Anatomic Changes

Until approximately the 12th gestational week, the uterus remains in the pelvis, and by 20 weeks and 34 to 36 weeks, it reaches the umbilicus and the costal margin, respectively. During the last 2 weeks of gestation, the fundus frequently descends as the fetal head engages the pelvis. The progressive enlargement of the uterus causes the bowel to be displaced cephalad and therefore keeps it relatively protected from blunt abdominal trauma, whereas the uterus and its contents become more vulnerable (Fig. 4.1).

During the second trimester, the uterus enlarges beyond its protected intrapelvic location, but the fetus remains mobile and protected by a generous amount of amniotic fluid; the amniotic fluid can be a source of embolism and disseminated intravascular coagulation following trauma if it gains access to the intravascular space.

By the third trimester, secondary to the location of the fetal head within the pelvis, pelvic fractures may result in fetal skull fracture or significant intracranial injury. Unlike the elastic myometrium, the placenta has little elasticity, which predisposes it to shear forces at the uteroplacental interface and placental abruption.

While interpreting pelvic x-rays, it is important to remember that the pubic symphysis widens to 4 to 8 mm and the sacroiliac joint spaces increase by the 7th month of gestation.

### Cardiovascular System

Maternal cardiac output begins to increase during the first 10 weeks of pregnancy, reaching a peak of 30% to 50% above nonpregnant levels by the latter part of the second trimester (22). After the 10th week of pregnancy, the cardiac output can be increased by 1.0 to 1.5 L per minute, due to the increase in plasma volume and decrease in vascular resistance of the uterus and placenta, which during the third trimester of pregnancy receive 20% of the patient's cardiac output. During the same period, the cardiac output may be transiently lowered by aortocaval compression by the gravid uterus, resulting in decreased placental perfusion. This phenomenon, known as the supine hypotension syndrome, may be observed clinically in otherwise normal pregnant patients (22,23). It is very important to remember while managing a pregnant trauma patient that changing the maternal position from the supine to the left lateral decubitus position may increase cardiac output by as much as 25% at term (23).

The average maternal heart rate increases 20% to 30% during pregnancy such that by term, the normal maternal pulse rate is 80 to 95 beats per minute, making borderline tachycardia difficult to evaluate (2,9,14,23). Mean arterial blood pressure gradually declines during the first two trimesters of pregnancy, reaching its nadir by approximately 28 weeks' gestation (22).

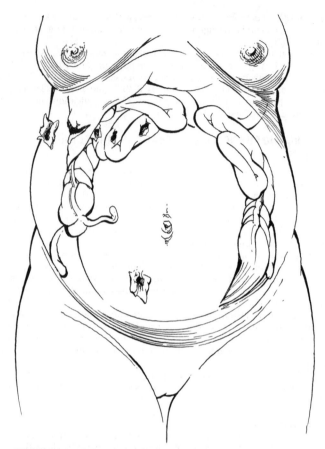

**FIGURE 4.1** Compartmentalization of intestines during pregnancy and sites of gunshot wounds above and below the umbilicus.

Systolic arterial pressure decreases by 0 to 15 mm Hg, whereas diastolic pressure declines by 10 to 20 mm Hg, creating a widened pulse pressure. These changes are the result of diminishing peripheral vascular resistance and should not be mistaken as evidence of hypovolemia during the first two trimesters of pregnancy. During the third trimester, blood pressure gradually increases, returning to pre-pregnancy levels near term (2,7,9,22,23). Hypertension, systolic or diastolic, is never expected during pregnancy and, if present, may either be a response to pain, anxiety, or injury or be the result of a direct complication of pregnancy such as pregnancy-induced hypertension (9).

Associated with the underlying decreased peripheral vascular resistance of the first two trimesters of pregnancy is a paradoxical response to stimuli that would normally cause vasoconstriction. This altered response causes the skin to be warm and dry, instead of cool and clammy which would be expected during hypovolemic shock (9). In addition, central venous pressure, normally approximately 9 cm $H_2O$ in the nonpregnant patient, gradually decreases throughout pregnancy until it reaches 4 to 6 cm $H_2O$ during the third trimester (4,7,14,24). Venous hypertension in the lower extremities is present during the third trimester.

Total maternal blood volume increases by as much as 50% at 34 weeks' gestation, improving maternal response to hemorrhage. A smaller increase in red blood cell (RBC) volume occurs, resulting in a decreased hematocrit (physiologic anemia of pregnancy) (1,22). The white blood cell (WBC) count increases, resulting in counts as high as 15K and 25K/mm$^3$ during pregnancy and labor, respectively (1,5,9). Levels of serum fibrinogen and other clotting factors are mildly elevated, leading to a hypercoagulable state (14,22). During periods of stress, the mother maintains homeostasis at the expense of the fetus. Acute maternal hemorrhage or maternal hypoxia induces uterine artery vasoconstriction, which can reduce uterine perfusion by 10% to 20% before clinical evidence of maternal hypovolemia occurs (1,4,5,9). Consequently, 30% to 35% of maternal blood volume may be lost before clinical signs of hypovolemia develop (1,6,7,9,14,24). This, combined with the sensitivity of the placental vasculature to catecholamines, places the fetus at risk during maternal hemorrhage that may, upon clinical examination of the mother, appear minimally significant. Early and adequate maternal volume replacement and thorough fetal evaluation, including fetal monitoring, are therefore critical in the management of the gravid trauma patient.

Electrocardiographic (ECG) changes in late pregnancy are not specific and reflect the leftward shift of the cardiac axis, by approximately 15 degrees, due to diaphragm elevation. The T waves may be flattened and inverted in lead III, and the Q waves may appear in leads III and aVF. Supraventricular ectopic beats may also be seen (9,14).

### Respiratory System

Minute ventilation increases by 40% to 50% over control values at term due to increases in tidal volume and respiratory rate (9,14,22,25). The metabolic effect of this change is a partially compensated respiratory alkalosis, with arterial blood gases showing a decrease in $PCO_2$ to approximately 30 to 34 mm Hg and a decrease in serum bicarbonate to 18 to 22 mEq/L. The net effect is to leave the pregnant woman with a decreased buffering capacity after trauma (1,9,22). A $PaCO_2$ of 35 to 40 mm Hg may indicate impending respiratory failure during pregnancy. Maternal arterial $PO_2$ increases by 10 mm Hg, but oxygen consumption increases by as much as 20% by term (9,14,25). Coupled with fetal oxygen demand and fetal sensitivity to hypoxia, these alterations place the pregnant trauma patient and her fetus at risk for hypoxic insult. Supplemental oxygen therefore becomes a priority in the pregnant trauma patient (9,25). Anatomic alterations in the thoracic cavity appear to account for the decreased residual volume, associated with diaphragmatic elevation, increased lung markings, and prominence of the pulmonary vessels noticed on chest x-ray. These should be kept in mind when considering chest tube placement in a pregnant trauma patient.

### Gastrointestinal System

The major physiologic alterations of the gastrointestinal system are those of increasing compartmentalization of the small intestine into the upper abdomen and a progesterone-induced decrease in gastrointestinal motility. The gravid uterus may protect the abdominal viscera from injury to the lower abdomen, but penetrating wounds to the upper abdomen may injure many loops of tightly crowded small intestine (Fig. 4.1). In addition, stretching of the abdominal wall alters the normal response to peritoneal irritation, at times masking significant intra-abdominal organ injury. Decreased gastric emptying increases the possibility of aspiration during trauma and intubation, therefore early gastric tube decompression is important in order to prevent aspiration of gastric contents (1,7,9,22,24,25). Position of the patient's spleen and liver is essentially unchanged by pregnancy.

### Urinary System

Progesterone-induced smooth muscle relaxation of the ureters and mechanical compression by the gravid uterus cause dilatation of the ureters and renal pelvises, which may appear as hydronephrosis on radiographic studies (14,22). In addition, ureteropelvic dilatation predisposes the urinary collecting system to stasis and subsequent infection, particularly after catheterization (14,22). Anatomically, the urinary bladder is displaced anteriorly and superiorly by the enlarging uterus, making it increasingly vulnerable to injury after the first trimester (1,2,8,22). Furthermore, the glomerular filtration rate and the renal plasma blood flow increase during pregnancy and the levels of creatinine and serum urea nitrogen drop to approximately one half of normal pre-pregnancy levels.

### Endocrine System

The pituitary gland increases in size and weight by 30% to 50% during pregnancy, and any significant drop in blood pressure can result in necrosis of the anterior pituitary gland and subsequent pituitary insufficiency.

### Neurologic System

One of the complications of late pregnancy is eclampsia, which can present with the same signs and symptoms as a head injury. It should always be considered in case of seizures associated with hypertension, hyperreflexia, proteinuria, and peripheral edema. It may be necessary to obtain expert neurologic consultation in these cases in order to differentiate between eclampsia and other causes of seizures.

Table 4.1 outlines the physiologic, anatomic, and laboratory changes associated with pregnancy.

## PATTERNS OF MATERNAL AND FETAL INJURY

### Blunt Abdominal Trauma

Following blunt abdominal trauma during the latter part of pregnancy, the gravid uterus is subject to direct injury, as well as to the shearing forces resulting from sudden deceleration. Most fetal morbidity is a result of catastrophic maternal trauma; however, some serious complications, including preterm delivery, abruptio placentae, fetal injury, fetal death, and massive fetomaternal hemorrhage (FMH), have occurred after seemingly minor injuries (5,11,26,27).

The abdominal wall, uterine myometrium, and amniotic fluid act as buffers to direct fetal injury from blunt trauma. Still, fetal injuries can occur when the abdominal wall strikes the dashboard or steering wheel, or in case, the pregnant patient is struck by a blunt instrument. Indirect fetal injury may take place secondary to rapid deceleration, contrecoup effect, or a shearing force leading to placental abruption.

| TABLE 4.1 | Physiologic and Anatomic Changes in Pregnancy | |
|---|---|---|
| **System** | **Physiologic Change** | **Effect** |
| Cardiovascular | ↑ Cardiac output | Tachycardia |
| | ↑ Blood volume | ↑ Maternal tolerance to hemorrhage |
| | ↓ Peripheral vascular resistance | ↓ Blood pressure; ↑ skin temperature |
| | ↓ Central venous pressure | 4–6 cm $H_2O$ during third trimester |
| | Aortocaval compression | Supine hypotension |
| | ↓ Uterine perfusion in response to hemorrhage | ↑ Fetal risk during hemorrhage |
| Pulmonary | ↑ Minute ventilation | Partially compensated respiratory alkalosis; ↓ tolerance to acidosis |
| | ↑ Oxygen consumption | ↓ Tolerance to hypoxia |
| | ↑ Fetal oxygen demand | |
| | Elevation of diaphragm 4 cm by term | Thoracostomies performed one to two interspaces higher than usual |
| Gastrointestinal | ↓ Motility; ↓ gastric emptying compartmentalization | ↑ Risk of aspiration |
| | | ↑ Risk of injury with upper abdominal trauma |
| | | ↓ Risk with lower abdominal trauma |
| Genitourinary | ↓ Motility of collecting system; ↓ bladder emptying | Physiologic abnormality of radiographic studies |
| | | ↑ Risk of infection with catheterization |
| | Displacement of bladder | ↑ Risk of injury |
| | ↑ Uterine size and blood flow | ↑ Risk of hemorrhage from abdominal wounds |
| Hematologic | ↑ Plasma volume without proportional ↑ in red cell mass | Dilutional anemia |
| | Leukocytosis | Normal WBC count can reach 18,000/mm³ in second and third trimester |
| | ↑ Factors VII, VIII, IX, and X and fibrinogen | Hypercoagulable state |

*Note*: ↑ Increased; ↓ decreased. WBC, white blood cell.

Abruptio placentae is a significant cause of fetal loss in both catastrophic and noncatastrophic trauma. While the exact mechanism of traumatic abruption is not known, the suggested mechanism is based on the fundamental differences in tissue characteristics between the relatively elastic myometrium of the uterus and the relatively inelastic tissue of the placenta.

When an external deforming force is applied to the abdomen, shearing of the uteroplacental interface occurs. Shearing is further aggravated by the increased intrauterine pressure that results from impact (10,15). Signs and symptoms suggesting abruption include vaginal bleeding, uterine tenderness or contractions, fetal heart rate abnormalities, and fetal death. Although the presence of these symptoms is significant, the absence of symptoms following trauma does not exclude the possibility of placental abruption (3,27–29). Most cases of significant abruption can be identified by clinical signs or electronic fetal monitoring within 4 to 6 hours of the traumatic event (15,23,30), however, even in minor abdominal trauma, significant placental abruption can occur without significant symptoms. This supports the importance of fetal monitoring after abdominal trauma (20). Cases of abruptio placentae have been reported to occur up to 5 days following severe trauma (29,31).

Uterine rupture may also result from blunt trauma. Uterine rupture complicates approximately 0.6% of traumatic events during pregnancy and tends to occur only with major blunt abdominal trauma (15,23). The presentation of uterine rupture ranges from subtle findings such as uterine tenderness and worrisome fetal heart rate patterns, without changes in maternal vital signs, to rapid onset of maternal hypovolemic shock associated with fetal and maternal death (15). Fetal mortality rate approaches 100%; maternal mortality is usually due to concurrent injury (23).

Amniotic fluid embolism is a rare complication of pregnancy characterized by poor response to treatment and high mortality. The incidence is between 1 in 8,000 and 1 in 80,000 live births with mortality ranging from 61% to 86%. While it most frequently occurs in the peripartum period, it has also been described after blunt abdominal trauma. It typically presents with sudden onset of hypoxia, altered mental status, hemodynamic compromise, and disseminated intravascular coagulation. The diagnosis remains largely a clinical one. Management is mainly nonspecific supportive therapy aimed at cardiopulmonary resuscitation, correction of coagulopathy, and treatment of hemorrhage. If delivery has not occurred, emergent cesarean section prevents further hypoxic insult to the fetus and facilitates treatment of the mother (32).

Premature uterine contractions are another common sequela of maternal trauma (1,3,30–31,33–36). Studies have shown that up to two thirds of traumatized gravidas experience frequent contractions during the initial 4 hours of monitoring (3,30,34). Postulated etiologies include placental abruption, uterine contusion, membrane ischemia, and membrane rupture (1). The use of tocolytics to halt premature contractions associated with trauma is controversial. Although some authors report successful cessation of preterm contractions with these agents (36,37), others discourage their use, believing that regular uterine activity after trauma will spontaneously subside during observation. In those cases in which contractions persist, placental abruption must be considered until proven otherwise (14,34). Although the mean abdominal abbreviated injury score (aAIS), a direct indicator of injury severity of intra-abdominal structures, is usually higher among patients who sustained acute termination of pregnancy and/or fetal loss, in some studies, a high aAIS (≥3) did not independently predict these complications (38).

Direct fetal injury complicates <1% of all pregnancies in which trauma occurs (15). The most common fetal injuries after blunt trauma are skull fractures and intracranial hemorrhage; these injuries are frequently fatal (5,6). The most commonly described mechanism of fetal head injury is that associated with fracture of the maternal pelvis late in gestation when the fetal head is engaged (39).

When evidence of serious or life-threatening hemorrhage is found, laparotomy should not be delayed because of pregnancy (26,37,40).

### Fetomaternal Hemorrhage

FMH, the transplacental passage of fetal blood into the maternal circulation, is reported to occur in 8.8% to 30.6% of victims of blunt abdominal trauma (14,30,34,36,41). The volume of blood lost from the fetus can range from as little as 5 mL up to approximately 70 mL, with the average volume of transfusion ranging from 12 to 16 mL (34,41,42). Although complications of FMH include Rh-D sensitization of the mother, neonatal anemia, and fetal death from exsanguination, detection of FMH has been shown to have little prognostic value in predicting adverse fetal or maternal outcome (3,27,30,33). Therefore, detection of FMH is not routinely indicated in maternal trauma (3,10,15,23,27,30). As little as 0.01 to 0.03 mL of transplacental fetal Rh D–positive blood may cause isoimmunization in the Rh D–negative mother, a complication easily prevented by the administration of Rh D immunoglobulin (RhIG) (14,15,22,27).

FMH detection can be attempted by using the Kleihauer–Betke (K–B) test, an acid-elution technique that identifies cells containing fetal hemoglobin in the maternal circulation. The K–B test can generally detect as little as 0.1 mL of fetal cells (14,22,43). Because the sensitivity of the K–B test varies among laboratories and may not be sufficient to detect small hemorrhages capable of sensitizing some Rh D–negative mothers, the standard dose of RhIG (300 $\mu$g) should be considered in all Rh D–negative women with a potentially Rh D–positive fetus who have sustained catastrophic or noncatastrophic blunt abdominal trauma (10,14,15,27,43). The K–B test is then used to further quantify FMH in excess of the amount covered by the standard dose of RhIG (14,15,22,36,43). One standard dose of RhIG (300 $\mu$g) neutralizes 30 mL of fetal whole blood or 15 mL of fetal RBCs in the maternal circulation (22,43). RhIG should be administered within 72 hours of injury (15,43).

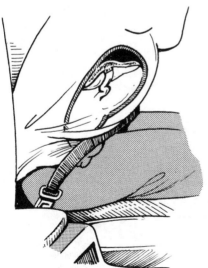

**FIGURE 4.2** Seat belt use without shoulder belt.

## Use of Restraints

The use of automobile restraints deserves special mention, because blunt vehicular trauma is the most common mechanism of injury among pregnant women (3,4,10–12,14,37,40,44). In a recent survey of pregnant women, less than three quarters admitted to noncompliance with restraint usage. The most common reasons cited were patient discomfort and failing to remember to utilize them. Still, one third of patients were unsure of the safety of restraints (20). When evaluating fetal outcome after motor vehicular crashes, crash severity, use of restraints, and maternal injury severity were predictors of fetal outcome. Unrestrained pregnant women involved in motor vehicle crashes are more likely to have major complications and adverse fetal outcomes (21). Seat belts decrease the severity of maternal injury and the frequency of maternal death by preventing ejection of the occupant from the vehicle (45). However, the type of restraint system affects the frequency of uterine rupture and fetal death. Lap belts worn too high allow enough forward flexion of the maternal abdomen and uterus over the belt during rapid deceleration for resultant compression to elevate intrauterine pressure and distort the size and shape of the uterus (Fig. 4.2) (45–48). This distortion predisposes the woman to placental abruption, uterine rupture, and direct fetal injury (45,46,48). The addition of shoulder restraints has been shown to improve fetal outcome, presumably by dissipating the deceleration force over a greater surface and preventing forward flexion of the mother (44,47). Three-point restraints are therefore preferable and recommended (14,15). If the lap belt alone is the only option, it should be secured low across the bony pelvis below the protuberant abdomen, rather than over the uterine fundus, to minimize abdominal compression during impact (Fig. 4.3) (14,46). Routine use of a lap and

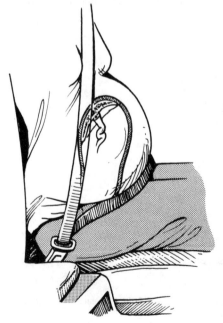

**FIGURE 4.3** Appropriate use of shoulder and lap belts.

shoulder belt reduces the chance of serious maternal injury and death by 50% (44) and has been associated with a significant decrease in fetal morbidity and preterm delivery (49). Studies have shown that unbelted women in crashes are more likely to have low birth weight infants than pregnant women who were not in crashes and are more likely to experience excessive maternal bleeding during delivery than belted women in crashes (50). The impact of airbags on maternal and fetal trauma appears to be positive and not associated with increased risk of fetal or maternal injury (15,22,51). Of note, only 37% of pregnant patients reported receiving information about seat belts during prenatal care in one study, emphasizing the need to focus on this important aspect of injury control (52). Greater public awareness and education are needed on safe driving habits and on the effectiveness of seat belts during pregnancy (50).

### Penetrating Abdominal Trauma

Gunshot and stab wounds are the most frequently encountered penetrating injuries (14,22). As with blunt trauma, pregnancy often changes the usual manifestations of penetrating abdominal trauma because the gravid uterus displaces other abdominal organs cephalad. When the route of entry is below the fundus, the gravid uterus will often protect maternal viscera by absorbing the force of the shell or instrument. In contrast, upper abdominal injuries may result in increased injury to bowel compressed into the upper abdomen (14,22).

Gunshot wounds to the abdomen are associated with a high rate of internal organ injury. When a bullet, particularly one of low velocity such as that commonly found in civilian injuries, strikes the pregnant uterus, much of its energy is dissipated in the dense uterine musculature, diminishing its velocity and ability to penetrate other maternal abdominal organs. Gunshot wounds to the pregnant abdomen therefore are associated with low maternal rates of morbidity and mortality (4,24,53). Fetal outcome, however, is generally poor, with reported rates of fetal injury varying from 59% to 78% and perinatal mortality ranging from 41% to 71% (1,22,24,39,53). Fetal mortality is caused by both prematurity and direct fetal injury (24). Although direct fetal injury portends a poor prognosis, cases have been reported in which a fetus having sustained a nonfatal injury later was successfully delivered alive (7,24,54). Because gunshot wounds to the abdomen have a high frequency of internal organ injury, surgical exploration remains the standard approach to this type of injuries (4,15,16,22).

Stab wounds to the abdomen are associated with a lower mortality rate than are gunshot wounds. As with gunshot wounds, the gravid uterus may protect the victim of a lower abdominal stab wound, whereas wounds to the upper abdomen carry a higher incidence of visceral injury (4,7,15,22). The trend toward conservative management of abdominal stab wounds extends to the pregnant patient. Clinical considerations influencing management include gestational age, condition of the mother and the fetus, and location of the wound in the abdomen. Management options include immediate surgical exploration, in case of diffuse abdominal tenderness or presence of peritonitis, or close observation and use of adjunctive imaging studies, which may provide information regarding potentially injured viscera and penetration or not of the abdominal fascia.

## EVALUATION AND MANAGEMENT

Initial evaluation and resuscitative efforts should be directed toward the mother, because the most common cause of traumatic fetal death is maternal death. Once maternal airway, respiratory, and hemodynamic stability are ensured, attention must be immediately directed to assessment and assurance of fetal health.

## Prehospital Management

Injured pregnant women, particularly those in the latter half of pregnancy, should be transported to an appropriately designated trauma center with facilities for adequate maternal and specialized neonatal care when possible (4,9). During the second and third trimesters, transport should be performed with the patient in the left lateral decubitus position or the spine must be immobilized, with the backboard tilted 15 degrees to the left (1,7,9,14). Listening for fetal heart tones may be performed en route but should not delay transport (7,14). The pneumatic antishock garment (PASG) may be used to control bleeding from pelvic or lower extremity fractures, but its use should not interfere with rapid reestablishment of intravascular volume by intravenous fluid infusion. If it is used during pregnancy, only the lower or leg compartments should be inflated. Inflation of the abdominal compartment is contraindicated in any patient with a potentially salvageable gestation because the PASG has a deleterious effect on uteroplacental blood flow, compromises maternal venous return, and has the potential to cause direct fetal injury (1,4,7,9,22,23).

Both in the prehospital setting and in the emergency department, oxygen therapy provides special benefit for the fetus. Although the maternal arterial blood is normally well saturated with oxygen when the mother is breathing room air, the oxygen hemoglobin dissociation curve of fetal blood is shifted such that increasing alveolar oxygen tension continues to improve fetal saturation and thereby fetal outcome (7,14). Maternal hemorrhage can reduce uterine blood flow 10% to 20% before signs of maternal hypovolemia appear (1,4,5,9). Therefore, early intravenous access and volume resuscitation are important for both the mother and the fetus. Vasopressors should be avoided, because they can further decrease uterine blood flow (4,7,15). The presence of initial maternal hypotension (defined as systolic blood pressure ≤90 mm Hg) has been shown to be associated with a higher risk of pregnancy loss. Toward the third trimester, maternal intravascular volume increases up to 50%. This improves maternal tolerance of hemorrhage and delays the appearance of signs and symptoms of shock, while the uterine circulation is reduced. Once obvious maternal hypotension ensues, the fetus has already been endangered by decreased uterine arterial blood flow (55).

## Evaluation of the Mother and the Fetus

Prehospital information is critical in ascertaining the mechanism of injury, vital signs, and patient condition in the field. Prenatal history is of particular importance, particularly in ascertaining the gestational age of the fetus and the presence of complicating medical conditions. Maternal perception of fetal movement may provide a very cursory indication of fetal health. The time of the last meal is more significant than in the nonpregnant patient because of the prolonged gastric emptying time associated with pregnancy (7,9).

Initial physical assessment of the mother is focused on the stability of the airway, adequacy of ventilation, effectiveness of the circulatory volume, and evaluation for occult injuries; there exist conflicting data regarding the relationship between the mother's Glasgow Coma Scale (GCS) and the fetal outcome (56). Supplemental oxygen should be administered to the mother throughout the initial resuscitation and evaluation, because minimal changes in maternal oxygenation result in appreciable changes in fetal oxygen content and reserve (4,14,25). Because of the increased potential for aspiration and importance of fetal oxygenation, endotracheal intubation should be pursued more aggressively than in the nonpregnant patient (4,15,22,25). The expanded maternal intravascular volume associated with pregnancy may delay the onset of clinical signs of shock, so fluid resuscitation should be more aggressive than in nongravid patients. Crystalloid fluid resuscitation and early type-specific blood administration are indicated to support the physiologic hypervolemia of pregnancy. Non–cross-matched type 0, Rh D–negative blood can be used if type-specific blood is not immediately available (16,23). Continuous uterine displacement, either manually or by placing the mother in the left lateral tilt position, is desirable after 20 weeks' gestation, because of the uterine compression of the inferior vena cava. Vasopressors should be avoided until appropriate volume replacement, including blood transfusion if indicated, has been administered (4,14,15,22).

Once maternal hemodynamic stability has been established and assessment of maternal injuries has begun, the condition of the fetus should be ascertained. Fetal evaluation includes determining fetal heart rate and fetal movement, evaluating uterine size and irritability, and examining the vagina for vaginal bleeding or leakage of amniotic fluid. Ideally, fetal heart rate and maternal contractions should be continuously monitored using external tococardiography. However, when this is not available, fetal heart tones should be auscultated at frequent intervals. Fetal heart rate abnormalities including tachycardia, late decelerations, and ultimately fetal bradycardia, even in the absence of vaginal bleeding and uterine tenderness or irritability, are highly suggestive of placental abruption (4,14).

Determination of fetal age and maturity may be critical in management decisions for the fetus. The quickest means of estimating gestational age is by palpation of the fundal height. At 12 weeks' gestation, the uterine fundus rises just above the symphysis pubis; at 20 weeks' gestation, it reaches the level of the umbilicus; and by 36 weeks of gestation, it lies just below the xiphoid process. The age of fetal viability is generally considered to be 24 to 26 weeks' gestation, depending, in part, on the neonatal facilities available (1,2,7). Palpation of the uterine fundus two to three finger-breadths above the umbilicus is consistent with the presence of a potentially viable fetus. Ultrasound is a more accurate tool and should be used if circumstances permit (4,14).

Asymptomatic patients with minor or insignificant abdominal trauma may be discharged with reassurance after 4 to 6 hours of fetal and maternal monitoring. Discharge instructions should include the need to return upon the development of abdominal pain, decreased fetal movement, vaginal bleeding, or leakage of fluid. Timely obstetric follow-up is advised (15,16).

### Routine Laboratory Studies

Urine $\beta$-human chorionic gonadotropin testing should be performed on all female trauma patients of childbearing age who are not obviously pregnant, as approximately 3% of females admitted to a trauma center are pregnant, and 8% of these pregnancies are newly diagnosed (57,58). Routine laboratory studies in the pregnant patient with significant trauma include type and cross-match; complete blood count with platelet count; electrolytes; and coagulation panel including prothrombin time, partial thromboplastin time, fibrinogen level, and fibrin degradation products (1,9,14,16,23). The finding of a normal nonpregnant value of fibrinogen (200 to 250 mg/dL) may be consistent with early disseminated intravascular coagulopathy (14), because normal fibrinogen levels during pregnancy may be twice that in nonpregnant women. Rh D–negative patients typically will undergo K–B testing to determine the volume of FMH that has occurred (14,15,22,36,43).

### Radiographic Procedures

The first trimester of intrauterine development is the time of greatest sensitivity to radiation (59). During the first 2 weeks of conception, the embryo is particularly sensitive to the lethal effects of radiation but has a low probability of sustaining teratogenic effects if implantation and continued development occur (60,61). During the period of embryonic development (2 to 8 weeks after conception), the embryo is particularly sensitive to the growth-retarding and teratogenic effects of radiation; from the 8th to the 15th week after conception, the fetal brain is undergoing rapid neuron development and is potentially vulnerable to radiation-induced mental defects. Throughout gestation, there is an increased risk of childhood malignancies, especially leukemia, in children exposed to radiation in utero (60–62). Determining the exact incidence of adverse effects, however, is difficult because of the prevalence of congenital malformations occurring in the general population and because of the other frequent biomedical and social factors that may influence pregnancy outcome (59,60). In general, fetal risk is considered negligible when the total radiation exposure is ≤5 rad and the risk of malformations is significantly increased above the control levels only at doses >10 to 15 rad (14,15,48,63). An increased risk of childhood cancers has been found at somewhat lower radiation doses (22,60,62). The dose of radiation absorbed by the fetus depends on several factors including the (a) energy and intensity of the x-rays, (b) proximity of the uterus to the anatomic area exposed, (c) extent of the area exposed, (d) patient positioning, (e) depth of the fetus, and (f) number of films acquired (64). If the uterus is outside the area radiographed, the dose of radiation to the conceptus is limited to that delivered by scatter and leakage radiation, declining rapidly farther the uterus is from the radiographed area. Pelvic shielding should be used whenever possible (9). Estimates of fetal radiation exposure from commonly used procedures are listed in Table 4.2. Routine diagnostic radiographs seldom result in significant radiation exposure to the fetus. Therefore, although unnecessary

**TABLE 4.2**    Estimated Radiation Dose to the Uterus From Commonly Used Radiographic Examinations

| Examination | Typical Dose (mrad/Examination)[a] | Range (mrad/Examination)[a] |
|---|---|---|
| Cervical spine | <0.5 | <0.5–3.0 |
| Chest | 1 | 0.2–43 |
| Abdomen | 250 | 25–1,900 |
| Extremities | <0.5 | <0.5–18 |
| Thoracic spine | 11 | <10–55 |
| Lumbar spine | 400 | 30–2,400 |
| Pelvis | 200 | 55–2,200 |
| Hips and femur | 300 | 73–1,400 |
| Intravenous urography | 600 | 70–5,500 |
| Computed tomography scans[b] | | |
| Head (10 slices) | <50 | |
| Chest (10 slices) | <100 | |
| Abdomen (10 slices) | 2,600 | |

[a]Typical doses adapted from Ref. 56 and based on Bureau of Radiological Health, FDA (1976), if available.
[b]Based on technique and equipment, doses may be well above or below typical values; values adapted from Ref. 61.

radiography should be avoided, necessary diagnostic studies should never be withheld out of concern for fetal irradiation (1,5,9,61,62). When possible, effective alternative imaging modalities such as ultrasonography should be used in evaluating the pregnant trauma patient and judicious shielding of the fetus should be used when feasible. Abdominal pelvic computerized tomography (CT), intravenous urography, and angiography may all be indicated and should be performed as necessary (4,15,16,61). The highest-dose radiologic studies are pelvic CT, pelvic angiography, and pelvic fluoroscopy, which may result in radiation doses of 2 to 5 rad (61). If such studies are necessary, CT scanning using a reduced number of slices or angiography with pelvic shielding and dose-reducing techniques should be considered (15,61). Although there are no reported deleterious effects from contrast agents, their potential effects have not been well studied, and therefore their use should be based on a well-considered risk–benefit analysis (61). Magnetic resonance imaging has not been associated with adverse fetal effects and may provide a safe and effective alternative to conventional radiography during pregnancy, but insufficient data currently exist to justify its routine use, particularly during the first trimester (9,60,62).

## Ultrasonography

Ultrasonography is indicated in all cases of significant trauma in pregnancy (1,2,4,8,34,37). Focused Assessment Sonography in Trauma (FAST) is a reliable screening modality for intra-abdominal and pelvic free fluid (1,4,16,34). Sonography is also a sensitive indicator of gestational age, presentation, amniotic fluid volume, and fetal movement, but it is not as sensitive as cardiotocographic monitoring for diagnosing early and clinically significant abruptio placentae (4,23). Although small abruptions are not easily seen, large abruptions, retroplacental clots, and some fetal fractures may be identified (1,2).

## Fetal Monitoring

Continuous fetal monitoring with a cardiotocodynamometer is recommended for all viable fetuses after 20 to 24 weeks' gestation. The normal range for fetal heart rate is between 120 and 160 beats per minute. An abnormal heart rate, repetitive decelerations, absence of accelerations or beat-to-beat variability, or frequent uterine activity may be a sign of impending maternal and/or fetal decompensation (1,2). The duration of monitoring remains controversial. Patients at risk for an adverse fetal outcome and for placental abruption require prolonged evaluation. Several studies have shown that most complications reveal themselves within 6 hours of the traumatic event. So, patients found to be at risk should undergo continuous monitoring for 6 hours. If there is no evidence of adverse fetal outcome, they may be discharged home with an instruction to return immediately in case of any signs of placental abruption, bleeding, contraction, or change in fetal movements. Patients with evidence of contractions, requiring general anesthesia and those at significant risk for unfavorable outcomes or placental abruption, must undergo 24 hours of continuous fetal monitoring. Any evidence of fetal distress should be managed aggressively with delivery by cesarean section, if necessary (21).

## Peritoneal Lavage

Diagnostic peritoneal lavage (DPL) has largely been supplanted by the FAST examination. However, DPL is a safe and accurate procedure in the pregnant trauma patient and can be considered in cases of blunt abdominal trauma as well as anterior abdominal and thoracoabdominal stab wounds (4,26). Open lavage, which allows direct visualization of the peritoneum at a site in the midline just above the uterine fundus, is usually recommended (4,5,7,15). Unless gross blood is obtained from the initial aspirate, a peritoneal dialysis catheter is placed above the umbilicus using the open technique, and it should be gently directed toward the pelvis and a liter of crystalloid infused through it. Fluid is returned by gravity drainage. Criteria for a positive lavage are identical to that in a nonpregnant patient (5). DPL does not assess retroperitoneal and intrauterine pathology, which may be better visualized by CT scanning in the stable patient with blunt abdominal trauma or penetrating wounds of the flank and back (4).

### Tetanus Prophylaxis

Transplacental transfer of tetanus antitoxin prevents neonatal tetanus (65). Therefore, tetanus immunization is recommended for both postexposure and routine administration during pregnancy. Indications, dose, and timing for postexposure tetanus prophylaxis with combined tetanus and diphtheria toxoids and passive immunization with tetanus immunoglobulin are identical to those in the nongravid female (65,66). Although there is no evidence that tetanus and diphtheria toxoids are teratogenic, routine administration of diphtheria toxoids should be performed during the second or third trimester to minimize concerns over teratogenicity (67).

### Injury Severity Score

The ISS is used frequently for injury severity assessment. Attempts to use the ISS to predict placental abruption or fetal death have had conflicting results, but the weight of evidence points to a correlation between a higher ISS and a higher risk of fetal death (53,68,69). Ejection from the vehicle, motorcycle crashes, pedestrian collisions, and maternal death do appear to be independent risk factors for fetal demise (70). Increased maternal age, loss of consciousness, and maternal pelvic fractures sustained during motor vehicle collisions contribute toward high ISS and impact fetal outcome (56). One study concluded that the only combination which could reliably exclude the possibility of fetal mortality was an ISS <9 in a near-third-trimester pregnancy; however, this conclusion was based on the data from only 17 cases (38). An ISS calculator can be found at the Web site www.trauma.org.

## SPECIFIC TRAUMA EPISODES

### Thoracic Injuries

Management of chest injuries in the gravid and nongravid patients is essentially the same. Early management of the airway and prompt treatment of pneumothorax and hemothorax are particularly important, because there is an increased risk of fetal hypoxia with maternal airway or ventilatory compromise. Thoracostomy tubes should be inserted one or two interspaces above the usual site, with careful digital exploration of the pleural space before insertion of the tube, owing to the elevation of the diaphragm by the gravid uterus (4,16).

### Pelvic Fractures

Pelvic and acetabular fractures have been shown to contribute to both high maternal (5% to 12.5%) and fetal (31% to 35%) mortality, especially during the first trimester. The most commonly documented fetal injury is skull fracture, associated with a 42% fetal death rate. However, in the evaluation of 101 reported cases of pelvic or acetabular fractures, fracture type (acetabular versus pelvic) and fracture designation (simple versus complex) had no influence on maternal or fetal mortality (19). Sixty-nine percent of women who presented in their third trimester went on to deliver within 21 days of injury, usually by vaginal delivery. Pelvic fractures during pregnancy are rarely treated with surgical intervention.

## Head and Spinal Cord Injuries

Management of the head-injured pregnant patient is similar to that of the nonpregnant. Cervical spine films and head CT scan should be obtained with abdominal shielding. A patient with an acute increase in intracranial pressure that results in herniation is treated with immediate airway protection, hyperventilation (only in the acute setting), and osmotic diuresis with mannitol, 1 g/kg. Head-up positioning at 20 degrees, provided that the cervical spine has been cleared, may marginally reduce hydrostatic pressure. Prompt neurosurgical consultation should be sought (22). Seizures or coma is frequently trauma induced, but any patient at >20 weeks' gestation who has these symptoms should be suspected of having eclampsia and should be treated as such, while undergoing evaluation and management for suspected head injury. Although hypertension, edema, proteinuria, and hyperactive reflexes are frequently present, they may not be prominent. When eclampsia is suspected, treatment with magnesium sulfate ($MgSO_4$) should be initiated immediately, per protocol. Urinary output, respiratory status, and the presence of patellar reflexes should be monitored during $MgSO_4$ infusion.

Injury to the spinal cord is not uncommon either as an isolated injury or in combination with other blunt or penetrating injuries. These injuries and the accompanying neurologic deficit or neurogenic shock may be difficult to diagnose in patients with an altered level of consciousness. A high index of suspicion should be maintained. Refractory hypotension unresponsive to proper patient positioning (15 degrees to the patient's left) or aggressive fluid replacement, without an identified ongoing source of blood loss, should raise the possibility of neurogenic shock.

## Thermal Burns

Although thermal burns do not commonly complicate pregnancy, it is estimated that between 5% and 10% of women of reproductive age admitted to burn units with significant burns are pregnant (39). Several observations have emerged from published studies of gravid patients who have sustained thermal injury (71–73). First, pregnancy does not appear to alter maternal outcome after thermal injury (14,22,71,73). Second, as might be expected, maternal and fetal survival are inversely related to the extent of the mother's burn (71–73), with burns covering >50% of the total body surface area portending a poor prognosis for the fetus (14,39,72). Premature labor or fetal death generally occurs within the 1st week after the burn injury and is often preceded by episodes of maternal hypotension, sepsis, or respiratory failure (39,72,73). As in other forms of trauma, fetal monitoring is indicated in the patient with a potentially viable fetus (22).

The basic principles of burn management that apply to the general population also apply to the pregnant patient (72,73). Uterine vasoconstriction accompanies maternal hypoxia and hypovolemia. These responses necessitate adequate oxygenation, including intubation at the first sign of respiratory compromise, aggressive fluid replacement with correction of electrolyte abnormalities, and prevention of sepsis to ensure satisfactory outcome for the mother and the fetus (4,39,71,72). Fetal survival is negligible when the maternal burn is >50% of the total body surface area, so some authors recommend expedited delivery if there is a good possibility of fetal survival (14,72). When possible, major burns should be treated in specialized burn units with obstetric consultation (4).

## Electrical Injury

Electrical injury during pregnancy is uncommon and there is little information regarding fetal outcome after such injury. Although most case reports tend to emphasize a poor fetal prognosis (74–76), one prospective study showed fetal outcome to be similar in women suffering electric shock during pregnancy and age-matched control subjects (77). Management of the pregnant patient after accidental electrical injury should address the well-being of both the mother and the fetus. Any woman with a history of significant electrical injury should have an ECG performed, followed by 24 hours of cardiac monitoring if the initial ECG is abnormal or there is a history of loss of consciousness (77). Fetal monitoring should be performed to detect fetal distress when the fetus is at least 24 to 26 weeks' gestation. In the previable fetus, simple auscultation of fetal heart tones will probably suffice (74). Unless previously documented, ultrasonography should be performed in all patients for assessment of gestational age and amniotic fluid volume to provide baseline parameters for following fetal growth (74,77).

## PERIMORTEM CESAREAN SECTION

Perimortem cesarean delivery is appropriate if massive trauma has resulted in maternal death and there is a chance of fetal viability. Perinatal outcome following this procedure is directly related to the gestational age of the fetus, the time from maternal death to delivery of the infant, the performance of cardiopulmonary resuscitation on the mother, and, to some extent, the availability of neonatal intensive care facilities (78–80). The fetus is most likely to survive if cesarean delivery is performed within 5 minutes of maternal arrest, but the procedure is justified regardless of elapsed time if fetal vital signs are present (23). In some cases, perimortem cesarean delivery has been shown to improve maternal hemodynamics through the relief of aortocaval compression, resulting in maternal survival (23,79,80). For further discussion on this topic, please see Chapter 6.

## DOMESTIC VIOLENCE

Domestic violence is a major cause of injury to women. Seventeen percent of injured pregnant patients are assaulted victims, and 60% of those experience repeated episodes of domestic violence. It is important to identify these cases and document them. Indicators that may suggest domestic violence include

1. Injuries inconsistent with stated history
2. Diminished self-image, depression, suicide attempts
3. Self-abuse
4. Frequent emergency department or doctor's office visits
5. Symptoms suggestive of substance abuse
6. Self-blame for injuries
7. Partner insists on being present for interview and examination and monopolizes discussion

The following three questions, when asked in a nonjudgmental manner and without the patient's partner being present, detect 65% to 70% of domestic violence victims (81):

1. Have you been kicked, hit, punched, or otherwise hurt by someone within the past year? If so, by whom?
2. Do you feel safe in your current relationship?
3. Is there a partner from a previous relationship who is making you feel unsafe now?

## SUMMARY

Trauma is the leading nonobstetric cause of death in women of reproductive age and requires an intense and highly specialized management approach involving emergency physicians, trauma surgeons, obstetricians, and pediatricians. Anatomic and physiologic changes that accompany pregnancy necessitate that adequate oxygenation and recognition of increased fluid requirements be the mainstay of initial resuscitative efforts. Once maternal stabilization is achieved, attention is rapidly directed to the fetus. For the previable fetus, assessment of fetal heart tones and observation for maternal complications of pregnancy may be all that is necessary. Once fetal age approaches that of viability, however, assessment of fetal health through ultrasonography and continuous external tococardiography becomes necessary. In general, the indications for diagnostic studies and operative intervention are similar to those in the nonpregnant patient. Fetal prognosis can be improved in hospitals with advanced neonatal and obstetric facilities, so transport to such a center is frequently appropriate. Such transport should not, however, take precedence over efforts directed toward maternal resuscitation and stabilization.

### *References*

1. Pimentel L. Mother and child: trauma in pregnancy. *Emerg Med Clin North Am.* 1991; 9:549–563.
2. Bocka J, Courtney J, Pearlman M, et al. Trauma in pregnancy. *Ann Emerg Med.* 1988;7:829–834.
3. Connolly AM, Katz VL, Bash KL, et al. Trauma and pregnancy. *Am J Perinatol.* 1997;14:331–336.
4. Esposito TJ. Trauma during pregnancy. *Emerg Med Clin North Am.* 1994;12:167–199.
5. Rothenberger D, Quattlebaum FW, Perry JF, et al. Blunt maternal trauma: a review of 103 cases. *J Trauma.* 1978;18:173–179.
6. Baker DP. Trauma in the pregnant patient. *Surg Clin North Am.* 1982;62:275–289.
7. Neufeld JDG, Moore EE, Marx JA, et al. Trauma in pregnancy. *Emerg Med Clin North Am.* 1987;5:623–640.
8. Farmer DL, Adzick NS, Crombleholme WR, et al. Fetal trauma: relation to maternal injury. *J Pediatr Surg.* 1990;25:711–714.
9. Sherman HF, Scott LM, Rosemurgy AS. Changes affecting the initial evaluation and care of the pregnant trauma victim. *J Emerg Med.* 1990;8:575–582.
10. Pearlman MD. Motor vehicle crashes, pregnancy loss and preterm labor. *Int J Gynecol Obstet.* 1997;57:127–132.
11. Poole GV, Martin JN, Perry KG, et al. Trauma in pregnancy—the role of interpersonal violence. *Am J Obstet Gynecol.* 1996;174:1873–1876.
12. Esposito TJ, Gens DR, Smith LG, et al. Trauma during pregnancy—a review of 79 cases. *Arch Burg.* 1991;126:1073–1078.
13. Kady DE, Gilbert WM, Anderson J, et al. Trauma during pregnancy: an analysis of maternal and fetal outcomes in a large population. *Am J Obstet Gynecol.* 2004;190(6):1661–1668.
14. Lavery JP, Staten-McCormick M. Management of moderate to severe trauma in pregnancy. *Obstet Gynecol Clin North Am.* 1995;22:69–90.
15. Obstetric aspects of trauma management. ACOG educational bulletin number 251—September 1998. *Int J Gynecol Obstet.* 1999;64:87–94.
16. Coleman MT, Trianfo VA, Rund DA. Nonobstetric emergencies in pregnancy: trauma and surgical conditions. *Am J Obstet Gynecol.* 1997;177:497–502.
17. Cokkinides VE, Coker AL, Sanderson M, Addy C, Bethea L. Physical violence during pregnancy: maternal complications and birth outcomes. *Obstet Gynecol.* 1999;93 (5, pt 1):661–666.
18. McAnena OJ, Moore EE, Marx JA. Initial evaluation of the patient with blunt abdominal trauma. *Surg Clin North Am.* 1990;70:495.
19. Leggon RE, Wood GC, Indeck MC. Pelvic fractures in pregnancy: factors influencing maternal and fetal outcomes. *J Trauma.* 2002;53:796–804.

20. Ikossi DG, Lazar AA, Morabito D, et al. Profile of mothers at risk: an analysis of injury and pregnancy loss in 1,195 trauma patients. *J Am Coll Surg.* 2005;200(1):49–56.
21. Curet MJ, Schermer CR, Demarest GB, et al. Predictors of outcome in trauma during pregnancy: identification of patients who can be monitored for less than 6 hours. *J Trauma.* 2000;49(1):18–24.
22. Hankin GDV. Trauma and envenomation. In: Clark SL, Cotton DB, Hankins GDV, et al. eds. *Critical Care Obstetrics.* 3rd Ed. Malden, MA: Blackwell Science; 1997: 597–628.
23. Pearlman MD, Tintinalli JE, Lorenz RP. Blunt trauma during pregnancy. *N Engl J Med.* 1990;323:1609–1613.
24. Buschbaum HJ. Diagnosis and management of abdominal gunshot wounds during pregnancy. *J Trauma.* 1975;15:425–430.
25. Walls RM. ed. *Manual of Emergency Airway Management.* Philadelphia, PA: Lippincott Williams & Wilkins; 2000.
26. Scorpio RJ, Esposito TJ, Smith LG, et al. Blunt trauma during pregnancy: factors affecting fetal outcome. *J Trauma.* 1992;32:213–216.
27. Dahmus MA, Sibai BM. Blunt abdominal trauma: are there any predictive factors for abruptio placentae or maternal-fetal distress? *Am J Obstet Gynecol.* 1993;169: 1054–1059.
28. Kettel LM, Branch W, Scott JR. Occult placental abruption after maternal trauma. *Obstet Gynecol.* 1988;71:449–453.
29. Lavin JP, Miodovnik M. Delayed abruption after maternal trauma as a result of an automobile accident. *J Reprod Med.* 1981;26:621–624.
30. Towery R, English P, Wisner D. Evaluation of pregnant women after blunt injury. *J Trauma.* 1993;35:731–736.
31. Higgins SD, Garite TJ. Late abruptio placenta in trauma patients: implications for monitoring. *Obstet Gynecol.* 1984;63:10S–12S.
32. Ellingsen CL, Eggebo TM, Lexow K. Amniotic fluid embolism after blunt abdominal trauma. *Resuscitation.* 2007;75:180–183.
33. Dhanraj D, Lambers D. The incidences of positive Kleihauer-Betke test in low-risk pregnancies and maternal trauma patients. *Am J Obstet Gynecol.* 2004;190(5): 1461–1463.
34. Pearlman MD, Tintinalli JE, Lorenz RP. A prospective controlled study of outcome after trauma during pregnancy. *Am J Obstet Gynecol.* 1990;162:1502–1510.
35. Williams JK, McClain L, Rosemurgy AS, et al. Evaluation of blunt abdominal trauma in the third trimester of pregnancy: maternal and fetal considerations. *Obstet Gynecol.* 1990;75:33–37.
36. Goodwin TM, Breen MT. Pregnancy outcome and fetomaternal hemorrhage after noncatastrophic trauma. *Am J Obstet Gynecol.* 1990;162:665–671.
37. Drost TF, Rosemurgy AS, Sherman HF, et al. Major trauma in pregnant women: maternal/fetal outcome. *J Trauma.* 1990;30:574–578.
38. Theodorou DA, Velmahos GC, Souter I, et al. Fetal death after trauma in pregnancy. *Am Surg.* 2000;66:809–812.
39. Dudley DJ, Cruikshank DP. Trauma and acute surgical emergencies in pregnancy. *Bemin Perinatol.* 1990;14:42–51.
40. Esposito TJ, Gens DR, Smith LG, et al. Evaluation of blunt abdominal trauma occurring during pregnancy. *J Trauma.* 1989;29:1628–1632.
41. Rose PG, Strohm PL, Zuspan FP. Fetomaternal hemorrhage following trauma. *Am J Obstet Gynecol.* 1985;153:844–847.
42. Bickers RG, Wennberg RP. Fetomaternal transfusion following trauma. *Obstet Gynecol.* 1983;61:258.
43. Doan-Wiggins L. Drug therapy for obstetric emergencies. *Emerg Med Clin North Am.* 1994;12:257–272.
44. Attico NB, Smith RJ, FitzPatrick MB, et al. Automobile safety restraints for pregnant women and children. *J Reprod Med.* 1986;31:187–192.
45. Crosby WM, Costiloe JP. Safety of lap-belt restraint for pregnant victims of automobile collisions. *N Engl J Med.* 1971;284:632–636.
46. Crosby WM, Snyder RG, Snow CC, et al. Impact injuries in pregnancy. *Am J Obstet Gynecol.* 1968;101:100–110.
47. Crosby WM, King AI, Stout LC. Fetal survival following impact: improvement with shoulder harness restraint. *Am J Obstet Gynecol.* 1972;112:1101–1106.

48. Pearlman MD, Klinich KD, Schneider LW, et al. A comprehensive program to improve safety for pregnant women and fetuses in motor vehicle crashes: a preliminary report. *Am J Obstet Gynecol*. 2000;182(6):1554–1564.
49. Wolf ME, Alexander BH, Rivara FP, et al. A retrospective cohort study of seatbelt use and pregnancy outcome after a motor vehicle crash. *J Trauma*. 1993;34:116–119.
50. Hyde LK, Cook LJ, Olson LM, et al. Effect of motor vehicle crashes on adverse fetal outcomes. *Obstet Gynecol*. 2003;102(2):279–286.
51. Moorcroft DM, Stitzel JD, Duma GG, Duma SM. Computational model of the pregnant occupant: predicting the risk of injury in automobile crashes. *Am J Obstet Gynecol*. 2003;189(2):540–544.
52. McGwin G, Russell SR, Rux RL, et al. Knowledge, beliefs, and practices concerning seat belt use during pregnancy. *J Trauma*. 2004;56(3):670–675.
53. Iliya FA, Han SN, Buchsbaum HJ. Gunshot wounds of the pregnant uterus: report of two cases. *J Trauma*. 1980;20:90–92.
54. Pierson R, Mihalovits H, Thomas L, et al. Penetrating abdominal wounds in pregnancy. *Ann Emerg Med*. 1986;15:1232–1234.
55. Baerga-Varella Y, Zietlow SP, Bannon MP, et al. Trauma in pregnancy. *Mayo Clin Proc*. 2000;75:1243–1248.
56. Aboutanos MB, Aboutanos SZ, Dompkowski D, et al. Significance of motor vehicle crashes and pelvic injury on fetal mortality: a five-year institutional review. *J Trauma*. 2008;65:616–620.
57. Bochicchio GV, Haan J, Scalea TM. Surgeon-performed focused assessment with sonography for trauma as an early screening tool for pregnancy after trauma. *J Trauma*. 2002;52(6):1125–1128.
58. Bochicchio GV, Napolitano LM, Haan J, et al. Incidental pregnancy in trauma patients. *J Am Coll Surg*. 2001;192(5):566–569.
59. Swartz HM, Reichling BA. Hazards of radiation exposure for pregnant women. *JAMA*. 1978;239:1907–1908.
60. Wagner LK, Lester RG, Saldana LR. Prenatal risks from ionizing radiations, ultrasound, magnetic fields, and radiofrequency waves. In: Wagner LK, Lester RG, Saldana LR, eds. *Exposure of the Pregnant Patient to Diagnostic Radiations—A Guide to Medical Management*. 2nd Ed. Madison, WI: Medical Physics Publishing; 1997:77–106.
61. Goldman SM, Wagner LK. Radiologic management of abdominal trauma in pregnancy. *Am J Radiol*. 1996;166:763–767.
62. Toppenberg KS, Hill AD, Miller DP. Safety of radiographic imaging during pregnancy. *Am Fam Phys*. 1999;59:1813–1818.
63. Mann FA, Nathens A, Langer SG, et al. Communicating with the family: the risks of medical radiation to conceptuses in victims of major blunt-force torso trauma. *J Trauma*. 2000;48(2):354–357.
64. Wagner LK, Lester RG, Saldana LR. The amount of radiation absorbed by the conceptus. In: Wagner LK, Lester RG, Saldana LR, eds. *Exposure of the Pregnant Patient to Diagnostic Radiations—A Guide to Medical Management*. 2nd Ed. Madison, WI: Medical Physics Publishing; 1997:43–76.
65. ACOG. Immunization during pregnancy. AGOG technical bulletin number 160: October 1991. *Int J Gynecol Obstet*. 1993;40:69–79.
66. ACIP. General recommendations on immunization: recommendations of the immunization practices advisory committee (ACIP). *Morbid Mortal Wkly Rep*. 1994; 43(RR-1):1–38.
67. ACIP. Update: vaccine side effects, adverse reactions, contraindications, and precautions. *Morbid Mortal Wkly Rep*. 1996;45(RR-12):1–35.
68. Goodwin H, Holmes JF, Wisner DH. Abdominal ultrasound examination in pregnant blunt trauma patients. *J Trauma*. 2001;50(4):689–693.
69. Schiff MA, Holt VL. The injury severity score in pregnant trauma patients: predicting placental abruption and fetal death. *J Trauma*. 2002;53(5):946–949.
70. Curet MJ, Schermer CR, Demarest GB, et al. Predictors of outcome in trauma during pregnancy: identification of patients who can be monitored for less than 6 hours. *J Trauma*. 2000;49(1):18–24. Discussion 24–25.
71. Amy BW, McManus WF, Goodwin CW, et al. Thermal injury in the pregnant patient. *Surg Gynecol Obstet*. 1985;161:209–212.

72. Rayburn W, Smith B, Feller I, et al. Major burns during pregnancy: effects on fetal well being. *Obstet Gynecol*. 1984;63:392–395.

73. Taylor JW, Plunkett GD, McManus WF, et al. Thermal injury during pregnancy. *Obstet Gynecol*. 1976;47:434–438.

74. Strong TH, Gocke SE, Levy AV, et al. Electrical shock in pregnancy: a case report. *J Emerg Med*. 1987;5:381–383.

75. Pierce MR, Henderson RA, Mitchell JM. Cardiopulmonary arrest secondary to lightning in a pregnant woman. *Ann Emerg Med*. 1986;15:597–599.

76. Lieberman JR, Mazor M, Molcho J, et al. Electrical accidents during pregnancy. *Obstet Gynecol*. 1986;67:861–863.

77. Einarson A, Bailey B, Inocencion G, et al. Accidental electric shock in pregnancy: a prospective cohort study. *Am J Obstet Gynecol*. 1997;176:678–681.

78. Katz VL, Dotters DJ, Droegemueller W. Perimortem cesarean delivery. *Obstet Gynecol*. 1986;68:571.

79. Strong TH, Lowe RA. Perimortem cesarean section. *Am J Emerg Med*. 1989;7:489–494.

80. Page-Rodriquez A, Gonzales-Sanchez JA. Perimortem cesarean section of twin pregnancy: case report and review of the literature. *Acad Emerg Med*. 1999;6:1072–1074.

81. Feldhaus KM, Koziol-McLain J, Amsbury HL, et al. Accuracy of 3 brief screening questions for detecting partner violence in the emergency department. *J Am Med Assoc*. 1997;277:1357–1361.

# 5 Cardiopulmonary Resuscitation During Pregnancy

**David Caro and Stephen Topp**

The incidence of maternal cardiopulmonary arrest during pregnancy is estimated to occur once in every 30,000 deliveries. Events leading to cardiopulmonary arrest in the pregnant patient (Table 5.1) include those found in the general population and those related specifically to pregnancy (1–6). Maternal arrest is a dramatic and difficult situation that requires the practitioner to make rapid decisions and take defined actions in order to maximize survivability. The approach to any cardiopulmonary arrest victim, including those who are pregnant, follows a set of defined algorithms designed to maximize the likelihood of recovery in the event of a cardiopulmonary arrest (7,8).

Cardiopulmonary resuscitation (CPR) refers to the application of both basic (BLS) and advanced (ALS) life support algorithms. Both BLS and ALS follow a streamlined format designed to intervene on life-threatening disorders that could potentially be reversed. A simple and easy-to-recall starting point is to approach each unstable or cardiopulmonary arrest victim in an "ABCDE" method, which is supported by multiple life support training courses (7,8). This ABCDE method becomes the basis for resuscitative evaluation, critical decision making, and intervention.

This chapter is designed to arm the practitioner with the tools necessary to manage the critically unstable patient or cardiopulmonary arrest victim. Cardiopulmonary physiology deserves special attention, especially in light of the dramatic alterations in cardiopulmonary physiology that accompany pregnancy and the unique fetal effects associated with maternal cardiac arrest and resuscitation. Discussion will then turn to BLS and ALS techniques, including critical equipment and medications. Finally, new resuscitation modalities will be reviewed to give a glimpse into recent advances in resuscitative technology.

## UNIQUE ANATOMIC AND PHYSIOLOGIC CONSIDERATIONS (SEE TABLES 5.2 AND 5.3)

Critical airway changes occur as the gravid patient approaches term. The most important is edema of the upper airway, causing a number of patients to go from a simple, straightforward laryngoscopic approach to a much more difficult one (9). The anesthesia method of analyzing airway difficulty includes the Mallampati assessment, which is a grading scale for a rapid assessment of the ease of laryngoscopy. Most women go from class 1 or 2 airways (easy intubations) to class 4 airways (most difficult intubations) by term (9). The practitioner must anticipate this during intubation attempts and have an alternative airway plan when attempting to control the airway.

The most critical respiratory concern is the contraction of maternal functional residual capacity as she nears term (9–11). The gravid uterus displaces abdominal contents superiorly and will encroach on the reserve of air in the lung bases. The result is lower vital capacity and lower physiologic oxygen reserve, even when fully pre-oxygenated with a nonrebreather mask for 5 to 8 minutes (9). This results in hypoxia developing more rapidly than expected and difficulty reoxygenating a pregnant patient, especially when lying flat (9).

Common Etiologies of Cardiac Arrest During Pregnancy

**Specifically associated with pregnancy**

Pregnancy-induced cardiomyopathy

Pregnancy-induced hypertension (preeclampsia and eclampsia)

Obstetric hemorrhage

Amniotic fluid embolism

Iatrogenic

Hypermagnesemia

Anesthesia during delivery

**Not specific to pregnancy**

Preexisting cardiovascular disease

Myocardial infarction

Congenital heart disease

Acquired valvular disease

Arrhythmia

Pulmonary disease

Pulmonary embolism

Asthma

Aspiration pneumonia

Anaphylaxis and angioedema

Intracranial hemorrhage

Sepsis

Trauma

Electrical injury

 Alterations in Pregnancy: Airway and Respiratory Systems

| Airway/Respiratory System Parameter | Alteration in Pregnancy |
| --- | --- |
| Airway patency | Most third-trimester patients with Mallampati four airways (most difficult) |
| Oxygen consumption | Increases by approximately 20% at term |
| Functional residual capacity (FRC) | Decreases due to decreased diaphragmatic excursion |
| $PCO_2$ | Diminished due to physiologic hyperventilation in pregnancy. Diminishes buffering capacity |

| TABLE 5.3 | Alterations in Pregnancy: Cardiovascular System |
|---|---|
| **Cardiovacular Parameter** | **Alteration in Pregnancy** |
| Blood volume (BV) | Increases up to 40% by 30 weeks' gestation |
| Hematocrit | Increase in RBC mass (20%–40%) is less than plasma volume (50%), causes dilutional anemia |
| Cardiac output (CO) | Increases 30%–50% by second trimester |
| Systemic vascular resistance (SVR) | Decreases due to uteroplacental unit in parallel (increases from 2% to 10% of cardiac output) |
| Venous return | Weight and size of uterus compress the inferior vena cava, reducing CO by >25%. |
| Aortic flow | Weight and size of uterus compress the abdominal aorta, resulting in diminished uterine blood flow |

Maternal blood volume increases during pregnancy and serves to protect maternal cardiovascular physiology in the face of hypovolemia (11). However, the uterine circulation is passive and dependent on normal maternal blood volume and flow, as it is in a parallel circuit with the maternal circulation (10). The gravid uterus also impacts maternal circulation by its size and weight. The uterus can compress the inferior vena cava and the distal aorta during later pregnancy. A critical maneuver to recall in the face of maternal shock or cardiac arrest is to either manually displace the uterus to the patient's left or to roll the patient into the left lateral decubitus position. These maneuvers will serve to decompress the great vessels and augment cardiac return (1–3,6,10–14). Poor venous return from infradiaphragmatic vessels makes the femoral and saphenous sites poor choices for administering drugs and fluids during CPR (6,15), and furthermore, therapeutic resuscitation doses of vasopressors, especially $\alpha$ -adrenergic or combined $\alpha$- and $\beta$-adrenergic agents, may produce uteroplacental vasoconstriction, thereby further compromising already diminished uteroplacental blood flow (10).

Some fetal physiologic changes are protected during maternal arrest. The oxyhemoglobin dissociation curve of fetal hemoglobin is shifted to the left when compared to maternal hemoglobin, yielding a greater oxygen saturation of fetal hemoglobin at any given partial pressure of oxygen (10,16). This enables the fetus to extract and carry a larger amount of oxygen at lower oxygen tension than the mother. The integrity of vital organs can be preserved for a limited period of time with this central redistribution of blood flow, but if asphyxia persists, such physiologic adjustments become inadequate, and neurologic damage or death of the fetus will occur (16,17).

It is also critical to remember that the best chance for fetal survival is with a resuscitated mother; however, experience with perimortem cesarean section indicates that fetal survival and neurologic outcome are best if delivery is performed within 5 minutes of maternal arrest (6,11,12,18,19). If CPR is unsuccessful, then rapid cesarean section is the only hope for fetal viability above 24 weeks' gestation (see Chapter 6).

## RESUSCITATION OVERVIEW

The approach to any unstable or unresponsive patient follows the ABCDE paradigm. Each letter in the mnemonic stands for a vital system that must be evaluated in the order that is designated. Any abnormality demands immediate intervention. The ABCDEs of resuscitation help identify reversible life threats that must be dealt with before moving on to the next system or a complete history and physical examination (Table 5.4).

## BASIC LIFE SUPPORT

Airway assessment in a crisis includes a quick check to hear if the patient can phonate. A phonating patient has a patent airway. Stridor, snoring, and/or gurgling respiratory sounds should raise concern that the airway is compromised. A cardiac arrest victim may have no spontaneous respirations and will then need BLS maneuvers and bag-mask ventilation to ensure airway patency. BLS airway maneuvers include the chin-lift and jaw-thrust techniques as well as the Heimlich maneuver in out-of-hospital arrest (8,20–22).

The chin lift consists of the use of index and long fingers to pull a supine patient's chin toward the ceiling, thereby pulling the base of the tongue off of the hypopharynx. The jaw thrust consists of using the index and long fingers of both hands to apply anterior pressure behind both angles of the mandible to cause the same effect (9,12). Use the jaw-thrust technique if there is a concern for cervical spine trauma. Either of these maneuvers helps to alleviate airway obstruction caused by loose pharyngeal musculature. The practitioner or an assistant then applies a bag-mask device attached to a high-flow oxygen source to the patient's face and delivers two breaths to determine if the patient has chest rise. Chest rise reassures that the airway is patent. No chest rise means that an airway obstruction is present and must be relieved; the initial maneuver would then be repositioning the airway, along with better bag-mask seal. If this is unsuccessful, then another airway-clearing maneuver should be considered.

The Heimlich maneuver consists of quick, forceful thrusts to the upper abdomen directed in a posterior/superior vector in an attempt to force air in the

| TABLE 5.4 | Immediately Reversible Life Threats |
|-----------|-------------------------------------|
| **Organ System** | **Life Threats Include (but not limited to)** |
| Airway | Obstruction |
| Breathing | Hypoxia, hypoventilation, tension pneumothorax, respiratory depression due to medications (magnesium, narcotics) |
| Circulation | Hypovolemia, tamponade, arrhythmia, sepsis, myocardial infarction, pulmonary or other embolus, CHF, aortic dissection |
| Disability (neurologic) | Drug overdose (narcotics, etc.), hypoglycemia, ischemic/thrombotic/hemorrhagic stroke, seizure |
| Exposure | Trauma, anaphylaxis, temperature |

lungs upward through the trachea to dislodge a foreign body. This maneuver is carried out with the rescuer standing behind a standing victim, with arms wrapped around the victim's abdomen and hands grasped in an overlapping fist. The fists are traditionally placed at a level superior to the umbilicus but below the xiphoid process. Quick, posterior/superior pulls then are applied in an attempt to clear the airway. Alternatively, a supine patient can be straddled, hands can be clasped with fingers interlocked, and the palm heels used to create quick pushes along the same vector. A practitioner with advanced airway equipment can also perform laryngoscopy accompanied by MaGill forceps when faced with an airway obstruction, with the MaGill used to extract any foreign body encountered (9,12,22,23).

Breathing assessment includes the observation of presence, speed, and depth of spontaneous respiration. Regular respiratory rates for the nonpregnant patient are from 12 to 16; in the gravid patient, the base respiratory rate increases above 20 (11). Patients without spontaneous respiration require oxygenation and ventilator support with bag-mask ventilation. Basic breathing support for spontaneously breathing patients might include oxygen by nonrebreather mask or bag-mask ventilation timed with ventilatory effort. Listen to both lung fields to determine that they are equal. Unequal breath sounds could identify a tension or spontaneous pneumothorax that would require needle decompression with a large-bore angiocath (12 or 14 gauge in the second intercostal space in the midclavicular line of the affected side) for relief (12).

Circulation assessment includes determination of pulse rate and rhythm along with blood pressure estimation. Patients will tend to lose peripheral pulses before femoral or carotid; if radial pulses are present, the patient has a minimum blood pressure of at least 70 mm Hg (24). An absence of pulses mandates the start of chest compressions.

Chest compressions should occur with the patient supine on a flat surface, with the uterus displaced to the right by an assistant (1,6,12). Alternatively, the patient can be placed in a 15- to 30-degree left lateral decubitus position. Although placing the patient in the true left lateral decubitus position will make manual chest compressions clumsy and ineffective, placing the patient in a 15-degree left lateral tilt position through the use of either a backboard or a tilt table may provide an acceptable alternative to manual uterine displacement without significantly compromising chest compressions (1,2,4,12). Compressions should be 1.5 to 2 in. deep and should be at a rate of approximately 100 bpm (8,25). Once started, compressions should continue with minimal interruption while ALS maneuvers occur (see below) (8,15,22).

Other BLS circulatory support activities include the establishment of large bore (18 gauge or higher) peripheral intravenous access sites, usually in the antecubital fossae. The patient should be attached to an automated external defibrillator (AED) if the practitioner is unfamiliar with defibrillation (21,26,27). The AED should be turned on and then compressions should stop temporarily, allowing the machine to analyze the patient's cardiac rhythm and deliver counter shock if required. A patient who has suffered cardiac arrest from ventricular fibrillation requires prompt electric countershock using current Basic (BCLS) and Advanced (ACLS) Cardiac Life Support guidelines (26,27). Current guidelines recommend either monophasic defibrillation at 200, 300, and then 360 J for the initial three shocks, with all subsequent shocks at 360 J or biphasic defibrillation at 100, 200, and 200 J for the first shocks, with all subsequent shocks at 200 J (26). Newer defibrillators (e.g., the LifePack 12®) are biphasic. There is no contraindication to external defibrillation during pregnancy, and direct current (DC) countershocks of up to 400 J have been used in pregnant patients without adverse fetal effects (6,28,29).

Neurologic assessment typically includes determination of unresponsiveness or level of alertness. If the patient is conscious, a quick determination of motor, verbal, and eye-opening responses to verbal and/or painful stimuli gives the team a baseline neurologic status to follow throughout the resuscitation (12,30,31). Reversible causes of neurologic depression can mimic cardiac arrest and should be investigated. Common reversible causes include hypoglycemia and drug overdoses (especially narcotics) (31).

Finally, as the resuscitation proceeds, a full examination of the patient is completed to ensure that obvious life-threatening hemorrhage, trauma, or other injuries do not exist.

## ADVANCED LIFE SUPPORT

A complete description of advanced airway techniques is beyond the scope of this chapter. The reader is referred to an alternative text for a full discussion of emergency airway management (9). Some specific tools and strategies bear mentioning, as full term patients are by definition difficult airways.

Emergent laryngoscopy and intubation are daunting tasks. Familiarity with intubation equipment is a necessity. A standard intubation in a pregnant patient must take into account the various physiologic changes that make laryngoscopy difficult. Paralytics can be used for intubation in the pregnant patient, but assessment of airway difficulty is important, as rapid decline in oxygenation can occur and intubation attempts might fail, necessitating a surgical airway (9).

A wide variety of alternative airway equipment exists, in addition to standard bag-mask devices and laryngoscopes. The most important for this discussion include the supraglottic airway devices and the bougie. Supraglottic devices are attractive alternative airways, as they require minimal training, can be inserted blindly, and provide a means for rapid oxygenation and ventilation (9,23). These devices include the laryngeal mask airway (LMA)®, the intubating LMA®, and the King LT airway®, among others. Each has an inflatable cuff at the end of the device designed to be seated over the glottis, which allows for ventilation when attached to a bag device. These devices have been included in the American Heart Association ACLS algorithm due to their ease of use and high success rates in establishing a means of oxygenation and ventilation (9,23).

The bougie is an aid to standard laryngoscopy and endotracheal intubation. Various forms of bougies exist. The two most common are made of solid plastic or of gum elastic. The bougie functions as an intubation guide to be used in difficult airways when the vocal cords are unable to be seen while performing direct laryngoscopy but some other glottis structure or the epiglottis is visualized. It has an angled tip that allows the practitioner to "hook" under the epiglottis and advance forward into the trachea. The practitioner then uses tactile sensation to feel the bougie gently bounce along the tracheal cartilage rings to confirm that it is in the airway, or alternatively, one can feed the bougie until it stops in a bronchus (and therefore confirms it is in the airway). Lack of tracheal ring "bumping" felt through the bougie as it advances or lack of defined endpoint as the bougie is inserted means that the device is not in the airway (9). An endotracheal tube can then be advanced over the bougie into the airway.

Advanced ventilatory support includes the use of medications, noninvasive positive pressure devices, and mechanical ventilation. Various combinations of advanced medications are employed for respiratory distress depending on the underlying cause of the problem. $\beta_2$-Agonists, anticholinergic agents, and steroids are employed in asthmatics. Nitroglycerin is employed in congestive heart failure patients. In severe respiratory difficulty, the use of noninvasive positive pressure devices for those requiring ventilatory support can at times avert intubation (9,12). Depending on the cause of respiratory distress, various medications can be employed in an attempt to help improve physiologic parameters. Once the decision to intubate has been made, mechanical ventilation becomes the mainstay of therapy. Various modes of ventilation exist. A frequently used mode immediately following intubation is synchronized intermittent mandatory ventilation (SIMV). The practitioner sets the rate of breaths to be given, the tidal volume to be given (5 to 7 mL/kg), the $FiO_2$ (usually started at 100%), and any pressure support (usually started at 10 cm $H_2O$) and positive end expiratory pressure (usually started at 5 cm $H_2O$) needed to maintain oxygenation (10,12). A full discussion of ventilator devices and parameters is beyond the scope of this chapter, and the reader is encouraged to further investigate a critical care textbook for a more in-depth discussion.

## CARDIAC RHYTHM ANALYSIS

Advanced cardiac life support measures require familiarity with cardiac rhythm analysis and the treatment of underlying rhythm abnormalities. Tachyarrhythmias, bradyarrhythmias, and cardiac arrest may occur during pregnancy and each has the ability to pose a substantial risk to the mother and the fetus. Although clinically significant or lethal arrhythmias are uncommon in the premenopausal female (32), when compared to their nongravid cohorts, pregnant females are more vulnerable to cardiac arrhythmias (33). Prompt identification and treatment of these rhythm disturbances are of utmost importance to both the mother and the fetus.

### Basic Rhythm Analysis

When attempting to analyze an EKG or rhythm on a bedside monitor, it is important to recognize a few key points about the rhythm's appearance. It is helpful to determine the rate of the rhythm ( fast versus slow) and if it is regular or irregular. A slow rate is <60 bpm. A fast rate is >100 bpm, but this will vary according to the stage of pregnancy. A rate >150 is definitely abnormal. The timing or intervals between the beats determine whether the rhythm is regular or irregular. Next, determine if the QRS complex is wide or narrow. The normal appearance of the QRS complex on an EKG or bedside monitor will be "narrow," meaning between 0.06 and 0.11 seconds, or three small boxes on the EKG paper. Any QRS greater than three small boxes is termed "wide complex" and is abnormal. Finally, the origin of the rhythm should be sought. A "sinus" rhythm originates in the SA node and correctly travels down the conduction system to the ventricles. This is denoted on the EKG by the P wave, normally a single, upward deflection just preceding the QRS complex. If no P wave is present, the rhythm has origin outside of the normal conducting system (i.e., foci within the atria or ventricles).

### Bradyarrhythmias

Symptomatic bradycardia is a rare occurrence during pregnancy (33). Sinus bradycardia is a slow (usually <60), regular, narrow-complex rhythm with a P wave before each QRS (Fig. 5.1). Common causes of sinus bradycardia include vasovagal events, hypothyroidism, hypothermia, myocardial ischemia, or the supine hypotensive syndrome of pregnancy (34). Treatment of sinus bradycardia is indicated for symptomatic patients—shock, hypotension, shortness of breath, chest pain, or altered mentation. Atropine is the treatment medication of choice, followed by transcutaneous cardiac pacing if not responsive to the atropine.

High-degree AV blocks (second- and third-degree AV blocks) are disorders of cardiac conduction in which the electrical impulse is not correctly transmitted from the AV node to the conduction branches of the ventricles. On the EKG or

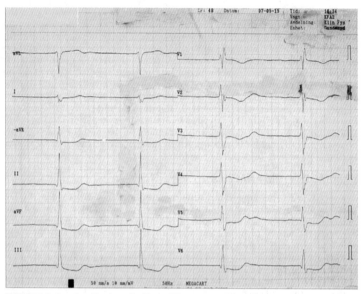

**FIGURE 5.1** Junctional bradycardia. Rate <60 bpm.

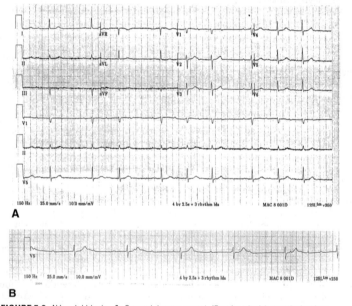

**FIGURE 5.2** AV nodal blocks. **A**: Second degree, type 1. (Reprinted with permission from Thaler MS. *The Only EKG Book You'll Ever Need*. 6th Ed. Philadelphia, PA: Lippincott Williams & Wilkins; 2010.). **B**: Third degree.

monitor, this can manifest as a slow to normal rate and can be regular or irregular. The hallmark of the AV blocks will be dissociation of the P waves from the QRS complexes, meaning the P waves will not precede the QRS complexes in a 1:1 fashion (Fig. 5.2). Two forms of second-degree blocks exist; type 1, also known as the "Wenckebach" phenomenon, is characterized by progressive lengthening of the PR interval until a QRS is dropped. This form of block is considered stable and does not warrant aggressive therapy. Type 2 second-degree block presents with no progressive PR lengthening, and QRS complexes are suddenly "dropped." Third-degree block is characterized by complete dissociation between atrial and ventricular impulses. These "high-degree" AV blocks (second degree type 2 and third degree) are treated with immediate transcutaneous pacing until transvenous or permanent pacing can be established, with case reports of successful cardiac pacing implemented during pregnancy without any risk to the mother or the fetus (34).

### Supraventricular Tachycardia

Supraventricular tachycardia (SVT), sometimes termed paroxysmal supraventricular tachycardia (PSVT), is a regular, narrow-complex tachycardia (Fig. 5.3). This arrhythmia is usually caused by a reentry loop or a bypass tract through the AV Node. Because of this fast reentry, propagation of the signal down the circuit can produce ventricular rates of 140 to 240 bpm. The patient will generally seek medical care with complaints of palpitations, light-headedness, or shortness of breath. Pregnancy increases the risk of new onset SVT and may additionally increase the frequency or severity of the preexisting disease (32). In the hemodynamically unstable patient (hypotensive, altered mental status, etc.), treatment consists of prompt, synchronized DC cardioversion with 10 to 50 J, up to 100 J with a biphasic device (29). However, in the stable patient, Vagal maneuvers (carotid massage, cold-water facial emersion, and Valsalva maneuver) may be sufficient to break this arrhythmia. When Vagal maneuvers are unsuccessful in the stable patient, adenosine may be safely administered in the standard doses with termination success rates of 89% to 100% reported (29,33,35).

### Atrial Fibrillation and Atrial Flutter

Atrial fibrillation (AFib) and atrial flutter occur infrequently in pregnant women, particularly in the absence of structural heart disease (34). In patients with structurally normal hearts, metabolic derangements such as thyroid disease or alcohol intoxication should be sought. Additionally, other acute cardiac conditions such as pericarditis, mitral stenosis, or pulmonary embolus should be considered. In general, AFib is a narrow-complex, irregularly irregular rhythm with a rate that can vary from normal to tachycardic. In contrast, atrial flutter is usually a narrow-complex, regular rhythm with a varying rate. As with SVT, unstable AFib and atrial flutter are safely treated with synchronized DC cardioversion. For stable patients, rate control is usually achieved with $\beta$-blockers, calcium channel blockers, or digoxin.

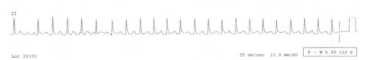

**FIGURE 5.3** Narrow-complex (AKA "supraventricular") tachycardia.

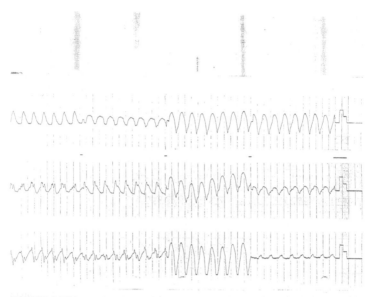

**FIGURE 5.4** Wide-complex tachycardia.

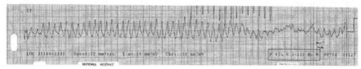

**FIGURE 5.5** Ventricular fibrillation.

## Ventricular Tachycardia

Ventricular tachycardia (VT) is a very fast, wide-complex ventricular rhythm (usually >150 bpm) and is usually dissociated from any underlying atrial rate (Fig. 5.4). In pregnant and nonpregnant patients with structurally normal hearts, VT is rare. During pregnancy, the occurrence of VT is often due to severe electrolyte or acid-base disorders or by maternal abuse of stimulant drugs. As with other arrhythmias, once VT is identified, the patient must be assessed for hemodynamic instability. For the unstable patient with a palpable pulse, VT is treated emergently with synchronized cardioversion at 100 J. If no pulse is palpable, treat like ventricular fibrillation (see next section) and defibrillate with 200 J. For hemodynamically stable VT, conservative management is indicated. Procainamide (class C) and Lidocaine (class B) appear safe during pregnancy and should be used in sustained, stable VT (36). The role of Amiodarone during pregnancy is limited by its teratogenic profile (class D), and its use should be limited to pharmacologic and shock resistant VT (32).

## Cardiac Arrest: Ventricular Fibrillation, Pulseless Electrical Activity, and Asystole

Ventricular fibrillation (VF) is caused by disorganized electrical activity originating in the ventricles. Because organized electrical activity is absent, the ventricles are not contracting effectively and the patient is without perfusion. This rhythm will appear as a fast, sinusoidal wave pattern with no normal, discernable QRS complex (Fig. 5.5). When this rhythm is encountered, the patient is by default unstable and chest compressions must be started immediately until defibrillation is available. Defibrillate at 200 J followed by chest compressions for at least 2 more minutes regardless of return of spontaneous circulation (ROSC). The 2005 American Heart Association ACLS guidelines stress the importance of minimal interruptions in chest compressions as each pause drastically reduces the coronary perfusion pressures (9). Early administration of vasopressors, either epinephrine or vasopressin, is standard but should not interfere with CPR and shocks. Little information exists about ACLS pharmacologic therapy in pregnancy. In theory, these adrenergic agents may reduce the uteroplacental blood supply. However, standard ACLS doses and protocols should be used in all pregnant resuscitations (1,15,37).

Pulseless electrical activity (PEA) is a rhythm defined by the presence of organized electrical activity (not VT or VF) as displayed on a cardiac monitor in the absence of a pulse. In contrast to unstable VT and VF, a PEA rhythm will not benefit from cardioversion or defibrillation. Minimally-interrupted chest compressions and pharmacologic therapy with vasopressors (epinephrine or vasopressin) and atropine are the foundation of PEA ACLS care. PEA is frequently caused by reversible etiologies and correction of these is the best chance for a successful resuscitation. It is helpful to remember the "Five H's and T's" when PEA is encountered: hypovolemia, hypoxemia, hydrogen ion (acidosis), hyper/hypokalemia, hypothermia and thrombosis (coronary and pulmonary embolus), tension pneumothorax, tamponade (cardiac), tablets (drug OD) (15). Pregnant patients are particularly vulnerable to pulmonary embolus and hypovolemia secondary to hemorrhage; however, consideration of all causes is prudent.

Asystole is the cardiac arrest rhythm with the most dismal prognosis. It is characterized by little to no cardiac electrical activity (usually a "flat line" on the monitor) and no pulse. As with PEA, asystole does not benefit from cardioversion or defibrillation. The best chance for successful resuscitation is to identify and treat the reversible cause. The treatment algorithm for asystole mirrors that of PEA, with quality, minimally interrupted chest compressions and pharmacologic therapy with vasopressors and atropine (15).

Clinical experience with the pharmacologic agents used in ACLS is limited in pregnancy. The general recommendation is that standard pharmacologic therapy be used without modification (6). Vasopressors such as epinephrine and dopamine generally are avoided during pregnancy because of their adverse effects on uteroplacental blood flow but should *not* be withheld during arrest when clinically indicated (6,38). Similarly, despite theoretical concerns about some drugs such as lidocaine inducing fetal acidosis and $\beta$-blocking agents inducing fetal bradycardia, no adverse fetal effects have been shown when these agents are used in maternal cardiac arrest (6,29,38,39). Table 5.5 lists the drugs commonly used during CPR and their application during pregnancy.

The initial minutes of a maternal resuscitation should focus on restoration of the maternal cardiorespiratory function. Optimum fetal care occurs in the setting of a resuscitated mother. However, if immediate resuscitative efforts do not restore spontaneous circulation, consideration should be given to the performance of a crash cesarean section. Most texts give a guideline of 3 to 5 minutes of maternal resuscitation before crash c-section is initiated (1,6,38,40). The reader is referred to the chapter in this text describing this technique. It is important to note that once the fetus is delivered, a resuscitative team should redirect attention to the mother, as case reports of ROSC have occurred following fetal delivery by crash c-section (6,41).

**TABLE 5.5** Medications used During CPR—Considerations in Pregnancy

| Drug | Indications | FDA Category | Considerations in Pregnancy |
|------|-------------|--------------|------------------------------|
| Amiodarone | Current role in cardiac arrest due to VF/VT being defined | D | Role in cardiac arrest during pregnancy not defined. Embryotoxic in animals may result in congenital hypothyroidism in the newborn. Associated with transient bradycardia and prolonged QT intervals in newborns. |
| Atropine | Symptomatic or relative bradycardia<br><br>Asystole | C | Crosses placenta but does not result in fetal abnormalities. May result in fetal tachycardia. |
| Calcium chloride/ gluconate | Special circumstances such as hyperkalemia, calcium channel blocker overdose, respiratory arrest due to $Mg_2$ toxicity | C | Calcium gluconate is the preferred agent for $Mg_2$ induced respiratory depression. |
| Dobutamine | Pulmonary congestion and low cardiac output | C | Has not been studied in human pregnancy. Animal studies have not revealed evidence of harm to the fetus. |
| Dopamine | Hemodynamically significant hypotension in the absence of hypovolemia | C | Limited experience in human pregnancy. Animal studies have not revealed evidence of teratogenicity or embryotoxicity. |

| Drug | Indication | Category | Comments |
|---|---|---|---|
| Epinephrine | VF or pulseless VT unresponsive to initial countershocks, asystole, or PEA | C | Teratogenic in some animal species but human teratogenicity has not been clearly demonstrated. Theoretically may lead to decrease in uterine blood flow. |
| Lidocaine | First-line antiarrhythmic for VF and VT | B | Teratogenicity and developmental abnormalities have not been shown. At lower doses associated with neonatal muscular weakness and decreased tone; higher doses associated with significant neonatal depression. |
| Sodium bicarbonate | Special circumstances such as preexisting metabolic acidosis, hyperkalemia, or trycyclic or phenobarbital overdose. Consider after confirmed therapy such as cardiopulmonary resuscitation and epinephrine have failed. | C | Animal reproduction studies have not been performed. Risk of fetal harm unknown. |

FDA, Food and Drug Administration; VF, ventricular fibrillation; VT, ventricular tachycardia; PEA, pulseless electrical activity.

*Sources:* Clinical Pharmacology [database online]. Tampa, FL: Gold Standard, Inc.; 2009. URL: http://cp.gsm.com.lp.hscl.ufl.edu Updated February 2009. MICROMEDEX® Healthcare Series, Copyright © 1974–2009. Thomson Reuters. All rights reserved.

## EMERGING TECHNOLOGIES

Resuscitative technologies continue to creatively explore methods of resuscitation that are just now being studied in human populations, including maternal cardiac arrests. Therapeutic hypothermia has been demonstrated to improve neurologic outcomes in cardiac arrest survivors (38,42). This technique has also been employed successfully in case reports of maternal arrest (43). Similarly, fibrinolytic therapy has been considered for use in cardiac arrest for patients with pulmonary embolism (38), but the use of this treatment would complicate emergent cesarean section.

## COMPLICATIONS OF CPR

Maternal complications of CPR include fractures of ribs and sternum, hemothorax, hemopericardium, and laceration or rupture of internal organs, most notably the liver, spleen, and uterus (10,12). Damaging fetal effects include central nervous system toxicity from medications, transient dysrhythmias from DC countershock, altered uterine activity, and reduced uteroplacental perfusion with possible fetal hypoxemia and acidemia (44,45).

## SUMMARY

Cardiopulmonary arrest during pregnancy occurs infrequently. Most resuscitative procedures require little alteration, with the exception of displacement of the gravid uterus during the latter part of pregnancy. Resuscitative attempts should be directed primarily toward the mother, with the best chance of fetal survival being maternal survival. Perimortem cesarean section should be considered after the age of fetal viability, in an attempt both to save the infant and to improve maternal hemodynamics.

### References

1. Atta E, Gardner M. Cardiopulmonary resuscitation in pregnancy. *Obstet Gynecol Clin North Am.* 2007;34:585–597, xiii.
2. Peters CW, Layon AJ, Edwards RK. Cardiac arrest during pregnancy. *J Clin Anesth.* 2005;17:229–234.
3. Mallampalli A, Powner DJ, Gardner MO. Cardiopulmonary resuscitation and somatic support of the pregnant patient. *Crit Care Clin.* 2004;20:747–761, x.
4. Whitty JE. Maternal cardiac arrest in pregnancy. *Clin Obstet Gynecol.* 2002;45: 377–392.
5. Einav S, Matot I, Berkenstadt H, Bromiker R, Weiniger CF. A survey of labour ward clinicians' knowledge of maternal cardiac arrest and resuscitation. *Int J Obstet Anesth.* 2008;17:238–242.
6. Part 10.8: Cardiac arrest associated with pregnancy. *Circulation.* 2005;112:IV-150–153.
7. Part 1: Introduction. *Circulation.* 2005;112:IV-1–5.
8. Part 3: Overview of CPR. *Circulation.* 2005;112:IV-12–18.
9. Walls RM, Murphy MF. *Manual of Emergency Airway Management.* Philadelphia, PA: Lippincott Williams & Wilkins; 2008.
10. Dildy GA. *Critical Care Obstetrics.* Malden, MA: Blackwell; 2004.
11. Cunningham FG, Williams JW. *Williams Obstetrics.* New York, NY: McGraw-Hill Professional; 2005.
12. Roberts JR, Hedges JR, Chanmugam AS. *Clinical Procedures in Emergency Medicine.* Philadelphia, PA: W.B. Saunders; 2004.
13. Kiefer RT, Ploppa A, Dieterich HJ. Aortocaval compression syndrome. *Der Anaesthesist.* 2003;52:1073–1083, quiz 1084.
14. Bamber JH, Dresner M. Aortocaval compression in pregnancy: the effect of changing the degree and direction of lateral tilt on maternal cardiac output. *Anesth Anal.* 2003;97:256–258, table of contents.

15. Part 7.2: Management of cardiac arrest. *Circulation.* 2005;112:IV-58–66.
16. Reece EA, Hobbins JC. *Clinical Obstetrics: The Fetus & Mother.* Malden, MA: Blackwell; 2007.
17. Jensen A, Garnier Y, Berger R. Dynamics of fetal circulatory responses to hypoxia and asphyxia. *Eur J Obstet Gynecol Reprod Biol.* 1999;84:155–172.
18. Stallard TC, Burns B. Emergency delivery and perimortem C-section. *Emerg Med Clin North Am.* 2003;21:679–693.
19. Yildirim C, Goksu S, Kocoglu H, Gocmen A, Akdogan M, Gunay N. Perimortem cesarean delivery following severe maternal penetrating injury. *Yonsei Med J.* 2004;45: 561–563.
20. Part 1: Introduction. *Circulation.* 2005;112:1–4.
21. Part 2: Adult basic life support. *Circulation.* 2005;112:5–16.
22. Part 4: Adult basic life support. *Circulation.* 2005;112:IV-19–34.
23. Part 7.1: Adjuncts for airway control and ventilation. *Circulation.* 2005;112: IV-51–57.
24. Deakin CD, Low JL. Accuracy of the advanced trauma life support guidelines for predicting systolic blood pressure using carotid, femoral, and radial pulses: observational study. *Br Med J* (Clinical Research Ed.). 2000;321:673–674.
25. Part 6: CPR techniques and devices. *Circulation.* 2005;112:IV-47–50.
26. Part 3: Defibrillation. *Circulation.* 2005;112:17–24.
27. Part 5: Electrical therapies: automated external defibrillators, defibrillation, cardioversion, and pacing. *Circulation.* 2005;112:IV-35–46.
28. Nanson J, Elcock D, Williams M, Deakin CD. Do physiological changes in pregnancy change defibrillation energy requirements? *Br J Anaesth.* 2001;87:237–239.
29. Page RL. Treatment of arrhythmias during pregnancy. *Am Heart J.* 1995;130: 871–876.
30. Anonymous. Advanced trauma life support for doctors ATLS: manuals for coordinators and faculty. Chicago, IL: American College of Surgeons; 2008.
31. Marx JA, Hockberger RS, Walls RM, Adams J, Rosen P. *Rosen's Emergency Medicine: Concepts and Clinical Practice.* Philadelphia, PA: Mosby/Elsevier; 2006.
32. Kron J, Conti JB. Arrhythmias in the pregnant patient: current concepts in evaluation and management. *J Intervent Card Electrophysiol Int J Arrhythmias Pacing.* 2007;19:95–107.
33. Li JM, Nguyen C, Joglar JA, Hamdan MH, Page RL. Frequency and outcome of arrhythmias complicating admission during pregnancy: experience from a high-volume and ethnically-diverse obstetric service. *Clin Cardiol.* 2008;31:538–541.
34. Trappe HJ. Acute therapy of maternal and fetal arrhythmias during pregnancy. *J Intensive Care Med.* 2006;21:305–315.
35. Elkayam U, Goodwin TM. Adenosine therapy for supraventricular tachycardia during pregnancy. *Am J Cardiol.* 1995;75:521–523.
36. Chow T, Galvin J, McGovern B. Antiarrhythmic drug therapy in pregnancy and lactation. *Am J Cardiol.* 1998;82:58I–62I.
37. Shapiro JM. Critical care of the obstetric patient. *J Intensive Care Med.* 2006;21: 278–286.
38. Part 4: Advanced life support. *Circulation.* 2005;112:25–54.
39. Part 7.3: Management of symptomatic bradycardia and tachycardia. *Circulation.* 2005;112:IV-67–77.
40. Bloom SL, Leveno KJ, Spong CY, et al. Decision-to-incision times and maternal and infant outcomes. *Obstet Gynecol.* 2006;108:6–11.
41. Finegold H, Darwich A, Romeo R, Vallejo M, Ramanathan S. Successful resuscitation after maternal cardiac arrest by immediate cesarean section in the labor room. *Anesthesiology.* 2002;96:1278.
42. Part 7.5: Postresuscitation support. *Circulation.* 2005;112:IV-84–88.
43. Rittenberger JC, Kelly E, Jang D, Greer K, Heffner A. Successful outcome utilizing hypothermia after cardiac arrest in pregnancy: a case report. *Crit Care Med.* 2008;36:1354–1356.
44. Littleford J. Effects on the fetus and newborn of maternal analgesia and anesthesia: a review. *Can J Anaesth.* 2004;51:586–609.
45. Dildy GA, Clark SL. Cardiac arrest during pregnancy. *Obstet Gynecol Clin North Am.* 1995;22:303–314.

# Perimortem Cesarean Delivery

**Deborah S. Lyon**

Perimortem cesarean delivery (PMCD) is rarely performed; fewer than 300 cases have been reported in the English literature. Two concepts make this an important topic nonetheless. One is the clear imperative to decide and act promptly when PMCD is indicated. As in all aspects of emergency medicine, the knowledge must precede the crisis rather than await it. Advanced Cardiac Life Support and other algorithmically driven resuscitation measures were, in fact, designed for those who do not often have to use them, in the hope that committing certain "drills" to memory will allow an uncommon medical event to be optimally managed. In addition, the indications for PMCD have broadened considerably since the 1980s, and the procedure may attain a more prominent role in the future.

## HISTORICAL BACKGROUND

Cesarean delivery is one of the oldest surgical procedures in history, with literature dating back to at least 800 BC (1). Before the 20th century, however, the phrase "postmortem cesarean" would have been redundant, because the procedure was essentially never undertaken in any but a dead or moribund mother (2). Initially, the Roman decree (*Lex Cesare*; law of Caesar) that unborn infants should be separated from their mothers' bodies was for purposes of religious ritual rather than with any real hopes of survival of either. It would appear that some infants did survive, because the law specified "with the hope of preserving citizens to the State" and failure to obey the mandate was grounds for "legal suspicion that a living child had been killed" (1). Indeed, several mythologic and ancient historical figures were reported to have been born in this fashion, including Apollos' son, the Greek physician Asklepios, "from the womb of dead Koronis" (3). Bacchus was supposedly born this way, as was Scipio Africanus (the Roman general who defeated Hannibal). Pliny the Elder dates this event at 237 BC (2). Pope Gregory XIV had this distinction, as did 15th century Genoese admiral Andrea Doria. Some attribute the birth of Edward VI as occurring after the death of the unfortunate Jane Seymour, although others claim she lived several days after the delivery. Shakespeare referred to this practice in *Macbeth* (4).

Judaic writings from the 1st century through the 3rd century AD identify this practice (and find the mother not liable for a sacrifice of purification, as were women who delivered vaginally) (5), and Christian leaders made it a religious issue in the 1280 Council of Cologne as a means of ensuring the infant's baptism (3).

The first documented record of maternal survival from a cesarean delivery is that of the Swiss sow gelder Jacob Nufer, who sectioned his own wife for the delivery of their firstborn in 1500 (2). None of the available references describe in detail what must surely have been desperate circumstances leading to this intervention, but this hearty lady survived to have five spontaneous vaginal deliveries, including a delivery of a set of twins. She, thus, became the first recorded successful postcesarean trial of labor patient, as well as the first survivor of the procedure.

By the time of the renaissance, PMCD had become such a standard practice that, in 1749, King Charles of Sicily ruled that failure to perform the procedure was punishable by death, and there is one recorded instance of the law being applied to a physician (2).

During the late 19th and early 20th centuries, case reports began to arise of PMCDs successfully salvaging the fetus, and the procedure began to be seriously entertained as a legitimate medical intervention. Well into the 20th century, the salvage rate was very low, and therefore, wisdom dictated that all possible attempts be made to resuscitate the mother with the infant still in utero unless the demise was clear-cut and inevitable.

During the 1980s, several authors reported unexpected maternal recoveries after "postmortem" cesarean deliveries (5,6). This led to a consideration of the possibility that PMCD might actually improve, rather than worsen, a mother's chance of survival during a collapse. Uteroplacental blood flow may require up to 30% of a woman's cardiac output during pregnancy (7), some of which may be retrieved for other visceral organ perfusion after delivery. Indeed, several animal and laboratory models, as well as a growing body of clinical evidence, suggest that, relieved of the caval compression associated with a term pregnancy and of the tremendous circulatory demands of a placenta and fetus, cardiac compressions are significantly more effective (5). There is a 30% decrease in stroke volume and cardiac output in a pregnant woman who lies supine, largely because there is a complete occlusion of the inferior vena cava (which occurs in 90% of women in late pregnancy). In addition, there is a 20% reduction in functional residual capacity at term, and there is a higher metabolic rate, leading to decreased oxygen reserves and faster onset of anoxia following apnea (4). Delivery of the near-term fetus provides a 30% to 80% improvement in cardiac output and, in conjunction with other resuscitative measures, may provide sufficient circulatory improvement to adequately support the central nervous system's function during an arrest (5). This has led to the current thinking that PMCD is an appropriate resuscitative intervention for both the mother and the infant. In this light, it is critical to intervene promptly and appropriately to maximize the survival possibilities for two patients simultaneously.

In summary, the perspective on PMCD has evolved through 23 centuries as a means of

- Providing appropriate burial and religious rituals for both the mother and the baby
- Saving a child's life when maternal death is inevitable
- Optimizing resuscitation for both the mother and the baby.

## CHANGES IN MATERNAL CAUSES OF DEATH

One of the reasons PMCD has become more realistic relates to the prevailing etiologies of maternal demise. In a 1986 review, Katz et al. (4) highlighted the shift over the past century from primarily chronic, mostly infectious causes of death to primarily acute, mostly cardiorespiratory causes of death. The chronically ill mother may be hypoperfusing or inadequately nourishing her unborn child for months, thus making a good outcome of any delivery less likely. An acute event such as pulmonary embolus, on the other hand, leaves the infant with some reserves and allows a less-than-optimal delivery setting to produce a good outcome.

In addition to changing diagnoses, the evolution of medicine itself allows more hope for success. The ability to monitor high-risk patients and intervene in advance of a crisis has developed largely over the past 50 years. Cardiac support and respiratory support are available, at least for the short term, in virtually every setting in which medicine is practiced. Emergency transport services allow prompt medical attention to life-threatening conditions, and when time is the single most critical factor determining success, this emergency transport may be the most important development in medicine.

## CONSIDERATIONS FOR UNDERTAKING POSTMORTEM CESAREAN DELIVERY

Several factors must be considered when deciding whether to undertake PMCD (2,4,5,8–10). The first is the estimated gestational age (EGA) of the fetus. This information is sometimes difficult to obtain in an emergency situation, and time for an ultrasonographic estimate is not practical. Thus, an "eyeball estimate" may be necessary. As a general rule, the uterus reaches the umbilicus at 20 weeks of gestational age and grows in length at the rate of approximately 1 cm every week thereafter. Thus, in a relatively thin woman, a fundal height of 8 cm above the umbilicus would likely represent a pregnancy of 28 weeks' gestation. Depending on the resources of the institution, the fetus may be salvageable, in ideal circumstances (availability of all skilled personnel and a controlled setting), at anywhere from 23 to 28 weeks of EGA and this should be considered in the decision regarding PMCD. If the fetus is known to be of 23 weeks' EGA and there has never been a survival of that gestational age in the institution's nursery, PMCD is probably not indicated for the sake of the fetus. It may be of less help to the mother as well, compared with a third-trimester intervention. Cardiovascular effects of pregnancy are less pronounced before 28 weeks and thus delivery will not achieve a cardiovascular improvement as dramatic as at a later EGA. Indeed, in the first and early second trimesters, aggressive maternal support is the only indicated intervention, and there has been at least one reported case of a complete maternal and fetal recovery after a prolonged arrest at 15 weeks of EGA (11).

The second concern relates to the length of time between arrest and delivery. The latest reported survival was of an infant delivered 45 minutes after documented maternal cardiac arrest with multiple knife injuries, and there are scattered case reports of deliveries 20 to 30 minutes after maternal cardiac arrest, with surprisingly good infant outcomes (12). However, most of the authors cited earlier support a 5-minute rule. Best outcomes in terms of infant neurologic status appear to occur if the infant is delivered within 5 minutes of maternal cardiac arrest. This means the decision to operate must be made and surgery begun by 4 minutes into the code. Although the evidence is not based on a huge number of cases, a compelling argument for prompt intervention can be made on both maternal and fetal grounds (13).

The third critical factor for success is adequacy of other resuscitative efforts in the interim. Although chest compressions may provide only 30% of the baseline cardiac output (4), some oxygenation is clearly better than none. Displacement of the uterus leftward until surgery is actually begun allows for better blood return from the inferior vena cava. The fetus lives on the steep portion of the oxygen dissociation curve; therefore, relatively minor changes in maternal oxygenation result in far more dramatic changes for the fetus.

The fourth critical factor is the availability of adequate neonatal resuscitation. It is tragic to successfully extract a 28-week infant only to have no qualified person available to assume resuscitation efforts. All infants in this setting may be presumed to require postdelivery support, and the emergency department team will most likely be fully occupied with the mother. Furthermore, the emergency department team may well be suboptimally experienced with neonatal resuscitation techniques.

Finally, a vital factor beyond the control of the delivery team is the nature of the maternal condition. Acute conditions enable better results than chronic conditions, and conditions that involve primarily cardiopulmonary collapse respond better than more systemic organ failures.

There is no requirement for documentation of fetal heart tones before PMCD, partly because it is time-consuming and may negatively impact the baby's outcome and partly because maternal indications for the procedure are pressing regardless of fetal status.

To summarize, conditions that affect the success of PMCD are as follows:

■ Gestational age of the infant (>24 to 28 weeks is optimal)
■ Length of time from arrest to delivery (5 minutes or less is optimal)
■ Adequacy of maternal resuscitative efforts
■ Availability of neonatal resuscitation experts
■ Nature of the underlying maternal condition

There is a special case relating to the "scheduled PMCD." This involves a woman who would be legally considered "brain dead" but is being maintained on artificial support solely for the purpose of allowing further fetal development. The emergency department is often involved only in the initial stages of this setting, that is, in the decision to initiate extraordinary life-extending measures in the face of a hopeless case. While successful cases of this sort have been reported at an EGA as early as 6 weeks (14), the ethical argument exists that extraordinary support measures for the sole purpose of providing a fetal incubator constitute experimental interventions and require fully informed consent of the next of kin (15). The most likely time frame for both successful support and ethical imperative to support is 24 to 27 weeks of EGA (16), when a few days make a large difference to fetal outcome. Support beyond likely fetal survival ex utero is controversial (17), as is support from a very early EGA. A strong distinction is made by Dillon and colleagues between true brain death and persistent vegetative state, and they argue that termination of support measures is ethically defensible only in the former case. With regard to emergency evaluation, they comment, "The objective of emergent and early management should be to preserve maternal life until fetal viability and prognosis can be assessed" (16).

## TECHNIQUE FOR PERFORMANCE OF PMCD

The niceties of preoperative preparation are unlikely to be practical in this setting. If a urinary drainage catheter has not already been placed, time should not be spared to place one. Likewise, a detailed assessment of fetal well-being is impractical. Even assessing for fetal heart tones is unnecessary because this can be difficult and fraught with error (in the large patient or in a noisy room) and because the delivery is done as much for maternal indications as for fetal. A "splash prep" of antiseptic solution across the abdomen is ritually satisfying but of uncertain clinical value. In essence, preparation consists of acquiring some basic equipment and baring the patient's abdomen.

Full cardiopulmonary resuscitation measures should continue during the delivery. This optimizes oxygen delivery to both patients.

Most young obstetricians perform Pfannenstiel incisions almost exclusively for cesarean deliveries. Although taught that midline incisions allow faster entry into the abdominal cavity, many have found that, with optimal lighting, equipment, and assistance, a Pfannenstiel incision takes little more time, if any, and produces a stronger, prettier scar.

This absolutely does not apply to the incision made under suboptimal conditions. The equipment available is likely to be minimal and not neatly laid out with a scrub technician standing by. While there may be many spectators, there are likely to be no real assistants. Lighting may be poor and not deployable where needed within the incision. Given these restrictions, a midline abdominal incision remains the appropriate choice for performance of PMCD.

Regard for surgical technique should not be abandoned, however, despite the limitations of the setting. Given the possibility of maternal survival, care should be taken to protect bowel and bladder from injury if possible. In any case, the fetus should be protected from the large laceration which is a probable consequence of reckless uterine entry. The infant should be delivered with attention to planes of anatomic function so that permanent nerve damage from overextension does not occur. Someone trained in neonatal resuscitation should be available to assume medical responsibility for the infant as soon as delivery is effected. If desired, a loop of cord may be clamped off at each end and saved for later evaluation of cord gases. The closed loop of cord may sit for up to 60 minutes without significant degradation of the gases (18). Cord blood should also be collected, as it is with all deliveries, so that routine neonatal hematologic studies can be performed without necessitating blood draws from the infant.

The placenta should always be removed before closure. If the mother survives the initial collapse, bleeding or infection with residual placenta as a nidus will worsen her chances of eventual survival. If she does not survive the initial episode, the placenta may deliver spontaneously in the morgue if not extracted at the time of surgery. This is inconvenient at best.

Closure should be undertaken based on maternal circumstances. If the cardiorespiratory resuscitation team thinks that there is any chance of survival, a careful, layered closure should be performed as with any cesarean delivery. In fact, attention to meticulous closure technique is vital, because suboptimal perfusion might not reveal areas of bleeding that could later become problematic when circulatory function is restored. In addition, disseminated intravascular coagulation is a common sequela of massive hemodynamic challenge and might create postoperative problems if closure is not meticulous. If the maternal condition is thought to be hopeless, then a rapid closure for purposes of aesthetics is indicated as a kindness to the family.

If maternal survival seems likely, and in light of the probable absence of sterile technique, consideration should be given to antibiotic prophylaxis. Although there are no series defining an optimal choice for this setting, the rules of "dirty" surgery should apply, and any broad-spectrum penicillin or cephalosporin should be adequate.

The person best suited to perform the PMCD is the most experienced obstetric surgeon available. It is probably no accident that the first reported cesarean success was in the hands of a sow gelder, presumably comfortable with the feel of live tissue and familiar with concepts of vascular control. Sow gelders are relatively unavailable these days, but most communities have obstetricians. Their expertise in estimating risk–success factors such as gestational age, as well as their operative experience, will serve both patients well. If the emergency department is informed that a pregnant woman who is seriously ill or injured is en route, it is prudent to immediately call for obstetric and pediatric support. Only if these resources are not available when the patient arrives and resuscitation efforts are under way, should the emergency physician consider undertaking the PMCD personally.

To recap PMCD technique, one should

- Have only what preoperative prep can be performed without delaying the procedure
- Perform a midline abdominal incision, umbilicus to pubis (longer if necessary), and extend it to and through the uterine wall
- Protect the bowel, bladder, and other maternal organs to the extent possible in the circumstances
- Provide due attention to the position of the fetus and deliver by careful, anatomically attentive extraction
- Extract the placenta before closure
- Close all layers as meticulously as maternal condition dictates
- Inspect carefully for unexpected damage and repair if indicated

■ Pay particular regard to hemostasis
■ If maternal survival seems likely, consider 24 hours of antibiotic prophylaxis

## EQUIPMENT NECESSARY FOR PMCD

The optimal setting for PMCD is the operating room with an open section pack and a trained operating room crew. Failing this, several equipment packages have been recommended. These can be quite elaborate (10) or as simple as a "precip tray" (normally available in emergency departments for precipitous vaginal deliveries). The essential items are, for the most part, readily available and include

■ Scalpel
■ Pack of laparotomy sponges
■ Bandage scissors or straight Mayos
■ Three or four Kelly clamps
■ Suture material, preferably number 0 or number 1 chromic or Vicryl
■ Needle driver
■ Forceps (preferably Russians, Bonneys, or heavy-toothed)
■ Bulb suction
■ Warmer for the infant
■ Full neonatal resuscitation support (e.g., drugs and endotracheal tubes)

## OUTCOMES

Unfortunately, it is virtually impossible to rigorously answer the question of maternal and neonatal outcome after this rare and catastrophic event. The American literature contains primarily case reports and very small series. The United Kingdom includes some data in their Confidential Enquiry into Maternal Deaths, but as the name suggests, the registry applies only to cesarean deliveries in which the mother did not survive. In the Confidential Enquiry registry, infants do not fare particularly well either. For the period 1994 to 1996, there were 13 deliveries classified as either postmortem or perimortem. Of these, only two babies were born alive, and one of these expired shortly thereafter. The registry strongly supports the concept of rapid choice for delivery, as the outcome of the group labeled "perimortem" (patient moribund or undergoing cardiopulmonary resuscitation) was significantly better than that of the group labeled "postmortem" (patient felt to have already expired) (19). In 10 years, 40 perimortem deliveries were registered, of which 25 resulted in neurologically intact surviving infants (62.5%).

## MEDICOLEGAL CONSIDERATIONS

Unfortunately, the practice of medicine has been irreversibly tainted by physicians' fear of being held liable for actions undertaken with the best possible knowledge and compassion, but having a bad outcome. This is in large part accountable for the flight of many obstetricians into gynecology-only practices, where litigation risk is much lower. It might also lead to withholding PMCD when it might be effective, in fear of failure leading to legal repercussions.

It is of some comfort that, according to the medical literature on the subject, there has never been a suit filed on the basis of wrongful performance of PMCD. There has, in fact, been only one legal penalty levied, the aforementioned death penalty in the 18th century for failure to perform the procedure.

Generally, PMCD is deemed to fall under the same guidelines as any emergency procedure in which consent is not possible. Although some medical literature opines that consent should be obtained if possible, it may be very difficult to determine who is legally qualified to grant consent. Roseate discussions of "talking to the husband" fail to consider the complexities of relationships in this day. It is true that a patient has the right to refuse a cesarean delivery, even if her baby is in extreme jeopardy. This is based on the ethical principle of maternal autonomy. Nonetheless, when maternal consent is not an issue, no other opinion should be deemed legally binding in the emergency setting. Clearly, when the issue is the ventilator-dependent brain-dead patient being kept alive solely in an incubator, next-of-kin decisions do become relevant, and legal as well as spiritual counsel should be sought.

## SUMMARY

PMCD should be undertaken as part of maternal as well as fetal resuscitation in any gestation advanced beyond 24 to 28 weeks. It should be undertaken within 4 minutes of full cardiac arrest if possible, and the technique should be subject to time and environmental constraints. The most experienced obstetrician available is the optimal person to perform the procedure, and someone trained in neonatal resuscitation should be available if possible. Medicolegal considerations have thus far been only theoretical, and the law is likely to support this procedure under the emergency care rubric if it is ever tried. Brain-dead mothers may have extraordinary support measures undertaken for prolonged periods of time, but this should involve extensive discussion with next of kin.

## *References*

1. Duer EL. Post-mortem delivery. *Am J Obstet Gynecol.* 1879;12:1.
2. Weber CE. Postmortem cesarean section: review of the literature and case reports. *Am J Obstet Gynecol.* 1971;110:158.
3. Ritter JW. Postmortem cesarean section. *JAMA.* 1961;175:715.
4. Katz VL, Dotter DJ, Droegemueller W. Perimortem cesarean delivery. *Obstet Gynecol.* 1986;68:571.
5. DePace NL, Betesh JS, Kotler MN. "Postmortem" cesarean section with recovery of both mother and offspring. *JAMA.* 1982;248:971.
6. Marx GF. Cardiopulmonary resuscitation of late-pregnant women. *Anesthesiology.* 1982;56:156.
7. Dildy GA, Clark SL. Cardiac arrest during pregnancy. *Obstet Gynecol Clin North Am.* 1995;22:303.
8. Lanoix R, Akkapedii V, Goldfeder B. Perimortem cesarean section: case reports and recommendations. *Acad Emerg Med.* 1995;2:1063.
9. Arthur RK. Postmortem cesarean section. *Am J Obstet Gynecol.* 1978;132:175.
10. Strong TH, Lowe RA. Perimortem cesarean section. *Am J Emerg Med.* 1989;7:489.
11. Selden BS, Burke TJ. Complete maternal and fetal recovery after prolonged cardiac arrest. *Ann Emerg Med.* 1988;17:346.
12. Capobianco G, Balata A, Mannazzu MC, et al. Perimortem cesarean delivery 30 minutes after a laboring patient jumped from a fourth-floor window: baby survives and is normal at age 4 years. *Am J Obstet Gynecol.* 2008;198(1):e15–e16.
13. Katz V, Balderston K, DeFreest M. Perimortem cesarean delivery: were our assumptions correct? *Am J Obstet Gynecol.* 2005;192:1916–1921.
14. Sampson MB, Peterson LP. Post-traumatic coma during pregnancy. *Obstet Gynecol.* 1979;53:2S.
15. Loewy EH. The pregnant brain dead and the fetus: must we always try to wrest life from death? *Am J Obstet Gynecol.* 1987;157:1097.
16. Dillon WP, Lee RV, Tronolone MJ, et al. Life support and maternal brain death during pregnancy. *JAMA.* 1982;248:1089.
17. Heikkinen JE, Rinne RI, Alahuhta AM, et al. Life support for 10 weeks with successful fetal outcome after fatal maternal brain damage. *Br Med J.* 1985;290:1237.
18. Cunningham FG, MacDonald PC, Gant NF, et al., eds. *Williams Obstetrics.* 20th Ed. Norwalk, CT: Appleton & Lange; 1997.
19. Whitten M, Irvine LM. Postmortem and perimortem caesarean section: what are the indications? *J R Soc Med.* 2000;93:6.

# 7

# Hypertensive Disorders of Pregnancy: Preeclampsia/ Eclampsia

**Luis Sanchez-Ramos**

Hypertensive disorders of pregnancy, including preeclampsia and eclampsia, are the second leading cause of maternal mortality in the United States. Preeclampsia is a disorder that affects women exclusively during pregnancy. It is a disease of unknown etiology that presents in pregnant women at both extremes of reproductive age. Reported incidences range from 2% to 30%, depending on the diagnostic criteria used and the population studied (1). Conditions associated with an increased incidence include previous preeclampsia, multifetal pregnancy, molar pregnancy, and triploidy. It is a clinical condition that comprises a wide spectrum of signs and symptoms that have been observed to develop alone or in combination. Complications resulting from preeclampsia are also a leading cause of perinatal morbidity and mortality.

The diagnosis of the disease is based on the presence of hypertension in association with significant proteinuria. Preeclampsia is usually classified clinically as mild or severe (2). However, even in a seemingly stable patient with minimal signs and symptoms, this disease can rapidly progress to life-threatening eclampsia, with seizures and complications that may include pulmonary edema, intracerebral hemorrhage, acute renal failure, disseminated intravascular coagulation, and abruptio placentae. The criteria for severe preeclampsia are summarized in Table 7.1.

There appears to be an increased incidence of preeclampsia in patients with minimal or no prenatal care and in those of low socioeconomic status (3). All these types of patients are frequently seen for the first time by physicians in the emergency department. Consequently, it is not unusual for such physicians to be the first to make the diagnosis and initiate appropriate management.

## PATHOPHYSIOLOGY

The basic disorder underlying preeclampsia is vasospasm. Constriction of the arterioles causes resistance to blood flow and subsequent arterial hypertension. Vasospasm and damage to the vascular endothelium in combination with local hypoxia presumably lead to hemorrhage, necrosis, and other end-organ disturbances of severe preeclampsia.

Vascular reactivity to infused angiotensin II and other vasopressors is decreased in normotensive pregnancy (4,5). The refractoriness to angiotensin II may be mediated by vascular endothelium synthesis of vasodilatory prostaglandins such as prostacyclin. There are data to suggest that preeclampsia may be associated with inappropriately increased production of prostaglandins with vasoconstrictor properties such as thromboxane. Several authors have shown increased vascular reactivity to pressor hormones in patients with early preeclampsia. The increased reactivity to vasopressors may be due to altered ratios of thromboxane and prostacyclin (6).

Pregnancy normally increases blood volume by as much as 40%, but the expansion may not occur in a woman destined to develop preeclampsia. Vasospasm contracts the intravascular space and leaves her highly sensitive

| TABLE 7.1 | Criteria for Severe Preeclampsia |
|---|---|

Blood pressure ≥160 mm Hg systolic or ≥110 mm Hg diastolic, recorded on at least two occasions at least 6 hr apart with the patient at bed rest

Proteinuria ≥5 g in 24 hr (3+ or 4+ on qualitative examination)

Oliguria (≤400 mL in 24 hr)

Cerebral or visual disturbances

Epigastric pain

Pulmonary edema or cyanosis

Impaired liver function

Thrombocytopenia (<100,000)

Intrauterine growth restriction

to fluid therapy or blood loss at delivery. The vascular contraction impairs uteroplacental blood flow, contributes to intrauterine growth restriction, and may lead to intrauterine fetal demise. Circulatory impairment reduces renal perfusion and glomerular filtration, and swelling of intracapillary glomerular cells and glomerular endotheliosis may result. Edema probably occurs because of maldistribution of extracellular fluid, since plasma fluid is not increased.

## DIAGNOSIS

The diagnosis of preeclampsia is usually straightforward: the blood pressure is at least 140/90 mm Hg on at least two occasions 6 or more hours apart. In the past, it was recommended that an increase of 30 mm Hg in systolic or 15 mm Hg in diastolic blood pressure be used as a diagnostic criterion, even when absolute values remained lower than 140/90 mm Hg. During the last decade, the former definition has been accepted by the Working Group on High Blood Pressure in Pregnancy, because the only available evidence shows that women with blood pressures meeting the old criterion are not likely to have adverse outcomes (7,8).

In addition to hypertension, the patient often presents with significant proteinuria, defined as the presence of at least 300 mg of protein in a 24-hour urine collection or a reading of 1+ or higher on random dipstick samples. The degree of proteinuria often fluctuates widely over a 24-hour period. Therefore, a single random sample may fail to detect significant proteinuria.

Although in the past, edema was an accepted criterion for the diagnosis of preeclampsia, it is such a common finding in pregnant women that its presence should not validate the existence of preeclampsia any more than its absence should rule out the diagnosis. However, significant edema of the hands and face associated with a sudden increase in weight may be a valuable warning sign (Fig. 7.1).

In addition to the classic findings of hypertension and proteinuria, other laboratory clues may be helpful in the diagnosis of preeclampsia. Thrombocytopenia may at times be an early warning in patients who subsequently will develop hypertensive disorders of pregnancy. Increased serum levels of uric acid may be of both prognostic and diagnostic values. Patients with preeclampsia have markedly decreased urinary excretion of calcium; in fact, hypocalciuria can be detected prior to the appearance of clinical signs and symptoms (9).

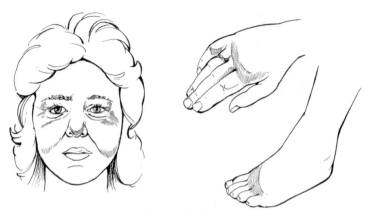

**FIGURE 7.1** Preeclampsia: edema of face, hand, and foot.

Hypertension and proteinuria, the two most important signs of preeclampsia, are often not obvious. By the time the patient has developed symptoms, such as epigastric pain and severe headache, the disorder may be far advanced. For this reason, prenatal care for early detection of this disorder is imperative (Fig. 7.2).

One of the earliest signs of preeclampsia may be a sudden increase in weight. Whenever weight gain exceeds 0.91 kg in any given week, or 2.73 kg in a month, early preeclampsia should be considered. Sudden and excessive weight gain may be attributed to abnormal retention of fluid and is demonstrable before significant edema of the face or upper extremities.

The most dependable warning sign of preeclampsia is hypertension. The diastolic blood pressure is a more reliable prognostic sign than the systolic, and a persisting diastolic pressure of ≥90 mm Hg is abnormal. Proteinuria varies greatly from case to case and, in the same patient, from hour to hour. This variability is likely due to intermittent renal vasospasm. Frequent urinary dipstick readings or a 24-hour urinary collection is often necessary to diagnose proteinuria.

Other signs and symptoms of preeclampsia, such as severe headache, epigastric pain, blurry vision, shortness of breath, and decreased urinary output, usually appear late and in severe cases (see Table 7.1). However, hemolysis, elevated liver enzymes, and low platelets (HELLP syndrome) may be an early portent of severe preeclampsia (10–12).

## PREPARTUM MANAGEMENT

The goal of therapy is to prevent eclampsia, as well as other severe complications of preeclampsia. The only definitive therapy for preeclampsia/eclampsia is delivery. Once this has been achieved in a form that assures maximum safety for both the mother and the newborn, the patient is usually on her way to full recovery. This decision is fairly simple in patients with mild preeclampsia at term or with severe preeclampsia at any time during gestation. However, the management of patients with mild preeclampsia far from term is very controversial (13). Some of the areas of controversy include the need for hospitalization, the use of antihypertensive agents, and the use of sedatives and anticonvulsants. Most obstetricians in this country usually advise bed rest in the hospital for the

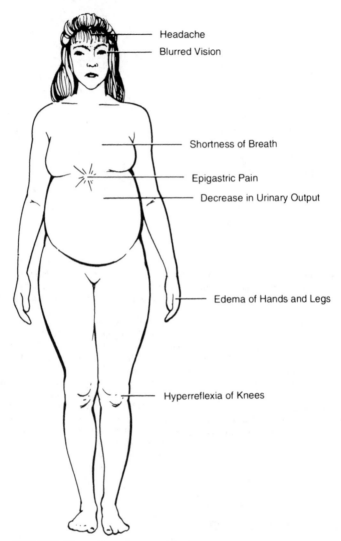

— Headache
— Blurred Vision

— Shortness of Breath

— Epigastric Pain
— Decrease in Urinary Output

— Edema of Hands and Legs

— Hyperreflexia of Knees

**FIGURE 7.2** Signs and symptoms of preeclampsia.

duration of the pregnancy. Ambulatory treatment may be appropriate for a minority of compliant private patients with very mild preeclampsia.

Preterm patients with mild preeclampsia are admitted to the hospital and placed on bed rest. Although this seems a reasonable form of therapy, its efficacy is not clearly established. Strict sodium restriction or diuretic therapy has no role in the prevention or treatment of preeclampsia. Patients are usually placed on a regular diet, although some authorities recommend a high-protein diet.

Close monitoring of both the mother and the fetus is initiated. Daily monitoring should include hematocrit and platelet count, frequent blood pressure checks, maternal weight estimation, and search for clinical evidence of severe disease. Important clinical signs and symptoms of severe disease include headache, epigastric pain, blurred vision, and shortness of breath.

If deterioration is progressive, as determined by laboratory findings, symptoms, and clinical signs, the decision to continue the pregnancy must be reevaluated daily. Important clinical signs that need to be monitored include blood pressure, urinary output, and fluid retention as evidenced by daily weight increase. Laboratory studies (24-hour urinary collection for total protein and creatinine clearance, complete blood count, serum uric acid, blood urea nitrogen, and creatinine) should be performed at intervals of no more than 48 hours. Once it has been determined that the patient has developed severe preeclampsia, steps should be taken for prompt delivery.

Fetal size, determined by ultrasonic biometry, is an accurate guide to the functional status of the fetus. Lack of growth suggests insufficient blood flow, which places the fetus in danger because of lack of placental reserve. Another indirect measure of altered maternal circulation is uterine artery Doppler velocimetry, which may serve as an early marker for preeclampsia.

Every effort should be made to deliver the baby as close to term as possible. Regardless of fetal maturity, however, delivery is indicated whenever the fetoplacental unit is shown to be failing, as documented by a lack of fetal growth or of reassuring tests of fetal well-being. In severe preeclampsia, neonatal survival reportedly ranges from 10% to 37%, depending on gestational age at delivery and birth weight.

The most important test of maturity is the lecithin/sphingomyelin ratio, which can be used to determine the risk of severe respiratory distress syndrome. The risk is high when the ratio is <1.5 but insignificant when the ratio is ≥2.

## INTRAPARTUM MANAGEMENT

When labor commences, either naturally or by induction, the patient is transferred to the labor and delivery suite, where a magnesium sulfate infusion is begun. This agent has long been considered the anticonvulsant of choice. Magnesium sulfate therapy should be started with an intravenous loading dose of 4 g of a 20% solution given slowly. The maintenance regimen is continuous infusion of 1 to 3 g per hour, beginning immediately after the loading dose. Magnesium sulfate is maintained until at least 24 hours after delivery. Magnesium toxicity should be avoided. At plasma levels of 7 to 10 mEq/L, the patellar reflex is lost, and severe respiratory depression sets in at 12 mEq/L. Fortunately, the therapeutic level is 4 to 7 mEq/L. A 10% solution of calcium gluconate should be readily available to be used as an antidote to magnesium toxicity. In addition to serum magnesium levels and the patellar reflex, urinary output should be monitored, since magnesium is cleared almost entirely by the kidneys.

Patellar reflexes and respiratory rate should be checked regularly. A respiratory rate of <16 breaths per minute is an early sign of magnesium toxicity. Urinary output should be maintained at a minimum of 25 mL per hour to ensure adequate magnesium clearance. In cases of magnesium toxicity, especially respiratory depression, a slow intravenous injection of 10 to 20 mL of 10% calcium gluconate should be infused slowly.

One of the more frequent complications of preeclampsia is severe hypertension. Hydralazine has long been the therapeutic agent of choice because it not only dilates arterioles but also increases cardiac output, renal blood flow, and placental blood flow. The goal is to lower diastolic pressure gradually to no <90 mm Hg. This pressure should maintain adequate uteroplacental perfusion while precluding the more serious complications of hypertension. The usual hydralazine regimen is an initial intravenous dose of 5 mg, followed by 5- to 10-mg doses at 20-minute intervals. The doses should be titrated to achieve the desired blood pressure level. Hydralazine may also be given as a continuous intravenous infusion of 80 mg in 500 mL of D5W beginning at a rate of 30 mL per hour (5 mg) and increased every 15 minutes as needed. Most patients will respond to 5 to 20 mg of hydralazine; an alternative agent should be considered if there is no response to a total dose of 30 mg of hydralazine. Parenteral labetalol has also been shown to be effective for the treatment of acute, severe hypertension during pregnancy. The drug may be administered as intravenous bolus injections of 20 or 40 mg or as a continuous intravenous infusion of 1 mg/kg as needed. This drug should be avoided in women with asthma and in those with congestive heart failure.

Alternative, rapid-acting antihypertensive agents are diazoxide and nitroprusside, but their use in pregnancy is controversial and they should be reserved for emergencies that do not respond to hydralazine. Diazoxide given as a standard 300-mL bolus may cause maternal hypotension, fetal hypoxia, and maternal and fetal hyperglycemia. Therefore, it should be administered in low doses, either 30 mg every 1 to 2 minutes or as a continuous infusion of 15 mg per minute to a total dose of 5 mg/kg.

Nitroprusside is a less desirable choice for the treatment of pregnancy-induced hypertension because it crosses the placenta and may cause cyanide toxicity in the fetus. It may be used, however, when hypertension is refractory to other agents. With short-term use, cyanide toxicity may be avoided. Infusion is started at a rate of 0.25 μg/kg per minute and increased by 0.25 μg/kg per minute every 5 minutes until the desired blood pressure is achieved.

Eclampsia occurs most frequently in a hospitalized patient being treated for preeclampsia. However, anyone who presents initially with eclampsia must be hospitalized and treated at once (14,15). The first priorities are to clear the patient's airway, aspirate mucus, give oxygen, and start anticonvulsant therapy with magnesium sulfate. The patient should be placed in the left lateral decubitus position and an indwelling catheter should be inserted.

Seizures usually stop minutes after the loading dose of magnesium sulfate, and within 2 hours a comatose patient should regain consciousness and be oriented to place and time. Patients whose seizures persist may be given a quick-acting barbiturate, such as sodium amobarbital, 250 to 500 mg as a slow intravenous injection.

## POSTPARTUM MANAGEMENT

Hypertension that persists after delivery may be reduced by intramuscular administration of hydralazine, 10 mg every 4 to 6 hours. A woman may be discharged while still hypertensive as long as her blood pressure appears to be falling and she is otherwise well. The patient must be reexamined within 2 weeks, by which time the pregnancy-induced hypertension should be gone. If hypertension persists after 8 weeks, essential hypertension is the likely cause.

## PREVENTION

Initial clinical trials had suggested that administration of low-dose aspirin (50 to 150 mg) in high-risk pregnant women reduced the incidence and severity of preeclampsia (16–19). More recently, a revised systematic review of 59 trials (3,756 women) showed a 17% reduction in the risk of preeclampsia associated with the use of antiplatelet agents (20). Further studies are needed to assess which women are most likely to benefit, when treatment is started, with the most appropriate dose. Several randomized trials of calcium supplementation in nulliparous women considered at risk have demonstrated significant reductions in the incidence of preeclampsia. These results have been confirmed by systematic reviews with metaanalysis (21–23). However, the old standbys of early and frequent prenatal checkups and good nutrition are still the most effective means of decreasing the incidence and severity of this disease.

## References

1. MacGillivray I. Some observations on the incidence of preeclampsia. *J Obstet Gynaecol Br Empire*. 1958;65:536.
2. Hughes EC, ed. *Obstetric–Gynecologic Terminology*. Philadelphia, PA: Davis; 1972:422.
3. Gant NF, Daley GL, Chand S, Whalley PJ, MacDonald PC. A study of angiotensin II pressor response throughout primigravida pregnancy. *J Clin Invest*. 1973;52:2682.
4. Talledo OE, Chesley LC, Zuspan FP. Renin–angiotensin system in normal and toxemic pregnancies. III. Differential sensitivity to angiotensin II and norepinephrine in toxemia of pregnancy. *Am J Obstet Gynecol*. 1968;100:218.
5. Sibai BM. The HELLP syndrome (hemolysis, elevated liver enzymes, and low platelets): much ado about nothing? *Am J Obstet Gynecol*. 1990;162:311.
6. Sibai BM, Taslimi MM, El-Nazer A, et al. Maternal perinatal outcome associated with the syndrome of hemolysis, elevated liver enzymes, and low platelets in severe preeclampsia–eclampsia. *Am J Obstet Gynecol*. 1986;155:501.
7. North RA, Taylor RS, Schellenberg JC. Evaluation of a definition of pre-eclampsia. *Br J Obstet Gynaecol*. 1999;106:767–773.
8. Levine RJ. Should the definition of preeclampsia include a rise in diastolic blood pressure ≥15 mm Hg? *Am J Obstet Gynecol*. 2000;182:225.
9. Sanchez-Ramos L, Jones DC, Cullen MT. Urinary calcium as an early marker for preeclampsia. *Obstet Gynecol*. 1991;77:685.
10. Cunningham FG, Leveno KJ. Management of pregnancy-induced hypertension. In: Rubin PC, ed. *Handbook of Hypertension, Vol 10. Hypertension in Pregnancy*. Amsterdam, the Netherlands: Elsevier; 1988:290.
11. Sibai BM, McCubbin JH, Anderson GD, et al. Eclampsia. I. Observations from sixty-seven recent cases. *Obstet Gynecol*. 1981;58:609.
12. Adams EM, MacGillivray I. Long-term effect of preeclampsia on blood pressure. *Lancet*. 1961;2:1373.
13. Fisher KA, Luger A, Spargo BH, Lindheimer MD. Hypertension in pregnancy: clinical-pathologic correlations and remote prognosis. *Medicine*. 1981;60:267.
14. Aarnoudse JG, Houthoff HJ, Weits J, Vellenga E, Huisjes HJ. A syndrome of liver damage and intravascular coagulation in the last trimester of normotensive pregnancy: a clinical and histopathological study. *Br J Obstet Gynaecol*. 1986;93:145.
15. Hinselmann H. Allgemeine Krankheitslehre. In: Hinselmann H, ed. *Die Eklampsie*. Bonn, Germany: Cohen; 1924:1.
16. Beaufils M, Uzan S, Donsimoni R, Colau JC. Prevention of pre-eclampsia by early antiplatelet therapy. *Lancet*. 1985;1:840.
17. Wallenburg HC, Dekker GA, Makovitz JW, Rotmans P. Low-dose aspirin prevents pregnancy-induced hypertension and pre-eclampsia in angiotensin-sensitive primigravidae. *Lancet*. 1986;1:1.
18. Schiff E, Peleg E, Goldenberg M, et al. The use of aspirin to prevent pregnancy-induced hypertension and lower the ration of thromboxane $A_2$ to prostacyclin in relatively high-risk pregnancies. *N Engl J Med*. 1989;321:351.
19. Benigni A, Gregorini G, Frusca T, et al. Effect of low dose aspirin on fetal and maternal generation of thromboxane by platelets in women at risk for pregnancy-induced hypertension. *N Engl J Med*. 1989;321:357.
20. Knight M, Duley L, Henderson-Smart D, King JF. Antiplatelet agents for preventing and treating pre-eclampsia. Cochrane Pregnancy and Childbirth Group. *Cochrane Database Syst Rev*. 2009;1.
21. Bucher HC, Guyatt GH, Cook RJ, et al. Effect of calcium supplementation on pregnancy-induced hypertension and preeclampsia: a meta-analysis of randomized controlled trials. *JAMA*. 1996;275:1113.
22 Melnikow JA. Calcium supplementation during pregnancy. *J Fam Pract*. 1996;43:115.
23. Lewis R, Sibai B. Recent advances in the management of preeclampsia. *J Matern Fetal Med*. 1997;6:6.

# 8 Bleeding in Pregnancy

**David C. Jones**

## BLEEDING IN PREGNANCY

Nothing provokes anxiety during pregnancy like vaginal bleeding. As a harbinger of miscarriage, any amount of bleeding in the first trimester, even spotting, can bring patients in for evaluation. While some will miscarry, many will go on to have successful pregnancies. Later in pregnancy, bleeding is more likely to be associated with a significant complication. In some of these cases, an expeditious workup and diagnosis will make the difference between a successful pregnancy and a loss. Having a systematic way to assess and triage these patients is important in optimizing outcomes. Throughout the entire process, the anxiety of the mother-to-be and family makes compassionate care one of the goals.

## VAGINAL BLEEDING BEFORE VIABILITY

Perhaps the first and most important question that must be addressed when a woman presents with early pregnancy bleeding is, "Is this an intrauterine pregnancy or could it be an ectopic pregnancy?" Consideration of this question and how to address it is covered in Chapter 3. Once an intrauterine pregnancy has been confirmed, a more in-depth investigation for the etiology of the bleeding may ensue. While it is considered abnormal to experience vaginal bleeding in the first trimester, about 15% of women who subsequently deliver healthy infants at term report they had some amount of early pregnancy bleeding. A similar number of recognized pregnancies experience early bleeding and miscarry. Another 15% of pregnancies miscarry but are unrecognized because they miscarry close to the time of the expected period (1). For a woman with somewhat irregular cycles, this cannot be distinguished from her normal cycle variation.

There are a number of etiologies for early pregnancy loss (Table 8.1). Aneuploidy is found in up to half of the miscarriage specimens, but after that, the incidence of the listed etiologies is low. In most instances, the etiology of the loss is not pursued. Even when an attempt is made to identify the cause of a miscarriage, it is frequently elusive. While women with recurrent miscarriages can benefit from a workup to look for an etiology such as Robertsonian translocations, the antiphospholipid antibody syndrome, uterine anomalies, and incompetent cervix, it is probably best to leave those studies to the obstetrician or reproductive endocrinologist who will be seeing them in a follow-up after the loss. The most important job the emergency room physician has is to identify women for whom early bleeding is related to ectopic pregnancy, women who are actually miscarrying, and women who have an incompetent cervix.

## ABORTION

Abortion is defined as a pregnancy loss prior to 20 weeks of gestation from the last menstrual period (LMP) or loss of a fetus weighing <500 g. Excluding abortions related to the active termination of a pregnancy, abortions are subdivided into five types (Table 8.2). Distinguishing between these five types is usually straightforward and is based on physical examination, speculum examination, and a transvaginal ultrasound examination.

**Etiology of Spontaneous Abortion**

Aneuploidy

Uterine abnormality
  Congenital
  Leiomyoma

Autoantibodies
  Antiphospholipid antibody syndrome
  Antithyroid antibodies

Infection

Incompetent cervix

Endocrine abnormalities
  Luteal-phase defect
  Poorly controlled diabetes mellitus
  Hyperprolactinemia
  Thyroid dysfunction

Uterine leiomyoma

Asherman syndrome

Unknown

 **Etiology of Bleeding in the First Half of Pregnancy**

Abortion
  Threatened
  Inevitable
  Missed
  Incomplete
  Complete

Ectopic pregnancy

Incompetent cervix

GTD

Cervical/vaginal infections and lesions

Friable cervix

### Threatened Abortion

Threatened abortion is the most common variety of abortion encountered. Any woman with early pregnancy bleeding who has a closed cervix and has an apparently viable intrauterine pregnancy is given this diagnosis. One does not know what will happen for sure, and the diagnosis of a "normal pregnancy" is only made retrospectively in these cases, but most of these women will maintain their pregnancy. If the fetus is visible on ultrasound and is appropriately grown with a heart rate over 100 beats per minute (bpm), the chance the pregnancy will miscarry is <10%. When a patient complains of cramping, the risk of miscarriage is somewhat increased, but many of these pregnancies end well. The acute loss of early-pregnancy nausea (morning sickness) may be more ominous, but when that change is related to a miscarriage, the fetus has usually already died.

When the diagnosis of a threatened abortion is made, women are usually counseled to limit their physical activity and avoid sexual activity. While this may seem logical, there is no scientific evidence that any particular behavior on the woman's part will hasten or prevent a miscarriage. Consequently, the patient must understand that these interventions are merely traditional recommendations. Helping the patient understand the lack of benefit of "bed rest" is important because when strict limitations are placed on activity, yet the patient is noncompliant and miscarries, she may be burdened with guilt thinking, "If only I had stayed in bed like I was told..." In truth, if a miscarriage is going to happen, there is nothing available to change that fact.

One question that does come up with early bleeding is whether Rh-negative women need prophylactic Rh immunoglobulin. Rh antigens appear on fetal red cells as early as 38 days of gestation, so sensitization is possible. Because fetomaternal hemorrhage has been documented as early as 7 weeks of gestation, some authorities have advocated the administration of a standard dose of Rh immunoglobulin (300 μg) to Rh-negative women with first trimester bleeding. Nonetheless, the incidence of Rh D alloimmunization related to threatened abortion is exceedingly small. Consequently, the American College of Obstetricians and Gynecologists (ACOG) have not taken a formal stand on this, and many practitioners do not offer any anti-D immune globulin to women with threatened abortions and live fetuses prior to 12 weeks of gestation (2). If one prefers to give prophylaxis, a 50-μg "minidose" of Rh immunoglobulin is sufficient. After 12 weeks', all at-risk women should be given the full 300-μg dose of Rh immunoglobulin.

## Missed Abortion

The diagnosis of "missed abortion" is made when ultrasound confirms the presence of a nonviable intrauterine pregnancy but the cervix is closed. This condition may be seen with an early fetal demise, with an obvious fetus on the ultrasound, or when there is no identifiable fetus. This latter case, which represents either an embryonic demise or failure of the embryo to form, is referred to as an "anembryonic gestation" and was formerly referred to as a "blighted ovum." Before the advent of ultrasound, this diagnosis was made when the uterus failed to grow in size over an 8-week period (3). The historical concept was that the uterus had not miscarried but had "missed" the fetal demise. When a missed abortion is diagnosed, women generally have three options (4). The first option is to manage the condition expectantly, commonly referred to as "letting nature take its course." This option is appealing to women who wish to manage the loss as naturally and "nonmedically" as possible. It is a reasonable option, particularly with first trimester losses. As the gestational age of the loss increases, the risk of disseminated intravascular coagulation increases, but this is not seen in the first trimester. The main disadvantage of this option is that a miscarriage may be more painful and involve more bleeding than a woman is comfortable with, and the timing of the event is uncertain. The second option would be a medical augmentation. Most commonly, misoprostol is prescribed for first trimester pregnancy failure. Misoprostol is a synthetic prostaglandin E1 analogue, which has been marketed for the treatment of gastric ulcers. It has been used by itself or in conjunction with other medications for a wide range of off-label indications in obstetrics including medical termination of pregnancy, management of early and late pregnancy loss, induction of labor, and cervical ripening at term. A number of regimens have been used for the completion of a missed abortion, such as misoprostol 600 to 800 $\mu$g intravaginally with a repeat dose given in 24° if the miscarriage had not occurred (5,6). ACOG recently recommended either 800 $\mu$g vaginally or 600 $\mu$g sublingually with the option of repeating the dose every 3° for two additional doses (7). The author's institution currently uses the 800-$\mu$g dose with a 24° repeat option. These methods carry an 80% to 90% success rate. The issues with pain and bleeding at home remain with this method, but the timing is more predictable for the patient. Failures of this medical method at 48° from the first dose are usually treated with a suction curettage. The dilation with suction curettage is also available as the third option. It carries a small risk of uterine perforation with potential bowel or bladder damage, but it is rare. Some patients feel this risk is balanced by the opportunity to avoid the discomfort, bleeding, and uncertain timing of a miscarriage. Misoprostol is often used to prepare the cervix preoperatively before suction curettage (e.g., misoprostol 400 $\mu$g 4° prior to the procedure). Any of the three options are reasonable in the first trimester, and women who choose a less invasive option can always later opt for a more invasive option. Once she is out of the first trimester, home medical management is generally not offered, and the choices are limited to expectant management, dilation and evacuation with suction or induction of labor in the hospital. If expectant management is chosen after the first trimester, platelet counts and fibrinogen should be measured weekly, especially as the gestational age of the loss approaches 20 weeks', as the risk of disseminated intravascular coagulation begins to increase at that gestational age.

### Inevitable Abortion
This diagnosis is made in the first trimester when the cervix is dilated or some of the products of conception (e.g., membranes, fetus, placenta) are visible at the dilated cervix. Once this diagnosis is made, there is no hope for retention of the pregnancy regardless of whether there is fetal heart activity or not. Women essentially have the same three options they have for a missed abortion, although less is published on the use of misoprostol for inevitable abortion. In some cases, the miscarriage may be completed simply by grasping the protruding products of conception with ring forceps and gently teasing them out of the uterus. The ring forceps may even be maneuvered into the uterine cavity blindly, though ultrasound guidance is preferred. In many cases though, suction curettage will be necessary. The use of a small uterine curette to gently scrape the sides of the endometrial cavity to confirm all the tissue has been removed is common; however, one must be very careful not to scrape too aggressively, because this may lead to Asherman syndrome. When the endometrium is scraped off by too aggressive a curettage, the anterior and posterior uterine walls may scar together, resulting in a small cavity and future infertility. The suction curettage may be performed in the operating room under IV sedation or deeper anesthesia, but in many emergency rooms, it is performed in the emergency department using IV sedation ± paracervical block.

### Incomplete Abortion
Incomplete abortion is diagnosed when a portion of the products of conception have been passed but there are still some retained. In this case, the patient may report that she has passed tissue (although sometimes blood clots are mistaken for tissue), and in some instances, she will have brought it in. Ultrasound is the primary means of determining whether all the tissue has passed or not. Misoprostol has also been used to complete an incomplete abortion with the best evidence suggesting a single dose of 600 $\mu$g (8). This dose has also been recommended by ACOG (7). However, in common practice in the United States,

the most frequent choice is to proceed with a suction curettage. As noted above, the suction curettage is often performed in the emergency department under IV sedation, and the patient is able to go home shortly thereafter.

## Complete abortion

This final type of abortion refers to a miscarriage that has been completed with all tissue passed. This is a frequent outcome up to about 6 weeks of gestation but less common afterwards. Women will notice a dramatic and relatively acute reduction in both cramping and bleeding when the abortion is complete. Once again, ultrasound is the primary means of confirming that all of the products of conception have been expelled from the endometrial cavity.

## Postabortion Care

After a pregnancy loss, it is important that women receive follow-up care. After the patient completes her miscarriage, she should be vigilant for evidence of infection or increased bleeding. Some physicians follow $\beta$-hCGs after the use of misoprostol to complete a miscarriage to provide additional reassurance that all of the products of conception have been passed. It is also reasonable to send the products of conception for pathologic examination to rule out gestational trophoblastic disease (GTD). Rh-negative patients should be given Rh immunoglobulin 300 $\mu$g for prophylaxis within 72° of their miscarriage if they are past 12 weeks' gestation. Prior to 12 weeks, while it is not clear that it is necessary, many practitioners give prophylaxis to be safe, and some use the 50-$\mu$g dose. The only exception to this is when the father of the pregnancy is known and is known to be Rh negative himself. Published estimates of mistaken paternity range widely (0.8% to 30%; median 3.7%), and inquiring about the chance of mistaken paternity can be quite sensitive (9). Consequently, given the risk of Rh sensitization is 2% to 4% after 12 weeks, prophylaxis is sometimes given as a matter of course without even testing the presumptive father.

Normally, women are seen for follow-up by their obstetrician, midwife or potentially in an emergency department follow-up clinic about 2 weeks after their miscarriage has completed.

# ADDITIONAL MARKERS

Ultrasound has become nearly indispensable in diagnosing the etiology of early pregnancy bleeding. But its usefulness goes beyond simply diagnosing a demise or a living fetus. The fetal crown–rump length, the main biometric measurement in the first trimester, should be appropriate for the expected gestational age. If the size is lagging and menstrual dating is reliable, it could represent an abnormal gestation. Trisomies 13 and 18 have been shown to exhibit growth restriction as great as 1 week in the first trimester. As noted before, a heart rate over 100 is reassuring. Conversely, a low heart rate is a cause for concern. At 7 weeks of gestation, a fetal heart rate ≤100bpm has a positive predictive value for miscarriage of 75%; this increases to 94% for a heart rate ≤80bpm (10). Assessment of fetal anatomy can also be helpful. An obvious cystic hygroma may suggest trisomy 21 (Down syndrome) or Turner syndrome (45,X). In centers with expertise in first trimester prenatal diagnosis, a number of markers that are associated with aneuploidy such as increased nuchal translucency, absent nasal bone, abnormal ductus venosus waveforms, tricuspid regurgitation, abnormal fetal mid-facial angle, and omphalocele may be identified. Even the yolk sac is somewhat predictive, as studies have shown that sac diameters outside the normal range (3.8 to 7mm) are associated with poor outcomes (11). When a fetal pole is not visualized, determination must be made as to whether it is likely the pregnancy is an early pregnancy that is not far enough along yet to reliably exhibit a fetal pole or whether it is an anembryonic pregnancy. In these cases, the size of the gestational sac is useful. A gestational sac exceeding a diameter of 25 mm (average of diameter in three planes) that does not exhibit a fetal pole is highly suggestive of a nonviable pregnancy (12,13). A follow-up ultrasound examination in 1 week and/or serial measurements of $\beta$-hCG levels are appropriate to confirm nonviability. When the ultrasound examination does not conclusively identify an intrauterine pregnancy in the presence of a positive urine pregnancy test, the diagnosis of an ectopic pregnancy must be considered, and referral to a gynecologist is appropriate. As noted before, this workup is covered in Chapter 3.

## CERVICAL INCOMPETENCE

When a woman presents with bleeding in the later stages of the second trimester, one of the important considerations is the diagnosis of an incompetent cervix. The primary symptoms reported may include spotting, bleeding, new onset vaginal discharge or change in a prior discharge, pelvic pressure, and cramping. Classically, the diagnosis of cervical incompetence was made after a woman had two or more losses in the second trimester associated with painless cervical dilation. More recently, consideration was given to making this diagnosis after one loss due to the increasing age at which many women are choosing to have children and the sense that "making" a woman suffer a second midtrimester loss in order to be eligible for some sort of treatment was perceived as cruel and insensitive. The advent of transvaginal ultrasound to monitor the cervix for changes before the appearance of frank incompetence has made it easier to manage women with a loss history that does not fit the classical definition. The main risk factors for cervical incompetence include cervical lacerations associated with a prior delivery, traumatic cervical dilation at the time of a dilation and curettage (D&C), dilation and evacuation (D&E), or dilation and extraction (D&X). It is unusual to see cervical incompetence after first trimester D&C in the contemporary era. A prior risk factor was exposure to diethylstilbesterol (DES) in utero. DES was taken in the 1950s and 1960s to prevent miscarriage, and female fetuses exposed to it have an increased incidence of congenital uterine anomalies and cervical incompetency. The last of the population of exposed women should be at the end of their reproductive years.

Women presenting with an incompetent cervix are often diagnosed when a sterile speculum examination shows either the external os of the cervix dilated with the membranes visible at the os or the membranes prolapsing through the cervix and filling the vagina (hourglassing membranes). Occasionally, this diagnosis is suspected or made based on a transvaginal ultrasound examination either showing the hourglassing membranes or the membranes protruding past the internal os and into the cervical canal. This is often characterized as membrane "beaking" or "funneling." Cervical incompetence carries a significant risk of fetal loss. It is often associated with chorioamnionitis, so the evaluation should include basic physical examination assessment such as temperature and abdominal tenderness, as well as a complete blood count with a differential.

In some cases, women will choose to end the pregnancy due to high risk of loss. In cases where the patient chooses to prolong the pregnancy, depending on the actual findings and gestational age, treatment may be expectant or may involve the use of progesterone or a cervical cerclage. When cervical incompetence is suspected or diagnosed, the patient should be placed in the Trendelenburg position and, if one is available, a fetal monitor should be used in screening for uterine contractions. An obstetrician/gynecologist should always be consulted. Further management and decision-making will be handled by the OBGYN service.

## PRETERM PREMATURE RUPTURE OF THE MEMBRANES

Sometimes women who present complaining of bleeding are actually leaking serosanguineous fluid after rupture of the amniotic membranes. The diagnosis is made when the examining physician sees a pool of fluid on sterile speculum examination, the fluid is "fern-positive" referring to the appearance of fern-like pattern of crystals on the glass slide when the fluid evaporates, and the fluid is also "nitrazine-positive" in that it turns nitrazine paper blue. However, both the fern test and the nitrazine test may be falsely positive when there is blood contaminating the fluid pool. A commercially available test identifies trace amounts of PAMG-1, a 34-kDa placental glycoprotein that is abundant in amniotic fluid (2,000 to 25,000 ng/mL) but is present in far lower concentrations in maternal blood (5 to 25 ng/mL) and in even lower concentrations in cervicovaginal secretions in the absence of ruptured membranes (0.05 to 0.2 ng/mL) (14–16). Since the test threshold is set at 5 ng/mL, significant blood contamination may also interfere with its results. So, none of the standard tests to detect ruptured membranes are foolproof in the setting of vaginal bleeding. The ultrasound finding of oligohydramnios, while not sufficient to diagnose rupture of the membranes, is supportive of the diagnosis.

This diagnosis is important because the outcome of these pregnancies is largely dependent on the gestational age at rupture and the amount of retained amniotic fluid. Although the perinatal survival for preterm premature rupture of the membranes (PPROM) at <20 weeks' has been reported to be up to 40%, there are frequently major impairments (17,18). When the largest vertical pocket of amniotic fluid that can be identified is <2 cm, there is a high risk of pulmonary hypoplasia (19). Consequently, PPROM prior to 24 weeks' and especially before 20 weeks', when the risk for pulmonary hypoplasia is particularly high, many women opt for induction of labor with oxytocin or prostaglandins to terminate the pregnancy. As was the case with cervical incompetence, PPROM is also associated with a significant incidence of chorioamnionitis. Similarly, attention must be paid to signs and symptoms of infection such as uterine tenderness, cramps or contractions, fever, and the white blood cell count and differential. Given all of these issues, consultation with an obstetrician or perinatologist is appropriate.

## GESTATIONAL TROPHOBLASTIC DISEASE

Women with GTD usually present with bleeding which can be quite heavy. This is commonly referred to as a molar pregnancy, and it is caused by the abnormal fertilization of an ovum. This may result from the fertilization of a defective ovum that lacks the haploid maternal genome by a single sperm, which then produces a diploid cell by endoreduplication. Less frequently, it is the consequence of fertilization of the defective ovum by two sperms (20,21). Thus, the chromosome complement of the complete mole is paternal, although the mitochondrial DNA is maternal.

This diagnosis is made by ultrasound. The fetus is absent, and the endometrial cavity is completely occupied by heterogeneous, cystic placental tissue. Classically, the ultrasound appearance was described as a "snowstorm." However, the vastly improved resolution of medical ultrasound has made that a historical artifact. The numerous cysts are now clearly seen, and individuals looking for a snowstorm might not recognize what they are seeing. Another clue to the diagnosis comes from the frequent presence of bilateral, large theca-lutein ovarian cysts, caused by stimulation from the high levels of $\beta$-hCG produced by molar pregnancies. If the diagnosis of GTD is suspected, consultation with an obstetrician/gynecologist or gynecologic oncologist is appropriate, and a $\beta$-hCG level should be obtained. In addition to a high $\beta$-hCG level helping to support the diagnosis, it also aids in prognosis of the risk of future malignant disease and is critical for follow-up as the levels drop during treatment. When women present with bleeding and are passing tissue, the tissue can be examined visually to see if it appears to be normal placenta or not. Molar tissue is frequently recognizable on gross examination due to the multiple clusters of small cysts, but pathologic confirmation is still required. A variant of GTD referred to as a "partial mole" is less common. Partial (or incomplete) mole is characterized by a triploid fetus, usually exhibiting growth restriction and often having anomalies. The extra set of chromosomes making up the triploid genome may be of maternal or paternal origin (22). In this case, the placenta usually appears grossly normal, but pathologic examination may reveal focal areas of cystic changes.

## CERVICAL AND VAGINAL INFECTIONS OR LESIONS

A lesion on the cervix or vaginal wall may occasionally cause bleeding. These lesions should be visible on speculum examination. Possible etiologies include herpetic lesions on the cervix or cervical ulcerations due to cervical cancer. Cervical lesions should lead to cultures for gonorrhea and Chlamydia. If the lesion is suggestive of herpes, those cultures should be taken as well. A referral for colposcopy and possible cervical biopsy is appropriate when a malignancy is suspected. Endometrial and cervical polyps are a less common cause of bleeding. They are usually visible protruding from the external os and usually appear as smooth, non-ulcerated, firm pieces of tissue. Management of protruding polyps is best left to the OBGYN consultant. Vaginal lacerations are a rare cause of vaginal bleeding. They are usually the result of traumatic sexual activity, though not always in the setting of sexual assault. A sensitive history usually leads to an explanation of the trauma, and if the contact was nonconsensual, appropriate steps should be taken. Finally, the cervix frequently becomes friable during pregnancy, which may lead to bleeding after intercourse or the insertion of sex toys into the vagina. This bleeding is usually best characterized as "spotting" but occasionally may be surprisingly heavy. A speculum examination and history can usually establish a friable cervix as a likely diagnosis.

## VAGINAL BLEEDING APPROACHING AND AFTER FETAL VIABILITY

The fetus is generally considered "viable" in the context of postdelivery survival at 24 weeks'. Nevertheless, there is a minority of fetuses who survive at 23 weeks', though surviving fetuses at these very early gestational ages do so with significant chronic deficits. As the pregnancy approaches 24 weeks' gestational age, in addition to the etiologies of bleeding described in the first trimester, other causes must be considered, some of which may be life-threatening to the mother and/or the fetus. Table 8.3 outlines this differential diagnosis. These conditions can often result in the loss of a very large amount of blood over a short time. Consequently, women may present with the signs and symptoms of shock. When there is evidence of hypovolemia, rapid initiation of fluid resuscitation is appropriate. Placement of two large bore IVs is appropriate, and if the hematocrit falls into the low 20s, replacement of blood products should commence. While the paramount concern is stabilization of the mother, the fetus should be assessed as soon as possible if the estimated gestational age is close to or beyond viability. Every emergency department should develop an understanding with their obstetrical service (surgery if no obstetrics are offered at that hospital), pediatric service, and tertiary care centers at what age they would consider delivering woman when her bleeding has stabilized, but fetal well-being cannot be maintained in utero. Many factors go into deciding when a patient should be delivered locally with the plan to stabilize the premature neonate for subsequent transport and when a patient is stable enough that she may be transported prior to delivery. These guidelines are best worked out prior to such a crisis than trying to figure out where local cutoffs are in the midst of an active case.

| TABLE 8.3 | Etiology of Bleeding in the Second Half of Pregnancy |
|---|---|

Labor
  Preterm
  Term

Placenta previa

Placental abruption (abruptio placentae)

Vasa previa

Incompetent cervix

Cervical/vaginal infections and lesions

Friable cervix

Non-vaginal source
  Rectal, hemorrhoids
  Urinary tract (e.g., urinary calculi)

Fetal assessment is usually evaluated by continuous external electronic fetal monitoring. Consultation with an obstetrician is appropriate, but the normal fetal heart rate is generally between 120 and 160 bpm across a broad range of gestational ages. The tracing should show variability in the heart rate (e.g., not a flat, unchanging rate) while not showing dramatic drops in the heart rate or a sinusoidal pattern. As soon as is possible, the patient should be transferred to a labor and delivery unit for further workup and monitoring if one is available. The initial goal with bleeding in the later second and third trimesters is to rule out a placenta previa.

### Placenta Previa
Prior to the widespread availability of ultrasound, placenta previa was divided into four categories based on a speculum examination and/or very gentle digital cervical examination. Digital examination was often performed in the delivery room as a "double setup" due to the risk that should a complete or partial previa be found the examination itself could dislodge the placenta further causing massive bleeding and the need for an immediate cesarean section. *Complete previa* referred to the case where the placenta completed covered the internal os. *Partial previa* referred to a placenta that partially covered the internal os. A *marginal previa* reached to the edge of the internal os and *low-lying placenta*, the least "severe" form of placenta previa, described a placenta that could be reached by the examiner's finger but did not reach the edge of the internal os.

The introduction of ultrasound and the ability to localize the placenta without knowing the dilation of the cervix have made application of the old phraseology inconsistent. When the placenta is centrally located over the internal os, the diagnosis of a complete placenta previa is relatively straightforward and unambiguous. However, a dilated cervix is still more of a "potential space" just as the vagina can accept two fingers during an examination but still looks "closed." So, considering that when the cervix is dilated <3 cm, it is still usually "closed" unless the examiner's fingers are in it, when the inferior margin of a placenta comes close to or only slightly overhangs the internal os, the sonologist is left to estimate just where the edge of that placenta would be where the cervix dilated to the point an examiner could assess the relationship of the placenta and internal os on speculum and/or digital examination. Some authors have suggested a more contemporary terminology based on ultrasound findings (23). When the placenta completely covers the internal os, it is a *complete previa*. When the edge of the placenta comes within 2 cm of the internal os but does not cover it, it is an *incomplete previa*. It is most helpful when the sonologist simply reports how close the inferior margin of the placenta comes to the internal os. This is a critical piece of information as it has been shown that so long as the inferior margin of the placenta is at least 2 cm from the internal os, there is not a significantly increased risk of bleeding during labor (24). Transabdominal ultrasound examination may require a full bladder to adequately evaluate the placental/cervical relationship. The transabdominal approach is best employed as a first step to show that the inferior margin of the placenta is far from the cervical os. If it is not obvious that such is the case, the transvaginal approach should be used. It should be noted that while there is no place for a digital examination of the cervix to assess placenta previa, transvaginal ultrasonography has been shown to be safe. Translabial ultrasound is also safe but may not provide images that are as clear as in transvaginal examinations. If there is a placenta previa, a gentle speculum examination may be used to estimate cervical dilation. Once a placenta previa has been ruled out, a normal digital cervical examination is appropriate to more adequately assess cervical dilation and effacement.

There is no treatment for a bleeding placenta previa other than delivery. A decision has to be made between an emergency cesarean section or whether temporizing measures such as blood transfusion and expectant management are feasible. Given the high risk that a patient will require a preterm delivery, when a placenta previa presents with significant bleeding, steroids are usually administered to enhance fetal maturity. These are given as betamethasone 12 mg IM × 2 given 24° apart, or if betamethasone is not available, dexamethasone 6 mg IM × 4 given 12° apart. Patients with a bleeding placenta previa usually report painless bleeding, but occasionally, there may be contractions. In some cases, administration of a tocolytic may be reasonable, but therapeutic decisions such as tocolytics are best left to obstetrical consultants. Appropriate lab work includes a complete blood count and a type and crossmatch for at least 2 units of packed red blood cells.

## Placental Abruption

When uterine bleeding is present and placenta previa has been ruled out, the most common diagnosis is placental abruption (Fig. 8.1). A placental abruption is simply the premature separation of a portion of the placenta from the uterine wall with concomitant bleeding. Women will usually present with bleeding and contractions, frequently painful. Ultrasound is not a sensitive technique to identify an abruption. When an abruption is large enough that it is obvious on ultrasound, it is a serious one (Fig. 8.2), and there are, usually, already signs of fetal compromise on fetal monitoring. Abruptions may arise from the edge of the placenta or may be more centrally located. The latter are more serious, because a central abruption may produce an expanding clot that dissects beneath the placenta, potentially shearing an increasing area of placental off the uterine wall. As more placenta separates, there is less placenta functioning as the primary respiratory organ for the fetus. This may eventually lead to fetal compromise, damage and demise. Smaller abruptions may not be as severe and are less commonly identified on ultrasound. Occasionally, terms such as a "marginal sinus bleed" or "peripheral placental separation" are used. While these are effectively synonyms for small abruptions, they are used to distinguish the lower risk of these bleeds from the sense of an imminent emergency that a larger abruption can entail. More recently, it is common to simply describe the abruption as one of three grades. In grade I, there is little bleeding, mild or no contractions, and no evidence of fetal compromise. In grade II, there is mild to moderate bleeding, contractions, and may be fetal heart rate changes. In grade III, there is moderate to severe bleeding or concealed bleeding, strong contractions or uterine tetany with severe abdominal pain, and obvious fetal compromise or death.

As with placenta previa, the management of abruption is largely expectant with supportive care consisting of fluid resuscitation with blood transfusions as necessary and deciding when to deliver based on signs of maternal and/or fetal compromise. The diagnosis of abruption at or beyond viability should also lead to the administration of steroids to enhance fetal maturation should delivery become necessary. Patients with grade III abruption may develop disseminated intravascular coagulation, so platelet counts and fibrinogen levels should be followed. A complete blood count and type and crossmatch for at least 2 units of packed red blood cells should also be one of the first steps due to the speed with which blood may be lost during a severe abruption. As was also the case with placenta previa, when this

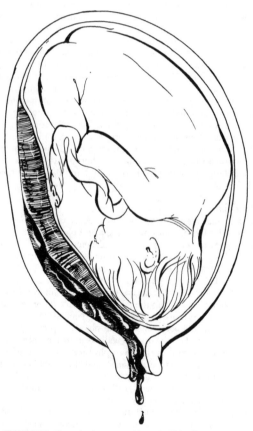

**FIGURE 8.1** Abruptio placentae with vaginal bleeding.

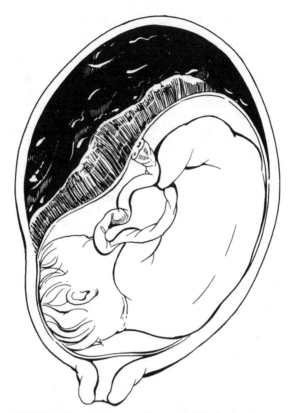

**FIGURE 8.2** Abruptio placentae with concealed bleeding.

diagnosis is suspected or confirmed, patients are best served by transfer to the labor and delivery unit under the care of an obstetrician or perinatologist. Risk factors for abruption include chronic hypertension, smoking, preeclampsia, connective tissue disorders such as lupus, antiphospholipid antibody syndrome, and familial thrombophilias. Cocaine use may also cause an abruption, so it is appropriate to get a urine toxicology screen when an abruption is diagnosed (25,26).

**Vasa Previa**

A rare cause of vaginal bleeding is bleeding from a vasa previa, when fetal vessels run in the membranes close to the internal cervical os. This may happen when there is a velamentous insertion of the umbilical cord, where the cord appears to insert directly into the membranes and the cord vessels then run to the placenta. It may also be seen when there is a succenturiate lobe of the placenta, and the vessels connecting the succenturiate lobe to the main placental mass pass close to the cervix. While benign for the mother, this condition is usually fatal for the fetus unless the diagnosis is suspected and made quickly. In either of these conditions, if the vessels break, the fetus may rapidly exsanguinate. The velamentous cord insertion variety is more dangerous, because the entire fetal blood volume is passing through the cord, and dividing fetal vessels closer to the cord involves a larger percentage of the circulating blood than the smaller portion that is circulating more "root branchings" away downstream in an accessory lobe. This abnormality can be identified by the ultrasound technician using color Doppler or power Doppler, but it is easily missed if the sonographer is not explicitly looking for it (27,28). If there is vaginal bleeding without a complete placenta previa, unless the placental cord insertion site is clearly seen, and there is no evidence of a succenturiate lobe, it is most appropriate to do a transvaginal ultrasound using power and/or color Doppler to rule out any fetal vessels in the vicinity of the internal os. Fetal heart rate abnormalities, such as late decelerations, bradycardia, or a sinusoidal tracing, will usually lead to a decision to deliver the fetus. In some cases though, particularly if bleeding is not severe and an ultrasound examination is unavailable, there may be time to determine whether bleeding is of maternal or fetal origin. A number of tests are available to make this determination, including some appropriate for bedside use (29). Perhaps the easiest and most convenient test given the chemicals readily available in most obstetrical units is to place a few drops of the blood into a test tube containing a 5% potassium hydroxide solution (the standard 10% KOH solution used for detecting yeast and diluted 50:50 with water). Fetal blood remains pink, but maternal blood turns greenish brown. Bleeding vasa previa is appropriately treated by delivery in almost all cases.

### Uterine rupture

Uterine rupture is quite rare in an unscarred uterus, and even then, it is usually restricted to the third trimester in women with a prior classical c-section or with multiple prior c-sections. However, when a history is taken, inquiries regarding the prior obstetrical history should not overlook asking whether any prior deliveries were by c-section, whether any of the c-sections were "classical" or had vertical uterine scars, and what the interval between her last c-section and her current pregnancy was. A prior vertical uterine incision, multiple c-sections, and labor all increase the risk of a uterine rupture. A short interdelivery interval also increases the risk of uterine rupture (30–32). Women will present with bleeding but surprisingly most do not have severe abdominal pain. Fetal monitoring will usually show obvious fetal compromise. Uterine rupture must be treated with emergency abdominal delivery of the fetus in order to minimize risk of neurologic compromise and stop maternal bleeding.

### Labor

Sometimes when patients present with bleeding and contractions, it is simply bleeding due to the cervical dilation of labor. This is often referred to as "bloody show" and is rarely heavy enough to be suggestive of an abruption. After placenta previa has been ruled out, a digital examination will help determine whether the woman is in labor. These patients are obviously best evaluated in the labor and delivery suite where fetal monitoring is more readily available. Unless delivery is imminent, it is best to transfer them to an appropriate unit or facility.

## NONVAGINAL SITES

Occasionally, women complain of vaginal bleeding when the vagina is not the source of the blood. The most likely complaint is of spotting or finding "blood on the toilet tissue after going to the bathroom." The most common etiology is bleeding from hemorrhoids, which are also more commonly seen during pregnancy. Bleeding from the urinary tract is rarely misidentified as vaginal bleeding. Urinary tract bleeding, such as may be seen with urinary calculi, is rarely grossly bloody, so women are more likely to complain of discolored urine or blood in their urine rather than bleeding per se.

## WOMEN ON ANTICOAGULANTS

When women present with excessive bleeding from a non-vaginal site, it is crucial to review their medications, as a considerable number of indications for anticoagulation during pregnancy exist. In addition to the indications for anticoagulation seen outside of pregnancy such as mechanical heart valves and recent thromboembolism, indications specific to treatment during pregnancy include certain past history of thromboembolism, antiphospholipid antibody syndrome, some familial thrombophilias if there is a history of a prior pregnancy complicated by intrauterine growth restriction, etc. Anticoagulation during pregnancy is usually maintained with unfractionated heparin or low molecular weight heparin but will occasionally include aspirin. Coumadin is rarely used during pregnancy due to teratogenic effects, but occasionally, it has been used after the period of embryogenesis in women with mechanical heart valves. As the use of unfractionated heparin is on the decline, the partial thromboplastin time is not automatically the test to order to evaluate coagulation status. It is important to identify the patient's anticoagulant so as to pick the correct test for evaluating the degree of anticoagulation. While most women will be able to provide their medication list, if there is any question or the patient is unable to provide a history, contact should be made with her obstetrician or midwife.

## SUMMARY

When a patient presents with vaginal bleeding, the triaging is relatively straightforward. One must confirm that the bleeding is really vaginal, rule out an ectopic pregnancy, and rule out a placenta previa. The next step varies based on gestational age. In early pregnancy, most of the workup deals with establishing the presumptive viability of the fetus and making management decisions accordingly. In the second half of pregnancy, more serious bleeding complications can directly harm the mother and otherwise normal fetus. Management decisions tend to focus on identifying the precise etiology of the bleeding and, if heavy, deciding when it is appropriate to deliver for maternal or fetal indications. In many instances of bleeding in all stages of pregnancy, consultation with the patient's (or on-call) obstetrician or midwife may be helpful or mandatory. Throughout the entire episode, the attendant must keep in mind that any degree of vaginal bleeding at any gestational age may be viewed by many patients as one of the most ominous signs for the health of their infant. A calm and sensitive approach will often provide the reassurance needed and in all cases will contribute to a positive perception of the clinical interaction.

## References

1. Wilcox AJ, Weinberg CR, O'Connor JF, et al. Incidence of early loss of pregnancy. *N Engl J Med.* 1988;319(4):189–194.
2. American College of Obstetricians and Gynecologists. Prevention of Rh D Alloimmunization. ACOG Practice Bulletin Number 4. 2008 Compendium of selected publications. Washington, DC: ACOG; 2008:573–580.
3. Hughes EC, ed. *Obstetric-Gynecologic Terminology.* Philadelphia, PA: F. A. Davis Company; 1972.
4. Chen BA, Creinin MD. Contemporary management of early pregnancy failure. *Clin Obstet Gynecol.* 2007;50(1):67–88.
5. Wood SL, Brain PH. Medical management of missed abortion: a randomized clinical trial. *Obstet Gynecol.* 2002;99(4):563–566.

6. Bagratee JS, Khullar V, Regan L, Moodley J, Kagoro H. A randomized controlled trial comparing medical and expectant management of first trimester miscarriage. *Hum Reprod.* 2004;19(2):266–271.

7. American College of Obstetricians and Gynecologists. ACOG Committee Opinion No. 427: misoprostol for postabortion care. *Obstet Gynecol.* 2009;113(2, pt 1):465–468.

8. Blum J, Winikoff B, Gemzell-Danielsson K, Ho PC, Schiavon R, Weeks A. Treatment of incomplete abortion and miscarriage with misoprostol. *Int J Gynaecol Obstet.* 2007;99(Suppl. 2):S186–S189.

9. Bellis MA, Hughes K, Hughes S, Ashton JR. Measuring paternal discrepancy and its public health consequences. *J Epidemiol Community Health.* 2005;59(9):749–754.

10. Merchiers EH, Dhont M, De Sutter PA, Beghin CJ, Vandekerckhove DA. Predictive value of early embryonic cardiac activity for pregnancy outcome. *Am J Obstet Gynecol.* 1991;165(1):11–14.

11. Cepni I, Bese T, Ocal P, Budak E, Idil M, Aksu MF. Significance of yolk sac measurements with vaginal sonography in the first trimester in the prediction of pregnancy outcome. *Acta Obstet Gynecol Scand.* 1997;76(10):969–972.

12. Nyberg DA, Filly RA, Filho DL, Laing FC, Mahony BS. Abnormal pregnancy: early diagnosis by US and serum chorionic gonadotropin levels. *Radiology.* 1986;158(2):393–396.

13. Nyberg DA, Laing FC, Filly RA. Threatened abortion: sonographic distinction of normal and abnormal gestation sacs. *Radiology.* 1986;158(2):397–400.

14. Petrunin DD, Griaznova IM, Petrunina Iu A, Tatarinov Iu S. Immunochemical identification of organ specific human placental alpha-globulin and its concentration in amniotic fluid. *Akush Ginekol (Mosk).* 1977;(1):62–64.

15. Cousins LM, Smok DP, Lovett SM, Poeltler DM. AmniSure placental alpha microglobulin-1 rapid immunoassay versus standard diagnostic methods for detection of rupture of membranes. *Am J Perinatol.* 2005;22(6):317–320.

16. Boltovskaia MN, Zaraiskii EI, Fuks BB, et al. Histochemical and clinical-diagnostic study of placental alpha 1-microglobulin using monoclonal antibodies. *Biull Eksp Biol Med.* 1991;112(10):397–400.

17. Dinsmoor MJ, Bachman R, Haney EI, Goldstein M, Mackendrick W. Outcomes after expectant management of extremely preterm premature rupture of the membranes. *Am J Obstet Gynecol.* 2004;190(1):183–187.

18. Farooqi A, Holmgren PA, Engberg S, Serenius F. Survival and 2-year outcome with expectant management of second-trimester rupture of membranes [see comments]. *Obstet Gynecol.* 1998;92(6):895–901.

19. Vergani P, Ghidini A, Locatelli A, et al. Risk factors for pulmonary hypoplasia in second-trimester premature rupture of membranes. *Am J Obstet Gynecol.* 1994;170 (5, pt 1):1359–1364.

20. Lawler SD, Pickthall VJ, Fisher RA, Povey S, Evans MW, Szulman AE. Genetic studies of complete and partial hydatidiform moles [letter]. *Lancet.* 1979;2(8142):580.

21. Jacobs PA, Wilson CM, Sprenkle JA, Rosenshein NB, Migeon BR. Mechanism of origin of complete hydatidiform moles. *Nature.* 1980;286(5774):714–716.

22. Szulman AE, Philippe E, Boue JG, Boue A. Human triploidy: association with partial hydatidiform moles and nonmolar conceptuses. *Hum Pathol.* 1981;12(11):1016–1021.

23. Dawson WB, Dumas MD, Romano WM, Gagnon R, Gratton RJ, Mowbray RD. Translabial ultrasonography and placenta previa: does measurement of the os- placenta distance predict outcome? *J Ultrasound Med.* 1996;15(6):441–446.

24. Oppenheimer LW, Farine D, Ritchie JW, Lewinsky RM, Telford J, Fairbanks LA. What is a low-lying placenta? *Am J Obstet Gynecol.* 1991;165(4, pt 1):1036–1038.

25. Dombrowski MP, Wolfe HM, Welch RA, Evans MI. Cocaine abuse is associated with abruptio placentae and decreased birth weight, but not shorter labor [see comments]. *Obstet Gynecol.* 1991;77(1):139–141.

26. Handler A, Kistin N, Davis F, Ferre C. Cocaine use during pregnancy: perinatal outcomes. *Am J Epidemiol.* 1991;133(8):818–825.

27. Catanzarite V, Maida C, Thomas W, Mendoza A, Stanco L, Piacquadio KM. Prenatal sonographic diagnosis of vasa previa: ultrasound findings and obstetric outcome in ten cases. *Ultrasound Obstet Gynecol.* 2001;18(2):109–115.

28. Lee W, Lee VL, Kirk JS, Sloan CT, Smith RS, Comstock CH. Vasa previa: prenatal diagnosis, natural evolution, and clinical outcome. *Obstet Gynecol.* 2000;95(4):572–576.

29. Odunsi K, Bullough CH, Henzel J, Polanska A. Evaluation of chemical tests for fetal bleeding from vasa previa. *Int J Gynaecol Obstet*. 1996;55(3):207–212.
30. Esposito MA, Menihan CA, Malee MP. Association of interpregnancy interval with uterine scar failure in labor: a case-control study. *Am J Obstet Gynecol*. 2000;183(5):1180–1183.
31. Shipp TD, Zelop CM, Repke JT, Cohen A, Lieberman E. Interdelivery interval and risk of symptomatic uterine rupture. *Obstet Gynecol*. 2001;97(2):175–177.
32. Bujold E, Mehta SH, Bujold C, Gauthier RJ. Interdelivery interval and uterine rupture. *Am J Obstet Gynecol*. 2002;187(5):1199–1202.

# Infections in Pregnancy

## C. David Adair, Shawn P. Stallings, and A. Ben Abdu

Despite numerous advances since the time of Semmelweis when infectious complications were the number one cause of maternal mortality, the obstetric community still faces challenges that remain a major cause of morbidity. We are reminded, as evident by the recent "swine flu" outbreak, that infections continue to remain a clinical and societal problem. Today, we face "super bug" resistance, increased nosocomial infections, and rapidly declining efficacy of antibiotics. These new challenges for the obstetric caregiver requires continued local surveillance of susceptibilities and resistance, organism identification, and adherence to established evidence based protocols that allow for optimal therapy and minimal contribution to microbiological ecology disruption.

## URINARY TRACT INFECTION

Urinary tract infections (UTIs) constitute one of the most common and costly infectious complications of pregnancy, most likely the result of several factors: a relatively short urethra, proximity to the vaginal–anal canal, and physiologic dilatory changes of pregnancy that result in urostasis and reflux. A recent article reported an independent association of maternal UTI with preterm delivery, preeclampsia, intrauterine growth restriction (IUGR), and cesarean delivery (1).

### Asymptomatic Bacteriuria

*Background*
Asymptomatic bacteriuria (ASB) is the presence of bacteria in the urine without concomitant specific urinary tract symptoms. The incidence is not influenced by pregnancy, and the prevalence remains 2% to 7% of all pregnancies, similar to the nonpregnant population, and tends to be more evident in the first trimester (2,3). Certain groups do appear to be at higher risk for ASB. These include patients with lower socioeconomic status, sickle cell trait and disease, diabetes, and chronic urinary retention (2–8). The American College of Obstetrics and Gynecology (ACOG) recommends routine screening for bacteriuria at the first prenatal visit. Recently, the US Preventive Services Task Force (USPSTF) reaffirmed screening for ASB in pregnant women by urine culture at the first prenatal visit or at 12 to 16 weeks' gestation (9).

*Diagnosis*
The diagnosis is made by bacterial culture revealing $\geq 10^5$ organisms of a single species per milliliter of urine without specific UTI symptoms. Because pyelonephritis may occur with lower colony counts (20k to 50k) in the presence of symptoms or specific isolates such as group B streptococcus or *Escherichia coli* should be considered positive findings, and patients should be provided treatment based on sensitivity of isolates. A single midstream clean-catch urine culture suffices for the diagnosis. *E. coli*, *Klebsiella*, and *Enterobacter* species account for more than 85% of the isolates. Group B streptococcus, although a rare isolate, when identified in the urine, should be aggressively treated to prevent transmission to the neonate and frank

progression to pyelonephritis. This patient will also require intrapartum GBS prophylaxis.

By identifying and treating ASB, a significant reduction in symptomatic infections can be achieved. Left untreated, approximately 40% of all cases of ASB will progress to acute symptomatic infection and 25% to acute pyelonephritis (AP) and its increased attendant morbidity. With adequate therapy, the risk is significantly decreased to only 3% (3,4).

### Management

Therapy should be directed by specific isolate identification and sensitivity; some authorities do not recommend C&S evaluation on initial positive cultures in uncomplicated pregnant individuals. Drugs that provide successful ASB treatment and have safe fetal profiles include sulfa-based drugs, first-generation cephalosporins, nitrofurantoin, and penicillin-based alternatives. The latter group should not be used empirically but rather for specific isolates with documented sensitivity because *E. coli* has high resistance to penicillin derivatives. It should be remembered that due to increased prevalence of antibiotic resistance the practitioner should use a community accepted first-line agent that presumes adequate coverage and then follow up with specific agents if culture and sensitivity dictates otherwise. In some areas of the country, up to a third of strains have resistance to penicillins and sulfonamides. Nitrofurantoin and trimethoprim–sulfamethoxazole have geographic resistance rates of 5% to 20%. Typically, in pregnant individuals, single-dose therapy is discouraged. A prolonged course of 7 days is recommended in this population with shorter duration of 3 days being reserved for nonpregnant patients. Suggested drug regimens are presented in Table 9.1. After completion of treatment, a test of cure culture should be obtained, because as many as one third of patients will have persistent bacteriuria. When persistence is confirmed, longer courses and/or suppressive therapy may be prudent.

## Acute Cystitis

Acute cystitis (AC) complicates 0.3% to 1.3% of all pregnancies. One third of the cases represent progression from ASB, and the remainder represent de novo infection and recurrence can be up to 1.3% (8). Patients with AC often present in the second trimester with complaints of urgency, frequency, dysuria, and pelvic pressure discomfort. A lower colony count (i.e., $\geq 10^2$) in the presence of the symptoms is usually sufficient to confirm diagnosis. In general, the same isolates as found in ASB are the culprits in AC such as *E. coli*, Gram-negative facultative organisms, Group B Streptococcus (GBS), and *Staphylococcus saprophyticus*. Therapy is largely empiric at first, then it is directed to specific agents as culture and sensitivities of isolates become available. Appropriate first-line therapies include nitrofurantoin macrocrystals or first-generation cephalporosporins. Therapeutic options are included in Table 9.1. Symptomatic abatement should occur between 48 and 72 hours, and the absence of symptom resolution should prompt reevaluation. Efficacy of therapy should be confirmed by conductance of a test of cure. From 17% to 25% of pregnant patients with AC experience a recurrent bout of AC or other UTI during pregnancy; importantly, AC does not increase the incidence of adverse pregnancy outcome like some of its counterparts (8).

## Acute Pyelonephritis

### Background

AP disorder complicates more than 1% to 2.5% of all pregnancies (10). Forty percent of pregnant women with AP have antecedent symptoms of lower UTI. Unlike

**TABLE 9.1**    Suggested Therapeutic Options for UTI in Pregnancy

Asymptomatic Bacteriuria and uncomplicated AC—7 d course
    Amoxicillin 500 mg orally t.i.d
    Ampicillin 250 mg orally q.i.d
    Cephalexin 250–500 mg orally q.i.d
    Nitrofurantoin 100 mg orally b.i.d
    Sulfisoxazole 2 g orally initially then 1 g q.i.d
    Trimethoprim–sulfamethoxazole 160/800 mg orally b.i.d

Complicated AC—7 d course
    Amoxicillin 500 mg orally t.i.d
    Ampicillin 250 mg orally q.i.d
    Cephalexin 250–500 mg orally q.i.d
    Nitrofurantoin 100 mg orally q.i.d
    Sulfisoxazole 2 g orally initially then 1 g q.i.d
    Trimethoprim–sulfamethoxazole 160/800 mg orally b.i.d

Suppressive therapy
    Nitrofurantoin 100 mg orally qHs until postpartum
    Trimethoprim–sulfamethoxazole 160/800 mg orally qHs until postpartum

AP in pregnancy
Outpatient ≤20 weeks' gestation, uncomplicated medical history, and not moderate or severe illness
    Amoxicillin 500 mg orally q.i.d
    Amoxicillin–clavulanate 875/125 mg orally b.i.d
    Trimethoprim–sulfamethoxazole 160/800 mg orally b.i.d
    Ceftriaxone 1–2 g intravenous q 24 hr

Intravenous for inpatient ≥20 weeks, complicated medical history, or moderate to severe illness
    Ceftriaxone 1–2 g IV daily
    Cefotetan 2 g IV q 12 hr
    Cefotaxime 1–2 g IV q 8 hr
    Ampicillin 2 g q 6 hr plus
    Gentamicin 3–5 mg/kg/d either daily or divided dosing q 8 hr
    Aztreonam 2 g IV q 6 hr (renal impaired patients)
    Ampicillin–sulbactam 1.5 g IV every hours

ASB and AC, pregnancy does seem to predispose to AP. Two thirds of cases arise in women with previously documented positive urine culture results and the remainder arise de novo. Most cases of AP in pregnant women occur in the second and third trimesters when significant and maximal physiologic changes have occurred (4,10). The disease is thought to result from the significant physiologic changes of the genitourinary system, namely, urethral dilation, mechanical obstruction of the gravid uterus, and significant glucosuria and aminoaciduria.

*Diagnosis*
The diagnosis of AP is based on the presence of systemic signs and symptoms that include fever, chills, nausea, vomiting, and costovertebral angle tenderness. Almost always, these cases are complicated by a fever and, in some cases, significant temperature elevation may occur ≥44°C (11). Costovertebral sensitivity

tends to be right sided in the predominance of cases but does not exclude the possibility of bilateral or left-sided tenderness.

Laboratory findings usually include an elevated white blood cell count, but occasionally, in mild or early infections, this may be normal. Some investigators have reported decreased hematocrit and transient renal dysfunction (10,12). Significant pyuria, hematuria, and ultimately positive urine cultures are mainstay findings. It is not unusual for a patient to have "sterile" urine despite having classic symptoms. When confronted with this clinical scenario, treatment should not be postponed.

Effects of AP are not limited to the kidney. These include hemolytic anemia, renal dysfunction, and pulmonary dysfunction including transient mild distress to frank adult respiratory distress syndrome (13,14). About 15% to 20% of women with AP also have bacteremia (2). As with any systemic infection combining with the immunocompromised status of pregnancy, septic shock may result. Unlike ASB and AC, AP is associated with increased occurrence of uterine contractions and preterm labor.

*Management*

The treatment of pyelonephritis consists of aggressive systemic intravenous antibiotics and judicious fluid management. All pregnant patients suspected of having pyelonephritis should be admitted to the hospital for treatment. The initial antimicrobial selection should be reflective of most common isolates and should be cost sensitive. Several regimens can be employed. These include gentamicin and ampicillin or first- or third-generation cephalosporins. A randomized controlled trial showed 95% efficacy of these regimens (15). This selection of the third-generation cephalosporins allows for the possibility of early discharge and outpatient therapy in gestations <20 weeks and absent complicating medical conditions (16). Significant cost savings have also been achieved with daily single-dose ceftriaxone use versus multi-dose regimens during inpatient therapy (17).

With antibiotic therapy selection, clinical resolution generally should be realized in 24 to 48 hours. If improvement is not achieved in 48 to 72 hours, clinical suspicion should be heightened, and a diligent search for other causes (e.g., renal calculi, abscess, or obstruction) commenced. Therapy should be continued until the patient is afebrile for 48 to 72 hours. A test of cure is mandatory. Up to 25% of patients will have recurrent pyelonephritis (10). This observation has led most authorities to recommend suppressive therapy for the duration of the pregnancy (18). The agent selected should differ from the treating agent, should be cost sensitive, and should have minimal normal flora impact. Therapeutic suggestions are provided in Table 9.1.

## INTRA-AMNIOTIC INFECTION

### Background

Intra-amniotic infection (IAI) is a bacterial infection of the chorion, amnion, and amniotic fluid usually diagnosed during prolonged labor. It complicates 0.5% to 2.0% of all pregnancies and, in special circumstances, can complicate up to 25% of pregnancies in certain high-risk populations (19–24). IAI is associated with increased maternal and neonatal morbidity, mortality, and long-term complications such as cerebral palsy.

### Diagnosis

Chorioamnionitis is technically a histologic diagnosis determined after delivery by a pathologist evaluating a microscopic specimen, whereas the term IAI is more appropriate, because it is a clinical diagnosis. IAI is diagnosed most commonly in the presence of maternal fever (temperature ≥37.8°C) with associated uterine tenderness, foul-smelling amniotic fluid, maternal and/or fetal tachycardia, or maternal leukocytosis in the absence of other obvious infectious sources (25).

Complications of IAI impact both elements of the maternal–fetal pair. IAI is commonly associated with dysfunctional labor. This results in a significant increase in cesarean deliveries. The less common circumstance is that of IAI associated with a precipitous delivery. Maternal mortality is fortunately a rare event. Neonatal morbidity can be significant and can lead to neonatal death. Neonates whose intrapartum course is complicated by IAI are at significantly increased risks of sepsis, congenital pneumonia, and cerebral palsy (26,27).

Numerous risk factors for the development of IAI have been elucidated. These include preterm labor, preterm rupture of membranes, dysfunctional labor, prolonged rupture of term membranes (>18 hours), meconium-stained amniotic fluid, presence of cervical pathogens, bacterial vaginosis, number of vaginal examinations, and presence of intrauterine fetal monitoring and contractile monitors (20,28–40). IAI most commonly is caused by bacteria found in the lower genital tract and is polymicrobial rather than related to a single pathologic isolate. The two most common isolates are group B streptococcus and *E. coli*.

## Management

The treatment of IAI is approached best by preventive measures, for example, by avoiding numerous or unnecessary vaginal examinations and intrauterine monitoring and by identifying and treating cervical pathogens before intrapartum presentation. When prevention proves inadequate, systemic antibiotic administration is required. Withholding antibiotics until after delivery is not prudent. IAI complicates both the maternal and the neonatal units. Thus, antibiotic selection and administration should be considered therapy for both the mother and the fetus. The selection should cover usual vaginal borne pathogens, especially group B streptococcus and enteric organisms. Although IAI alone is not an indication for cesarean delivery, when c-section is required in the face of IAI, coverage should also include antimicrobial activity directed to anaerobes.

Even though risk factors and common isolate epidemiology are well-known, the optimal "gold standard" therapy remains less well defined. Historically, penicillin or ampicillin, paired with the aminoglycoside gentamicin, has been favored. Single broad-spectrum therapeutic agents have also been advocated. The selection is empiric and should be broad enough to cover usual suspected pathogens (20–23).

Some commonly recommended drug regimens in the treatment of IAI are presented in Table 9.2. Again, IAI is not in and of itself an indication for cesarean delivery, but rather the mode of delivery should follow standard obstetric guidelines. With close fetal monitoring and the provision of good antibiotic coverage, no particular "rush" for delivery is indicated. There is accumulating evidence that respiratory distress syndrome, periventricular leukomalacia, and cerebral palsy are increased in both term and preterm infants. A thorough discussion of this is beyond the scope of this text. Once delivery has occurred, the decision to continue antibiotics postpartum remains controversial. One reasonable approach is to continue antibiotics in the presence of a cesarean delivery or for the patient who appears clinically ill. Otherwise, antibiotic discontinuance and close observation are practical (24).

| | Suggested Antibiotic Regimens for IAI or PPE |
| --- | --- |

Gentamicin 3–5 mg/kg/d IV either single dosing or divided q 8 hr

Plus ampicillin 2 g IV q 6 hr and/or clindamycin 600–900 mg IV q 8 hr for penicillin allergy, post-cesarean section, or obvious severe sepsis

Extended spectrum penicillins add gentamicin 3–5 mg/kg/d if unresponsive to monotherapy

## POSTPARTUM ENDOMETRITIS

### Background

Postpartum endometritis (PPE) complicates 1% to 3% of all vaginal deliveries and is much more frequent following cesarean delivery (41–43). This wide range of incidence depends on socioeconomic, delivery route, and labor parameters. PPE can be a continuation of IAI or arise de novo. The microbiologic isolates, like for IAI, the infection tends to be polymicrobial rather arising from a specific species. A mixed aerobic–anaerobic population is expected, especially after cesarean delivery (43,44). Single-species PPE should be suspected when the patient has received the benefit of prophylactic antibiotics (45–48).

### Diagnosis

PPE is diagnosed in the patient with fever ≥38°C, uterine tenderness, foul-smelling lochia, abdominal pain, leukocytosis, and, most importantly, the absence of other discernible causes of infection (e.g., pyelonephritis or pneumonia). Some cases of IAI, without question, are severe enough that despite delivery of the infected placenta or membrane, persistent infection accompanies the puerperium, particularly in cases complicated by cesarean delivery. In those cases, antibiotic administration should be extended into the puerperium. However, in the patient with low-grade IAI or suspected de novo PPE, a clinical examination and evaluation are mandatory. The temptation to empirically administer antibiotics should be restrained until the diagnosis is firmly established.

Clinical risk factors parallel those of IAI. Chiefly, the factors include the duration of membrane rupture and labor, internal monitoring, numerous vaginal examinations, cesarean delivery, IAI, lower socioeconomic status, and the presence of meconium staining (49–62).

### Management

The evaluation of the patient includes a detailed history and review of the labor record to ascertain the presence of risk factors and whether the patient has mitigating circumstances, such as antibiotic prophylaxis, immunosuppressive disorders, and drugs. A physical examination should exclude other likely sources. Most cases of endometritis are relatively straightforward in diagnosis; occasionally, the clinician encounters a postpartum fever with absent pinpoint focal findings. After thorough evaluation is inconclusive, it is reasonable to provide supportive measures, that is, antipyretics, and to observe the non-ill-appearing patient. However, if the patient's temperature is ≥38°C, particularly when following a cesarean delivery, antibiotics are generally indicated.

Antibiotic selection should be broad enough to cover all of the usual pathogens and should be aimed at a polymicrobial infection. Several recommended regimens are presented in Table 9.2. With appropriate selection, clinical symptoms and fever begin to abate in 24 to 48 hours. Blood cultures are generally reserved for patients with complicated underlying medical conditions or very ill appearing. For those with relatively straight forward PPE, omission of blood culture is acceptable. Failure to respond by 72 hours should prompt a reevaluation of the patient and antibiotic coverage to ensure no existence of a therapeutic gap in the chemotherapy. Pelvic ultrasound or computed tomography (CT) scan may assist in identifying hematoma, abscess, and retained placental products or instruments and in excluding septic pelvic thrombophlebitis.

If a hematoma is identified, CT-guided drainage may be beneficial. When septic pelvic thrombophlebitis is present, intravenous heparinization therapy for 7 days is recommended. When confronted with a pelvic abscess, unresponsive to antibiotics and nonamenable to needle drainage, surgical intervention is required. The surgical approach must be aggressive, because, left unchecked, the abscess may lead to myonecrosis and subsequent death.

Preventive measures to diminish PPE include several modalities. The foremost example is that of prophylactic antibiotic administration at the time of the cesarean delivery. Usually, a first-generation cephalosporin such as cefazolin is administered at the time of the cord clamping or in some series administered within 1 hour of surgical incision. For true allergic response to penicillins, those individuals are generally recommended to be treated with both gentamicin and clindamycin. Amnioinfusion has been suggested to reduce PPE in patients undergoing cesarean delivery with clear amniotic fluid and membrane rupture of >6 hours' duration (63,64), although this is not universally embraced. This approach seems to be not beneficial in cases with meconium staining (65).

PPE is more common after cesarean delivery than vaginal delivery. Because of the increased cesarean rates, PPE has become one of the most common causes of maternal morbidity. However, the use of single-dose perioperative antibiotic prophylaxis is likely the single greatest intervention to reduce the rates of postcesarean pelvic infections in the past 25 years (66). Prevention is the most prudent approach to PPE morbidity. However, when simple measures fail and active infection occurs, aggressive therapy aimed at the most common isolates is indicated. The clinician should be cognizant of the polymicrobial nature of PPE and, if therapy becomes unresponsive, more serious etiologies should be considered.

## HERPES INFECTION

Herpes simplex virus (HSV), cytomegalovirus (CMV), and varicella are specific viral pathogens that all belong to the family Herpesidae, all contain double-stranded DNA, and all have significant adverse maternal and fetal/neonate effects.

### Herpes Simplex Virus

*Background*
HSV-1 and -2 serotypes invade neural roots through mucosal membrane defects. Infection may be primary or, after acquisition, may remain dormant with recurrent episodic outbreaks. Acquisition can be by genital:genital, oral:genital, or anal:genital sexual contact. Serotypes previously were site specific, but each serotype may be associated with acute or recurrent HSV infection at oral, genital, or nongential sites. However, HSV-2 is more likely to be associated with recurrence regardless of site selection (67–69). Approximately 45 million adolescent and adult Americans are infected with HSV (70). Therefore, it may be a frequently encountered issue to be addressed in the pregnant female.

*Diagnosis*
The diagnosis of HSV infection is largely clinical. A history of vesicular, painful, burning ulcers prompts the decision to seek medical evaluation. During this

evaluation, the clinician should attempt to distinguish primary from recurrent HSV infection. Primary HSV acquisition is associated with flulike symptoms, lymphadenopathy, fever, and malaise. These viral syndrome symptoms typically are absent with recurrent HSV flare-ups. Exposure to onset of viral disease is >2 to 7 days (67,71).

Viral culture may be of assistance in providing absolute confirmation. However, clinically, if primary HSV infection is suspected, therapy should not be withheld pending culture results. Serum immunoglobulin M (IgM) and IgG antibodies may be of assistance in confirming the absence of previous infection. Papanicolaou smear test and Tzanck test have also been used to suggest HSV infection by identification of viral cytologic effects, but they lack sensitivity to be used for routine clinical care.

Recent evidence has suggested important prognostic values of primary versus recurrent HSV infection in pregnancy. Pregnancy per se does not influence the course of HSV infection, either in primary or recurrent episodes; however, both may result in hepatitis, meningitis, or pneumonia. Systemic manifestations require prolonged intravenous therapy with acyclovir. Disseminated HSV infection is associated with increased risk of maternal and neonatal mortality.

Neonatal vertical transmission remains the paramount concern for HSV infection complicating pregnancy. Most significant neurologic and severe adverse outcomes develop in those neonates with infection at or near the time of maternal primary disease, whereas infants born to mothers with recurrent disease have the least chance of acquisition and less morbidity (72).

### Management

Obstetric management remains supportive and directed to symptomatic management. The clinician should counsel women on possible transmission to partners and screen for other sexually transmitted diseases. Cesarean delivery is necessary for the patient in labor who has active disease or has the prodromal symptoms in cases of known recurrence. Cesarean delivery will not necessarily provide 100% prevention of HSV transmission to the neonate. Approximately 25% of affected neonatal cases were delivered by cesarean delivery (67,73,74). Vertical transmission rates are 30% to 60% when there is a primary HSV outbreak at the time of delivery (75). The rates are 3% if having a recurrent genital outbreak at the time of delivery, and only 2 per 10,000 in a patient with a history of HSV but no active lesions at the time of delivery (76).

There is currently no universally accepted screening guideline for HSV in pregnancy. Therapy is with any of the synthetic acyclic purine nucleoside analogues such as acyclovir, valacyclovir, and famciclovir. These agents (Category B) have no evidence of teratogenic or adverse effects on the human fetus. They should be used in doses similar to those used in a nonpregnant patient. Prophylactic suppression has been reputed to be successful in reducing recurrence of HSV infection at term. Generally, prophylaxis is initiated at 36 weeks (77,78). ACOG currently recommends offering suppressive viral therapy for women with active recurrent genital herpes at or beyond 36 weeks' gestation (79). However, a recent Cochrane review suggests that the overall risk of neonatal herpes is low, and there is insufficient evidence to determine if antiviral prophylaxis reduces the incidence of neonatal herpes (80).

### Cytomegalovirus

#### Background

CMV is the most common perinatally transmitted viral infection, occurring in 1% to 2% of all neonates. Like HSV, it can be transmitted to the fetus by either primary or reactivation of CMV infection. More than 85% of patients in low socioeconomic status have evidence of previous CMV infection and about 50% of the adult sexually active population. Fetal transmission in these cases is <1%, whereas maternal seroconversion during pregnancy is associated with high fetal transmission rates, generally 30% to 40% and as high as 90% in some series. These cases of transmission result in symptomatic infections in 10% to 15% of patients, whereas most will remain asymptomatic and continue to develop normally in the neonatal period. The transmission can be primarily through maternal viremia of autoinfection and cervical secretion (81).

### Diagnosis and Management

The diagnosis of CMV infection is made by observation of seroconversion of a seronegative patient. The patient is usually asymptomatic, but flulike symptoms, fever, and malaise may occur. Rarely, hepatitis, pneumonia, meningitis, and anemia may complicate the primary course. This diagnosis is fraught with difficulties in that more than one half of pregnant women are positive for IgG CMV. Furthermore, IgM antibodies may persist far past the initial infection and may remain positive at the time of recurrent infection. Fetal infection has been confirmed by polymerase chain reaction (PCR) and CMV culture of amniotic fluid, chorionic villus sampling (CVS), and percutaneous umbilical cord blood sampling. Sonographic findings are nonspecific but include periventricular calcifications, ventriculomegaly, and microcephaly. Neonatal infection is confirmed by CMV IgM and IgG antibodies and/or PCR CMV viral culture. No specific therapeutic modality exists. For severe infections in the neonatal period, ganciclovir may be used (82–88).

One recent development to the treatment regimen has been the use of hyperimmune globulin as both treatment and prophylaxis for congenital CMV (89). This approach is controversial and requires individuals with specialized expertise to care for these fetuses.

## Varicella Zoster

### Background

Varicella zoster (VZ) infection is a major infectious complication for the obstetric practitioner. VZ infection results in the classic "chicken pox" symptoms, but in pregnancy, these simple nuisance symptoms can result in grave morbidity and even death. Varicella also has the ability to cross the placenta, and fetal infection can result in congenital anomalies. Neonates born to mothers who have not had time to produce IgG have significant risk of morbidity and mortality.

More than 90% of adults have serologic titers consistent with previous varicella infection despite a negative clinical history. Varicella complicates 1 to 7 per 10,000 pregnancies and 25% of maternal infection results in evidence of fetal infection (90,91). Viral transmission is by viral respiratory droplets and incubation requires approximately 2 weeks.

### Diagnosis and management

The diagnosis of VZ infection is fairly straightforward. Most patients have a history of recent exposure of acute vesicular maculopapular rash of the scalp and trunk with progression to the extremities and other body areas. These lesions are commonly accompanied by flulike symptoms, myalgia, headaches, and fever. Each new lesion has active viral shedding for 6 days with "crusting" persisting for 1 week. Fever generally persists until cessation of lesion formation.

VZ infection usually is self-limiting and treatment is thus largely symptomatic. VZ infection complicating pregnancy, however, presents unique challenges to the clinician. Complications are usually more frequent and severe when accompanying pregnancy. These include meningitis, encephalitis, arthritis, acute glomerulonephritis, and pneumonia. Pneumonia is the most frequent complication and is of the most concern. Varicella pneumonia may result in respiratory insufficiency, edema emphysema, superimposed bacterial infections, and even death. Pulmonary insult and injury lead to maternal and fetal hypoxia.

Varicella has been associated with an embryopathy (91). However, no increased adverse perinatal outcome has been reported, such as spontaneous abortion, prematurity, growth restriction, or death (92–95). The embryopathy syndrome was originally described by LaForest and Lynch (91). Characteristics are skin scarring, limb hypoplasia, and CNS and eye abnormalities. Developmental abnormalities appear to be limited to exposure at 12 weeks or less and occur in 2% to 3% of pregnancies.

The risk of congenital anomalies occurring secondary to varicella has been estimated to be approximately 2% (94–99). These anomalies include cicatrix skin deformities, ocular scarring, cataracts, chorioretinitis, and limb shortening (91,93,96,100–102).

The exposure to varicella requires documenting the antibody status of women who have uncertain varicella history. The majority of women who have no prior history of varicella infection will have serologic evidence of varicella exposure and IgG conversion. The patient who has negative IgG titers should receive VZ immunoglobulin (VZIG). The dose is 125 units/10 kg intramuscularly with a maximum of 625 units or five vials intramuscularly and is ideally administered within 96 hours of exposure. Once varicella infection is established, care is directed at symptomatic relief, prevention of community spread, especially to other pregnant women, and close surveillance for complications of disease progression. Acyclovir can be used to provide some symptom relief in mild to moderate cases, although this is largely an empiric treatment. Cases of severe disease of pneumonia mandates intravenous acyclovir at 10 mg/kg administered every 8 hours. The patient with any pulmonary complaint should be given acyclovir and observed closely in a negative airflow room.

Labor, whether it is preterm or term, frequently accompanies severe varicella infection. Caution should be used in administering tocolytics and glucocorticosteroids. Maternal viremia results in antibody production within 4 to 5 days of rash development. Thus, the infant at highest risk of neonatal varicella acquisition is born within 2 to 5 days of rash development. If labor begins during this interval, consideration of tocolysis may be prudent until 5 days after the appearance of the rash, even in term fetuses. Neonates born during this time interval have the highest risk of adverse complication and should therefore receive VZIG and acyclovir (92,103,104). Of interest is the increasing number of varicella vaccinated females that are approaching reproductive age and how the vaccine will impact varicella in pregnancy.

### References

1. Mazo-Dray E, Levy A, Schlaeffer F, Sheiner E. Maternal UTI: is it independently associated with adverse pregnancy outcome? *J Matern Fetal Noenatal Med.* 2009;22(2): 124–128.
2. Creasy RK, Resnik R, Iams JD, Lockwood CJ, Moore TR. Maternal and fetal infections. In: *Creasy and Resnik's Maternal Fetal Medicine.* 6th Ed. St. Louis, MO: Saunders-Elsevier,2009.
3. Whalley; P. Bacteriuria of pregnancy. *Am J Obstet Gynecol.* 1967;97:732.
4. Turck M, Goff BS, Petersdorf RG. Bacteriuria in pregancy: relation to socioeconomic factors. *N Engl J Med.* 1962;266:857.

5. Whalley PJ, Mrtin RG, Pritchard JA. Sickle cell trait and urinary tract infection during pregnancy. *JAMA*. 1964;189:9036.
6. Baker ER, Cardenas DD, Benedetti TJ. Risks associated with pregnancy in spinal cord-injured women. *Obstet Gynecol*. 1992;80:4258.
7. Lye WC, Chan RK, Lee EJ, et al. Urinary tract infections in patient with diabetes mellitus. *J Infect*. 1992;24:16974.
8. Harris RE, Gilstrap LC. Cystitis during pregnancy: a distinct clinical entity. *Obstet Gynecol*. 1981;57:578–580.
9. USPSTF. *Ann Intern Med*. 2008;149(1):43–47.
10. Gilstrap LC, Cunningham FG, Whalley PJ. Acute pyelonephritis in pregnancy: an anterospective study. *Obstet Gynecol*. 1981;57:409–413.
11. Stenqvist K, Standberg A, Lidin-Janson G, et al. Virulence factors of *Escherichia coli* in urinary isolates from pregnant women. *J Infect Dis*. 1987;156:870–877.
12. Whalley PJ, Cunningham FG, Martin FG. Transient renal dysfunction associated with acute pyelonephritis of pregnancy. *Obstet Gynecol*. 1974;46:17–47.
13. Cunningham FG, Lucas MJ, Hankins GDV. Pulmonary injury complicating antepartum pyelonephritis. *Am J Obstet Gynecol*. 1987;156:797–807.
14. Cunningham FG, Leveno KJ, Hankins GDV, et al. Respiratory insufficiency associated with pyelonephritis during pregnancy. *Obstet Gynecol*. 1984;63:12–15.
15. Wing DA, Hendershott CM, Debesque L, et al. A randomized controlled trial of three antibiotic regimens for the treatment of pyelonephritis in pregnancy. *Am J Obstet Gynecol*. 1998;92:249.
16. Millar LK, Wing DA, Paul RH, et al. Outpatient treatment of pyelonephritis in pregnancy: a randomized controlled trial. *Obstet Gynecol*. 1995;86:560–564.
17. Sanchez-Ramos L, McAlpine KJ, Adair CD, et al. Pyelonephritis in pregnancy: once-a-day ceftriaxone versus multiple dose cefazolin: a randomized, double-blind trial. *Am J Obstet Gynecol*. 1995;172:129–133.
18. Zinner SH, Kass EH. Long-term (10–14 years) follow-up of bacteriuria of pregnancy. *N Engl J Med*. 1971;285:820–822.
19. Koh KE, Chan FH, Monfared AH, et al. The changing perinatal and maternal outcome in chorioamnionitis. *Obstet Gynecol*. 1979;53:730.
20. Gibbs RS, Castillo MS, Rogers PJ. Management of acute chorioamnionitis. *Obstet Gynecol*. 1980;136:709.
21. Hauth JC, Gilstrap LC III, Hankins GDV, et al. Term maternal and neonatal complications of acute chorioamnionitis. *Obstet Gynecol*. 1985;66:59.
22. Gilstrap LC III, Leveno KJ, Cox SM, et al. Intrapartum treatment of acute chorioamnionitis: impact on neonatal sepsis. *Am J Obstet Gynecol*. 1988;159:579.
23. Satin AJ, Maberry MC, Leveno KJ, et al. Chorioamnionitis: a harbinger of dystocia. *Obstet Gynecol*. 1992;79:91–93.
24. Wendel PJ, Cox SM, Roberts SW, et al. Chorioamnionitis: association of nonreassuring fetal heart rate patterns and interval from diagnosis to delivery on neonatal outcome. *Infect Dis Obstet Gynecol*. 1994;2:162.
25. Gibbs RS, Suff P. Progress in pathogenesis and management of clinical intraamniotic infection. *Am J Obstet Gynecol*. 1991;164:1317.
26. Duff P, Sanders R, Gibbs RS. The course of labor in term pregnancies with chorioamnionitis. *Am J Obstet Gynecol*. 1983;147:391.
27. Yoon BH, Romero R, Kim CJ, et al. High expression of tumor necrosis factor-alpha and interleukin-6 in periventricular leukomalacia. *Am J Obstet Gynecol*. 1997;177:406–411.
28. Newton ER. Chorioamnionitis and intraamniotic infection. *Clin Obstet Gynecol*. 1993;36:795.
29. Looff JD, Hager WD. Management of chorioamnionitis. *Surg Gynecol Obstet*. 1984;158:161.
30. Guzick DS, Winn K. The associate of chorioamnionitis with preterm delivery. *Obstet Gynecol*. 1985;65:11.
31. Sturchier D, Menegaz F, Dialing J. Reproductive history and intrapartum fever. *Gynecol Obstet Invest*. 1986;21:182.
32. Newton ER, Prihoda TJ, Gibbs RS. Logistic regression analysis of risk factors for intra-amniotic infection. *Obstet Gynecol*. 1989;73:571.
33. Soper DE, Mayall CG, Dalton HP. Risk factors for intraamniotic infection: a prospective epidemiologic study. *Am J Obstet Gynecol*. 1989;161:562.

34. Edwards LA, Barrada MI, Hamann AA, et al. Gonorrhea in pregnancy. *Am J Obstet Gynecol*. 1978;132:637.
35. Regan JA, Chao SJ, James SL. Premature rupture of the membranes, preterm delivery and group B streptococcal colonization of mother. *Am J Obstet Gynecol*. 1981; 141:184.
36. Hillier S, Krohn MA, Kiviat NB, et al. Microbiologic causes and neonatal outcomes associated with chorioamnion infection. *Am J Obstet Gynecol*. 1991;165:955.
37. Gibbs RS. Chorioamnionitis and bacterial vaginosis. *Am J Obstet Gynecol*. 1993; 169:460.
38. Romero R, Hanaoka S, Mazor M, et al. Meconium-stained amniotic fluid: a risk factor for microbial invasion of the amniotic cavity. *Am J Obstet Gynecol*. 1991;164:859.
39. Adair CD, Ernest JM, Sanchez-Ramos L, et al. Meconium-stained amniotic fluid-associated infectious morbidity: a randomized double-blind trial of ampicillin-sulbactam prophylaxis. *Obstet Gynecol*. 1996;88:216.
40. Piper Jm, Newton ER, Berkus MD, et al. Meconium: a marker for peripartum infection. *Obstet Gynecol*. 1998;91:741.
41. Gilstrap LC III, Cunningham FG. The bacterial pathogenesis of infection following cesarean section. *Obstet Gynecol*. 1979;53:545–549.
42. Sweet RL, Ledger WJ. Cefoxitin: single agent treatment of aerobic-anaerobic pelvic infections. *Obstet Gynecol*. 1979;54:193–198.
43. Gibbs RS. Clinical risk factors for puerperal infection. *Obstet Gynecol*. 1980;55(s): 178–183.
44. Phillips LE, Faro S, Martens MG, et al. Post cesarean microbiology of high-risk patients treated for endometritis. *Curr Ther Res*. 1987;42:1157–1165.
45. Faro S, Cox SM, Phillips LM, et al. Influence of antibiotic prophylaxis on vaginal microflora. *Am J Obstet Gynecol*. 1986;6(S):54–56.
46. Stever HG, Forward KR, Tynell DC, et al. Comparative cervical flora-microflora shift after cefoxitin or cefazolin prophylaxis against infection following cesarean section. *Am J Obstet Gynecol*. 1984;149:718–721.
47. Gilstrap LC III. Puerperal infection. In: Faro S, ed. *Diagnosis and Management of Female Pelvic Infection in Primary Care Medicine*. Baltimore, MD: Williams & Wilkins; 1985:151–167.
48. Gilstrap LC III. Prophylactic antibiotics for cesarean section and surgical procedures. *J Rep Med*. 1988;33:588–590.
49. Gibbs RS, Castillo MS, Rogers PJ. Management of acute chorioamnionitis. *Obstet Gynecol*. 1980;136:709–713.
50. Newton ER. Chorioamnionitis and intraamniotic infection. *Clin Obstet Gynecol*. 1993; 36:795.
51. Looff JD, Hager WD. Management of chorioamnionitis. *Surg Gynecol Obstet*. 1984; 158:161.
52. Guzick DS, Winn K. The associate of chorioamnionitis with preterm delivery. *Obstet Gynecol*. 1985;65:11.
53. Sturchler D, Menegaz F, Dialing J. Reproductive history and intrapartum fever. *Gynecol Obstet Invest*. 1986;21:182.
54. Newton ER, Prihoda TJ, Gibbs RS. Logistic regression analysis of risk factors for intra-amniotic infection. *Obstet Gynecol*. 1989;73:571.
55. Soper DE, Mayall CG, Dalton HP. Risk factors for intraamniotic infection: a prospective epidemiologic study. *Am J Obstet Gynecol*. 1989;161:562.
56. Edwards LA, Barrada ML, Hamann AA, et al. Gonorrhea in pregnancy. *Am J Obstet Gynecol*. 1978;132:637.
57. Regan JA, Chao SJ, James SL. Premature rupture of the membranes, preterm delivery and group B streptococcal colonization of mother. *Am J Obstet Gynecol*. 1981; 141:184.
58. Hillier S, Krohn MA, Kiviat NB, et al. Microbiologic cases and neonatal outcomes associated with chorioamnion infection. *Am J Obstet Gynecol*. 1991;165:955.
59. Gibbs RS. Chorioamnionitis and bacterial vaginosis. *Am J Obstet Gynecol*. 1993; 169:460.
60. Romero R, Hanaoka S, Mazor M, et al. Meconium-stained amniotic fluid: a risk factor for microbial invasion of the amniotic cavity. *Am J Obstet Gynecol*. 1991;164:859.

61. Adair CD, Ernest JM, Sanchez-Ramos L, et al. Meconium-stained amniotic fluid-associated infectious morbidity: a randomized double-blind trial of ampicillin-sulbactam prophylaxis. *Obstet Gynecol.* 1996;88:216.

62. Piper JM, Newton ER, Berkus MD, et al. Meconium: a marker for peripartum infection. *Obstet Gynecol.* 1998;91:741.

63. Moen MD, Besinger RE, Tomich PG, et al. Effect of amnioinfusion of the incidence of postpartum endometritis in patients undergoing cesarean delivery. *J Reprod Med.* 1995;40:383–386.

64. Monahan E, Katz VL, Cox RL. Amnioinfusion for preventing puerperal infection: a prospective study. *J Reprod Med.* 1995;40:721–723.

65. Adair CD, Weeks JW, Johnson G, et al. The utility of amnioinfusion in the prophylaxis of meconium-stained amniotic fluid infectious morbidity. *Infect Dis Obstet Gynecol.* 1997;5:366–369.

66. Cunningham FG, Leveno KJ, Bloom SL, et al. Puerperal infection. In: *Williams Obstetrics.* 22nd Ed. New York, NY: McGraw-Hill; 2005.

67. Cook CR, Gall SA. Herpes in pregnancy. *Infect Dis Obstet Gynecol.* 1994;1:298–304.

68. Reeves W, Corey L, Adams H, et al. Risk of recurrence after first episodes of genital herpes. *N Engl J Med.* 1981;305:315–319.

69. Corey L, Adams H, Brown Z, et al. Genital herpes simplex virus infections: clinical manifestation, course and complications. *Ann Intern Med.* 1983;98:958–972.

70. Fleming DT, McQuillan GM, Johnson RE, Nahamias AJ, Aral SO, Lee FK. Herpes simplex virus type 2 in the United States, 1976 to 1994. *N Engl J Med.* 1997;337: 1105–1111.

71. Maccato M. Herpes in pregnancy. *Clin Obstet Gynecol.* 1993;36:869–877.

72. Brown ZA, Selke S, Zeh J, et al. The acquisition of herpes simplex virus during pregnancy. *N Engl J Med.* 1997;337:509–515.

73. Whitley R, Corey L, Arvin A, et al. Changing presentation of herpes simplex virus infection in neonates. *J Infect Dis.* 1988;158:109–116.

74. Stone KM, Brooks CA, Guinan ME, et al. National surveillance for neonatal herpes simplex virus infections *Sex Transm Dis.* 1989;16:152–156.

75. Brown ZA, Selke S, Zeh J, et al. The acquisition of herpes simplex virus during pregnancy. *N Engl J Med.* 1997;337:509–515.

76. Brown ZA, Benedetti J, Ashley R, et al. Neonatal herpes simplex virus infection in relation to asymptomatic maternal infection at time of labor. *N Engl J Med.* 1991; 324:1247–1252.

77. Burroughs Wellcome Company. Pregnancy outcomes following systemic prenatal acyclovir exposure. June 1, 1984 to June 30, 1993. *Morbid Mortal Wkly Rep.* 1993;42: 806–809.

78. Scoff LL, Sanchez PJ, Jackson GL, et al. Acyclovir suppression to prevent cesarean section after first episode genital herpes in pregnancy. *Obstet Gynecol.* 1996;87:69–73.

79. Managing Herpes in Pregnancy. ACOG Practice Bulletin. No. 82, June 2007.

80. Hollier LM, Wendel GD. Third trimester antiviral prophylaxis for preventing maternal genital herpes simplex virus recurrences and neonatal infection. *Cochrane Database Syst Rev.* 2008;1:CD004946.

81. Stagno S, Whitely RJ. Herpes virus infection of pregnancy, Part 1. Cytomegalovirus and Epstein-Barr virus infection. *N Engl J Med.* 1986;313:1270–1274.

82. Raynor BD. Cytomegalovirus infection in pregnancy. *Semin Perinatol.* 1993;17:394–402.

83. Sison AV, Sever JL. Cytomegalovirus infections in pregnancy. In: Queenan JT, ed. *Management of High Risk Pregnancy.* Boston, MA: Blackwell Scientific Publications; 1994:315–321.

84. Donner C, Liesnard C, Content J, et al. Prenatal diagnosis of 52 pregnancies at risk for congenital cytomegalovirus infection. *Obstet Gynecol.* 1993;82:481–486.

85. Dong W, Yan C, Yi W, et al. detection of congenital cytomegalovirus infection by using chorionic villi of the early pregnancy and polymerase chain reaction. *Int J Gynecol Obstet.* 1994;44:229–231.

86. Catanzaarite V, Dankner WM. Prenatal diagnosis of congenital cytomegalovirus infection: false negative amniocentesis at 20 weeks' gestation. *Prenat Diagn.* 1993;12: 1021–1125.

87. Hogge WA, Buffone GJ, Hogge JS. Prenatal diagnosis of cytomegalovirus (CMV) infection: a preliminary report. *Prenat Diagn.* 1993;13:131–136.

88. Twickler DM, Perlman J, Maberry MC. Congenital cytomegalovirus infection presenting as cerebral ventriculomegaly on antenatal sonography. *Am J Perinatol.* 1993;10:404–406.
89. Nigro G, Adaler SP, LaRorre R, et al. Passive immunization during pregnancy for congenital cytomegalovirus infection. *N Engl J Med.* 2005;353:1350–1362.
90. Stagno S, Whitely RJ. Herpes virus infection of pregnancy. Part II. Herpes simplex virus varicella-zoster virus infections. *N Engl J Med.* 1985;313:1327–1332.
91. LaForest E, Lynch CL. Multiple congenital defects following maternal varicella. *N Engl J Med.* 1947;126:534–537.
92. Brunell PA. Varicella zoster-infections. In: Amstey MS, ed. *Virus Infection in Pregnancy.* Orlando, FL: Grune & Stratton; 1984:131–145.
93. Paryani SG, Arvin AM. Intrauterine infection with varicella-zoster virus after maternal varicella. *N Engl J Med.* 1986;314:1542–1546.
94. Preblud S, Cochi S, Orenstein W. Varicella-zoster infection in pregnancy. *N Engl J Med.* 1986;315:14–15.
95. Enders G. Varicella-zoster virus infection in pregnancy. *Prog Med Virol.* 1984;29:166.
96. Srabstein JC, Morris N, Larke RP, et al. Is there a congenital varicella syndrome? *J Pediatr.* 1974;84:239–243.
97. Siegal M, Fuerst HT. Low birth weight and maternal viral diseases: a prospective study of rubella, measles, mumps, chicken pox, and hepatitis. *JAMA.* 1966;197:88.
98. Seigel M, Fuerst HT, Pareso NS. Comparative mortality in maternal virus diseases: A prospective study on rubella, measles, mumps, chicken pox, and hepatitis. *N Engl J Med.* 1966;274:76–78.
99. Fox MJ, Krumpiegel ER, Teresi JL. Maternal measles, mumps, and chicken pox as a cause of congenital anomalies. *Lancet.* 1972;2:62–69.
100. McKendry JBJ, Bailey JD. Congenital varicella associated with multiple defects. *Can Med Assoc J.* 1977;108:66–67.
101. Charles NC, Bennett TW, Margolis S. Ocular pathology of the congenital varicella syndrome. *Arch Ophthalmol.* 1977;95:2034–2037.
102. Coftier E. Congenital varicella cataract. *Am J Ophthalmol.* 1978;86:627.
103. Raine DN. Varicella infection contracted in utero: sex incidence and incubation period. *Am J Obstet Gynecol.* 1966;94:1144–1145.
104. Steen J, Pederson RB. Varicella in a newborn girl. *J Oslo City Hosp.* 1959;9:36–45.

# 10 Pregnant Women and Chemical–Biological Warfare

Shawn P. Stallings, Jason Joseph, Joseph H. Kipikasa, and C. David Adair

There has been increased concern and heightened awareness regarding the possibility of deliberate attacks against susceptible civilian populations with agents of chemical or biological warfare. One such population that would be a value-added target to such a group would be that of pregnant women. Pregnant women represent a unique population that may differ from the populace at large in both susceptibility to certain agents and their management.

## GENERAL PREPARATION

All medical facilities and personnel since September 11, 2001 have made preparation for an attack on the general population. While most patients will likely be encountered first by emergency services personnel and first responder physicians, the obstetrician should be ready to participate and/or advise in the care of the exposed pregnant patient. Local hospitals, tertiary care centers, and government agencies have developed a plan for the triage of victims near the site of contact with the harmful substance or for the containment of persons who may have been in contact with a hazardous substance and are now at risk for spreading the problem to a wider area. Protocols have been prepared for possible transfer of patients to tertiary care centers. In the case of pregnant women, requiring intensive care and having sufficient gestational age for infant survival will likely require facilitation to a tertiary care center. However, this does not alleviate the need for local facilities to be prepared for care and for the possibility that transfer may not be possible due to damage in communication lines or transportation modes. Often, the disaster management will be run by a state or local law enforcement head, fire chief, or person in charge of emergency services in cases of natural disaster or industrial accident. In the case of a terrorist event, the Federal Bureau of Investigations will take control of managing these events and the Federal Emergency Management Agency (FEMA) will also become involved to mobilize federal resources (1).

In a major event such as bioterrorism, it is important to have protocols for identifying triage victims who are exposed and showing symptoms versus those who are exposed but asymptomatic and may require little intervention or prophylaxis only. Particularly in a delivery setting, this may be difficult to arrange logistically. This may be further complicated by the fact that most labor and delivery units have little or no facility for negative-pressure respiratory isolation. These negative flow units are usually in medical/surgical floors or ICUs, thus placing the emphasis of care on excellent interteam communication and cooperation. Labor and delivery unit managers need to be prepared to provide fetal monitoring to multiple patients in these remote settings. Such monitoring must be accompanied by preparation of instruments and surgical staff to accomplish emergent deliveries if necessary. Neonatal and anesthesia consultations are required given the increased likelihood of an emergent situation in an area unfamiliar and nontraditional for the delivery of child.

## BIOLOGICAL AGENTS

Biological agents have received the most attention from the news media as potential weapons of terrorism. The Centers for Disease Control and Prevention (CDC) has designated three different categories for agents that are potential threats for bioterrorism. Category A agents have been chosen because of their ease of dissemination and high morbidity and mortality rates or, alternatively, for their potential to cause widespread panic or disruption. These agents include anthrax, small pox, plague, botulism, hemorrhagic fevers, and tularemia. Category B agents are considered relatively high in priority because of their ease in dissemination; however, they may not cause as widespread injury. These agents might include ricin, threats to food safety such as *Escherichia coli* 0157:H7, typhus, brucellosis, or Q fever. Category C agents are agents that have not been used in the past for acts of terrorism or mass destruction, but their high morbidity and mortality rates make them potential targets for engineering to make them more widely disseminated. These agents would include various hemorrhagic viruses, tick-borne encephalitides, and multidrug resistant tuberculosis (2–4). More recently, the "Swine Flu" H1N1 demonstrates the susceptibility of our population and the relative ease at which a native or an engineered virus might wreak widespread disease and panic.

### Anthrax

Anthrax is the transmittable disease arising from infection with the Gram-positive, spore-forming bacterium *Bacillus anthracis*. Humans acquire naturally occurring disease from contact with infected animals or contaminated animal products. The disease more commonly infects herbivores, which ingest the spores from the soil. Animal vaccination is a common practice and has decreased animal mortality from the disease (5). There are three main illnesses in humans depending on the route of contact—cutaneous, inhalational, and gastrointestinal. The cutaneous form is the most common natural disease, although outbreaks of gastrointestinal anthrax are occasionally reported due to the consumption of undercooked, contaminated meat. Inhalational anthrax is rare but has raised the most concern as a bioterrorist threat because of its high mortality rate and ease of dissemination (5).

The spores of *B. anthracis* are stable for many years; are resistant to sunlight, heat, and disinfectants; and can be dispersed as a dry or moist aerosol cloud. It is reported that weaponized spores may be disseminated throughout an entire building even after delivery by a contained letter (6). As an example of the deadly nature of the spores, it was reported from the former Soviet Union that an outbreak near one of its weapons facilities in 1979 resulted in 77 cases of inhalational anthrax with 66 deaths (85% mortality) (4,6). In the fall of 2001, 22 cases of anthrax infection occurred following delivery of spores through the US Postal Service. Eleven of the cases were inhalational with five deaths occurring in that group, while the rest of the cases were cutaneous (4–6). The knowledge that strains of *B. anthracis* have been modified and may potentially be released creates a whole new outlook in public health policies. It is estimated that more than 30,000 potentially exposed persons were placed on postexposure prophylaxis during the US outbreak of 2001 (6). The direct and indirect costs of handling a limited contamination such as the 2001 mailed attacks are undoubtedly high.

The spores germinate in an environment rich in amino acids, nucleic acids, and glucose, such as in mammalian tissues or blood. The bacteria multiply rapidly and will only form spores again when the nutrients are depleted, such as when contaminated body fluids are discharged and encounter ambient air. The vegetative bacteria do not survive long in ambient conditions unlike their spore form which may remain stable for many years.

Inhalational anthrax begins when inhaled spore particles sized 1 to 5 $\mu$m enter alveolar spaces and are subsequently ingested by macrophages. Spores that survive and are not lysed may travel to the mediastinal lymphatic tissue where they germinate and multiply. The incubation period varies. Most often, incubation occurs within 1 to 7 days but can be delayed as much as 43 days (2,4–6). The replicating *B. anthracis* produces toxins that carry on cellular damage even if all living bacteria are eradicated with antibiotics (4,5). This ongoing damage results in hemorrhagic lymphadenitis, hemorrhagic mediastinitis, necrosis, and pleural effusions. The patient may present initially with fever, cough, dyspnea, and malaise. An initial chest radiograph may be abnormal with widened mediastinum, infiltrates, and effusion. The more fulminant case progresses rapidly with a continued rise in fever, worsening dyspnea, chest pain, and respiratory failure. Blood culture will usually show the characteristic colony formation, but direct communication with the lab is important when *B. anthracis* is suspected as such colonies may be mistaken for contaminant normal flora (2,5). Neurological complications, such as hemorrhagic meningitis, cerebral edema, parenchymal brain hemorrhages, vasculitis, and subarachnoid hemorrhage, can be associated with the three different forms of anthrax exposure. The aforementioned should be considered a fourth type of presentation that prompts investigation for bioterrorism (7). The organism may be identified readily in the cerebrospinal fluid in the presence of absence of CNS symptomatology.

Cutaneous anthrax occurs following the deposition of the spores in cuts or abrasions of the skin. Subsequently, germination occurs in the skin, and toxin production proceeds to local tissue edema and necrosis. A skin vesicle typically forms which then dries to form a black eschar. Antibiotic therapy will not alter the course of skin destruction and eschar resolution, but it will decrease the localized edema and the risk of systemic spread. Systemic spread may be possible, and untreated mortality is reported to be as high as 20% (4–7). Gastrointestinal anthrax may be contracted from ingestion of contaminated meat. Spores may germinate in either the upper or the lower intestinal tract. Ulcer formation in the mouth or esophagus may lead to regional lymphadenitis. In the lower tract, intestinal anthrax may lead to nausea, vomiting, acute abdomen, ascites, mesenteric lymphadenopathy, bowel edema, and bloody diarrhea. In both cases, death may occur due to systemic illness, and mortality as high as 25% to 60% has been reported (2,5–7). Unfortunately, there is limited information available on anthrax infection during pregnancy, but in general, usual nonpregnant therapeutic guidelines are employed given the high morbidity and mortality to the untreated patient let alone the treated individual (8).

It is important to remember that casual contact or respiratory droplets from coughing or sneezing do not spread anthrax. While person-to-person respiratory transmission does not occur, caution should be used when caring for patients with nonintact skin from cutaneous anthrax (2). Treatment consists of a combination therapy that usually includes ciprofloxacin and doxycycline and may also include clindamycin, rifampin, vancomycin, or chloramphenicol (5). The recommendations for appropriate antibiotic therapy are the same for pregnant women or children as for nonpregnant adults. One should check with an infectious disease consultant or the CDC website for the latest recommended drug combination. Supportive end organ therapy such as ventilator assistance is usually required for severe cases.

Prophylactic antimicrobial therapy is not needed unless law enforcement and public health officials document an actual exposure. It is recommended that the primary care women's health provider not initiate the therapy unless directed to do so by the appropriate public health officials (9). Screening may be performed by way of nasal swab, but due to potential error, postexposure prophylaxis is recommended only after a confirmed exposure or high-risk encounter (9).

The current CDC guidelines were based on susceptibilities determined from anthrax isolates from the intentional exposures in 2001 (7). These isolates were found to be sensitive to penicillin, amoxicillin, ciprofloxacin, doxycycline, chloramphenicol, clindamycin, tetracycline, rifampin, clarithromycin, and vancomycin. Adult exposure prophylaxis is typically given with ciprofloxacin 500 mg orally every 12 hours for 60 days or doxycycline 100 mg orally every 12 hours for 60 days (2). The recommendation is the same for pregnant and lactating women. The potential morbidity and mortality from anthrax are felt to outweigh the historical and theoretical concerns regarding these medications (9). If the anthrax isolate in a current case is found to be sensitive to penicillin, the pregnant or lactating patient should be switched to amoxicillin 500 mg orally three times a day for the remainder of the prophylaxis period (9).

Vaccination against anthrax may be performed. The vaccine, called anthrax vaccine adsorbed (AVA), is a cell-free product given in a six-dose series over 18 months (5). While there has been significant media coverage of concerns over side effects of the vaccine following the US military's mandated vaccination of active-duty and reserve-duty personnel, AVA is thought to be acceptably safe (5). Due to the potential for spores to remain dormant in tissues for prolonged periods despite antibiotic prophylaxis, there has been interest in the use of AVA for postexposure prophylaxis in conjunction with antibiotics (5,8). The vaccine should theoretically be safe for use during pregnancy due to a lack of an active organism. No published experience is available on the use of the vaccine during pregnancy, but the potential benefits may outweigh the risk associated with systemic diseases in the event of a large-scale exposure. Experience from the military vaccination program suggests no adverse effect on pregnancy outcomes for women vaccinated prior to becoming pregnant (10).

## Smallpox

Smallpox is caused by the DNA virus known as variola. It is easily transmitted from person to person by respiratory droplets. In addition, the virus may remain stable on fomites for up to 1 week (6). The virus replicates in respiratory epithelia and then migrates to regional lymph nodes. An initial viremia, accompanied by mild fever and malaise, will lead to introduction of the virions to a variety of tissues, resulting in localized infections in the kidneys, lungs, intestines, skin, and lymphoid tissues. After an incubation of 7 to 17 days, a second viremia occurs with high fevers, headache, backache, rigors, and vomiting. A rash is usually apparent within 48 hours of this new phase. The rash is initially maculopapular but changes soon to a vesicular eruption. The characteristic smallpox appearance is reached when the vesicles become pustules. Viral shedding may occur from the time of the rash until the lesions have crusted and separated. Death may occur in this phase due to overwhelming viremia and multiple organ failure (6).

Historical series of pregnant women affected by smallpox describe very high rates of prematurity and fetal loss (11). In addition, pregnant women appear more susceptible to the disease, with case-fatality rates as high as 61% among unvaccinated individuals and mortality rates of 27% even among vaccinated pregnant women. This compares with commonly reported mortality rates in nonpregnant adults of 3% when vaccinated and 30% among unvaccinated patients (2,11). Pregnant women develop the hemorrhagic form of the disease with increased frequency compared with nonpregnant women and men (8,11). This hemorrhagic form of smallpox is characterized by fever, backache, abdominal pain, and a diffuse red rash. Historically, spontaneous epistaxis, ecchymoses, and bleeding into various organs led to rapid patient deterioration. The case-fatality rate among women with hemorrhagic smallpox was 100% in one series. Congenital smallpox among live born infants has been reported to occur in as many as 9% to 60% cases, with a very high mortality rate (8,11).

Infected patients should be isolated in negative-pressure rooms. Anyone who has had direct contact with and infected person should undergo strict quarantine with respiratory isolation for 17 days (4). Especially in the setting of large numbers of infected individuals, quarantine and separate physical facilities may be required to minimize further disease spread. Airborne and body fluid contact precautions must be utilized. All discarded laundry or waste should be placed in biohazard bags and autoclaved prior to disposal (6). A certain number of hospital personnel may need to be vaccinated in advance in order to provide care in the event of a deliberate infection. Hospitals with maternity services should anticipate the need to designate obstetrical and neonatal physicians and nurses for a team response.

Cidofovir has been tried with success against other pox viruses and has been reported to show in vitro activity against variola, but it cannot yet be recommended as treatment (2,4). The principles of managing an outbreak of smallpox will be isolation and supportive care of infected patients and postexposure vaccination for contacts. Vaccination against smallpox is by inoculation of the related *Orthopoxvirus*, vaccinia. Vaccination is moderately effective at aborting or attenuating the disease if given within 4 days of an exposure (2,4). Complications from widespread vaccination with vaccinia in the past included localized dermal reactions, vaccinia gangrenosa (with local extensive skin necrosis at the site of inoculation), eczema vaccinatum (a super infection of eczema with the vaccinia virus), progressive vaccinia, and postvaccinial encephalitis (11). While pregnant mothers may be vaccinated, there is a low risk of a potentially fatal fetal infection from the vaccinia virus. Therefore, routine vaccination of pregnant women in nonemergent settings is not recommended. In the event of an actual bioterrorism event, a pregnant woman at risk for exposure must weigh the risks of adverse effect from the vaccine against the devastating outcomes associated with smallpox infection in pregnancy (11).

### Tularemia

Tularemia is a bacterial zoonosis first isolated by McCoy and Chapin in Tulare County, CA, in 1912 while searching for the causative agent of a disease affecting ground squirrels in the region. Documentation of this disease dates back to the 16th century in Norway and has been described throughout the northern hemisphere. Shortly after its isolation, Tularemia was recognized as a potential agent of severe and possibly fatal disease. A number of countries have done extensive research on its possible application as a biological weapon including Japan, Russia, and the United States. In the 1950s and 1960s, the US military developed weapons that could deliver aerosolized *Francisella tularensis* (12). Along with stock piling of weaponized *F. tularensis*, a live attenuated vaccine was developed that could partially protect against the virulent SCHU S4 strain and research was performed with various antibiotic regimens including streptomycin, tetracyclines, and chloramphenicol. With the termination of its biological weapons development program by executive order in 1970, all supplies were subsequently destroyed by 1973. Parallel efforts by the former Soviet Union continued into the 1990s with strains engineered that are resistant to vaccines and antibiotics (12). The impact of a weaponized release of Tularemia was estimated by the WHO in 1969 that aerosol dispersal of 50 kg of virulent *F. tularensis* over a metropolitan area with 5 million inhabitants would result in 250,000 incapacitation casualties including 19,000 fatalities (12).

The epidemiology of Tularemia is extremely complex. The organism has been isolated from over 200 animal species, including warm- and cold-blooded vertebrates, invertebrates, and numerous arthropods (13). Transmission can occur through several routes, including direct contact with the infected animals, arthropod vectors such as fleas and ticks, inhalation, and ingestion. In the United States, ticks are responsible for 75% of cases (14). Inhalational tularemia is extremely rare in the United States and should raise the suspicion of intentional use via aerosolized attack. Any case of tularemia is reportable to the CDC, but the inhalational form should be extremely concerning (14).

Clinically, tularemia can present in several forms, including ulceroglandular, oculoglandular, oropharyngeal, inhalational, typhoidal, and septic forms (12–14). Manifestations of the disease vary and are dependent on the route of exposure, dose, and virulence. In general, infection occurs 3 to 5 days after exposure with symptoms including abrupt onset of fever, chills headache, coryza, sore throat, myalgia, arthralgia, and fatigue (12). Hematogenous spread may also occur, causing meningitis, pericarditis, pneumonia, hepatitis, peritonitis, endocarditis, ataxia, osteomyelitis, sepsis, rhabdomyolysis, and acute renal failure (13). Ulceroglandular disease is the most common form of naturally presenting infection. Usual presentation includes the development of a tender pruritic papule at the site of infection. Progression to a painful ulcer and regional lymphadenitis occurs several days later. Over time, if not treated, spontaneous drainage of lymph nodes will occur. Oropharyngeal tularemia should be suspected in patients developing ulcerative pharyngitis or tonsillitis. Oculoglandular disease presents as a unilateral conjunctivitis with periauricular lymphadenitis. Inhalational tularemia will present like other pnuemonias with symptoms such as fever, nonproductive cough, dyspnea, and pleuritic chest pain. Radiographic examination of the chest may find peribronchial infiltrates, bronchiolar pneumonia in one or two lobes, pleural effusions, and hilar lymphadenopathy. Typhoidal tularemia describes systemic illness in the absence of localizing symptoms. Sepsis from tularemia is potentially fatal. Nonspecific findings of fever, abdominal pain, diarrhea, and vomiting may be present early. An individual with sepsis from tularemia will appear toxic and may develop confusion and coma. Prompt treatment is imperative with the possibility of shock, DIC, ARDS, and multisystem organ failure if treatment is delayed.

Diagnosis is first and foremost accomplished by a physician with a high index of clinical suspicion. Physicians that suspect tularemia should promptly collect specimens of respiratory secretions and blood. Specimens should be handled with care by laboratory personnel. Microscopic identification of *F. tularensis* may be accomplished with fluorescent-labeled antibodies. This is a rapid diagnostic procedure that is performed by laboratories in the National Public Health Laboratory Network (12). Culture is the definitive means of confirmatory testing and can be performed from pharyngeal washings, sputum, fasting gastric aspirates, and rarely from blood.

In the event of encountering a release of aerosolized tularemia, standard precautions can be used due to the highly unlikely transmission from human to human. Decontamination of spills or areas containing infected persons can be accomplished with a 10% bleach solution followed by a solution of 70% alcohol (13). Persons with exposure to aerosols containing tularemia should wash themselves and contaminated clothing with soap and water. Municipal water sources should remain safe secondary to their standard levels of chlorine. Public education should include avoidance of sick or dead animals and include precautions to take appropriate measures to avoid arthropod bites (13).

Antibiotic therapy for the general population can be determined by the classification of the cases as either contained- or mass-casualty situation.

For isolated cases in adults, a regimen of streptomycin 1 g IM or gentamicin 5 mg/kg should be administered for 10 days. With a mass-casualty exposure, doxycycline 100 mg orally twice daily for 14 days and ciprofloxacin 500 mg orally for 10 days are recommended. In the pregnant population, a course of gentamicin is recommended in the contained-casualty situation and is likely to pose a low risk to the fetus. In the event of a mass-casualty exposure, the recommended regimen consists of oral ciprofloxacin. Prophylactic antibiotic treatment is recommended to persons who are asymptomatic. In the pregnant female, a 14-day course of ciprofloxacin is recommended.

## Plague
Plague has held a special place in world history with multiple pandemics, leading to the death of millions of people. The bacillus, *Yersinia pestis*, is generally transmitted to humans from a rodent host by way of a flea vector. However, direct host-to-host transmission may occur by way of an infectious aerosol from affected individuals. This makes the disease extremely contagious. The disease is rapidly fatal in the absence of an appropriate antibiotic treatment (6). There have been attempts in the past to create a weapon out of plague; however, most such attempts have met with limited success. Still, plague represents a potential bioterrorism threat by way of an aerosol or inhalational route.

Typical bubonic plague is acquired from the bite of a flea, which regurgitates the *Y. Pestis* from its foregut. The organisms rapidly multiply and spread to regional lymph nodes within 1 to 8 days. The infection of lymph nodes creates a characteristic bubo, which is a large tender area of inflammation within the regional lymph node. From there, the patient may become septic within several days. Some patients will develop pneumonia and begin to shed *Yersinia* organisms in their cough droplets. Patients typically develop a productive cough with blood-tinged sputum within 24 hours of the onset of symptoms (6). Plague can also be ingested from a contaminated food source. The gastrointestinal form of the disease also follows a rapid course with the buboes developing in mesenteric drainage sites. Persons infected by the inhalation route may not develop the typical buboes but may progress rapidly to septicemia.

The definitive diagnosis is made by a sputum Gram stain showing Gram-negative coccobacilli with bipolar "safety pin" staining. The chest radiograph may show consolidating lobar pneumonia. Further tests include an IgM enzyme immunoassay, antigen detection, and polymerase chain reaction (2). These tests are available typically through state health departments and the CDC. This approach requires a high index of suspicion to obtain these tests early enough to involve state organizations in containment. Patients with suspected bubonic plague should be separated from other patients, preferably under negative-pressure conditions, and body fluid precautions followed until at least 3 days of appropriate antibiotics have been completed (6). Patients who are suspected of being septic, having respiratory symptoms, or are diagnosed with pneumonic plague should be maintained under respiratory droplet precautions including negative-pressure isolation until the completion of at least four or more days of antibiotic therapy (6).

Standard therapy is 10 days of intravenous antibiotic, which may be switched to oral therapy when patients begin to improve. For nonpregnant adults, the recommended treatment is streptomycin 1 mg intramuscularly twice a day or gentamicin 5 mg/kg IM or IV every 24 hours. Other choices include chloramphenicol or fluoroquinolones. For patients with suspected meningitis, chloramphenicol is considered mandatory because of its superior penetration of the CNS. The dose is 50 to 75 mg/kg per day (2,6).

It is thought that the major determinant of outcome for the mother and child is the timing of antibiotic administration (6). The fetus is susceptible to exposure to *Y. pestis* in utero or through contact with maternal blood. Historically, plague acquired during pregnancy led to nearly universal fetal loss and could be especially severe in the pregnant woman (8). Gentamicin should be substituted for streptomycin in the case of pregnancy. Chloramphenicol should be used with caution in pregnant women due to potential adverse effects on fetus and newborn. Doxycycline and ciprofloxacin have also been considered as alternative regimens. Their use in this situation would represent a choice between benefits from treating the infection and potential risks of medication exposure to the fetus (8). Empiric treatment of the newborn following delivery of an infected mother should also be considered. In the event of a bioterrorist attack, it is thought that postexposure prophylaxis would be necessary to prevent rapid spread of the disease within the population. The decision would have to be made whether or not to place pregnant patients on the recommended prophylaxis of doxycycline 100 mg twice a day based on the risk of exposure and spread of the disease (8). Again, timely treatment with the appropriate antibiotics is very important in affecting the maternal outcome in pregnancy. Untreated, the mortality from plague is estimated at close to 100%. Even in treated cases, pneumonic plague is highly lethal with up to 50% to 60% mortality despite appropriate antibiotic therapy. In general, given the immunosuppressed state and normal physiological adaptations of pregnancy, a higher mortality would be anticipated. Thus, the dilemma of treating pregnant women with medications such as doxycycline, which are not typically used in the pregnant population, emphasizes the importance of carefully evaluating the exposure risk and the need for ongoing assessment and coordination of the disaster event with local, state, and federal authorities.

## Q Fever

Q fever is caused by a small intracellular bacterium known as *Coxiella burnetii*. This agent would be attractive for use in bioterrorism because of the ease with which it causes infection since a single viable organism is adequate (4). Most immunocompetent persons have a self-limited infection without serious long-term complications, although chronic infection and endocarditis may occur in a small portion of infected individuals and can be debilitating. Hepatic transaminase levels are frequently elevated and the peripheral white blood cell count is normal (4). An intentional release of Q fever would more likely be intended to cause disruption and psychological effects rather than mass casualties with overall mortality as low as 2.4% (4). The organism has long been known for its association with infection leading to abortion in animals. More recent information suggests that an effect on fetal loss is true in humans as well.

Q fever is generally obtained through inhalation of *Coxiella* organisms. The organisms are carried in body fluids such as the amniotic fluid of farm animals. A spore-like form can survive heat and drying with the capability to spread in the air (4). The incubation period is between 2 and 14 days. The clinical manifestations are similar to other nonspecific viral illnesses with fever, chills, and headache. The patient may also experience malaise, anorexia, and weight loss. More serious complications include neurological derangements in at least 23% of acute cases (2).

The diagnosis is generally made by the clinical complaints along with patchy infiltrates on chest x-ray, no cough, and a history consistent with exposure (4). Serology for IgG and IgM to *Coxiella* can be identified with antibodies appearing during the 2nd week of the illness. Convalescent titers usually show a fourfold increase after 2 to 3 months (4). The typical treatment for uncomplicated infections or prophylaxis for a nonpregnant adult is with doxycycline twice a day for 5 to 7 days. Chronic infections may require prolonged combination therapy (4). Fluoroquinolones may also be considered for empiric therapy. The disease is not thought to be contagious from person to person (2). A vaccine is extensively used in Australia, but it is not approved for use in the United States (15).

While Q fever has long been implicated as a cause of low birth weight and abortion in farm animals, more recent data from France suggest that it has a significant role in human pregnancy as well (16). Acute infection during the first trimester leads to a very high rate of spontaneous abortion in untreated patients. Acute infection in the second or third trimester is less commonly associated with fetal loss but can be associated with low birth weight and premature delivery. The recommended treatment is trimethoprim 320 mg with sulfamethoxazole 1,600 mg daily for the duration of the pregnancy. Chronic infection is more common in women who develop the acute infection during pregnancy as compared to acquisition in the nonpregnant patient. This is thought to be related to the relatively immunocompromised state of pregnancy (16). The use of trimethoprim/sulfamethoxazole during pregnancy reduces the frequency of abortion as well as reduces the number of women with identifiable *Coxiella* in the placenta at delivery (16). Such treated patients are still at risk for early delivery and low birth weight. Long-term treatment after delivery for the woman is also recommended to resolve the chronic infection. The recommended postpartum regimen is doxycycline 100 mg twice daily and hydroxychloroquine 600 mg daily for 1 year following the pregnancy. For women who are appropriately treated, subsequent pregnancies seem to be unaffected. Similarly, women who acquire and resolve the acute infection prior to becoming pregnant also do not show a lasting effect on pregnancy outcomes (16). Breastfeeding is not recommended for women with acute Q fever.

### Ricin

Ricin is a potent toxin easily derived from the beans of the castor plant (*Ricinus communis*). The toxin received media attention as an agent of bioterrorism through the arrest of six persons in Manchester, England, in December of 2002, who allegedly produced the toxin in their apartment as part of a potential attack. The discovery of powdered ricin in the mailroom serving former US Senate Majority Leader Bill Frist's office in February, 2004, resulted in renewed fears regarding vulnerability to an attack with this toxin. The potential for ricin to be a weapon of mass destruction rests in the ease of producing the toxin and its stability, which allows for relatively easy dissemination with low risk of detection. The amount of ricin necessary to produce the effects is also very small.

The protein is derived in the processing of castor beans, the oil of which is used in industrial settings, including a component of brake or hydraulic fluid (17). The waste mash or aqueous phase of the oil production is 5% to 10% ricin, which can then be isolated through the common technique of chromatography. The toxins RCL III and RCL IV are relatively small dimeric proteins consisting of an "A" chain and a "B" chain. After entry to the cell by binding to cell surface glycoproteins, the toxins inhibit the 60S ribosomal subunit, preventing continued protein synthesis. The interruption of protein synthesis eventually leads to cell death (17).

In the event of inhalational exposure, symptoms are related to irritation of the lungs. Respiratory symptoms will begin usually 4 to 8 hours after the exposure. Early symptoms can include fever, chest tightness, cough, and dyspnea. Within 1 to 2 days, severe inflammation of the respiratory tract, cell death, and the development of acute respiratory distress syndrome may be expected. The treatment consists only of respiratory support with mechanical ventilation.

(2,3). There has been fear that ricin might be used also to contaminate the water or food supply. This seems to be more difficult considering the large lethal dose extrapolated for humans (15). In the event of a gastrointestinal exposure, symptoms would be expected from necrosis of the gastrointestinal epithelium as well as damage to spleen, liver, and kidneys. Symptoms might manifest as abdominal cramps and nausea, as well as high output gastrointestinal fluid loss. Ricin is thought to be much less toxic when ingested rather than inhaled, although a large gastrointestinal exposure could lead to enough necrotic multiorgan damage to produce hemorrhage and hypovolemic shock (2,3).

The diagnosis may be confirmed by ELISA testing, although this is not widely available (4). Patients should be treated by decontamination with removal of garments and cleansing with soap and water. Outside of contact with residual, undetected toxin remaining on the victim, there is thought to be little secondary risk to emergency department personnel; however, as with all patients, the observation of universal contact precautions is prudent. There is no direct antidote to the toxin, although gastric decontamination with charcoal has been reported to be potentially of benefit in some cases (2–4,15). Supportive care is the main approach to management. In the case of a pregnancy, the size of the toxin makes it unlikely to readily cross with ease to the fetus. The outcome for the baby will depend on the supportive care of the mother.

## TOXINS OR CHEMICALS

There are several compounds that may be encountered as either the result of an intentional release, such as in the case of the release of nerve gas on a Japanese subway, or in the event of an industrial accident. For the most part, care of the pregnant patient will differ little from the nonpregnant patient. The lethal agents are classified into four categories: nerve agents or anticholinesterases, vesicants or blistering agents, choking or pulmonary agents, and cyanogens or "blood" agents (18).

### Nerve Agents—Acetylcholinesterase Inhibitors

These are organophosphorus compounds and include tabun, sarin, soman, GF, and VX. Their primary mechanism of action is through the inhibition of acetylcholinesterase at synapses and neuromuscular junctions. The tyrylcholinesterase in plasma and acetylcholinesterase in the red blood cell are also inhibited. The result is an excess of acetylcholine leading to hypersecretion and bronchoconstriction in airways, mental status changes, nausea, vomiting, and muscle fasciculation and weakness (18). A large exposure may be rapidly fatal with loss of consciousness, seizures, and apnea from respiratory muscle paralysis and central nervous system depression. The agents are usually clear and colorless and may be disseminated as either a vapor or a liquid. Exposure may be through skin absorption, inhalation, or gastrointestinal ingestion. Inhalation is more effective than absorption through intact skin (19).

Patients with a large exposure or significant symptoms should be treated with atropine and pralidoxime (2-PAM) (18). Atropine competes with the accumulated acetylcholine and diminishes the cholinergic effects. Pralidoxime dissociates the nerve agent from the cholinesterase and is excreted in the urine as a complex with the agent (19). Atropine is commonly given as a 2-mg intramuscular or intravenous dose and is sometimes available for self-administration via an auto-injector. The patient should be reevaluated every 10 to 15 minutes, and a repeat dose given until secretions decrease or breathing becomes easier (19). Pralidoxime also can be given as 600 to 1,000 mg intramuscularly or as a slow intravenous dose. Timing of administration is important as the cholinesterase enzyme will dissociate less easily from the organophosphate as time passes.

The aging time is different for each nerve agent (19). If severe respiratory distress is apparent, intubation should be accomplished. In addition, severely injured victims should be given a benzodiazepine (diazepam, lorazepam, or midazolam) to raise the seizure threshold and help prevent secondary anoxic brain injury (18,19). Successfully treated patients should begin to recover within a few hours, but neurological symptoms may persist for weeks.

There is little information available on the fetal effects of such an exposure. The fetus will be particularly susceptible to any respiratory depression or anoxia in the mother. Theoretically, the compounds may be able to reach the fetal brain with some behavioral depression likely, which may alter fetal biophysical or non-stress testing or maternal perception of fetal activity. Ultimately, fetal survival will depend on the expeditious and appropriate care of the mother.

### Vesicants and Pulmonary Agents

The vesicants, such as mustard gas and lewisite, are easily absorbed through the skin and mucous membranes. The damage may not be evident until 2 to 12 hours after contact (19). Damage is caused by cross-linking and methylation of DNA. Blisters may form on the skin in the early stages. Skin sloughing will later place the patient at risk for secondary infection. Wounds should be cared for the same way as scald burns; systemic antibiotics are not necessary (19). Similarly, the damage to lung tissues results in a chemical pneumonia that may also lead to secondary infection. Mortality is generally low from an acute attack with overall mortality rates at 2% to 5%, but the number of people affected may be high and caring for the high morbidity will consume a large amount of medical resources and health care dollars (18,19).

Similarly, pulmonary agents, such as phosgene and chlorine, lead to damage in the respiratory tract within hours of exposure. Hydrolysis of the inhaled gas produces hydrochloric acid that mediates the local tissue toxicity (19). The effect with this agent involves damage to the alveolar–capillary membrane and subsequent reactionary pulmonary edema. The lung's ability to clear the excess fluid will be overcome and dyspnea will result. There can be a delay in the onset of lung failure up to 48 hours. Victims usually require mechanical ventilation, but survival past 48 hours generally suggests that recovery is likely and purports a favorable long-term outcome (18,19). Care is supportive and early tracheotomy is advisable for severe exposure. Preventive antibiotics are not indicated and will only result in microbial selection. Some degree of lung fibrosis and pulmonary restriction can be seen in severe cases (19).

## RADIATION

Public concern over radiation exposure has been elevated by worries about the safety of nuclear power facilities, the transport and disposal of nuclear waste, or the threatened use of radiation-contaminated weapons—so-called dirty bombs. Much is known about the consequences of inadvertent exposure. Damage can range from skin reddening to cancer induction and death. Particularly relevant to pregnancy is the fact that rapidly growing fetuses and children are more susceptible to the subtle effects of radiation exposure than are adult tissues (20,21). Damage is also cumulative, with increasing or repetitive exposures resulting in more severe damage (20).

"Dirty bombs" are typically intended to spread radiation in such a way as to make areas unusable. Depending on the source, the amount of radiation released from such a weapon is unlikely to cause severe forms of acute radiation syndrome (20). From the United Nations' report of Iraq's testing of dirty bombs in 1987, the Iraqis deemed that radiation levels achieved were too low to cause

Biological Effects of Total Body Irradiation

| Amount of Exposure | Effect |
|---|---|
| 50 mGy (5 rad) | No detectable injury |
| 1 Gy (100 rad) | Nausea and vomiting for 1–2 d, temporary drop in new blood cell production |
| 3.5 Gy (350 rad) | Nausea and vomiting initially, followed by periods of apparent wellness. At 3–4 weeks, may see deficiencies of white blood cells and platelets |
| >3.5 Gy | May be fatal |

*Source*: Ref. 20.

significant damage and the project was abandoned. In a modern context, such weapons would likely be used to disrupt routines and generate fear in the general public (Table 10.1).

The management of the initial exposure to radiation adheres to the principles of decreasing the time near the source, increasing the distance from the source, and the use of physical barriers, such as glass or concrete to shield an individual from exposure (20,22). In the event of an exposure, it is recommended to leave the area on foot. Do not take cars or public transit that may harbor contaminated dusts. Make use of barriers by entering buildings. Clothes are to be removed and bagged for later disposal. A shower may remove contaminated dust or debris from the skin (20).

Radiation exposure can result in significant dysfunction to many organs within the body. Depending on the dose and length of time of exposure, as well as the mechanism of exposure, injury may range from a local injury such as a burn to a more widespread injury such as the acute radiation syndrome (ARS) (22,23). A local injury often involves exposed contact areas like the hands and face. Patients may present with erythema, blistering, desquamation, and ulceration of the skin. The patient may or may not realize when the exposure might have occurred. For example, handling an unknown metallic object might be the source of exposure. Such injuries generally evolve slowly and the full extent of injury may not be known for several weeks. Conventional wound management may be ineffective (23).

The ARS is a quickly developing illness caused by a total body exposure to radiation. It is characterized by damage of several organ systems due to the effect of ionizing radiation, leading to a deficiency in cell numbers or cell function. Radioactive sources provoking ARS might consist of machines that emit gamma rays, x-rays, or neutrons. There are four phases of ARS (23). The first is a prodromal phase in which a patient might experience nausea, vomiting, and loss of appetite. Generally, these symptoms disappear within 1 to 2 days and a symptom-free latency period may follow. The length of the latent period may vary depending on the radiation dose. A period of full-blown illness may then follow with electrolyte imbalances, diarrhea, hematologic abnormalities, and even CNS changes. The overt illness results either in death or in slow, eventual recovery (23). Severe organ dysfunction that may be noticed includes low white blood cell count leading to immunodeficiency. A gastrointestinal syndrome also may occur with loss of the cells lining the gut, leading to water and electrolyte loss through vomiting, diarrhea, and impaired nutrient absorption. The patient may also demonstrate confusion and disorientation resulting from the dramatic changes in dehydration and electrolyte imbalance. These mental status changes, including periods of unconsciousness, are generally considered a poor prognostic sign (22,23). Full recovery is possible and may occur over a prolonged period of time, from several weeks to 2 years.

The initial management of a large radiation exposure includes treating traumatic injuries (fractures, lacerations) as they would normally be managed. In addition, care should be taken to remove external contaminants. The history should focus on details of the source of exposure including the type of radiation, the proximity to the source, and the length of time of the exposure (23). A careful medical history should be obtained and, in the case of pregnant women, an estimate of the gestational age and a summary of pregnancy history included. Diagnosis of ARS may be aided by following the complete blood count every 4 to 6 hours. A significant drop in the absolute lymphocyte count and platelet count may aid in timing the exposure (22,23). Suspected exposures <2 Gy may not need to be hospitalized. Prospective evaluation of the white blood cell count with differential over the course of the next few days may be appropriate. Nausea and vomiting in the early phase might not be present for someone with <7.5 to 8.0 Gy of exposure (22,23) (Table 10.2).

For more severe ARS with a known higher exposed dose, supportive care should be the rule. Initial care of nausea and vomiting can be managed with selective serotonin $5HT_3$ receptor antagonists (23). Admission to the hospital is required. The anticipated drop in blood cell count merits consideration of antiviral prophylaxis and possibly neutropenic precautions. Management should be performed in conjunction with a hematologist or someone knowledgeable in radiation illness (23).

Potassium iodide has been considered as a means of protecting thyroid function in the event of an acute population exposure to radiation (24). This becomes useful primarily in the event of exposure to radioactive iodine, which is typically present early in a nuclear explosion and decays rapidly. Radioactive iodine is potentially taken up by the thyroid gland and leads to destruction of the normal glandular tissue. Potassium iodide salt taken with the first 3 to 4 hours of an event saturates the thyroid gland's iodine uptake mechanism, blocking the uptake of the radioactive form. Due to the quick decay of the radioactive iodine, usually only a single dose is needed (24).

Because of the relatively greater activity of the thyroid gland in children, potassium iodide is the recommended treatment for children, as well as adults up to age 40. Adults are to receive one tablet or 130 mg. Children between the ages of 3 and 18 are to receive one half tablet (65 mg). Children 1 to 3 years of age receive 32 mg, and under 1 year of age, 16 mg is the recommended dose. The adult dose therapy is recommended for pregnant women, as the fetus is also susceptible. Women who are breastfeeding should also be given the usual adult dose, and the child should receive the appropriate dose based on age (24).

In conclusion, the practitioner is recommended to always consult the CDC and governing authorities for the most up-to-date recommendations and treatments (Table 10.3). In general, most threats are dealt with in the pregnant patient as in the nonpregnant patient. Therapy largely is supportive with some individualized therapeutic choices for certain biological and other terroristic acts. Fetal effects may vary but are almost always correlated with maternal status. A coordinated plan with authorities and general common sense measures of minimizing exposure, good decontamination procedures, and appropriate universal precautions remain the stalwarts of therapy and prevention of further spread. In almost all cases, breastfeeding would be contraindicated. Plan of care should be coordinated with first response providers, obstetrical care team, and tertiary referral centers (25–27).

**Acute Radiation Syndrome (Whole Body or Extensive Partial Body)**

| Dose (Gy) | Clinical Status | Description |
|---|---|---|
| 0–1 | Generally asymptomatic | White blood count normal or minimally depressed below baseline levels at 3–5 weeks postaccident. |
| 1–8 | Hematopoietic syndrome | Main prodromal signs and symptoms include anorexia, nausea, vomiting, and, occasionally, skin erythema, fever, mucositis, and diarrhea. Laboratory analysis in cases with whole-body exposure >2 Gy can show an initial granulocytosis, with pancytopenia evident 20–30 d postaccident. Subsequent systemic effects of the hematological phase of ARS include immunodysfunction, increased infectious complications, possible hemorrhage, sepsis, anemia, and impaired wound healing. |
| 8–30 | Gastrointestinal syndrome | Symptoms may include early, severe nausea, vomiting, and watery diarrhea, often within hours postaccident. In severe cases, the patient may present with shock, and possibly renal failure and cardiovascular collapse. Death from gastrointestinal syndrome usually occurs 8–14 d postaccident. Hematopoietic syndrome occurs concomitantly. |
| >20 | Cardiovascular/central nervous syndrome | Patients may experience a burning sensation within minutes of exposure, nausea and vomiting within the first hour postaccident, prostration, and neurological signs of ataxia and confusion. Death is inevitable and usually occurs with 24–48 hr. |

*Source*: Adapted from Medical preparedness and response subgroup of the Homeland Security Department working group on Radiological Dispersal devices (RDD) and Preparedness (p. 15), December 9, 2003 update. Available at: http://www1.va.gov/emshg/docs/Radiological_Medical_Countermeasures_Indexed-Final.pdf. Cited April 12, 2009. Ref. 22.

| TABLE 10.3 | Useful Web Links |

**American College of Physicians—Bioterrorism Resources**
http://www.acponline.org/clinical_information/resources/bioterrorism/?chapinc

**Agency for Healthcare Research and Quality—Bioterrorism Planning and Response**
http://www.ahrq.gov/prep

**American Academy of Pediatrics**
http://www.aap.org/disasters/index.cfm

**American Hospital Association—Disaster Readiness**
http://www.aha.org/aha_app/issues/Emergency-Readiness/index.jsp

**American Medical Association—AMA Center for Disaster Preparedness and Emergency Response**
http://www.ama-assn.org/ama/pub/physician-resources/public-health/center-public-health-preparedness-disaster-response.shtml

**Anthrax**
Anthrax as a biological weapon, 2002: updated recommendations for management. *JAMA*. 2002 May;287(17):2236–2252.
http://jama.ama-assn.org/cgi/content/short/287/17/2236

Anthrax as a biological weapon: medical and public health management. *JAMA*. 1999 May;281(18):1735–1745.
http://jama.ama-assn.org/cgi/content/short/281/18/1735

**Botulism**
Botulinum toxin as a biological weapon: medical and public health management. *JAMA*. 2001 Feb;285(8):1059–1070.
http://jama.ama-assn.org/cgi/content/short/285/8/1059

**Plague**
Plague as a biological weapon: medical and public health management. *JAMA*. 2000 May;283(17):2281–2290.
http://jama.ama-assn.org/cgi/content/short/283/17/2281

**Smallpox**
Smallpox as a biological weapon: medical and public health management. *JAMA*. 1999 June;281(22):2127–2137.
http://jama.ama-assn.org/cgi/content/short/281/22/2127

**Tularemia**
Tularemia as a biological weapon: medical and public health management. *JAMA*. 2001 June;285(21):2763–2773.
http://jama.ama-assn.org/cgi/content/short/285/21/2763

**American Red Cross—Preparing for Events—Terrorism**
http://www.redcross.org/portal/site/en/menuitem.53fabf6cc033f17a2b1ecfbf43181aa 0/?
vgnextoid = d8d1779a32ecb110VgnVCM10000089f0870aRCRD&vgnextfmt = default

**Association for Professionals in Infection Control and Epidemiology—Bioterrorism Resources**
http://www.apic.org/Content/NavigationMenu/PracticeGuidance/Topics/Bioterrorism/Bioterrorism.htm

*(continued)*

TABLE
10.3    Useful Web Links *(continued)*

**Center for Biosecurity of the University of Pittsburge Medical Center (UPMC)**
http://www.upmc-biosecurity.org

**National Center for Environmental Health**
http://www.cdc.gov/nceh

**National Center for Immunization and Respiratory Diseases**
http://www.cdc.gov/vaccines

**National Center for Preparedness, Detection, and Control of Infectious Diseases**
http://www.cdc.gov/ncpdcid

**National Center for Zoonotic, Vector-Borne, and Enteric Diseases**
http://www.cdc.gov/nczved

**Public Health Emergency Preparedness and Response**
http://www.bt.cdc.gov

**Anthrax**
http://www.bt.cdc.gov/agent/anthrax

**Botulism**
http://www.bt.cdc.gov/agent/botulism

**Plague**
http://www.bt.cdc.gov/agent/plague

**Smallpox**
http://www.bt.cdc.gov/agent/smallpox

**Tularemia**
http://www.bt.cdc.gov/agent/tularemia

**Department of Energy**
http://www.energy.gov

**Lawrence Berkeley National Laboratory**
http://securebuildings.lbl.gov/printer.html

**DisasterHelp**
http://www.disasterhelp.gov

**Disaster Preparedness and Emergency Response Association**
http://www.disasters.org

**Doctors for Disaster Preparedness**
http://www.ddponline.org

**Federal Emergency Management Agency**
http://www.fema.gov

**Are You Ready: A Guide to Citizen Preparedness**
http://www.fema.gov/areyouready

*(continued)*

**TABLE 10.3**    Useful Web Links *(continued)*

***Food and Drug Administration—Center for Drug Evaluation and Research (CDER)***
http://www.fda.gov/cder

**CDER Drug Preparedness and Response to Bioterrorism**
http://www.fda.gov/cder/drugprepare/default.htm

***Johns Hopkins University—Bloomberg School of Public Health—Center for Public Health Preparedness***
http://www.jhsph.edu/preparedness

**National Library of Medicine**
http://www.nlm.nih.gov

**MEDLINEplus Health Information—Biodefense and Bioterrorism**
http://www.nlm.nih.gov/medlineplus/biodefenseandbioterrorism.html

**MEDLINEplus Health Information—Chemical Weapons**
http://www.nlm.nih.gov/medlineplus/chemicalemergencies.html

**MEDLINEplus Health Information—Disaster Preparation and Recovery**
http://www.nlm.nih.gov/medlineplus/disasterpreparationandrecovery.html

**Wireless Information System for Emergency Responders**
http://wiser.nlm.nih.gov

***PrepareNow.org***
http://www.preparenow.org

## References

1. Bleck TP. Fundamentals of disaster management. In: Farmer JC, Jimenez EJ, Talmor DS, Zimmerman JL. *Fundamentals of Disaster Management.* Des Plaines, IL: Society of Critical Care Medicine; 2003:1–8.
2. Agrawal AG, O'Grady NP. Biologic agents and syndromes. In: Farmer JC, Jimenez EJ, Talmor DS, Zimmerman JL. *Fundamentals of Disaster Management.* Des Plaines, IL: Society of Critical Care Medicine; 2003:71–93.
3. Moran GJ. Threats in bioterrorism II: CDC category B and C agents. *Emerg Med Clin North Am.* 2002;20:311–330.
4. Moran, GJ, Talan, DA, Abrahamian, FM. Biological terrorism. *Infect Dis Clin North Am.* 2008;22:145–187.
5. Inglesby TV, O'Toole T, Henderson DA, et al. Anthrax as a biological weapon, 2002; updated recommendations for management. *JAMA.* 2002;287(17):2236–2252.
6. Darling RG, Catlett CL, Huebner KD, Jarrett DG. Threats in bioterrorism I: CDC category A agents. *Emerg Med Clin North Am.* 2002;20:273–309.
7. Kyriacou, DN, Adamski, A, Khardori, N. Anthrax: from antiquity and obscurity to a front-runner in bioterrorism. *Infect Dis Clin North Am.* 2006;20:227–251.
8. White SR, Henretig FM, Dukes RG. Medical management of vulnerable populations and co-morbid conditions of victims of bioterrorism. *Emerg Med Clin North Am.* 2002;20:365–392.
9. Management of asymptomatic pregnant or lactating women exposed to anthrax. ACOG Committee Opinion No. 268. American College of Obstetricians and Gynecologists. *Obstet Gynecol.* 2002;99:366–368.

10. Wiesen AR, Littell CT. Relationship between prepregnancy anthrax vaccination and pregnancy and birth outcomes among US army women. *JAMA*. 2002;287(12): 1556–1560.

11. Suarez VR, Hankins GDV. Smallpox and pregnancy: from eradicated disease to bioterrorist threat. *Obstet Gynecol*. 2002;100:87–93.

12. Dennis, D, Inglesby, T, Henderson, D, et al. Tularemia as a biological weapon: medical and public health management. *JAMA*. 2001;285(21):2763–2773.

13. Eliasson, H, Broman, T Forsman, M, Back, E, Tularemia: current epidemiology and disease management. *Infect Dis Clin North Am*. 2006;20:289–311.

14. Kman N, Nelson R. Infectious agents of bioterrosim: a review for emergency physicians. *Emerg Med Clin North Am*. 2008;26:517–547

15. Pappas, G, Panagopoulou, P, Christou, L, Akritidis, N. Category B. Potential bioterrorism agents: bacteria, viruses, toxins, and foodborne and waterborne pathogens. *Infect Dis Clin North Am*. 2006;20:396–421.

16. Raoult D, Fenollar F, Stein A. Q fever during pregnancy. *Arch Intern Med*. 2002;162: 701–704.

17. Mirarchi FL, Allswede M. CBRNE—Ricin. *e-medicine* 2004. In: Mothershead JL, Talavera F, Darling RG, Halamka J, Roberge RJ. Available at: http://www.emedicine. com/emerg/topic889.htm. Cited May 15, 2009.

18. Lantz G, Talmor DS. Chemical agents and syndromes. In: Farmer JC, Jimenez EJ, Talmor DS, Zimmerman JL. *Fundamentals of Disaster Management*. Des Plaines, IL: Society of Critical Care Medicine; 2003:57–70.

19. Fry DE. Chemical threats. *Surg Clin North Am*. 2006;86:637–647.

20. Oak Ridge Institute for Science and Education, Radiation Emergency Assistance Center/ Training Site. Guidance for radiation accident management. Types of radiation exposure. Available at: http://www.orau.gov/reacts/injury.htm. Cited May 19, 2009.

21. Guidelines for diagnostic imaging during pregnancy. ACOG Committee Opinion No. 299. American College of Obstetricians and Gynecologists, 2004. Available at: http://www.acog.org/publications/committee_opinions/co299.cfm. Retrieved May 25, 2009.

22. Flyn DF, Goans, nuclear terrorism: triage and medical management of radiation and combined-injury casualties. *Surg Clin North Am*. 2006;86:601–636.

23. Oak Ridge Institute for Science and Education, Radiation Emergency Assistance Center/Training Site. Guidance for radiation accident management. Managing radiation emergencies: acute radiation syndrome. Available at: http://www.orau.gov/ reacts/syndrome.htm#Acute. Retrieved March 7, 2004.

24. Centers for Disease Control. Emergency preparedness & response. Radiation emergencies: potassium iodide. Available at: http://www.bt.cdc.gov/radiation/ki.asp. Cited May 25, 2009.

25. Mushtaq, A, El-Azizi, M, Khardori N. Category C potential bioterrorism agents and emerging pathogens. *Infect Dis Clin North Am*. 2006;20:423–441.

26. Koirala, J. Plague: disease, management, and recognition of act of terrorism. *Infect Dis Clin North Am*. 2006;20:273–287.

27. Cono J, Cragan JD, Jamieson DJ, Rasmussen SA. Prophylaxis and treatment of pregnant women for emerging infections and bioterrorism emergencies. Medscape published 11/21/2006. Cited May 25, 2009.

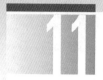

# Mosquito-Borne Illnesses: Western Nile Virus

## Carlos Torres, Allison H. Luper, and C. David Adair

West Nile virus (WNV) is a mosquito borne single-stranded RNA flavivirus, which targets the human nervous system, and can generate viral infections ranging in severity from a mild flu-like presentation known as West Nile fever (WNF) up to an acute neuroinvasive form of illness known as West Nile meningoencephalitis (WNME).

For those infected, cases of WNV generally remain clinically unapparent or present mild flu-like symptoms subsiding before treatment is ever sought. For patients who do require treatment, options are limited, as neither a vaccine nor direct treatment has been fully devised to combat human cases of WNV; the only means of decreasing the morbidity and the mortality of the disease remains mosquito management and avoidance. For this reason, careful planning is necessary especially in the case of immunocompromised individuals, who are at greater risk of contracting more severe forms of the disease.

The immunosuppressive accommodations made by a mother's body on the behalf of a fetus during pregnancy may leave expectant mothers more susceptible to WNV than people with full immunocompetence (1,2). There are data from animal models that support this concept (3). There have also been several documented cases of the virus being capable of maternal fetal transmission but not automatic (1,4–6).

## EXPOSURE

Less than 1% of the people bitten by mosquitoes will ever be exposed to WNV and only approximately 20% of WNV-exposed individuals will ever develop the symptoms associated with WNF according to the Center for Disease Control's (CDC) records (7). Of those people infected who become symptomatic, it is estimated that 10% will seek medical attention for their illness.

The more severe neuroinvasive expression is far less common than 1 in 10 exposed and occurs in only 1 in 150 exposed individuals (<1%) (7). In the group that does contract WNME, there is a documented death rate of 8% to 14%, with deaths occurring only in the United States and Israel (8) (Table 11.1).

## EPIDEMIOLOGY

WNV is a mosquito-borne single-stranded RNA flavivirus of the Japanese encephalitis antigenic serocomplex, which targets the human nervous system (9). Although similar to other members of its serocomplex, WNV shares its greatest similarities with St. Louis encephalitis, Murray Valley encephalitis, Kunkin, and Japanese encephalitis, with which it can be easily confused (9).

WNF infection was first documented as early as 1937 in a febrile adult woman in the West Nile District of Uganda. The more severe WNME first came to light in an Israeli nursing home in 1957 (8,10). Despite WNV's long-standing history throughout Africa, Europe, and western Asia, outbreaks have been mild until 1990; however, since 1990, there has been a disturbing trend toward more

| TABLE 11.1 | Percentage Outcomes of Individuals Exposed to WNV |
|---|---|
| WNF | 20.00% |
| Seek Care | 10.00% |
| WNME | 0.67% |

| TABLE 11.2 | Case Figures of Domestic WNV Infection From 1999 Through August 22, 2004 (1,5,7,15–18) | | | |
|---|---|---|---|---|
| **Year** | **Total Cases** | **Neuroinvasive** | **Deaths** | **Pregnant Cases** |
| 1999 | 62 | *a* | 7 | *a* |
| 2000 | 21 | *a* | 2 | *a* |
| 2001 | 66 | *a* | 9 | *a* |
| 2002 | 4,156 | 2,942 | 284 | 5 |
| 2003 | 9,862 | 2,866 | 210 | 72 |
| 2004[b] | 703 | 267 | 20 | *a* |

[a]Records unavailable.
[b]Figures available as of August 22, 2004.
*Source*: 1999–2001 figures from Ref. 18.

severe outbreaks in eastern Europe and central Africa, as well as new expansion of the virus to Canada and the United States in 1999 (11).

Recent outbreaks of WNV encephalitis include those in Algeria in 1994, Romania in 1996 to 1997, Czech Republic in 1997, the Democratic Republic of the Congo in 1998, Russia in 1999, Israel in 2000, and the current outbreaks in the United States from 1999 to 2004 (10,12–14) (Table 11.2).

### Case Experience with WNV-Complicated Pregnancies
Five verified reports of pregnant mothers exposed to WNV were documented in 2002, with the first confirmed case of intrauterine transmission on August 29, 2002 (1,5,7,15–19).

In 2003, there were 72 confirmed cases of WNV-infected pregnancy, four of which concluded with infants showing evidence of WNV infection (5) (Table 11.3).

### VECTORS

#### Mosquitoes
WNV is maintained through an enzootic cycle involving a number of different mosquito carrier species and up to 130 avian reservoir species (20,21). Mosquitoes acquire the virus while feeding on avian reservoirs and then transfer the virus to other birds during subsequent blood meals, maintaining the cycle as well as occasionally transmitting the virus to humans and horses.

Of the transmitting and maintaining species, mosquitoes of the Culex species and birds of the Corvidae family are thought to be the largest contributors to their respective roles in WNV's maintenance cycle (22) (Figs. 11.1 and 11.2).

| TABLE 11.3 | WNV-Infected Infant Results (5) | | | | | |
|---|---|---|---|---|---|---|
| **Maternal Age** | **Description** | **Fever Onset** | **Delivery** | **Infant Delivery** | **Additional Considerations** | **Infant 2 m/o** |
| 18 | Native American, G4P3 | 33 | 37 weeks, emergency C-section | Facial skin tags | Cord blood WNV IgM positive | Normal |
| 32 | Native American, G3P3 | 37 | 40 weeks, vaginal | Normal-appearing | CSF, 300 WBCs, WNV IgM positive; lissencephaly, cerebral calcifications, cystic changes, infant death 6 w/o | Death |
| 32 | Caucasian, G2P1 | 39 | 39 weeks, induced vaginal | Afebrile, mild nuchal rigidy, macular rash on face and trunk | Afebrile, maculopapular rash, group B streptococcus positive, normal amnio | WNV + H1 IgM/ PRNT positive |
| 19 | Caucasian, G2P1 | 37 | 38 weeks, vaginal | Normal-appearing | Maternal IgM negative 3 weeks predelivery and positive 6 weeks postdelivery; breast milk WNV IgM positive/PCR negative 4 weeks postdelivery | Normal |

*Source:* Based largely upon Dr. O'Leary's presentation at the Fifth National Conference on West Nile Virus in the United States. Available at: www.cdc.gov/ncidod/dvbid/westnile/conf/pdf/Oleary_2_04.pdf (accessed May 2, 2009).

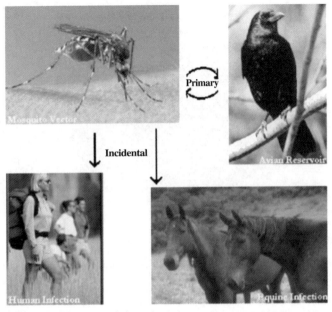

**FIGURE 11.1** Primary transmission cycle.

### Additional Modes of Communication

Human-to-human WNV transmission has been limited thus far to isolated cases of intrauterine transmission, transmission through breast milk, blood transfusion, and organ donation (1,23–25). These reports are exceedingly rare especially in the case of blood transfusion and organ transplantation, where new screening methods are continuously being refined. Of the approximately 1 million donations screened in 2004 as of August 5, a total of 329 (~0.03%) were found reactive for WNV infection by using the NAT format and were excluded from use (26).

The virus is not spread through casual contact with a WNV-infected person. Normal interaction or kissing is not shown to spread the disease.

There is also no evidence that a person can get WNV from handling live or dead infected birds nor is there evidence of dogs or cats having ever communicated the disease (21).

### PROPHYLAXIS

The best way to avoid WNV is to avoid the mosquitoes that carry the disease.

### DIAGNOSIS—CLINICAL

WNV infections are largely asymptomatic and are generally described as a rapid onset febrile illness with temperature in excess of 102.2°F (39°C) frequently accompanied by headache and/or gastrointestinal symptoms (1,7,20) (Table 11.4).

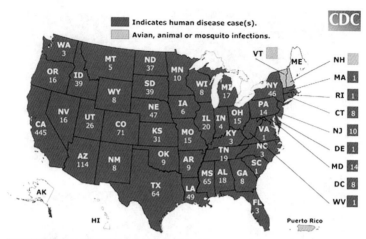

**FIGURE 11.2** Final 2008 WNV activity in the United States.

This map reflects surveillance findings occurring between January 1, 2008 through December 31, 2008 as reported to CDC's ArboNET system for public distribution by state and local health departments.

The map shows the distribution of avian, animal, or mosquito infections occurring during 2008 with number of human cases if any, by state. If WNV infection is reported to CDC from any area of a state, that entire state is shaded.

**Data Table**

Avian, animal or mosquito WNV infections have been reported to CDC ArboNET from the following states in 2008: Alabama, Arizona, Arkansas, California, Colorado, Connecticut, Delaware, District of Columbia, Florida, Georgia, Idaho, Illinois, Indiana, Iowa, Kentucky, Louisiana, Maryland, Massachusetts, Michigan, Minnesota, Mississippi, Missouri, Montana, Nebraska, Nevada, New Hampshire, New Jersey, New Mexico, New York, North Dakota, Ohio, Oklahoma, Oregon, Pennsylvania, Puerto Rico, Rhode Island, South Carolina, South Dakota, Tennessee, Texas, Utah, Vermont, Virginia, Washington, West Virginia, Wisconsin, and Wyoming.

Human cases have been reported in Alabama, Arizona, Arkansas, California, Colorado, Connecticut, Delaware, District of Columbia, Florida, Georgia, Idaho, Illinois, Indiana, Iowa, Kansas, Kentucky, Louisiana, Maryland, Massachusetts, Michigan, Minnesota, Mississippi, Missouri, Montana, Nebraska, Nevada, New Jersey, New Mexico, New York, North Carolina, North Dakota, Ohio, Oklahoma, Oregon, Pennsylvania, Rhode Island, South Carolina, South Dakota, Tennessee, Texas, Utah, Virginia, Washington, West Virginia, Wisconsin, and Wyoming.

**USGS:** http://diseasemaps.usgs.gov/

Mild forms of the infection, which are referred to as WNF, generally set in within 3 to 14 days of being exposed to an infected mosquito. Symptoms can include nausea, vomiting, anorexia, backache, neck ache, malaise, rash, myalgia, and lymphadenopathy (7).

Signs of confusion, muscle weakness, arthralgias, paresis, and abnormal sensory or reflex responses are elements that may be found in the more severe neuroinvasive expression of WNME. The full neurological presentation of WNV's

| TABLE 11.4 | Symptomatic Frequency of WNV Infection in Hospitalized Patients (8,10,12–14) |
|---|---|

| Symptom | Incidence (%) |
|---|---|
| Fever | 93 |
| Headache | 61 |
| Weakness (New York 1999 only) | 56 |
| Nausea (New York 1999 only) | 53 |
| Vomiting | 45 |
| Stiff neck | 35 |
| Change in mental status | 15 |

severe form including those documented by the CDC may include ataxia and extrapyramidal signs, abnormalities of the cranial nerve, optic neuritis, polyradiculitis, myelitis, seizures, or coma. Meningitis, encephalitis, and flaccid paralysis are also possible with meningoencephalitis more common than meningitis alone (7).

Patients presenting with several of the aforementioned symptoms

- In a highly mosquito active region
- With inexplicable meningitis or encephalitis especially from May to September (Summer and early Fall months)
- With a recent history of mosquito bites
- Who have recently traveled to mosquito-prone areas of the world including jungle and/or tropical environments, where mosquitoes are more prevalent
- Who have a relative (particularly over the age of 50) with a newly acquired case of meningitis or encephalitis

should arouse additional suspicion of a possible WNV infection.

## DIAGNOSIS—LABORATORY

As signs and symptoms of WNV cannot be reliably distinguished from either arboviral infections or many of the tick-borne encephalitides, identification is made by the detection of IgM antibody in acute-phase serum or cerebrospinal fluid (CSF) through serologic analysis (20). Rapid testing is available through usage of a TaqMan® reverse transcriptase–PCR assay, yet detection of IgM antibody to WNV in serum or CSF using MAC-ELISA is the most efficient method for verifying the presence of WNV (7, 27). Since IgM antibodies do not cross the blood–brain barrier, IgM antibody in CSF strongly suggests CNS infection (7).

## TREATMENT

Although treatments and vaccines are currently under development, there is no recognized treatment or cure for WNV in either adults or children (28). Generally, treatment consists of supportive care tailored to address particular symptoms and the risk of secondary infection with severe cases commonly requiring respiratory support as well as IV fluids. Antipyretics and analgesics may help in symptomatic treatment. The rest of the knowledge currently available on potential treatments deals principally with the use of ribavirin, interferon $\alpha$-2b, and intravenous WNV antibodies, which have all yet to be examined in controlled studies (29).

Of the experimental treatments currently under development—including a killed whole virus vaccination, a live attenuated chimeric virus vaccination, and passive immunization—attenuated chimeric virus offers perhaps the most promising results (30,31).

The use of intravenous immunoglobulin (IVIG) with a high titer of WNV antibodies has yet to be studied in pregnant women but has been successfully used in a case of an immunosupressed lung transplant patient (32). IVIG has also been studied along with pooled human plasma (PP) for treatment of WNV-infected mice demonstrating prophylactic and therapeutic efficacy (33).

While unfortunately adults and children to this point have no comprehensive treatment, a treatment for in vitro WNV infections may have two very promising options, including the use of nucleoside analogue ribavirin or interferon $\alpha$-2b.

Insofar as an infected mother is concerned, high does ribavirin nor interferon $\alpha$-2b has shown effectiveness in combating WNV in adults (34). Ribavirin and interferon have however been linked to a variety of hematologic complications including anemia, bone-marrow suppression, neutropenia, and thrombocytopenia under different combinations of circumstances.

## CONCLUSION

Obstetricians as well as other doctors should remain mindful of the potential hazard that WNV may pose to pregnant women as well as their unborn children, particularly in mosquito-endemic areas. As there is no established treatment, preventative measures involving mosquito avoidance and management remain the best measure for combating the morbidity and the mortality associated with WNV until vaccinations and direct cures become available for wide scale usage. Health care providers should be highly suspicious of cases which present with a number of symptoms consistent with West Nile viral infections during the mosquito season, summer months (35,36).

### *References*

1. Chappa J, Ahn J, DiGiovanni L, Ismail M. West Nile virus encephalitis during pregnancy. *Obstet Gynecol.* 2003;102:229–230.
2. Bruno J, Rabito FJ, Dildy GA. West Nile virus meningoencephalitis during pregnancy. *J La State Med Soc.* 2004;156(4):204–205.
3. Cordoba L, Escribano-Romero E, Garmendia A, Saiz JC. Pregnancy increases the risk of mortality in West Nile virus-infected mice. *J Gen Virol.* 2007;88(pt 2):476–480.
4. Carles G, Peiffer H, Talarmin A. Effects of dengue fever during pregnancy in French Guiana. *Clin Infect Dis.* 1999;28:637–640.
5. O'Leary DR, Kuhn S, Kniss KL, et al. Birth outcomes following West Nile virus infection of pregnant women in the United States: 2003–2004. *Pediatrics.* 2006;117: e537–e545.
6. Skupski DW, Eglinton GS, Fine AD, Hayes EB, O'Lery DR. West Nile virus during pregnancy: a case study of early second trimester maternal infection. *Fetal Diagn Ther.* 2006;21(3):293–295.
7. CDC. *Epidemic/Epizootic West Nile Virus in the United States: Guidelines for Surveillance, Prevention, and Control.* 3rd Revision 2003.
8. Petersen L, Marfin A. West Nile virus: a primer for the clinician [Review]. *Ann Intern Med.* 2002;137:173–179.
9. CDC. Virology: classification of West Nile virus. Available at: www.cdc.gov/ncidod/ dvbid/westnile/virus.htm (accessed May 23, 2009).
10. CDC. Background: virus history and distribution. Available at: www.cdc.gov/ncidod/ dvbid/westnile/background.htm (accessed May 27, 2009).

11. Petersen L, Roehrig J. West Nile virus: a reemerging global pathogen. *Emerg Infect Dis*. 2001;7:611–614.

12. Tsai T, Popovici F, Cernescu C, et al. West Nile encephalitis epidemic in southeastern Romania. *Lancet*. 1998;352:767–771.

13. Platonov A, Shipulin G, Shipulina O, et al. Outbreak of West Nile virus infection, Volgograd Region, Russia, 1999. *Emerg Infect Dis*. 2001;7:675–678.

14. Weinberger M, Pitlik S, Gandacu D, et al. West Nile fever outbreak, Israel, 2000: epidemiologic aspects. *Emerg Infect Dis*. 2001;7(4):686–691.

15. CDC. 2008. West Nile virus activity in the United States. Available at: www.cdc.gov/ncidod/dvbid/westnile/Mapsactivity (accessed May 27, 2009).

16. CDC. 2003. West Nile virus activity in the United States. Available at: www.cdc.gov/ncibod/dvbid/westnile/activity.htm (accessed May 27, 2009)

17. CDC. Statistics, surveillance and control: West Nile virus disease 2003 human cases by clinical syndromes as of May 25, 2009. Available at: www.cdc.gov/ncidod/dvbid/westnile/prevention_info.html (accessed July 15, 2004).

18. Asnis DS, Conetta R, Teixeira AA, et al. The West Nile virus outbreak of 1999 in New York: the Flushing Hospital experience. *Clin Infect Dis*. 2000;30(3):413–418.

19. CDC. Interim guidelines for the evaluation of infants born to mothers infected with West Nile virus during pregnancy. *MMWR*. 2004;53:154–157.

20. Surveillance and reporting guidelines for West Nile virus. Washington: Department of Health; 2004. Available at: www.doh.wa.gov/Notify/giudelines/wnv.html (accessed May 18, 2009).

21. CDC. Vertebrate ecology. Available at: www.cdc.gov/ncidod/dvbid/westnile/birds&mammals.htm (accessed May 26, 2009).

22. Solomon T, Ooi M, Beasley D, et al. West Nile encephalitis. *Br Med J*. 2003;326:865–869.

23. CDC. Possible West Nile virus transmission to an infant through breast feeding-Michigan, 2002. *MMWR*. 2002;51:877–878.

24. CDC. Update: investigations of West Nile virus infections in recipients of organ transplantation and blood transfusion. *MMWR*. 2002;51:879.

25. CDC. Update: West Nile virus screening of blood donations and transfusion-associated transmission—United States, 2003. *MMWR*. 2004;53:281–284.

26. CDC. Detection of West Nile virus in blood donations—United States, 2003. *MMWR*. 2003;52;769–772.

27. Halstead S, Jacobson J. Japanese encephalitis. *Adv Virus Res*. 2003;61:103 138.

28. Monath TP. Prospects for the development of a vaccine against the West Nile virus. *Ann N Y Acad Sci*. 2001;951:1–12.

29. http://www.turner-white.com/memberfile.php?PubCode = hp_may04_nile.pdf

30. Monath T, Arroyo J, Miller C, et al. West Nile virus vaccine. *Curr Drug Targets Infect Disord*. 2001;1:37–50.

31. Jordan I, Briese T, Fischer N, Lau JYN, Lipkin WI. Ribavirin inhibits West Nile virus replication and cytopathic effect in neural cells. *J Infect Dis*. 2000;182:1214–1217.

32. Hamdan A, Green P, Mendelson E, et al. Possible benefit of intravernous immunoglobulin therapy in a lung transplant recipient with West Nile virus encephalitis. *Transpl Infect Dis*. 2002; 4:160–162.

33. Ben-Nathan D, Lustig S, Tam G, et al. Prophylactic and therapeutic efficacy of human intravenous immunoglobulin in treating West Nile virus infection in mice. *J Infect Dis*. 2003;18:5.

34. Chowers MY, Lang R, Nassar F, et al. Clinical characteriscs of the West Nile fever outbreaks, Israel, 2000.*Emerg Infect Dis*. 2001;344:1807–1814.

35. CDC. Intrauterine West Nile Virus infection—New York, 2002. *MMWR*. 2002;51:1135–1136.

36. Hinckley AF, O'Lery DR, Hayes EB. Transmission of West Nile virus through human breast milk seems to be rare. *Pediatrics*. 2007;119(3):666–671.

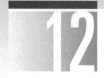

# Delivery in the Emergency Department

**Isaac Delke**

In the United States, 99% of all births have been in hospitals over the past several decades (1). In many areas, the emergency department (ED) is where the obstetric patient enters the hospital. These patients are subsequently sent to the labor and delivery suite if the hospital has an obstetric service. Sometimes, however, emergency medical system (EMS) personnel and/or ED staff are faced with a gravida ready to deliver, and they must be prepared to handle such a situation. The apprehension experienced by emergency birth attendants is not simply due to the lack of expertise with normal deliveries but also is due to the awareness of the potential for serious maternal and perinatal complications.

This chapter presents basic steps in the management of imminent delivery. It focuses on (i) EMS preparedness, (ii) normal spontaneous vaginal delivery, and (iii) complications of vaginal delivery (shoulder dystocia, breech presentation, cord prolapse, and postpartum hemorrhage and/or perineal lacerations). Preparedness and knowledge of the management of obstetric emergencies that commonly confront the ED staff maximize the potential for effective intervention and optimal outcome.

## EMS PREPAREDNESS

EMS personnel must be trained to recognize and manage precipitate delivery appropriately. This requires knowledge by EMS personnel of available obstetric and neonatal units in the system's catchment area for appropriate transport. The transport team should be trained to assist in the precipitate delivery of an infant and skilled in the use of basic obstetrical kits. Prehospital protocols should be reviewed often so that EMS personnel remain prepared for the rare and potentially catastrophic pregnancy-related events. Whether patients deliver in the prehospital setting or on immediate arrival to the ED, every ED should be ready for emergency delivery by preparing a basic delivery kit, along with resources for the initial care and potential resuscitation of the newborn (Table 12.1). Because of the relatively infrequent delivery in the prehospital setting or ED, extra care should be taken to educate EMS and ED personnel through educational programs, annual in-services, and equipment orientation sessions.

## SPONTANEOUS VAGINAL DELIVERY

The initial step in the management of a woman in active labor is to obtain vital signs and initiate supportive therapy, including obtaining venous access and monitoring the mother and fetus. Pelvic examination should reveal fetal presentation, including visible or palpable head or, in the case of breech presentation, the fetal buttock or extremity. Sometimes, confirmation of fetal cardiac activity and presentation may be accomplished using portal ultrasound. The stage of labor and the parity of the patient should be taken into account when considering transport of a patient in labor to another facility or to the labor and delivery suite.

| TABLE 12.1 | Basic Emergency Delivery Kit |
|---|---|

Sterile gloves

Sterile towels and drapes

Two surgical scissors

Hemostats

Syringes (10 mL)

Needles (25 gauge)

Gauze sponge (4 × 4)

Rubber suction bulb

Neonatal airways

Cord clamps

Towels (infant)

Placenta basin

## Delivery of the Head

If delivery of the head is already well on its way, the attending physician should prepare for the delivery after a stat call to obstetric and pediatrician staff. Ideally, the patient should be on the delivery table in the lithotomy position. If the patient is on a bed or stretcher, her legs should be supported. As time allows, the perineum may then be prepared by washing with mild soap and water and swabbing with povidone-iodine or chlorhexidine topical solution. Drapes should be placed over the patient, and the birth attendant should use gowns, masks, and gloves. The mother should be informed, assured, and instructed to enhance maternal cooperation to accomplish a controlled delivery. If the fetus is dead, there is no risk of further fetal trauma, and focus is totally on the mother.

### The Ritgen Maneuver

As the head becomes increasingly visible, the vaginal outlet and vulva are stretched until they ultimately encircle the largest diameter of the baby's head (*crowning*). As the infant's head emerges from the introitus, the perineum should be supported by placing a sterile towel along the inferior portion of the perineum. Forward pressure should be extended on the chin of the fetus through the perineum just in front of the coccyx, while the other hand exerts mild counterpressure superiorly against the occiput to prevent rapid expulsion of the fetal head, which may lead to perineal or periurethral tears (Fig. 12.1). It also favors extension of the head, so that delivery occurs with its smallest diameters passing through the introitus and over the perineum. The head is delivered slowly, with the base of the occiput rotating around the lower margin of the symphysis pubis as a fulcrum, while the bregma (anterior fontanel), brow, and face pass successively over the perineum (2,3). The mother is then asked to breathe through contractions rather than bearing down and attempting to push the baby out rapidly.

The use of routine episiotomy for a normal spontaneous vaginal delivery has been discouraged in recent years, because it has been demonstrated to

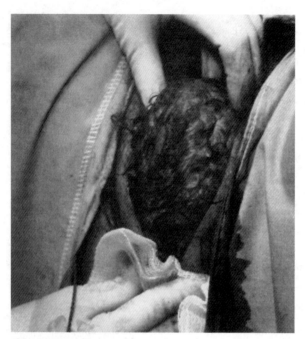

**FIGURE 12.1** The Ritgen maneuver.

increase the incidence of third- and fourth-degree perineal lacerations occurring at the time of delivery. If an episiotomy is necessary, it may be performed as follows: 5 to 10 mL of 1% lidocaine solution is injected with a 25-gauge needle into the posterior fourchette and perineum. While protecting the fetal head, a 2 to 3 cm midline cut is made with scissors to extend the vaginal opening. The incision must be supported with manual pressure from below, taking care not to allow the incision to extend into the rectum.

### Delivery of the Shoulders

After delivery of the head, the occiput promptly turns toward one of the maternal thighs, so that the head assumes a transverse position. The successive movements of restitution and external rotation indicate that the bisacromial diameter (transverse diameter of the thorax) has rotated into the anteroposterior diameter of the pelvis. The anterior shoulder should then be delivered by *gentle* downward traction in concert with maternal expulsive efforts. Traction should be exerted only in the direction of the long axis of the infant, because, if applied obliquely, it causes bending of the neck and excessive stretching of the brachial plexus. The posterior shoulder is then delivered by upward traction. Some practitioners, including the author, prefer to deliver the anterior shoulder prior to its external rotation (head-and-shoulder delivery) to avoid potential shoulder dystocia. The rest of the body almost always follows the shoulders without difficulty. A point of practical concern is the need to maintain control of the newly born infant such that inadvertent dropping does not occur.

## Clearing the Nasopharynx

To minimize the likelihood of aspiration of amniotic fluid debris, meconium, and blood that might occur once the thorax is delivered and the infant can inspire, the face is quickly wiped and the nares and mouth are aspirated (Fig. 12.2). A soft rubber ear syringe or its equivalent, inserted with care, is suitable for this purpose.

## Nuchal Cord

After delivery of the head and anterior shoulder, check for a nuchal cord by passing a finger around the fetal neck. A nuchal cord occurs in about 25% of cases and ordinarily does no harm. If a cord is felt, it should be drawn down between the fingers and, if loose enough, slipped over the infant's head. If it is applied too tightly to the neck to be slipped over the head, it should be cut between two clamps *only after delivery of the anterior shoulder* and the infant should be delivered promptly.

## Clamping the Cord

The timing of cord clamping should be dictated by convenience, and cord clamping is usually performed immediately after delivery of infant. The cord is clamped after thoroughly clearing the infant's airway, which usually takes about 30 seconds. The infant is not elevated above the introitus at vaginal delivery. The umbilical cord is cut between two clamps placed 4 or 5 cm from the fetal abdomen. Later, an umbilical cord clamp is applied 2 or 3 cm from the fetal abdomen. A segment of the umbilical cord is saved for blood gas analysis.

## Delivery of the Placenta

The placenta should be allowed to separate spontaneously. Immediately after delivery of the infant, the height of the uterine fundus and its consistency are ascertained. As long as the uterus remains firm and there is no unusual bleeding, the usual practice is to watch carefully for any of the following signs of placental separation.

1. The uterus becomes globular and firm. This sign is the earliest to appear.
2. There is often a sudden gush of blood.
3. The uterus rises in the abdomen because the placenta, having separated, passes into the lower uterine segment and vagina, where its bulk pushes the uterus upward.
4. The umbilical cord protrudes farther out of the vagina, indicating that the placenta has descended.

These signs usually appear within 5 minutes. The mother may be asked to bear down, and the intra-abdominal pressure so produced may be adequate to expel the placenta. If these efforts fail, the attendant, again having made certain that the uterus is contracted firmly, lifts the fundus cephalad with the abdominal hand, keeping the umbilical cord slightly taut (Brandt-Andrews method). Aggressive traction on the cord risks uterine inversion, tearing of the cord, or disruption of the placenta, which can result in severe vaginal bleeding (2,3). As the placenta passes through the introitus, pressure on the uterus is stopped. The placenta is then gently lifted away from the introitus. Care is taken to prevent the membranes from being torn off and left behind. If the membranes start to tear, they are grasped with a ring forceps and removed by gentle traction. After removal of the placenta, the uterus should be massaged gently to promote contraction. The placenta, membranes, and umbilical cord should be examined for

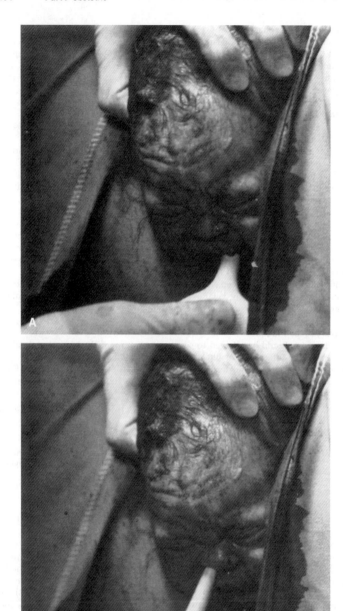

**FIGURE 12.2 A:** Aspiration of mouth. **B:** Aspiration of nose.

abnormalities of cord insertion, confirmation of a three-vessel cord, and completeness of removal of placenta and membranes.

## Oxytocin Agents

After delivery of the placenta, the primary mechanism by which hemostasis is achieved at the placental site is by a well-contracted myometrium. Oxytocin (Pitocin, Syntocinon, etc.), ergonovine maleate (Ergotrate), methylergonovine maleate (Methergine), and misoprostol (Cytotec) are used in various ways in the conduct of the third stage of labor, principally to stimulate myometrial contractions and thereby reduce the blood loss (Table 12.2).

Oxytocin, ergonovine, methylergonovine, and misoprostol are all used widely in the conduct of the normal third stage of labor, but the timing of their administration differs at various institutions. Oxytocin, and especially ergonovine, given before delivery of the placenta will decrease blood loss somewhat. However, the use of oxytocin, and especially ergonovine or methylergonovine, before delivery of the placenta may entrap an undiagnosed, and therefore undelivered, second twin. This may prove injurious, if not fatal, to the entrapped fetus. In most cases following uncomplicated vaginal delivery, the third stage of labor can be conducted with reasonably little blood loss.

| | TABLE 12.2 | Medications for Emergency Delivery and Indications for Use |

| Medication | Route/Dose | Frequency | Indication and Comment |
|---|---|---|---|
| Oxytocin (Pitocin) | IV infusion: 10–40 units in 1 L normal saline or lactated Ringer's solution IM: 10 units | Continuous | Give routinely for uterine contraction and hemostasis immediately postpartum |
| Methylergonovine (Methergine) | IM: 0.2 mg IM or orally | q 2–4 hr | Control of postpartum hemorrhage Avoid if the patient is hypertensive |
| Misoprostol (Cytotec) | Rectally: 800–1,000 µg | Single dose | Control of postpartum hemorrhage |
| Terbutaline sulfate 1 mg/mL | SC: 0.25 mg | q 3 hr | Tocolysis during transport |
| Lidocaine 1% solution | Locally: 1–10 mL | Single dose | Local anesthetic for episiotomy and/or perineal laceration repair |

IM, intramuscular; IV, intravenous; SC, subcutaneous.

If an intravenous (IV) access has been established, oxytocin 10 to 20 units in 500 mL normal saline, already premixed, is administered after delivery of the placenta at a rate of 10 mL per minute for a few minutes, until the uterus remains firmly contracted and the bleeding is controlled. Then the infusion rate is reduced to 2 mL per minute until the mother is ready for transfer from ED to the labor and delivery suite or the postpartum unit. In instances where there is no IV access, oxytocin can also be given as 10 units intramuscularly. The use of nipple stimulation in the third stage of labor also has been shown to increase uterine pressures and to decrease the duration of the third stage of labor and blood loss (2,3).

### Infant Care
Once the cord has been divided, the infant is immediately placed supine with the head lowered and turned to the side in a heated unit that has appropriate thermal regulation.

After delivery, the infant should be held securely or placed on the mother's abdomen and wiped dry, while any mucus remaining in the airway is suctioned. The infant's clinical status should be assessed at 1 and 5 minutes after delivery. In the setting of an uncomplicated delivery, the mother may hold the child immediately while the cord is being cut, provided that the child has responded well to initial stimulation and has a clear airway and good respiratory effort (2,3).

### Breastfeeding
If both mother and baby are stable and no medical contraindications exist, breastfeeding should be encouraged as soon as possible after birth. Benefits include promotion of uterine contractions that control hemorrhage at the placental insertion site, encouragement of maternal–newborn bonding, provision of easily digestible and balanced nutritional support for the baby, and transmission of antibodies (immunoglobulin A) that protect the enteric mucosa against invasion by colonizing bacteria.

## COMPLICATIONS OF EMERGENCY VAGINAL DELIVERY

### Shoulder Dystocia
Shoulder dystocia is an obstetric emergency that can lead to significant neonatal morbidity (brachial plexus injury, fractured humerus or clavicle, etc.) and mortality (severe asphyxia), if not managed appropriately. The major maternal consequence of shoulder dystocia is postpartum hemorrhage, usually from uterine atony but also from vaginal and cervical lacerations.

Shoulder dystocia is first recognized after delivery of the fetal head, when gentle downward traction is insufficient to deliver the anterior shoulder. After delivering the infant's head, it retracts tightly against the perineum (the turtle sign). Shoulder dystocia is the impaction of fetal shoulders at the pelvic outlet after delivery of the head. Typically, the anterior shoulder is trapped behind the pubic symphysis, leading to a delay of delivery of the rest of the infant. It usually occurs in the delivery of larger infants with disproportionately large shoulders compared with the fetal head. *Shoulder dystocia also occurs with an extremely rapid delivery of the head, or as a result of overzealous external rotation of the fetal head by the birth attendant. Shoulder dystocia cannot be predicted from clinical characteristics or labor abnormalities.*

The reported incidence varies from 0.2% to 3.0% of all vaginal deliveries. The lack of uniformly accepted definition or criteria for the diagnosis of shoulder dystocia contributes to its varying incidences (4,5).

Various maneuvers have been described to free the anterior shoulder from its impacted position beneath the maternal symphysis pubis. Unfortunately, there is no one superior algorithm to manage shoulder dystocia. The specific maneuver used is probably not as critical as a careful, quick, and organized action to relieve the shoulder dystocia and avoid desperate and potentially traumatic traction of the fetal head.

### Management
**Key Management Points:** A previously uncompromised fetus/infant may be able to withstand 5 to 7 minutes of shoulder dystocia without suffering permanent injury from lack of oxygen (5). Once you recognize shoulder dystocia:

- Call for help: obstetric, pediatric, and anesthesia teams.
- Designate a care-team member as a timekeeper. Tracking the time is necessary both to allow periodic reassessment of the situation in case of severe shoulder dystocia and for documentation after delivery.
- Inform patient/family as to why certain actions are being taken—*communication points*:
  - "The baby's shoulders are stuck"
  - "I'm going to need to focus on getting the baby out"
  - "I may need to ask for your help"
- Empty the patient's bladder.
- McRoberts position plus suprapubic pressure.
- Delivery of the posterior arm after an episiotomy.
- Rotational maneuvers: Woods/Rubin.
- All-fours position (Gaskin maneuver).
- Fracture clavicle.
- Zavanelli maneuver.
- Abdominal rescue.

The most popular techniques include the following:

   **1. McRoberts Position and Suprapubic Pressure.** This consists of sharply flexing the woman's legs on her own abdomen (Fig. 12.3). This has been

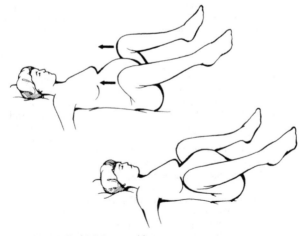

**FIGURE 12.3** The McRoberts position.

shown to straighten the sacrum relative to the lumbar vertebrae, with accompanying rotation of the symphysis pubis toward the patient's head and a decrease in the angle of pelvic inclination. This position does not increase the dimensions of the pelvis, but the cephalic rotation of the pelvis frees the impacted anterior shoulder. The bladder should be drained if this has not been done already. Then, moderate suprapubic pressure is applied obliquely by an assistant while downward traction is applied to the fetal head by the attendant. The success rate of McRoberts position in resolving shoulder dystocia, used either alone or in combination with suprapubic pressure, is reported between 42% and 58% (5).

**2. Delivery of the Posterior Arm.** If McRoberts position and suprapubic pressure fail to effect delivery, attempt to deliver the posterior arm. Posterior arm extraction, when successful, will replace the bisacromial diameter with the axilloacromial diameter, thereby reducing the obstructing diameter in the pelvis. Insert a hand along the posterior shoulder, grasp and flex the forearm at the elbow, sweep it across the chest, and bring it through the vagina. It is usually easy to do this using your hand that is opposite the fetal face. The mother should not be pushing during this maneuver.

If the head is tightly retracted against the maternal perineum, it may be necessary to perform episiotomy or proctoepisiotomy in order to insert your hand into the vagina to deliver the posterior arm.

After delivery of the posterior arm, gentle downward traction on the fetal head will usually result in delivery of the anterior shoulder and the baby. If delivery of the anterior shoulder and baby cannot be accomplished, perform rotation of the posterior shoulder 180 degrees to the anterior position. If the fetus is facing the mother's right side, rotation should be attempted in a counterclockwise direction as a first step. Some birth attendants prefer to attempt rotational maneuvers before attempting to deliver the posterior arm. Two types of rotational maneuvers are generally attempted.

**3. Rotational Maneuvers: Woods Corkscrew and Rubin Maneuvers.** The Woods corkscrew maneuver is rotating the fetal posterior shoulder by placing your index and middle fingers on the ventral surface (that facing the fetal face) and rotating the entire fetal body. If the fetus is facing the mother's right side, this would be accomplished with your left hand and rotation would be in a counterclockwise direction. Often after a 90-degree rotation, it will be necessary to replace your left hand with your right hand to complete a 180-degree rotation.

The first Rubin maneuver is accomplished by rotating the anterior shoulder under the symphysis pubis. If the fetus is facing the mother's right side, you would use your right hand to perform this maneuver. The second Rubin maneuver is rotating the posterior shoulder in a clockwise direction by placing pressure on the dorsal surface of the posterior shoulder.

If neither delivery of the arm nor rotational maneuver is possible, bilateral shoulder dystocia may be present, in which the anterior shoulder is lodged behind the symphysis pubis and the posterior shoulder is lodged high in the pelvis at or near the sacral promontory. In this case, *"all-fours"* position (Gaskin maneuver) could be attempted.

**4. All-Fours Position (Gaskin Maneuver).** The mother is now positioned on her hands and knees. This allows rotation of the maternal pelvis with disimpaction of the anterior shoulder under the symphysis. This position exploits the effects of gravity and increased space in the hollow of the sacrum to facilitate delivery of the posterior shoulder and arm. An attempt is now made to deliver the posterior shoulder by gentle downward traction followed by delivery of the anterior shoulder by gentle upward traction. If this is not successful, an attempt can be made to deliver the posterior arm as described above. If the mother cannot assume the "all-fours" position or delivery cannot be accomplished in this position, *deliberate fracture of the clavicle, cephalic replacement* and cesarean delivery, or *abdominal rescue* may be necessary in rare cases.

**5. Deliberate Fracture of the Clavicle.** The anterior clavicle is deliberately fractured by pressing against the ramus of the pubis so that the shoulder is freed of impaction. The fracture heals rapidly and is not nearly as serious as a brachial nerve injury, asphyxia, or death.

**6. The Zavanelli Maneuver (Cephalic Replacement).** The first part of this maneuver consists of returning the head to the occipitoanterior or occipitoposterior position. If the head has rotated from either position, the second step is to flex the head and slowly push it back into the vagina. Once the fetal head is reintroduced into the vagina, emergency cesarean delivery should be performed. A fetal heart should be documented, if at all possible, before performing cesarean delivery.

**7. Abdominal Rescue.** If all maneuvers have been attempted and you are unable to replace the fetal head, low transverse uterine incision can be performed, the anterior shoulder manually rotated into the oblique diameter by the surgeon, and vaginal delivery performed by the birth attendant.

*Maneuvers to Avoid*

- Avoid aggressive *fundal pressure*, because it may further worsen the impaction of the shoulder and also may result in uterine rupture.
- Any nuchal cord, if unable to be reduced over the fetal head, should not be clamped and cut until delivery of the anterior shoulder, if at all possible.

**Breech Presentation**

Vaginal breech deliveries are associated with a morbidity rate three to four times greater than that of cephalad presentations. Risks to the fetus inherent in vaginal breech delivery include (i) prolapse of the umbilical cord, (ii) entrapment of the aftercoming head by the incompletely dilated cervix, and (iii) trauma resulting from extension of the head or nuchal position of the arms (6,7).

A major current dilemma is that of obtaining sufficient experience at vaginal breech delivery. Little or minimal experience is gained in many training programs. Thus, many recently trained obstetricians may have great difficulty when faced with imminent vaginal breech delivery at a facility unable to perform an emergency cesarean delivery.

*Management*

1. The patient who enters the ED with a breech presentation with buttocks crowning or legs showing through the introitus requires rapid mobilization of personnel for delivery.

2. Generally, there is time for transfer to the labor and delivery suite. Give 0.25 mg subcutaneous terbutaline to inhibit uterine activity before transfer of the patient.

3. Call for an obstetrician, a nurse assistant, a pediatrician, and anesthesia personnel. If possible, a quick ultrasound (portal) examination to determine the presence of fetal cardiac activity, fetal head, its attitude, and

possible hydrocephaly would be ideal and helpful in the management decision. If the fetus is dead, there is no risk of further fetal trauma, and concern is totally for the mother.

4. If a leg is presenting at the vaginal introitus, it should not be pulled down because the patient may not be ready to deliver. This may be a footling presentation through a cervix that is not fully dilated. There is time to transfer the patient to the labor and delivery unit, preferably in the knee–chest position to avoid possible cord compression.

5. Avoid artificial rupture of membranes (AROM) in breech presentations. As the amniotic sac balloons into the birth canal, it helps to dilate the cervix completely. This facilitates descent of the baby, providing a lubricated smooth surface against which the body can freely move, and cushions the umbilical cord against compression in the birth canal.

6. If the fetus is already delivered to the umbilicus, the attendant should wrap the fetal trunk with a towel to provide support to the body while further descent results from expulsive forces from the mother only.

7. Delivery of the aftercoming head: The index and middle fingers of one hand are applied over the maxilla (not mandible) to flex the head, while the fetal body rests on the palm of the hand and forearm. The forearm is straddled by the fetal legs. Two fingers of the other hand then are hooked over the fetal neck, and grasping the shoulders, downward traction is applied until the suboccipital region appears under the symphysis. Gentle suprapubic pressure simultaneously applied by an assistant helps keep the head flexed (Fig. 12.4). The body then is elevated toward the maternal abdomen, and the mouth, nose, brow, and eventually the occiput emerge successively over the perineum.

8. Entrapment of the aftercoming head: Occasionally, especially with small preterm fetuses, the incompletely dilated cervix will not allow delivery of the aftercoming head. With gentle traction on the fetal body, the cervix, at times, may be manually slipped over the occiput. If this is not successful, then *Dührssen incisions* (incisions of the cervix at 2 and 10 o'clock positions) are usually necessary. Another option is replacement of the fetus high into the vagina and uterus, followed by cesarean delivery.

## Umbilical Cord Prolapse

The reported incidence of umbilical cord prolapse (UCP) varies between 0.2% and 0.6% of births. The major etiologic categories of UCP are (i) fetal malpresentation (50%), (ii) preterm labor (30% to 50%), and (iii) AROM (10% to 15%) (7).

*Management*

- In the event that vaginal examination reveals palpable, pulsating cord alongside the presenting part or in the cervix or vagina, the examiner's hand should not be removed but rather should be used to elevate the presenting fetal part to reduce compression on the cord. Call for obstetric, pediatric, and anesthesia personnel.
- Cesarean delivery is the treatment of choice in almost all cases if there is fetal cardiac activity.
- Fetal cardiac activity should be confirmed by portal ultrasound rather than cord palpation only.
- Give terbutaline 0.25 mg subcutaneously to inhibit uterine activity.
- Transfer the patient to the labor and delivery unit or operating room in Trendelenburg or the knee–chest position, and the presenting part should be manually elevated as far out of the pelvis as possible and held there until delivery is accomplished.

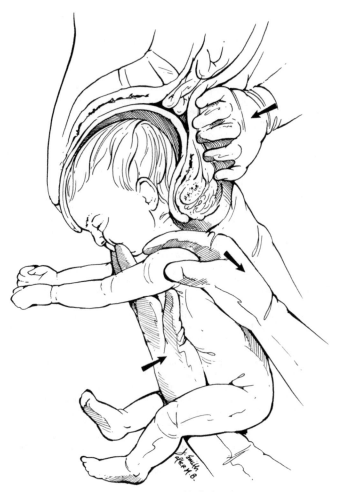

**FIGURE 12.4** Delivery of the aftercoming head by flexion.

### Neonatal Resuscitation

- Dry the baby thoroughly, keep the baby warm, and clear the nose and mouth of excess fluid.
- Assess the respiratory effort and heart rate (by auscultation or palpation at the base of the umbilical cord).
- Keep the baby warm and observe if the baby is breathing spontaneously with a pulse rate >100 beats per minute.
- Improve ventilation if the pulse falls below 100 beats per minute and the respiratory effort is poor.
- Ventilatory support: If stimulation of the baby by rubbing with a towel or flicking the heels fails to elicit improvement in respiratory effort and

pulse, apply positive-pressure ventilation with a neonatal mask and Ambu bag (preferably with oxygen).
- Assess the infant for any bony (fracture of clavicle or humerus) and/or brachial plexus injury.

## Postpartum Hemorrhage

Hemorrhage is one of the leading causes of maternal death in women delivering after 20 weeks' gestation. Postpartum hemorrhage is caused by uterine atony, genital tract lacerations, or retained placenta. Uterine atony or genital tract lacerations may follow an emergency delivery and may lead to excessive vaginal bleeding (8,9).

### Management

- Transfer the patient to the labor and delivery unit for management of the third stage of labor.
- Medical management pertains primarily to the treatment of uterine atony. Many clinicians utilize a prophylactic infusion of oxytocin consisting of 10 to 20 units of oxytocin in 1,000 mL of normal saline or Ringer's lactate administered at 10 to 20 mL per minute to prevent uterine atony (Table 12.2).
- If the signs of placental separation have appeared, expression of the placenta should be attempted by manual pressure on the fundus of the uterus. If bleeding continues, manual removal of the placenta is mandatory.
- In the presence of any external hemorrhage during the third stage, the uterus should be massaged if it is not firmly contracted.
- Oxytocin is the first-line agent. Additional oxytocin may be administered, as well as methylergonovine 0.2 mg intramuscular (IM) (not IV), or misoprostol 800 to 1,000 μg per rectum. With significant postpartum hemorrhage, vigorous bimanual massage should be continued while administering contractile agents (Table 12.2).
- The hour immediately following delivery of the placenta is critical. Even though oxytocics are administered, postpartum hemorrhage as the result of uterine relaxation is most likely to occur at this time. It is mandatory that the uterus be evaluated frequently throughout this period by a competent attendant who places a hand frequently on the fundus and massages it at the slightest sign of relaxation. At the same time, the vaginal and perineal regions are also inspected frequently to allow prompt identification of any excessive bleeding.

## Lacerations of the Genital Tract

- Lacerations to the perineum occur commonly following a rapid, uncontrolled expulsion of the fetal head. Perineal lacerations due to birth trauma are categorized into four groups. First-degree lacerations are limited to the mucosa, skin, and superficial subcutaneous and submucosal tissues. Second-degree lacerations penetrate deeper into the superficial fascia and transverse perineal musculature. In addition to these structures, a third-degree laceration disrupts the anal sphincter, whereas a fourth-degree laceration extends into the rectal lumen (2,3,9).
- After delivery of the placenta, the cervix, vagina, and perineum should be carefully examined for evidence of lacerations. Perineal injuries, either spontaneous or with episiotomy, are the most common complications of spontaneous vaginal deliveries.

■ Perineal laceration repair fundamentally involves the sequential anatomic reapproximation, using absorbable suture material, of the rectal mucosa, anal sphincter, transverse perineal musculature, vaginal mucosa, and skin. *In precipitate ED deliveries, the repair of the episiotomy and/or perineal lacerations can often be performed by the obstetric staff, the details of repair being beyond the scope of this book* (3).

## SUMMARY

Management of spontaneous vaginal delivery is an essential skill for EMS and ED personnel, particularly in settings where obstetric staff is not immediately available. Protocol or guidelines should therefore be in place and should include provisions for the availability of appropriate equipment, medications, trained support personnel, necessary forms for documentation, and universal precaution material (masks, gowns, gloves, goggles, wall suction, etc.) needed for the prevention of human immunodeficiency virus and hepatitis B virus transmission.

Key factors for successful management of emergent vaginal delivery and its complications include constant preparedness, a team approach, and appropriate documentation.

## DOCUMENTATION

■ Clear documentation in the chart of the exact events that have taken place during delivery of an infant after shoulder dystocia, breech presentation, or cord prolapse is essential. *If the infant has suffered permanent birth injury, there is a high likelihood of malpractice litigation. The best defense can be mounted if there is a clearly documented description of the efforts made to deliver the fetus.*

■ The events of the delivery must be documented by all care-team members involved.

### Postdelivery Note

■ Type of delivery
■ Position of the fetal head on restitution (e.g., facing the mother's right or left thigh)
■ Description, sequence, and result of maneuvers used to relieve shoulder dystocia; delivery of the aftercoming head in breech presentation; and management of cord prolapse
■ Delivery date/time
■ Time elapsed from diagnosis to delivery
■ Complete umbilical cord blood gases
■ Condition of the infant with particular attention to Apgar scores and signs of bony and/or brachial plexus injury
■ Information provided to the patient/family members

### *References*

1. Martin JA, Kung H-C, Mathewsa TJ, et al. Annual summary of vital statistics: 2006. *Pediatrics.* 2008;121:788–801.
2. Cunningham FG, Leveno KL, Bloom SL, Hauth JC, Gilstrap LC III, Wenstrom KD. Conduct of normal labor and delivery. In: Cunningham FG, Leveno KL, Bloom SL, Hauth JC, Gilstrap LC III, Wenstrom KD, eds. *Williams Obstetrics.* 22nd Ed. New York, NY: McGraw-Hill; 2005:429–434.
3. Kilpatrick S, Garrison E. Normal labor and delivery. In: Gabbe SG, Niebyl JR, Simpson JL, eds. *Obstetrics: Normal and Problem Pregnancies.* 5th Ed. New York, NY: Churchhill Livingstone Elsevier; 2007:317–319.

4. Benedetti TJ. Shoulder dystocia. In: Queenan JT, Hobbins JC, Spong CY, eds. *Protocols for High-Risk Pregnancies*. 4th Ed. Malden, MA: Blackwell Publishing; 2005:565–569.
5. Gottlieb AG, Galan HL. Shoulder dystocia: an update. *Obstet Gynecol Clin North Am*. 2007;34:501–531.
6. Lanni SM, Seeds JW. Malpresentations. In: Gabbe SG, Niebyl JR, Simpson JL, eds. *Obstetrics: Normal and Problem Pregnancies*. 5th Ed. New York, NY: Churchhill Livingstone Elsevier; 2007:436–446.
7. Klatt TE, Cruikshank DP. Breech, other malpresentations and umbilical cord complications. In: Gibbs RS, Karlan BY, Haney AF, Nygaard I, eds. *Danforths Obstetrics and Gynecology*. 10th Ed. Philadelphia, PA: Lippincott Williams & Wilkins; 2008: 413–414.
8. American College of Obstetricians and Gynecologists. Postpartum hemorrhage. Practice Bulletin No. 76. *Obstet Gynecol*. 2006;108:1039–1048.
9. Gilstrap LC, Yeomans ER. Complications of delivery. In: Gibbs RS, Karlan BY, Haney AF, Nygaard I, eds. *Danforths Obstetrics and Gynecology*. 10th Ed. Philadelphia, PA: Lippincott Williams & Wilkins; 2008:452–458.

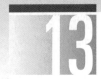

# Transport of the Pregnant Patient

**Pam Adams and C. David Adair**

The main objective of obstetric transports is to provide safe and rapid transport of the high-risk obstetrics (HROB) patient to a facility most appropriate to meet the needs of the mother and the fetus (1). This is accomplished by careful assessment, stabilization, and transport by *skilled* personnel who are comfortable dealing with obstetric and neonatal crisis and emergencies. There is definitive evidence that perinatal and neonatal outcomes are significantly improved when delivery occurs in a tertiary referral center that includes a Level 3 NICU. In utero transport results in reduced morbidity for infants of high-risk pregnancies. There is a 90% survival rate for infants transported in utero versus an 81% survival rate of out-born infants transported after delivery, proving that in most cases the mother is truly the best transport incubator (2).

There are many factors that must be considered when caring for a pregnant patient in the transport environment. Foremost is an understanding that two patients are being transported. The fetus cannot be visually assessed; therefore, the crew must be trained in assessment of the fetus in utero. This includes training in reviewing and interpreting fetal monitoring tracings as well as having knowledge of antepartum testing. The teams must understand that all treatments and interventions provided to the mother have the potential to adversely or positively affect the status of the unborn fetus.

Interfacility transfers are classified as either one-way transports or two-way transports. A one-way transport involves moving the patient using a local transport vehicle (ground ambulance or helicopter) that can respond promptly and move the patient from one facility to another. During a one-way transport, the referring physician calls for a transport vehicle and then usually remains responsible for the patient's care until she reaches the receiving facility. This type of transfer can be tricky as many referral facilities turn the patient over to a transport crew that they assume will provide the same level of care that was given at the referring facility. The reality is that many times the level of care is actually decreased in transport, without the knowledge of the referral physician who is still ultimately responsible for that patient throughout the transfer. If the patient's condition worsens en route, appropriate evaluation and intervention are dependent on the skill level and expertise of the transport personnel. In an effort to address this potential problem, referring facilities may desire to send one of their nurses or physicians with the patient. This can lead to added problems, as those persons are often unfamiliar with the uniqueness of transport medicine. They are not accustomed to working in the unstable environment of a moving transport vehicle where vibration, motion, noise, and a cramped, poorly lit workspace make it challenging to continually assess and alter patient care. In addition, should the patient originate from a small community facility, the facility may not be able to function well with one less caregiver or ambulance for several hours while they are on a transport (3).

A two-way transport usually involves using the transport system that is associated with or contracted by the receiving facility. With a two-way transport, the receiving facility accepts responsibility of the patient when their transport team arrives and assumes her care. This type of transport is usually preferable for the receiving facility, as the caregivers on this transport team often originate from and are viewed as an extension of the receiving facility. They work under standing protocols designed to meet the needs of this type of obstetric patient. Should a situation arise where they have questions or concerns regarding care, they will contact their medical director, thereby releasing the referral physician from any further liability. A disadvantage of this type of transport is the length of time it can take for the team to arrive to assume care of the patient. That is often the reason that referring hospitals use local transport providers.

Prior to using either type of transport team, it is wise for the referral facilities to have full knowledge of exactly what training and experience each team has received for HROB patients and what equipment they use and what treatments they can provide. It is also important that written letters of agreement are made between both the referral and receiving facilities clearly stating each institution's responsibility to assure compliance with local, state, and federal laws.

## TEAM CONFIGURATION

All EMS and transport crew members will eventually be called upon to transport a pregnant medical, trauma, or laboring patient. When this request occurs in the pre-hospital environment, the crews will follow the standing orders of their field medical director.

Transport teams that accept the responsibility of caring for HROB patients must be capable of meeting the needs of the most critical OB and neonatal patients. For transporting HROB patients from one facility to another (interfacility transport), the teams' training should encompass triage, assessment, stabilization, and decision making regarding how and when to safely move these patients. Suggested

**TABLE 13.1** Team Qualifications

The configuration of the team may vary based on local and state guidelines as well as facility medical direction. There must be a core crew consisting of two team members meeting the minimal qualifications, with the primary team leader meeting both minimal and optimal team qualifications.

Minimal Maternal Transport Team Qualifications
- Registered nurse and/or paramedic licensed in the state of the base of operation.
- Respiratory therapist and/or EMT must be licensed in the state of the base of operation to function as a secondary team member.
- BLS (Basic life support) certified.
- NRP certified.
- Successful completion of a flight safety and orientation course as specified by organizational protocols and meeting state and federal guidelines.
- Completion of a ground transport orientation in compliance with state guidelines.
- Other non-team members such as obstetrician, OB fellow, certified nurse, midwife, OB nurse practitioner, or critical care transport nurse may be added to the core transport team on a case specific basis.

Optimal Maternal Transport Team Qualifications (primary leader must complete)
- Completion of a high-risk obstetrical transport course.
- Completion of maternal transport competency skills checklist with proficiency.
- ACLS certified.

Team configuration should be based on consideration of the following:
- Established local and state guidelines.
- Legal scope of practice of team members.
- Program policies and protocols.
- Medical director approval.

minimal and optimal qualifications for each team member should be considered while keeping in compliance with his or her scope of practice as well as local and state guidelines (Table 13.1). The level of care that team members can provide is then categorized according to their individual performances defining them as either primary or secondary team members (Table 13.2). The team members must have completed or must be in the process of completing the skills competency checklist and should possess complete knowledge and understanding of the standing orders mandated by their institutions' medical director (Table 13.3) (4).

Beginning with the initial report received, the patient can be placed into a Priority 1, 2, or 3 status based on her acuity (Table 13.4) (4). This priority level is

| TABLE 13.2 | Performance Objectives |

The primary team leader must be proficient in all aspects of high-risk maternal transport. Proficiency shall be based on individual performance of the following:

- Technical and clinical competencies.
- Critical thinking and leadership skills.
- Competent in community relations and interpersonal communication.

The secondary team member must be capable of assisting the primary team leader with assessment and stabilization, as well as comfortable with assuming care of the mother or neonate in the event of an emergency delivery.

**Primary team leader**
- Completed transport skills competency list (must meet with medical director approval and fall within the scope of practice of the individuals' licensing bureau).
- Consistently proficient with all levels of care including triage, stabilization, patient packaging, transport, and follow-up. Proficiency in maternal assessment and stabilization should include the following:
  - Performance of a complete maternal physical examination
  - Advanced airway management including intubation
  - IV access and medication stabilization
  - Advanced cardiac life support certification
  - Accurate vaginal examinations including sterile speculum (when applicable)
  - Testing of amniotic fluid for nitrazine and ferning
  - Ultrasound identification for fetal positioning
  - Fetal heart rate monitoring and interpretation
  - Administration of tocolytic medication
  - Emergency delivery if necessary
  - Proficiency in neonatal resuscitation

**Secondary team member**
- Completed or working to complete transport skills competency list.
- Completion of helicopter/ground vehicle orientation. Aware of transport safety issues.
- Proficiency in assistance of maternal assessment and stabilization to include
  - IV access.
  - Fetal monitor interpretation.
  - Basic life support certified.
  - NRP certified.
  - Competent to assist with emergency delivery and initial resuscitation.

TABLE

13.3  Team Education Competency

The items included in the transport competency checklist of each individual program will be based on the program's protocols and medical direction. Primary team members must demonstrate competency in all of the areas listed on the transport checklist. Secondary team members must be working toward completion of competencies for their position on the team.

A. Triage
- Accept verbal report from sending facility.
- Categorize transport according to severity and mode of transport.
- Estimate ETA for referral facility.
- Activate appropriate transport personnel and vehicle.
- Notify medical director, NICU, perinatal center of new admission.
- Prepare appropriate equipment for departure.
B. Vaginal examinations
- Perform vaginal examinations on laboring women in controlled setting with a preceptor. Differentiate between normal and abnormal rate of cervical dilation, effacement, and descent of presenting part.
- Must show competency by consistently demonstrating 90% accuracy when determining dilation, effacement, and station as well as fetal presentation and position.
- Examination competency includes showing proficiency in determining all dilation stages from a closed/thick cervix to complete dilation.
C. Speculum examinations for PROM
- Demonstrate proficiency in proper insertion of speculum.
- Assess color, amount, and odor of the amniotic fluid.
- Visualize cervix to assess dilation when applicable.
- Confirm rupture of membranes with nitrazine or fern test.
D. Ultrasound identification of fetal position
- Proficiency in utilizing ultrasound examination to determine fetal position (in accordance with institutional policy and nurse practice act).
- Confirmation of correct fetal position vital prior to transport.
E. Fetal heart rate monitoring and interpretation
- Completion of basic fetal monitoring course or equivalent.
- Passing of fetal monitoring test with 90% or higher.
- Recognize normal and abnormal fetal heart rate patterns and identify non-reassuring tracings.
- Promptly initiate appropriate nursing interventions for non-reassuring FHR tracings and notify appropriate physician.
- Recognize normal and abnormal contraction patterns.
- Initiate appropriate nursing interventions for abnormal contraction status and notify appropriate physician.
- Apply direct fetal monitoring devices in accordance with nurse practice act, institution policy, and medical direction when necessary
F. Obstetrical pharmacology administration
- Competency validation of medication knowledge including medication desired effect, route, dosage, adverse effect, interactions, and considerations.
- Monitor the mother and the fetus for desired and deleterious effects of administered medications. Prepare for medication discontinuance and reversal if necessary.
G. Medical directing standing orders
- Competency validation of knowledge of standing orders.
- Requesting of further orders from medical direction when completion of standing orders achieved if needed.

*(continued)*

**TABLE 13.3** Team Education Competency *(continued)*

H. Equipment
  - Competency validation of safe usage of equipment in multiple transport settings.
  - Yearly or more frequent equipment updates or in-service.
I. Neonatal resuscitation procedures
  - Current neonatal resuscitation procedure—(NRP) certification.
  - Advanced procedures—Intubation, UVC insertion, medication administration in accordance with medical direction, institution policy, and nurse practice act.
J. Transport vehicle safety competency
  - Safety orientation of ground vehicle or air ambulance to include location of emergency exits, fire extinguishers, securing of self and equipment, life vests and floats, emergency oxygen, survival kits, radio usage and ELT activation for air ambulance.
  - Function as air crew member with rotor wing transport using safety instruction such as rotor safety, obstacle watch, participation in take off and landing safety checklist, etc.
  - Knowledge and adherence to safety rules for each type of transport vehicle.
  - Location of vehicle oxygen, suction, and emergency telecommunication transmitting ability.

The transport coordinator and/or medical director of the transport team shall evaluate the skills and clinical competencies. Methods of evaluation and documentation may include any or all of the following:

- Written examination
- Skills labs
- Case presentations with oral examination

---

different than that of current trauma criteria where the Priority 1 patient has no vital signs, yet the HROB Priority 1 patient is still the sickest and most acute of the pregnant patients requiring transportation. In some circumstances, the teams may want to reconfigure their team members based on the priority status of the patient and the training level of the team currently in place. This allows for more qualified personnel to be added to, or changed out, based on: patient acuity, possibility of delivery prior to returning to the receiving facility, etc.

## TRANSPORT TEAM PRELIMINARY ASSESSMENT

The transport of the HROB patient is very challenging in many aspects (5,6). The team members must appreciate that two patients are being transported. It is imperative to perform an accurate assessment on both patients and begin stabilization efforts prior to moving the patients. The evaluation begins with the initial report received from the referring facility. This report helps both the referring facility and the transport team to determine if additional stabilization techniques should be implemented by the referral physician while the team is en route and allows the team to prepare a preliminary care plan prior to their arrival.

To ensure that the patient report is provided in a clear and concise manner, it is helpful to use a specialized "triage form." When both the referral facility and the team have a copy of this form, report flow is much smoother and ensures that nothing is forgotten in the process.

### Priority Status

**Definitions**

- **Primary team leader**—defined as a team member proficient in all aspects of HROB transport (completed transport skills checklist).
- **Secondary team leader**—defined as a team member who is capable of assisting with the primary team leader with assessment and stabilization as well as comfortable with assuming care of the mother or the neonate in the event of an emergency delivery (working to complete transport skills checklist).

**Priority 1 Team Configuration**

At least one primary team leader and either a second primary team member or a very skilled secondary team member must accompany all Priority 1 patients.

**Examples of Priority 1 Patients**

This patient is usually the most severe patient and can become unstable rapidly. Examples of this type of patient include

- Multipara with ruptured or bulging membranes.
- Multipara with >3 cm and regular contraction pattern.
- Primigravida @ 4 cm or greater.
- Preeclampsia, eclampsia, or HELLP syndrome
- Premature labor with regular contraction pattern (<36 weeks' gestation or with an estimated fetal weight of <2,000 g).
- Premature rupture of membranes (same as above).
- Third-trimester bleeding (placenta previa, placental abruption, etc.)
- Maternal conditions which may affect fetus or precipitate premature delivery such as
  - Poorly controlled diabetes
  - Maternal heart disease
  - Drug or alcohol abuse
  - Trauma or surgical conditions beyond the capability of the referral facility possibly resulting in premature labor
  - Febrile or hypermetabolic conditions
  - Pyelonephritis or renal conditions
  - Hepatitis
  - Influenza or pneumonia

**Priority 2 Team Configuration**

A primary team leader should accompany all Priority 2 patients and a secondary team member of either status may be used.

**Examples of Priority 2 Patients**

This patient is usually more stabile or more easily stabilized. Examples of this patient include

- Ruptured membranes with no contractions
- Multipara with <2 cm dilation and no contractions
- Mild preeclampsia (stabilized)
- Primigravida <4 cm not in active labor
- Stable maternal conditions

**Priority 3 Team Configuration**

Priority 3 patients should be accompanied by two team members (with either primary or secondary team qualifications).

*(continued)*

**TABLE 13.4** Priority Status *(continued)*

**Examples of Priority 3 Patients**
This patient is usually stable. Examples of this patient include

- Primigravida <2 cm
- Multipara <1 cm
- Gestation of <21 weeks without labor
- Patients above with absent or mild contractions and intact membranes

## PRIMARY AND SECONDARY OBSTETRIC EVALUATION

Transport members who provide care to the HROB patient must be able to do a rapid primary and secondary survey and provide intervention as the need arises. Life-threatening situations noted for the mother must be treated immediately with assessment and intervention for the fetus secondarily. The effects of all treatments provided to the mother will likely directly impact the fetus as well. The maternal secondary survey should include a complete head to toe examination. Areas of assessment should include

| System | Assessment Parameters |
|---|---|
| Cardiac | Cardiac rhythm, skin color and temperature, hydration, capillary refill, edema, pulses equality in arms and legs |
| Respiratory | Respirations (rate, depth, and quality), breath sounds, chest rise and symmetry, presence of cough or sputum |
| Neurologic | Orientation, Glasgow Coma score, best motor and verbal responses, pupil dilation, strength in arms and legs, DTRs/Clonus, sensitivity to light or noise |
| Gastro | Bowel sounds, abdomen rigidity or tenderness |
| Genitourinary | Voiding or catheterization, intake and output |

Assessment parameters to specifically focus on depend largely on the chief diagnosis. For example, a patient with preeclampsia, eclampsia, or HELLP syndrome may present with c/o of headache, blurred vision, or epigastric pain. It is important to determine the patient's vital signs, lung sounds and $SaO_2$, DTRs and Clonus, hourly intake and output, and specific labs such as platelet count and liver enzymes. Knowing specific intakes and urine outputs or if the patient has any renal compromise if they are being stabilized on $MgSO_4$ is extremely important, so as not to fluid overload the patient or cause $MgSO_4$ toxicity.

Vital signs including blood pressure, pulse, and respirations should be taken initially and repeated every 15 minutes or more often as needed during transportation of all HROB transports (temperature every 2 hours if ruptured membranes). Patients on $MgSO_4$ should have continuous cardiac and $SaO_2$ readings as well as hourly DTRs and lung sounds evaluated in the transport environment.

Determination of cervical dilation either through a digital or a sterile speculum examination should most often be reassessed prior to departure, as each case warrants. Also, notation should be made on quantity and color of amniotic fluid, if present, and whether any bloody show is noted.

Once the secondary survey is completed, the initial plan of care is revised to accommodate any changes. At this time, any additional stabilization should be performed, and all monitoring equipment should be transferred onto the patient. Packaging of the patient should be done in preparation for transport and the receiving facility alerted as to the ETA, if any additional assistance might be needed upon arrival.

## FETAL ASSESSMENT AND SURVEILLANCE

In addition to assessing the mother, fetal assessment must be done by careful review of the bedside fetal monitor tracing at the referring facility. Fetal monitor tracings provide a "window" for evaluating the unborn fetus in a noninvasive manner. They provide the transport team with a great deal of information on not only the fetus but indirectly reflect the condition of the mother much like a "barometer." Fetal monitors document FHR and contraction patterns that allow transport personnel to identify potential problems and provide stabilization techniques prior to and during transport (if transport team carries a fetal monitor). Regardless of whether the team carries a fetal monitor en route, evaluating the FHR tracing at the bedside is imperative to determine "fetal well-being" or noting a "reassuring FHR pattern" prior to moving the patient. Parameters that should be evaluated and charted include the following (7):

### NICHD Terminology for Fetal Heart Rate Characteristics (7)
*Baseline*

- Rate—mean FHR rounded to increments of 5 bpm during a 10-minute segment excluding periodic or episodic changes, periods of marked variability, and segments of baseline that differ by >25 bpm. Duration must be ≥2 minutes.
- Bradycardia—baseline rate of <110 bpm for ≥10 minutes
- Tachycardia—baseline rate of >160 bpm for ≥10 minutes

*Variability*
Fluctuations in the baseline FHR of two cycles per minute or greater. Visually quantitated as the amplitude of the peak to trough in beats per minute—classified as absent, minimal, moderate, and marked

- Absent variability—amplitude from peak to trough undetectable.
- Minimal variability—amplitude from peak to trough more than undetectable and ≤5 bpm.
- Moderate variability—amplitude from peak to trough 6 to 25 bpm.
- Marked variability—amplitude from peak to trough >25 bpm.

*Acceleration*
Visually apparent abrupt increase (onset to peak is <30 seconds) of FHR above baseline. Peak is ≥15 bpm. Duration is ≥15 bpm and <2 minutes. In gestations <32 weeks, peak of 10 bpm and duration of 10 seconds are acceleration.

**Prolonged acceleration**—acceleration >2 minutes and <10 minutes duration.
**Early deceleration**—visually apparent gradual decrease (onset to nadir is ≥30 seconds) of FHR below baseline. Return to baseline associated with a uterine contraction. Nadir of deceleration occurs at the same time as the peak of the contraction. Generally, the onset, nadir, and recovery of the deceleration occur at the same time as the onset, peak, and recovery of the contraction.
**Variable deceleration**—visually apparent abrupt decrease (onset to nadir is <30 seconds) in FHR below baseline. Decrease is ≥15 bpm. Duration is ≥15 seconds and <2 minutes.
**Late deceleration**—visually apparent gradual decrease (onset to nadir is ≥30 seconds) of FHR below baseline. Return to baseline associated with a

uterine contraction. Nadir of deceleration occurs after the peak of the contraction. Generally, the onset, nadir, and recovery of the deceleration occur after same time as the onset, peak, and recovery of the contraction.

**Prolonged deceleration**—visually apparent abrupt decrease (onset to nadir is <30 seconds) in FHR below baseline. Decrease is ≥15 bpm. Duration is ≥2 minutes but <10 minutes.

*Contractions*

**Frequency**—timed from beginning of one contraction to beginning of the next (e.g., 2 to 4 minutes)

**Duration**—timed from beginning to end of each contraction. Charted in range (e.g., 60 to 80 seconds)

**Intensity**—classified as mild, moderate, or strong based on uterine palpation.

**Resting tone**—softness of uterus noted between contractions noted as present or absent.

According to the 2008 NICHD recommendations, the following is the new Uterine Activity Assessment—uterine contractions are quantified as the number of contractions present in a 10-minute window, averaged over a 30-minute period of time. Contraction frequency alone is a partial assessment of uterine activity. Other factors such as duration, intensity, and relaxation time between contractions (resting tone) are equally important in clinical practice (7).

## Interventions for Abnormal FHR Patterns

The overall goal is to improve the uterine/placental blood flow and fetal oxygenation by

- Repositioning maternal patient to the extreme lateral left or right side, modified Trendelenburg (mom's hips higher than her head) or knee–chest position in the presence of fetal distress to improve uterine blood flow and oxygenation. Vaginal examination may be done to exclude cord prolapse.
- $O_2$ via face mask at 100% (high-flow non-rebreather).
- IV fluid hydration (500 to 1,000 mL LR or NS) to prevent maternal hypotension/dehydration.
- Reducing uterine contractions with medications such as tocolytics.
- Reevaluating and repeating above interventions until fetal distress is resolved.
- Notifying MD—being done simultaneously with above treatments.
- Considering delivery at outlying facility if transport is lengthy or unexpected delays anticipated.
- Continual fetal monitoring during transport of fetus with abnormal FHR pattern.

## Standard of Care in the Transport Industry Regarding Fetal Monitoring

Unfortunately, a majority of transport programs do not use continuous fetal monitoring in transport. There are some critical care transport programs that have adopted using fetal monitors, but it has not yet been universally adopted.

The current standard of care in the transport industry regarding fetal assessment in transport is the use of "Doppler FHR" noted every 15 minutes in early labor and every 5 minutes in active labor. There are, however, limitations in the transport environment making it very difficult to manually achieve Doppler FHR as listed above. These include the inability to note FHR due to the noise and continuous movement in a transport vehicle as well as the inability to adequately palpate uterine contractions in a moving vehicle.

The most common reason for transporting a HROB patient is that the mother or the fetus needs a higher level of care than can be provided by the referring facility. Any information that can be obtained through continuous monitoring of the fetal status is imperative to the continuity of care. Taking a HROB patient off continuous fetal monitoring has been compared to taking a cardiac patient off a cardiac monitor for the transport. That would never be done as is a violation of a standard practice, and it would change the way in which that cardiac patient was being assessed. Yet, the cardiac patient could still be visualized, something that cannot be achieved even when using fetal monitoring. It takes away the only source of information on the changes happening in utero.

There is ongoing controversy as to the necessity of fetal monitoring during transport. Some view it as a "decrease" in the level of care that was provided at the referring facility when the fetal monitor is not being continued on a patient being cared for by an ACLS or critical care transport team. The feeling is that the team should at least continue to maintain if not increase the level of care provided by the referral facility but certainly not decrease it. Many things can change in the time frame between auscultating an FHR every 15 minutes

Others feel that auscultating a FHR every 15 minutes is adequate. Those advocates state that a c-section cannot be performed en route, so what could be done if there is a problem? Fly faster? As noted in the stabilization section, there are many interventions that can be successfully accomplished in transport while getting the patient to definitive care.

A final concern is that teams that are properly trained to interpret fetal monitor tracings but chose to discontinue continuous surveillance of the fetus have been subject to intense scrutiny by attorneys in medical malpractice cases. This can be considered a breach of duty and abandonment in some transport situations.

## CONDITIONS WARRANTING TRANSPORT

The majority of maternal transports will be carried out due to concern for a sick mother or a potentially compromised fetus. The following conditions usually require that the pregnant mother be transported to a regional center for high-risk care (Level 3 NICU) (1,8).

A. Common maternal transports
   - Preterm labor (PTL)—occurring before 34 weeks or with a fetus estimated to weigh <2,000 g
   - Premature rupture of membranes (PPROM)—occurring before 34 weeks or with a fetus estimated to weigh <2,000 g
   - Hypertensive disorders—preeclampsia, HELLP syndrome, or eclampsia
   - Bleeding disorders—placenta previa, placental abruption, postpartum hemorrhage
   - Diabetes—poorly controlled gestational diabetes or severe diabetes mellitus
   - Multiple gestation
   - Intrauterine growth restriction (IUGR)
   - Oligohydramnios, polyhydramnios
   - Rh isoimmunization
   - Maternal conditions which may affect the fetus or precipitate delivery such as transplant candidate, cancer, lupus, infection, heart disease, renal disease or dialysis, trauma, drug abuse

- Surgical complications—trauma, acute abdomen, previous C/S, thoracic emergencies
- Fetal conditions requiring specialized neonatal treatment upon delivery such as diaphragmatic hernia, omphalocele, neural tube defects, fetal heart dysrhythmias, fetal hydrops, etc.

B. Emergency childbirth

Emergency delivery may be necessary at the referral facility if stabilization attempts are unsuccessful. Emergency childbirth situations may include

- Breech presentation
- Shoulder dystocia
- Umbilical cord prolapse
- Meconium stained amniotic fluid delivery
- Prolonged fetal non-reassurance
- Nuchal cord
- Potential for delivery in confined spaces in transport
- Postpartum hemorrhage
- Uterine inversion
- Uterine rupture

**Preterm Labor (PTL) and/or Preterm Premature Rupture of Membranes (PPROM)**

Premature births are the number one obstetric problem in the United States. Approximately 70% of all maternal transports are secondary to complications of preterm labor and/or premature rupture of membranes. According to the National Center for Health Statistics, 543,000 babies were born prematurely in the United States in 2006 (9). This is a 36% increase since the 1980s. While medical facilities and NICUs have excellent success rates with very premature infants, approximately 12 babies die daily due to prematurity. While organizations such as March of Dimes provide fund-raising and education for the prevention of prematurity, the United States was given a "D" on an overall report card for this condition (9).

Some methods of stabilization of the preterm patient should include (10–12)

- Prompt identification by rapid assessment of preterm labor patients.
- Prompt interventions using stabilization techniques beginning with the least invasive and working in a progressive manor:
    - Dehydration can cause contractions that mimic labor
    - Give IVF bolus of 500 to 1,000 mL of LR or NS to a healthy patient with adequate urine outputs (>30 mL per hour) and no underlying disease processes, and repeat prn
    - Ensure patient bladder remains empty; use of Foley Catheter recommended for transport
    - Infection may cause contractions; consider antibiotics following completion of blood draws and cultures dependant on medical direction protocols
    - Avoid repeated vaginal exams unless patient appears more active or c/o urge to have bowel movement or push, especially if already PPROM in which case vaginal exam should be especially avoided
    - Consider starting tocolytics immediately coinciding with the IV fluid bolus. Although there is controversy with regard to continuing using these tocolytics once at the receiving facility, most transport teams and receiving physicians will agree that having the ability to administer rapid-acting tocolytics during transport is a huge benefit in getting the patient from point A to point B.
    - Tocolytics

- Brethine (Terbutaline Sulfate)—a $\beta$-sympathomimetic. Decreases smooth muscle contractility, resulting in uterine and bronchial relaxation

    Dosage—0.25 mg SQ—may repeat every 20 minutes for three doses

    Side effects—tremors, light-headedness, flushed feeling, restlessness, maternal and fetal tachycardia, palpitations, nausea and vomiting

    Contraindications—hold for maternal pulse >120 bpm. Active bleeding, insulin-dependent diabetes, cardiac or chronic HTN

    Is one of three drugs that when used together can increase chances of pulmonary edema (MgSO4 and steroids are the other two)

- Magnesium sulfate ($MgSO_4$)—relaxes smooth muscle of uterus by substituting itself for calcium. Often first-line drug for PTL/PPROM and HTN. Is a smooth muscle relaxer used to relax the uterus.

    Loading dose: 4 to 6 g loading dose over 30 minutes (unless contraindicated—lower dose with decreased renal clearance). Administered IVPB only, never mainlined. Never give IM.

    Maintenance dose: 1 to 4 g per hour

    Therapeutic level: 4 to 7 mEq/L

    Side effects—**flushing, sweating, nausea and vomiting**, drowsiness. Lower doses should be given in renal impairment or decreased urine output/preeclamptic patients. **Must maintain urine output >30 mL per hour** to prevent possible toxicity as $MgSO_4$ is excreted through urine

    Frequent assessment of vitals, pulse ox, DTRs, lung sounds

    **Toxicity:** weakness, visual disturbances, general muscle relaxation, loss of DTRs, respirations <12 per minute

    Antidote—**turn off MgSO$_4$**, for reversal of $MgSO_4$ effect: calcium gluconate, 1g of 10% solution IVP over 3 minutes

    Interventions: monitor VS every 15 minutes, DTRs hourly or more often. Continuous pulse oximeters, strict I&Os, Mag levels every 6 to 12 hours

- Prostaglandin inhibitors—indomethacin (Indocin)

    Dosage—50 mg orally or rectal followed by 25 mg every 4 hours for 48 hours maximum

    Side effects—premature closure of the ductus arteriosus, neonatal pulmonary hypertension if used longer than 48 hour, oligohydramnios (too little amniotic fluid)

    Do not use after 32 weeks' gestation. Only used for 48 hours maximum

- Procardia—used in some institutions in place of other meds above for tocolysis, but not currently used as a standard in the transport industry

    Dosage—10 mg initially PO followed by 10 mg in 30 minutes

    Repeat with lowest effective dose of 10 to 20 mg PO every 4 hours × 48 hours

    90 systolic and/or <40 diastolic or pulse <60 or >120

**Steroid therapy—Betamethasone or Dexamethasone**

- Use: Decreases the risk of respiratory distress syndrome in the premature neonate. Given for gestation of 24 to 34 weeks

    Dosage: Dexamethasone—6 mg IM every 12 hours × 4 doses; Betamethasone (Celestone)—12 mg IM every 24 hours × 2 doses

- Side effects: Increased risk of infection, watch for increased risk of pulmonary edema when used with tocolytics.
- Special care and considerations for transport of these pregnant patients
  - Delineation of the total clinical picture for this patient such as number of pregnancies, how fast previous labors went, current dilation/effacement/station /presenting part/ ruptured or intact membranes, FHR and contraction status, etc.
  - Appropriate placement of tocometry or palpation of contractions
  - Does patient understand description of contractions? She may not be feeling "contractions" but may c/o a backache, cramping, tightening, or lower abdominal pain
  - Can patient be stabilized and transported successfully from point A to point B?
  - Is this patient adequately stabilized for transport? Are her contractions slowing down without further cervical dilation?
  - Could this be a COBRA (Consolidated Omnibus Budget Reconciliation Act) violation to transport patient in active labor? Is it safer for the patient to deliver there and can a NICU team transfer the infant?
- Determining mode of transport
  - Categorize patient into priority status based on current evaluation (Table 13.4).
  - Determine if the appropriate mode of transport is being used for this patient.
  - Fastest and safest transport modality should be used.
  - Patient condition may change the course of original mode of transport.
  - Team may originally plan on ground transport and need to change to flight due to changes in maternal or fetal status, weather or traffic delays, etc.
  - Unforeseen circumstances may warrant a planned flight to go by ground as well.
- Evaluating safety of transport
  - Consider reason for maternal transport
  - Consider adequacy of fetal monitoring techniques and interventions en route
  - Fetal stress may warrant reconsideration of moving the patient
  - Unexpected delays in transport time may change transport modality
  - Need for specialized equipment or advanced expertise including surgical intervention will determine if and when the patient should be moved
- Air versus ground (pros and cons) (11–14)
  - Air: pro—rapid response to patient and rapid return to receiving facility
  - Air: con—weather, patient fear of flight, too confined a space for some HROBs
  - Ground: pro—more room for reconfiguring team to include taking additional staff, ability to transport isolette and mother together in some instances
  - Ground: con—vibrations in ambulance are adverse for many OB patients especially advanced dilation or bulging amniotic sac, traffic delays, slower response to patient, and return of patient
- Care and considerations en route (13,14)
  - Patient positioning in vehicle (Trendelenberg, lateral, knee–chest)
  - Is position providing maximal uterine perfusion?
  - Can both ends of the patient be accessed (head and abdominal area)?
  - Is the facility equipped for emergency delivery/neonatal resuscitation?

- Prepare to give additional tocolytics en route
- Consider premedicating all HROB with antinausea, antianxiety medications to prevent nausea/vomiting secondary to medications and motion sickness
- Fetal and uterine surveillance en route
  - Continuous fetal and uterine monitoring preferable
  - Consider inability to note FHR due to noise
  - Consider inability to palpate uterine contractions in moving vehicle
  - Consider ignoring surveillance as breach of standard of care
- When to say NO to maternal transport
  - Sometimes safer to assist referring facility than move the patient
  - Active and advanced labor—is it an EMTALA violation?
  - Maternal hemorrhage, severe hypotension, shock
  - Fetal compromise with repetitive late decelerations, non-reassuring FHR tracings
  - Ensure the referral physician understands possible need to keep the patient

## LEGAL CONSIDERATIONS

The transfer of a pregnant patient from one facility to another raises some medicolegal considerations. The largest area of concern is the liability issue of who assumes patient responsibility during the transport. Prior to any transfer, the risks and benefits of the transport should be discussed with the patient and the family as well as documented extensively. According to the COBRA laws, the referral physician must discuss the patient status with the receiving physician, who then accepts the patient transfer (15,16). Evaluation and stabilization of the patient should be performed prior to moving the patient to ensure that no harm will come to the patient as a result of the transfer and that the benefits of transfer clearly outweigh the risks (14,17).

It is important that both the referral and the receiving facilities understand that not all transport teams are created equally with regard to obstetric transport knowledge and expertise. According to a 2001 article in the *Air Medical Journal*, 203 air medical transport programs were surveyed, with 133 programs responding to a series of questions regarding the air medical transport of HROB patients. It was concluded that "many programs appeared poorly prepared for these patients" (HROB). This study also showed that only 52% of the programs required their staff to have neonatal resuscitation certifications (18). There is NO universally mandated training required for teams who perform maternal transport, regardless of whether they are a local ambulance called for a one-way transport or a team sent from a receiving facility providing a two-way transport.

While there has been some discussion amongst specialty transport organizations to develop suggested maternal transport guidelines or protocols, none have been adopted as of yet. This leaves it up to the individual transport agencies to decide what, if any, type of training they wish for their employees to have. Some transport team administrators feel that OB transports are a low-volume type of transport (overall <5% of their total transports) and that their education funds are better served in other areas, leaving OB transport education open for the individual transport member to seek out if interested.

## SUMMARY

The transport of the HROB patient is one of the more challenging types of transfers that teams will be called to do. Because they tend to be low volume, HROB's calls often elicit several types of responses from team members. They appear overconfident or conversely exhibit anticipatory despair.

Admittedly, there is very little training done in nursing, paramedic, or respiratory therapy schools that focuses on how to assess, stabilize, and transport the high-risk obstetrical patient. The reader is encouraged to review each state guideline for specific requirements regarding personnel, equipment, and protocols.

The first step is to receive adequate training from someone who has done HROB transports on a regular basis and can provide education which is appropriate for the transport environment. Didactic training (lectures) combined with hands-on skills training that comes from spending time in an L&D doing hands-on skills is much more effective than spending one shift a year in L&D watching a baby being delivered. Birthing is important but so is developing skills such as fetal and maternal assessment parameters as well as putting all the pieces together to determine whether the patient would be stable enough to be transported from one facility to another.

Due to the fact that maternal transports are interfacility transports to a higher level of care, it should be recognized that there are times when it may be safer to say NO to the maternal transport than to risk the lives of the mother or the unborn fetus. When faced with a very sick pregnant patient and/or fetal distress, many factors must be figured into the decision to transport or divert to another facility that can handle the crisis situation. Consideration should include whether the referring facility has a functional operating room, anesthesia, and a surgeon or if it is safer to package and go with the patient using the fastest mode of transport. The time of transport including any unexpected delays should be considered thoroughly prior to moving the patient as well as any special equipment or expertise that is necessary for this impending delivery.

Some areas where it may be safer to assist with delivery and neonatal resuscitation at the referral facility than to move the patient may include

- Active or advanced labor (potential EMTALA violation)
- Maternal hemorrhage, severe hypotension, or shock
- Fetal compromise such as repetitive late decelerations or non-reassuring FHR patterns

When in doubt, it is always better to err on the side of caution than to take a patient from a "stable" environment into a "less stable" transport environment.

### References

1. Gilstrap LC. *Guidelines for Perinatal Care.* 6th Ed. Elk Grove Village, IL: American Academy of Pediatrics and American College of Obstetricians and Gynecologists; 2007.
2. Anderson CL, Aladjem S, Ayuste O, et al. An analysis of maternal transport within a suburban metropolitan region. *Am J Obstet Gynecol.* 1981;140:499–504.
3. Pon SP, Nodderman DA. The organization of a critical care pediatric transport program. *Pediatric Clin North Am.* 1993;40:241.
4. Adams P. O.B. STAT, Inc. Maternal Transport Manual, Copyrighted 1992, 2002.
5. Elliott J, Sipp T, Balazs K. Maternal transport of patients with advanced cervical dilation—to fly or not to fly? *Obstet Gynecol.* 1992;79(3).
6. James DK, Steer PJ, Weiner CP, Gonik B. (eds.). *High Risk Pregnancy, Management Options.* 3rd Ed. New York, NY: Saunders; 2005.
7. NIHCD Standardized Nomenclature for Electronic Fetal Monitoring, Joint ACOG, AWHONN, NICHD publication; 2008.
8. Creehan P, Simpson K. *Perinatal Nursing.* 2nd Ed. Washington, DC: AWHONN; 2001.
9. Source National Center for Health Statistics for 2006, released January 7, 2009.
10. Management of Preterm Labor. ACOG Practice Bulletin. Number 43, May 2003.

11. Nelson M. The high-risk obstetric patient. In: *Air Medical Crew Core Curriculum.* Pasadena, CA: US Department of Transportation; 1988:177–190.

12. AAMS. *Guidelines for Air Medical Crew Education* Dubuque, IA: Kendall Hunt Publishing; 2004.

13. National Flight Nurses Association, *Flight Nursing Core Curriculum.* "Obstetrical Transport" Chapter 16 & "Neonatal Transport" Chapter 17; 1997.

14. Lee G. *Flight Nursing principles and practice.* 1st Ed. St. Louis, MO: Mosby; 1991.

15. Cady R., Rostant D. *Liability Issues in Perinatal Nursing.* Washington, DC: AWHONN; 1999.

16. Frew SA, Roush WR, LaGreca, K. COBRA: implications for emergency medicine. *Ann Emerg Med* 1988;17:835.

17. Mandeville L., Troiano, N. *High-risk & Critical Care Intrapartum Nursing.* 2nd Ed. Philadelphia, PA: J.B. Lippincott; 1999.

18. Jones AE, Summers RL, Deschamp C, Galli RL. A national survey of the air medical transport of high-risk obstetric patients. *Air Med J.* 2001;20(2):17–20.

# 14

## Human Immunodeficiency Virus (HIV) Infection and Pregnancy: Labor and Delivery Management

**Isaac Delke**

Adult and adolescent females accounted for 27% of persons living with HIV infection in the United States at the end of 2007. By region, 40% resided in the South, 29% in the Northeast, 20% in the West, and 11% in the Midwest. African American and Hispanic women account for 80% of cases (1). The majority of these women are of childbearing age and approximately 6,000 to 7,000 HIV-infected women deliver children in the United States each year. Approximately 15% to 30% of these women would be expected to give birth to infected infants, in the absence of specific interventions aimed to decrease perinatal transmission. Perinatal HIV transmission may occur in utero, during delivery, or through breastfeeding (2).

Treatment of HIV infection has evolved with an increasing proportion of women receiving highly active antiretroviral therapy (HAART) throughout pregnancy. With the implementation of universal prenatal HIV counseling and testing, antiretroviral prophylaxis, scheduled cesarean delivery, and avoidance of breastfeeding, perinatal HIV infection has dramatically diminished to <2% in the United States over the last 25 years (2–5).

The emergency department (ED) continues to be the site of entry into the hospital for obstetric patients. The ED staff could be faced with an HIV-infected patient in labor ready to deliver and must know how to handle such a situation. This chapter focuses on (a) the identification of HIV-infected women in labor and (b) interventions for the prevention of perinatal HIV transmission—antiretroviral prophylaxis, cesarean delivery, and avoidance of breastfeeding. Various scenarios that commonly occur in clinical practice are presented, and the factors that influence treatment considerations are highlighted.

## IDENTIFICATION OF HIV-INFECTED WOMEN IN LABOR

Since many women with HIV infection (over 75% at our center) enter pregnancy with a known diagnosis, a confidential review of maternal history and prenatal record for HIV serostatus on admission to the ED is vital. This has been enhanced by the availability of electronic medical record (including prenatal) in many hospitals.

Any woman without documented HIV status at the time of labor should be screened with rapid HIV testing unless she declines (opt-out screening) (6,7). Currently, there are six rapid HIV screening tests that are approved by the US Food and Drug Administration (FDA) (6) and commercially available for use in the United States (Table 14.1). Rapid HIV tests are relatively simple to use, and they make it possible to provide information on HIV antibody status at the point of care. Statutes and regulations in this area vary from state to state (8). Rapid HIV testing is also recommended for women who present in labor with a negative HIV test early in pregnancy, but who are known to be at increased risk for HIV acquisition or who deliver in locations with elevated incidence or prevalence of HIV infection. Rapid HIV antibody testing should be available on a 24-hour basis at all facilities with a maternity service and/or neonatal intensive

**TABLE 14.1** FDA-Approved Rapid HIV Antibody Screening Tests

| Test Kit Name (Approval Date) | Specimen Type | CLIA Category | Sensitivity (95% CI) | Specificity (95% CI) | Manufacturer (Web Site) |
|---|---|---|---|---|---|
| OraQuick ADVANCE Rapid HIV-1/2 Antibody Test (Nov 2002) | Oral fluid Whole blood Plasma | Waived Waived Moderate complexity | 99.3% (98.4–99.7) 99.6% (98.5–99.9) 99.6% (98.9–99.8) | 99.8% (99.6–99.9) 100% (99.7–100) 99.9% (99.6–99.9) | Orasure Technologies, Inc. (http://www.orasure.com/) |
| Reveal Rapid HIV-1 Antibody Test (Apr 2003) | Serum Plasma | Moderate complexity Moderate complexity | 99.8% (99.2–100) 99.8% (99.0–100) | 99.1% (98.8–99.4) 98.6% (98.4–98.8) | MedMira, Inc. (http://www.medmira.com) |
| Uni-Gold Recombigen HIV-1 Test (Dec 2003) | Whole blood Serum and Plasma | Waived Moderate complexity | 100% (99.5–100) 100% (99.5–100) | 99.7% (99.0–100) 99.8% (99.3–100) | Trinity BioTech, plc (http://www.trinitybiotech.com/EN/index.asp) |
| MultiSpot HIV-1/HIV-2 Rapid Test (Nov 2004) | Serum Plasma | Moderate complexity Moderate complexity | 100% (99.94–100) 100% (99.94–100) | 99.93% (99.79–100) 99.91% (99.77–100) | BioRad Laboratories (www.biorad.com) |
| Clearview HIV 1/2 STAT-PAK (May 2006) | Whole blood Serum and plasma | Waived Nonwaived | 99.7% (98.9–100) 99.7% (98.9–100) | 99.9% (99.6–100) 99.9% (99.6–100) | Inverness Medical Professional Diagnostics (www.invernessmedicalpd.com) |
| Clearview COMPLETE HIV-1/2 STAT-PAK (May 2006) | Whole blood Serum and plasma | Waived Nonwaived | 99.7% (98.9–100) 99.7% (98.9–100) | 99.9% (99.6–100) 99.9% (99.6–100) | Inverness Medical Professional Diagnostics (www.invernessmedicalpd.com) |

*Note:* CLIA, Clinical Laboratory Improvement Amendments.
*Source:* Ref. 6.

care unit. Women with a positive rapid antibody test should be presumed to be infected until standard HIV antibody confirmatory testing clarifies their status. All women with a positive rapid HIV test in labor should have interventions started immediately to prevent perinatal HIV transmission, as discussed below.

## INTERVENTIONS TO REDUCE PERINATAL HIV TRANSMISSION

In 1994, use of zidovudine (ZDV) in pregnancy, beginning at 14 weeks' gestation and continuing through completion of delivery, was studied in the Pediatric AIDS Clinical Trials Group Protocol (PACTG) 076. A three-part regimen, beginning at 14 weeks' gestation, with intravenous (IV) infusions of ZDV throughout labor and delivery, and subsequent use of oral ZDV for 6 weeks by the infant, resulted in a decrease in transmission rate by approximately 70%, from 25% to 8% (9). At present, there are over 20 FDA-approved antiretroviral drugs in the United States (Table 14.2) (5).

Current recommendations for the prevention of perinatal HIV transmission include the use of combination antiretroviral therapy during pregnancy, as would ordinarily be indicated for the mother's own care, with the addition of ZDV during labor and delivery (Table 14.3) (5). However, abbreviated courses of ZDV and/or other antiretroviral drugs have also been shown to be effective in reducing perinatal HIV transmission to infants whose mothers never received antiretroviral drugs during pregnancy or labor (Table 14.4) (5).

The short-term toxicity of antiretroviral drugs appears to be acceptable, in terms of both mother and infant. The long-term toxicities of in utero exposure to antiretroviral agents are not yet known. It is thus imperative that all HIV-infected pregnant women be educated and counseled prior to making decision regarding the use of antiretroviral agents during the antepartum and intrapartum periods. The ultimate decision regarding the use of antiretroviral agents in pregnancy must reside with the patient herself, after careful and nonjudgmental discussion with her health care providers (5).

Additional means to decrease perinatal transmission include avoidance of artificial rupture of the membranes during labor, scheduled cesarean delivery when the HIV RNA level close to delivery is $\geq$1,000 copies/mL or unknown, and avoidance of breastfeeding. Each of these interventions poses particular problems in resource-poor regions of the world, where standard guidelines for the prevention of perinatal HIV infection must, of practical necessity, be altered. Early recognition of HIV infection will be important in these areas, as well as prenatal care and the use of antiretroviral therapy in late pregnancy, in delivery, and/or given to the newborn. *Clearly, primary prevention of maternal infection is still the best intervention.*

HIV-infected women in labor who have received antiretroviral drugs during pregnancy should be managed as outlined in Table 14.3. Women who are receiving an antepartum combination antiretroviral treatment regimen should continue this regimen on schedule as much as possible during the intrapartum period, regardless of the route of delivery, to provide maximal virologic effect, but consultation with the attending anesthesiologist should be obtained before administering in the preoperative period. If maternal antiretroviral therapy must be interrupted temporarily (i.e., for <24 hours) in the peripartum period, all drugs (except for intrapartum intravenous ZDV) should be stopped and reinstituted simultaneously to minimize the chance of resistance development (5).

HIV-infected women in labor who have had no prior antiretroviral therapy should be managed as outlined in Table 14.4. All HIV-infected women who have not received antepartum antiretroviral therapy, as well as those with a positive rapid HIV test in labor, should have intravenous ZDV started immediately to prevent perinatal HIV transmission. In addition to intravenous intrapartum ZDV, if intrapartum single-dose NVP is given to mother, administration of

**TABLE**
**14.2**    Antiretroviral Drugs and FDA Pregnancy Category

| Antiretroviral Drug Class and Generic Name (Brand and Other Name) | FDA Pregnancy Category[a] |
|---|---|
| ***Nucleoside and nucleotide analogue reverse transcriptase inhibitors (NRTIs)*** | |
| Abacavir (Ziagen, ABC) | C |
| Didanosine (Videx, Videx EC, ddl) | B |
| Emtricitabine (Emtriva, FTC) | B |
| Lamivudine (Epivir, 3TC) | C |
| Stavudine (Zerit, d4T) | C |
| Tenofovir DF (Viread, TDF) | B |
| Zidovudine (Retrovir, AZT, ZDV) | C |
| ***Nonnucleoside reverse transcriptase inhibitors (NNRTIs)*** | |
| Efavirenz (Sustiva, EFV) | D |
| Etravirine (Intelence, Celsentri, TMC125) | B |
| Nevirapine (Viramune, NVP) | B |
| ***Protease inhibitors*** | |
| Atazanavir (Reyataz, ATV) | B |
| Darunavir (Prezista, TMC114) | C |
| Fosamprenavir (Lexiva, FFV) | C |
| Indinavir (Crixivan, IDV) | C |
| Lopinavir/Ritonavir (Kaletra, LPV/r) | C |
| Nelfinavir (Viracept, NFV) | B |
| Ritonavir (Norvir, RTV) | B |
| Saquinavir (Fortovase, SQV) | B |
| Tipranavir (Aptivus, TPV) | C |
| ***Entry inhibitors*** | |
| Enfuvirtide (Fuzeon, T-20) | B |
| Maraviroc (Selzentry, MVC) | B |
| ***Integrase inhibitors*** | |
| Raltegravir (Isentress, MK-0518) | C |

[a]FDA pregnancy categories: A: Adequate and well-controlled studies of pregnant women fail to demonstrate a risk to the fetus during the first trimester of pregnancy (and there is no evidence of risk during later trimesters); B: Animal reproduction studies fail to demonstrate a risk to the fetus and adequate and well-controlled studies of pregnant women have not been conducted; C: Safety in human pregnancy has not been determined, animal studies either are positive for fetal risk or have not been conducted, and the drug should not be used unless the potential benefit outweighs the potential risk to the fetus; D: Positive evidence of human fetal risk based on adverse reaction data from investigational or marketing experiences, but the potential benefits from the use of the drug in pregnant women may be acceptable despite its potential risks; X: Studies in animals or reports of adverse reactions have indicated that the risk associated with the use of the drug for pregnant women clearly outweighs any possible benefit.
*Note*: Combinations antiretroviral drugs: Combivir (lamivudine + zidovudine); Trizivir (abacavir + lamivudine + zidovudine); Truvada (emtricitabine + tenofovir DF); and emtricitabine, tenofovir, and efavirenz are included as a fixed-dose combination in Atripla.
*Source*: Ref. 5.

| | Intrapartum Maternal and Neonatal Zidovudine Dosing for Prevention of Mother-to-Child HIV Transmission |

| Drug | Dosing | Duration |
|---|---|---|
| **Maternal** | | |
| ZDV plus other antiretroviral agents | • 2 mg/kg body weight intravenously over 1 hr, followed by continuous infusion of 1 mg/kg body weight per hour<br>• Other antiretroviral agents are continued orally | • Onset of labor until delivery of infant<br>• Evaluate the need for continuation of maternal therapy postpartum |
| **Neonatal** | | |
| ZDV (>35 weeks' gestation) | 2 mg/kg body weight per dose given orally (or 1.5 mg/kg body weight per dose given intravenously) started as close to birth as possible (by 6–12 hr of delivery), then q 6 hr[a] | Birth to 6 weeks |
| ZDV (<35 but >30 weeks' gestation) | 2 mg/kg body weight per dose given orally (or 1.5 mg/kg body weight per dose given intravenously) q 12 hr, advanced to q 8 hr at 2 weeks of age | Birth to 6 weeks |
| ZDV (<30 weeks' gestation) | 2 mg/kg body weight per dose given orally (or 1.5 mg/kg/dose given intravenously) q 12 hr, advanced to q 8 hr at 4 weeks of age | Birth to 6 weeks |

*Note*: ZDV, zidovudine

[a]ZDV dosing of 4 mg/kg body weight per dose given q 12 hr has been used for infant prophylaxis in some international perinatal studies. While there are no definitive data to show equivalent pharmacokinetic parameters or efficacy in preventing transmission, a regimen of ZDV 4 mg/kg body weight per dose given orally twice daily instead of 2 mg/kg body weight per dose given orally four times daily may be considered when there are concerns about adherence to drug administration to the infant.

*Source*: Ref. 5.

intrapartum oral 3TC followed by the administration of ZDV and 3TC for 7 days postpartum to reduce the development of NVP-resistant virus is recommended. Although intrapartum/neonatal antiretroviral medications will not prevent perinatal transmission that occurs before labor, most transmission occurs near to or during labor and delivery. Pre-exposure prophylaxis for the fetus can be provided by giving the mother a drug that rapidly crosses the placenta to produce systemic antiretroviral drug levels in the fetus during intensive exposure to HIV in maternal genital secretions and blood during birth. In general, ZDV and other NRTI drugs as well as NNRTI drugs cross the placenta well, while the protease inhibitor drugs do not (5).

## INTRAPARTUM CARE FOR ALL HIV-INFECTED WOMEN IN LABOR

1. Identify HIV-infected women in labor.
2. Implement universal body fluid/substance precautions for *all* births to prevent nosocomial infection.

| | Intrapartum Maternal and Neonatal Dosing for Additional Antiretroviral Drugs for Prevention of Mother-to-Child HIV Transmission | |
|---|---|---|
| **Drug** | **Dosing** | **Duration** |
| **Maternal intrapartum/postpartum** | | |
| NVP (as single dose intrapartum)[a] | 200 mg given orally as single dose | Given once at onset of labor |
| ZDV + 3TC (given with single-dose NVP as "tail" to reduce NVP resistance) | ZDV: intravenous infusion intrapartum (as per Table 13.3); then after delivery, 300 mg orally twice daily; 3TC: 150 mg orally twice daily starting at labor onset | Through 1 week postpartum |
| **Neonatal** | | |
| NVP (as single dose)[b] | 2 mg/kg body weight given orally as single dose | Single dose between birth and 72 hr of age If maternal dose is given <2 hr before delivery, infant dose should be administered as soon as possible following birth |
| ZDV + 3TC (given with single-dose NVP as "tail" to reduce NVP resistance) | ZDV: neonatal dosing (as per Table 13.3); 3TC: 2 mg/kg body weight given orally twice daily | ZDV: Birth to 6 weeks; 3TC: birth to 1 week |

*Note*: NVP, nevirapine; ZDV, zidovudine; 3TC, lamivudine.
[a]Given *in addition* to intravenous intrapartum ZDV; if intrapartum single-dose NVP is given to mother, administration of intrapartum oral 3TC followed by the administration of ZDV and 3TC for 7 days postpartum to reduce the development of NVP-resistant virus is recommended.
[b]Given *in addition* to 6 weeks of infant ZDV; addition of 7 days of 3TC may be considered to reduce the development of NVP-resistant virus.
*Source*: Ref. 5.

3. Delay artificial rupture of membranes (AROM).

4. Avoid fetal scalp electrodes and scalp pH sampling.

5. Administer intrapartum IV ZDV plus other oral antiretroviral agents (Tables 13.3 and 13.4).

6. Offer the option of CD for patients with viral loads ≥1,000 copies/mL close to delivery or unknown.

7. Artificial rupture of membranes or invasive monitoring should be considered only when obstetrically indicated and the length of time for ruptured membranes or monitoring is anticipated to be short.

8. Operative delivery with forceps or the vacuum extractor and/or episiotomy should be performed only in select circumstances.

9. Suction the baby with a bulb or wall suction apparatus.

10. Wash off maternal secretions from the infant as soon as possible after birth.

11. Consultation with a pediatric HIV specialist is recommended.

12. Postpartum hemorrhage, antiretroviral drugs, and methergine use: Methergine should not be coadministered with drugs that are potent CYP3A4 enzyme inhibitors, including protease inhibitors and the NNRTI drugs such as EFV. The concomitant use of ergotamines and protease inhibitors has been associated with exaggerated vasoconstrictive responses. When uterine atony results in excessive postpartum bleeding in women receiving protease inhibitors or NNRTIs as a component of an antiretroviral regimen, oxytocin and/or misoprostol are safe to use (5).

Infants born to mothers who have received no antiretroviral therapy during pregnancy or labor (5):

■ The 6-week neonatal ZDV component of the ZDV chemoprophylaxis regimen should be discussed with the mother and offered for the newborn. ZDV should be initiated as soon as possible after delivery—preferably within 12 to 24 hours of birth.

■ Some clinicians may choose to use ZDV in combination with other antiretroviral drugs.

■ HIV infection in infants should be diagnosed using HIV DNA PCR or RNA virologic assays. Maternal HIV antibody crosses the placenta and will be detectable in all HIV-exposed infants up to 18 months of age and should not be used for HIV diagnosis in newborns.

## POSTPARTUM CARE

■ Evaluate the need for continuation of maternal antiretroviral therapy postpartum.

■ Woman with a positive rapid antibody test in labor: Along with confirmatory HIV antibody testing, the woman should have appropriate assessments (e.g., CD4 count and HIV RNA copies/mL) in the immediate postpartum period to determine maternal health status and whether antiretroviral therapy is recommended for her own health.

■ Arrangements for establishing HIV care and providing ongoing psychosocial support after discharge should also be provided.

## SUMMARY

It is essential that women presenting in active labor to the ED have confidential review of maternal history and prenatal record for HIV serostatus. Women with known HIV infection should continue their combination antiretroviral therapy with the addition of intravenous ZDV during labor and delivery. Counseling and rapid HIV testing should be performed in the intrapartum and/or postnatal periods if serostatus has not been previously determined. Women identified as HIV infected in labor should be treated with (a) intravenous ZDV in labor and ZDV for 6 weeks to the neonate and/or (b) nevirapine, a single dose in labor, with a single dose to the neonate. In addition to intravenous intrapartum ZDV, if intrapartum single-dose NVP is given to mother, administration of intrapartum oral 3TC followed by the administration of ZDV and 3TC for 7 days postpartum to reduce the development of NVP-resistant virus is recommended. CD should be recommended to all women when the most recent viral load is ≥1,000 copies/mL or unknown. It is recognized that strategies to prevent perinatal transmission and concepts related to management of HIV infection during pregnancy are rapidly evolving. The most recent information is available at the Public Health Service Web site (http://www.aidsinfo.nih.gov), which provides a regularly updated, practical, and thorough guide to the management of HIV infection (5).

### References

1. Centers for Disease Control and Prevention. HIV/AIDS Surveillance Report, 2007. Vol. 19. Atlanta: U.S. Department of Health and Human Services, Centers for Disease Control and Prevention; 2009:8–10. Available at: http://www.cdc.gov/hiv/topics/surveillance/resources/reports/. Retrieved May 10, 2009.
2. Centers for Disease Control and Prevention (CDC), Mofenson LM, Taylor AW, et al. Achievements in public health: reduction in perinatal transmission of HIV infection–United States, 1985–2005. *MMWR Morb Mortal Wkly Rep.* 2006;55(21): 592–597.
3. Cooper ER, Charurat M, Mofenson LM, et al. Combination antiretroviral strategies for the treatment of pregnant HIV-1 infected women and prevention of perinatal HIV-1 transmission. *J Acquir Immune Defic Syndr Hum Retrovirol.* 2002;29(5): 484–494.
4. Jamieson DJ, Clark J, Kourtis AP, et al. Recommendations for human immunodeficiency virus screening, prophylaxis, and treatment for pregnant women in the United States. *Am J Obstet Gynecol.* 2007;197(3 Suppl.):S26–S32.
5. Perinatal HIV Guidelines Working Group. Public Health Service Task Force Recommendations for use of antiretroviral drugs in pregnant HIV-infected women for maternal health and interventions to reduce perinatal HIV transmission in the United States. 2009 April;1–90. Available at: http://aidsinfo.nih.gov/contentfiles/perinatalgl.pdf. Retrieved May 20, 2009.
6. Centers for Disease Control and Prevention. FDA-approved rapid HIV antibody screening tests. Atlanta (GA): CDC; 2008. Available at: http://www.cdc.gov/hiv/topics/testing/ rapid/rt-comparison.htm. Retrieved May 20, 2009.
7. American College of Obstetricians and Gynecologists. Prenatal and perinatal human immunodeficiency virus testing: expanded recommendations. Committee Opinion No. 418. *Obstet Gynecol.* 2008;112:739–742.
8. National HIV/AIDS Clinician's Consultation Center. Compendium of State HIV Testing Laws - 2009. Available at: http://www.nccc.ucsf.edu/statelaws/index.html. Retrieved May 10, 2009.
9. Connor EM, Sperling RS, Gelber R, et al. Reduction of maternal-infant transmission of human immunodeficiency virus type 1 with zidovudine treatment. *N Engl J Med.* 1994;31:1173–1180.

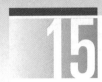

# Postpartum Emergencies

**David C. Jones**

## POSTPARTUM EMERGENCIES

Most pregnancies conclude successfully, and when postpartum complications arise, they usually arise prior to discharge from the hospital. However, occasionally, complications arise after discharge or are noted in women who have home births, and in the latter case, the emergency department physician may be faced with complications that are normally seen in labor and delivery suites (Table 15.1). Family members may become quite worried about relatively minimal complications or may dismiss signs and symptoms of significant disease as normal postpartum complaints. The emergency department physician may need to sort out the serious conditions from those that are self-limited. For that reason, this chapter will review some of the critical postpartum emergencies seen immediately postpartum as well as those normally seen in women discharged from the hospital following uncomplicated deliveries.

## SEIZURES

Eclampsia is the most common etiology for postpartum or peripartum seizures. While most eclamptic seizures occur prior to or during labor, 20% occur postpartum. Most of those occur within the first 48 hours, but they may be seen as late as a week after birth and have even been reported 23 days after delivery. If there is no history of a prior seizure disorder, the diagnosis of eclampsia should be assumed until proven otherwise. The first priority in these cases is to stop the seizure, and the drug of choice for this is magnesium sulfate. There are several protocols for administration, but a reasonable choice with eclampsia is to load with 6 mg intravenously over 20 minutes and then begin an infusion of 2 mg per hour, aiming for a therapeutic level of 5 to 8 mg/dL. This infusion is continued for 24 to 48 hours, although this will most likely be managed by the admitting obstetrician. If the magnesium fails to control the seizure, secondary medications that may be used include thiopental 100 mg administered slowly intravenously or diazepam 2 to 10 mg intravenously.

Since eclampsia is usually accompanied by the standard signs of preeclampsia, the presence of hypertension and proteinuria as well as the symptoms of a severe headache, blurred vision, and scotoma would help support that diagnosis. The physical examination may also reveal right upper quadrant pain (due to swelling of the liver within the capsule), hyperreflexia, edema (particularly of the hands and face), and clonus. Laboratory studies may show an elevated uric acid, and possibly elevated liver functions, and elevated serum creatinine or thrombocytopenia. While eclampsia is the most likely diagnosis, once the seizure is controlled, other possible etiologies should be considered. A CT scan is indicated in the evaluation as the differential diagnosis includes cerebral venous thrombosis, hemorrhagic stroke, CNS tumors, and the syndrome of inappropriate antidiuretic hormone secretion. If associated symptoms such as hypertension are found, they should be controlled with relatively rapidly acting agents such as beta-blockers (e.g., labetalol) or calcium channel blockers (e.g., nifedipine). These patients are usually admitted to the labor and delivery suite or to a monitored floor where the magnesium infusion is continued for at least 24 hours and monitoring for further seizures is maintained.

| TABLE 15.1 | Primary Medical Problems of the Postpartum Patient seen at the Emergency Department |
|---|---|

**Infection**
  Genital tract
    Endometritis
    Parametritis
    Pelvic cellulitis (including infected vaginal lacerations and repaired episiotomies)
    Necrotizing fasciitis, toxic shock syndrome
    Septic pelvic thrombophlebitis
  Mastitis
  Urinary tract
    Cystitis
    Pyelonephritis

**Postpartum hemorrhage**
  Early
  Late

**Thrombosis and thrombophlebitis**
  Superficial thrombophlebitis
  Deep venous thrombosis
  Pulmonary embolism
  Ovarian torsion

**Postpartum seizures**
  Eclampsia
  Other

**Postpartum psychological reactions**
  Initial maternal indifference
  Postpartum "blues"
  Postpartum depression
  Postpartum psychosis

## POSTPARTUM HEMORRHAGE

Blood loss exceeding 500 mL at a vaginal delivery is generally considered a postpartum hemorrhage (PPH); however, studies have shown that the average blood loss at a delivery is about 600 mL. It is clear that blood loss is usually underestimated at uncomplicated deliveries. PPH is divided into two categories based on timing with "immediate" PPH occurring within 24 hours of delivery and "delayed" PPH occurring more than 24 hours of delivery. This distinction has a limited usefulness in terms of the differential diagnosis. The bleeding seen after delivery comes primarily from the placental implantation site and, to a lesser extent, from lacerations of the genital tract such as vaginal, introital, periurethral, and labial lacerations. The primary mechanism to control this bleeding from the placental implantation is the contraction of the myometrium. Normal hemostatic mechanisms are responsible for control of bleeding from lacerations and are the secondary means of controlling bleeding from the uterus.

    Immediate PPH is usually due to uterine atony, but other etiologies must be considered including lacerations, retained placenta, uterine rupture (if the patient has a history of prior c-section), and coagulation abnormalities. When a patient is seen emergently after a delivery outside the hospital, heavy bleeding can potentially lead to a state of shock, and fluid resuscitation must be pursued in parallel to the workup of the bleeding. Obstetric hemorrhage requiring a transfusion generally requires many units of blood, so getting units of packed cells typed and crossmatched should be done at the first thought a transfusion may be necessary. Late hemorrhage is more likely caused by retained placenta or membranes, infection, subinvolution of the placental site, coital trauma, or breakdown of genital tract laceration repairs.

## Workup and Treatment

When a patient presents with bleeding, initial assessment must include vital signs, complete blood count, and obviously physical examination. The initial vital signs may suggest the need for fluid resuscitation, and placing one or two large-bore IVs is appropriate. The initial focus of the physical examination is the uterus. Palpation of the uterine fundus should suggest whether it is firm and well-contracted or boggy and soft, suggesting atony. Uterine atony is initially treated with an intravenous infusion of oxytocin (40 units of oxytocin/L of lactated ringers solution or normal saline). Examination of the uterus also has a secondary role. When the uterus is atonic, blood and clot build up in the uterine cavity, which by their presence can make uterine contraction difficult, causing more bleeding and clot. The atonic uterus should be massaged to squeeze out the clots, and occasionally, a manual sweep of the clots is necessary. If oxytocin alone is insufficient to maintain uterine contraction, a number of other options can be tried. The prostaglandin E1 analogue misoprostol has been successfully used to control PPH. The dosage has ranged widely and the route of administration has included rectal, oral, sublingual, and buccal (1–3). Reasonable dosing would include up to 1,000 $\mu$g rectally or 600 $\mu$g sublingual or buccally. This is an off-label use for misoprostol. Prostaglandin E2 is also available (20 mg given rectally), but it is more likely to cause fever, nausea, and diarrhea. Prostaglandin E2 is also not heat stable, so if it has not been stored properly, it will loose efficacy. Prostaglandin F2$\alpha$ (Hemabate) is also used (250 $\mu$g given intramuscularly, intracervically, or intramyometrially) but can cause bronchoconstriction in asthmatics, so a past medical history must be obtained that specifically asks about asthma and reactive airway disease. This dose may be repeated every 10 minutes up to a total of three doses. These prostaglandins have largely replaced the former second-line agent, the ergot alkaloid methylergonovine maleate (Methergine). Methylergonovine maleate is usually given as 0.2 mg intramuscularly, but it may be administered at the same dose orally. If the atony persists despite these treatments, other etiologies must be considered, particularly retained placenta or membranes. In the setting of delayed PPH, ultrasound may be a useful modality to examine the cavity, and if retained products of conception are seen, a gentle dilation and curettage, often with suction, should be performed. One must recognize that an overly aggressive curettage of the endometrial cavity after a delivery is the main risk factor for Asherman syndrome, so these procedures must be performed with great care. In the setting of an immediate PPH, ultrasound is less useful because it frequently looks like there is significant debris in the cavity after an uncomplicated delivery. Instead, the evaluation consists of carefully examining the placenta and membranes (if available) to look for evidence of a retained portion of the placenta or a succenturiate lobe. Direct evaluation of the cavity may be performed by a digital examination with palpation once adequate anesthesia is available. If that examination is suggestive of retained products that cannot be manually removed, then a gentle curettage should be performed with care.

If there is no evidence of retained products of conception or uterine bleeding persists despite their removal, other nonsurgical approaches are available. Intrauterine balloon tamponade is an effective treatment for PPH, particularly those related to bleeding from the lower uterine segment such as a relative low placental implantation (4). This balloon is useful both in terms of treating atony and also as a means of deciding who will probably need surgical management (4). In centers that have interventional radiology services available, embolization of the uterine arteries or hypogastric arteries will frequently control bleeding and avoid surgery. The interuterine balloon may also be placed to decrease hemorrhage while the IR team is being assembled. If these nonsurgical methods fail and it is clear that the etiology of the bleeding is uterine rather than from another site, a laparotomy will be required. Surgical ligation of the uterine or hypogastric arteries may decrease the pulse pressure and control the bleeding adequately. If uterine atony persists, the B-Lynch Brace suture has been shown to be an effective measure. This stitch uses rapidly absorbable sutures to squeeze the uterus in an attempt to simulate the ongoing uterine massage or compression. The B-Lynch has been combined with an intrauterine balloon tamponade to maximize compression in a technique referred to as the "uterine sandwich" (5). If all of these surgical measures fail, hysterectomy may be required. This is usually performed as a supracervical hysterectomy because it can be difficult to identify the cervix after a vaginal delivery, and the surgeon usually leaves the cervix to make sure none of the vaginal is taken.

Because chorioamnionitis and endometritis may increase the likelihood of uterine atony, signs such as an elevated white blood cell count, c-reactive protein, uterine fundal tenderness, and fever should be evaluated. If there is suspicion of infection, appropriate treatment includes admission to the hospital for inpatient intravenous antibiotics.

In an immediate PPH, evaluation for other etiologies would include a careful examination of the vagina and the cervix for lacerations. Bleeding lacerations should be repaired with an intermediate-duration absorbable suture. In a delayed PPH when the bleeding is from a prior repair, antibiotic coverage is appropriate. If the repair does not appear infected, a few stitches can be placed to address the bleeding. If the repair is broken down and appears badly infected, a full repair is best postponed until the infection is well-controlled with antibiotics.

Finally, in some patients, there may be coagulopathies, either because of inherent bleeding disorders or because of disseminated intravascular coagulation secondary to their ongoing PPH. Coagulation parameters should be measured, and blood product components replaced as necessary. A number of obstetrical disorders, including familial thrombophilias with a bad obstetric history, a history of thromboembolism, and antiphospholipid antibody syndrome, are now treated with anticoagulation, at both prophylactic and therapeutic doses. A careful history of past medical conditions and medications once again plays an important role here.

## THROMBOEMBOLISM

The risk of thromboembolism is increased during pregnancy. In fact, a number of factors come together to make pregnancy and the postpartum period perhaps the highest-risk period in a woman's life. Stasis, vessel wall injury, and altered clotting factors promoting clotting, the classic triad leading to intravascular thrombosis that was proposed by Virchow, are all present. All of the clotting factors except XI and XIII are increased in pregnancy, and there is mixed evidence that activity of the fibrinolytic system may be decreased during pregnancy. Venous stasis occurs in maternal leg veins primarily through two mechanisms. First, the gravid uterus compresses the inferior vena cava and iliac veins. This leads to both venous stasis and the lower extremity edema commonly experienced by pregnant women in the third trimester. Venous dilation also plays a role, most likely due to progesterone, allowing for more pooling in the leg veins. After delivery, decreased mobility, particularly after a c-section, may play an additional role in promoting stasis. Blood vessel damage may occur directly from delivery. These factors all come together after delivery and put the woman at high risk for thrombosis. Thromboembolism in pregnancy is often the first clue that a patient has a familial or acquired thrombophilia, and a workup to identify these is appropriate (Table 15.2).

## Superficial Thrombophlebitis

Superficial thrombophlebitis is the most common thrombosis identified during pregnancy occurring in 11 per 1,000 deliveries (6). Patients present with pain, redness, and warmth over the affected area. The affected vein may be swollen, but this may be hard to identify. Occasionally, the clot itself is palpable as a "cord." Superficial thrombosis poses no direct risk to the patient beyond discomfort. It is usually treated with heat, elevation, analgesics (especially aspirin), and occasionally, anticoagulation. If there is evidence of cellulitis, prescription of an antibiotic with coverage for skin flora (e.g., *Staphylococcus* and *Streptococcus*) such as dicloxacillin is appropriate. Superficial thrombophlebitis, particularly of the saphenous vein, can progress to deep venous thrombosis, so if there is any question of the extent of the clot, appropriate studies to rule out deep vein thrombosis must be obtained.

## Deep Venous Thrombosis

Unlike the more benign superficial thrombophlebitis, DVT poses a direct risk to the patient because it may lead to a pulmonary embolism (PE). Consequently, it is of utmost importance to accurately identify and expeditiously treat this condition. The main complaint women present with is pain and leg swelling. This is usually unilateral leg swelling, which helps distinguish it from the normal lower extremity swelling of pregnancy. If a clot reaches the inferior vena cava, bilateral swelling may occur, which can lead to the false

| TABLE 15.2 | Thrombophilia Panel |
| --- | --- |

Activated partial thromboplastin time

Anticardiolipin antibodies

Lupus anticoagulant

Protein S

Protein C

Antithrombin III

Leiden factor V mutation screen

Prothrombin G20210A mutation screen

Hyperhomocysteinemia (fasting homocysteine level)

Activated protein C resistance

attribution of the swelling to normal postpartum swelling. The challenge in making this diagnosis is that there are no signs or symptoms (including pain and swelling) that are sensitive or specific. Homan's sign, the classic sign for DVT of pain in the calf with dorsiflexion of the foot, is not sensitive nor specific. The clinician's main tool is a high index of suspicion. When history and physical examination findings allow for DVT to be in the differential diagnosis, it must be ruled out as best as possible. The standard means for assessing this is a venous Doppler flow study. This is a noninvasive study that looks for alterations in flow that suggest an obstruction and has a sensitivity of up to 90% with a specificity of 98% (6). An alternative noninvasive procedure, impedance plethysmography, examines changes in resistance in tissue. This evaluation tool has largely been replaced by Doppler due to its lower sensitivity and specificity (77% and 93%, respectively), but it still may be useful in some centers because it is a relatively automated study and does not require the skilled examiner needed for a Doppler study (7). Traditionally the gold standard, venography has been replaced by the noninvasive tests. One of the reasons for this shift is not only that venography is invasive, but also that one of its complications is venous thrombosis. Because of this, it is reasonable to check other lab studies prior to moving forward with venography. d-Dimer and fibrinopeptide A are both highly sensitive (but not specific) for venous thrombosis. Normal d-dimer and fibrinopeptide A levels all but rule out thrombosis. In cases where noninvasive tests are inconclusive and the index of suspicion remains high with abnormal d-dimer or fibrinopeptide A levels, venography is still a useful option. [$^{125}$I] fibrinogen is given intravenously and is taken up into the clot. Isotope scanning is useful for clots that are at, or distal to, the midthigh.

Pulmonary embolization arises mostly from DVT above the knee. While DVTs below the knee were once treated less aggressively, the realization that 20% will propagate above the knee has led to the treatment being uniform despite precise location. Up to 25% of untreated DVTs will embolize to the lung, leading to death in up to 15% of patients. By contrast, when patients are appropriately anticoagulated, <1% of DVT leads to embolization, with a mortality rate <1% as well (7). Treatment not only decreases the risk of embolization but also speeds resolution. Treatment is primarily with low molecular weight heparin (LMWH) or fondaparinux (8–10). Several preparations are on the market, and the dosing varies with each product. The main benefits of LMWH are easier dosing, limited need for monitoring, lower risk of heparin-associated thrombocytopenia, and convenience for the patient since the preparations are prefilled syringes. The main drawback for LMWH is the cost, and unfractionated heparin, the traditional treatment for DVT, is cheaper and may be the only treatment covered by a patient's insurance. Unfractionated heparin is given as a 5,000 to 7,500 unit bolus (100 units/kg) followed by a continuous intravenous infusion of about 1,000 units per hour (20 units/kg per hour). This infusion is adjusted to maintain an activated partial thromboplastin time (aPTT) 1.5 to 1.5 times the control and a plasma heparin level of 0.2 to 0.4 U/mL protamine sulfate or 0.3 to 0.6 U/mL by an amidolytic anti-Xa assay (11). Note that one of the risk factors for thromboembolism, the lupus anticoagulant, may itself prolong the aPTT, so one of the other two assays should be followed in cases where patients have this factor present. When LMWH is used, it is administered subcutaneously. There are several different products, and each is dosed differently, so the package inserts should be consulted. Patients should be on anticoagulation for 3 months, because recurrences are increased in women going off anticoagulants before that. It is possible to switch the patient to warfarin after 5 days of heparin. However, some women find the heparin less of a hassle than the increased monitoring necessary to get the warfarin dosing established. When warfarin is desired, the heparin should be continued until the INR $\geq 2$ for at least 24 hours. The target INR is 2.5.

### Pulmonary Embolism

As noted previously, it is of primary importance to treat DVTs because in about 15% of untreated cases in pregnancy, PE results. Heparin therapy for PE is critical, as shown in the only randomized, controlled trial of heparin for PE (12). The authors found a 26% mortality rate in the untreated group and a 0% mortality in the treated group. More recently, thrombolytic therapy has been recommended for PE with hemodynamic compromise (10). When a PE is highly suspected, anticoagulation should be instituted before confirming the diagnosis.

## OVARIAN TORSION

The incidence of ovarian torsion is increased during the postpartum period as well as in early pregnancy. This seems to be related to the relatively rapid movement of the ovaries as the uterus increases or decreases in size during those time periods and is primarily limited to ovaries with cysts or other masses. Women generally present with a history of steadily worsening unilateral lower abdominal or pelvic pain. A mass may be felt on an abdominal or a bimanual pelvic examination. The most useful diagnostic study is ultrasound, which will usually demonstrate a dramatically enlarged ovary on the painful side. The ovary will be edematous, and there may be decreased venous outflow noted on Doppler ultrasound examination. A CT scan may occasionally be useful. Ovarian torsion is treated with surgery. Preservation of the ovary is frequently possible, despite relatively necrotic looking tissue (13,14). When the ovary has a large associated mass, it may be difficult to save the ovary either because it is hard to identify the normal ovary or because there is a concern regarding a malignant neoplasm. The surgeon must use his or her best judgment whether to perform a cystectomy or an oophorectomy. For a more complete discussion, see chapter 23.

## INFECTION

Puerperal infection is defined as a "temperature above $38.0\,^{\circ}\text{C}$ ($100.4\,^{\circ}\text{F}$) maintained over 24 hours or recurring during the period from the end of the first to the end of the tenth day after childbirth or abortion" in the International Classifications of Diseases (ICD-10). Similarly, the Joint Commission on Maternal Welfare in the United States defines a puerperal fever as used for reporting puerperal morbidity as an "oral temperature of $38.0\,^{\circ}\text{C}$ ($100.4\,^{\circ}\text{F}$) or more on any 2 of the first 10 days postpartum" (15). The most frequent etiology of postpartum fever is infection of the genital tract. The rate of postpartum infection is estimated at 1% to 8% (16). Most risk factors for postpartum infection are related to events taking place during labor and delivery. These include chorioamnionitis, use of an interuterine fetal monitor (e.g., scalp electrodes, intrauterine pressure catheter), multiple cervical examinations, duration of labor, duration of rupture of the membranes, obesity, diabetes, manual removal of the placenta, vaginal lacerations (particularly fourth-degree lacerations), and postpartum anemia. Endometritis is frequently seen after c-section but may occur after vaginal delivery as well. While it normally presents prior to discharge from the hospital, it may present later. A number of terms are synonymous for this infection including lendometritis, endomyometritis, metritis, and endoparametritis. The diagnosis is usually straightforward and is based on the finding of fever, abdominal pain, and uterine tenderness without another obvious source. Other diagnoses that should be considered include infections of other sites such as a pelvic abscess, wound infection (e.g., vaginal laceration after vaginal delivery or abdominal wound after a c-section), appendicitis, septic pelvic thrombophlebitis, pyelonephritis, mastitis, and pneumonia. If a woman presents only with low-grade fevers, breast engorgement may be the etiology. Instrumental delivery may be associated with an increased risk of infection, and c-section, particularly after labor, is perhaps the strongest risk factor for infection.

The initial workup includes a thorough review of the history of the labor and delivery, including length of labor and length of rupture of the membranes, mode of delivery, and type of anesthesia (pudendal blocks may predispose to infected pelvic hematomas). The past medical history should assess risk factors such as conditions predisposing to infection such as diabetes, HIV infection, or sickle cell disease. Vital signs are taken to document fever and heart rate, as tachycardia may be present. Physical examination, particularly of the abdomen, pelvis, and costovertebral angle, often narrows the differential diagnosis. While uterine tenderness is always present with endometritis, it may be hard to differentiate post-cesarean operative pain from endometritis. After c-section, inspection of the skin incision is important. Erythema or induration suggests a wound infection. A fluctuant or draining incisional wound may represent an infected hematoma or abscess. After a vaginal delivery, inspection of the perineum is important to look for an infection or breakdown of a vaginal laceration repair. While a bimanual pelvic examination may be uncomfortable, particularly after a vaginal delivery, it may be necessary unless the source of the fever is obvious. In that instance, it should be gently performed to palpate for a pelvic abscess or hematoma. Hematomas and abscesses are more common with operative vaginal deliveries and when a pudendal block has been given for anesthesia. A rectovaginal examination may also be required to palpate for a hematoma or abscess, especially if there was a fourth-degree laceration. While a speculum examination is of limited use in this evaluation, if the patient had a third-degree laceration, it should be carefully examined to make sure that there was not actually a fourth-degree laceration that was missed and consequently not repaired. Pelvic and rectovaginal examinations must be performed very gently both to minimize discomfort for the woman and to minimize the risk that any repairs will be disrupted by the examination. Costovertebral angle tenderness is suggestive of pyelonephritis, and costovertebral angle ecchymosis is a sign of a dissecting pelvis hematoma. Occasionally, other parts of the examination produce useful clues. One of the infrequent complications seen after pudendal or paracervical block is a subgluteal or a retropsoas abscess. These abscesses commonly produce significant pain for the patient during ambulation, and she limps, favoring the affected side. On physical examination, extension and abduction of the hip is painful. When this abscess is suspected, CT scan may reveal gas formation. Immediate assessment for possible surgical intervention with drainage and debridement should be arranged when this is suspected.

While physical examination usually makes these diagnoses, ancillary tests that may be supportive include complete blood count, urinalysis, urine culture, and occasionally, a cervical swab for GC/Chlamydia. If there is a concern regarding possible sepsis, blood cultures may be helpful. Otherwise, wound and endometrial cultures are not useful. Ultrasound and CT scan may be helpful in identifying an abscess, particularly in obese patients where it may be difficult to examine adequately to palpate an abscess. Ultrasound may also help identify retained placenta associated with endometritis; however, there is commonly a small amount of debris retained after a vaginal delivery, and this should not be misconstrued as retained placenta (17).

### Treatment of Endometritis and Pelvis Abscess

As is the case with pelvic inflammatory disease, these infections tend to be polymicrobial. They are generally ascending infections caused by aerobes and anaerobes from the lower genital tract. The list of specific organisms cited as causative agents includes group A and group B streptococci, enterococci, *Staphylococcus aureus*, *Gardnerella vaginalis*, *Escherichia coli*, *Enterobacter*, *Proteus mirabilis*, *Bacteroides bivius*, and other *Bacteroides* species, peptococci and peptostreptococci, *Ureaplasma urealyticum*, and *Mycoplasma hominis*. Of note, while *Chlamydia trachomatis* is not usually thought of as a possible agent, it has been associated with late-onset postpartum endometritis, which should therefore not be overlooked in the emergency department (18). Appropriate antibiotic regimens need to cover both Gram-positive and Gram-negative aerobes and also anaerobes. Frequently used combinations include ampicillin, gentamicin, and clindamycin; ampicillin, gentamicin, and metronidazole; ampicillin plus sulbactam; ticarcillin plus clavulanic acid, etc. Fever curves usually trend downward within 48 hours, and once a patient is afebrile for 48 hours they may usually be discharged without further antibiotics. Although cure rates with initial therapy exceed 95%, failures may be due to abscesses or septic pelvic thrombophlebitis, and imaging should be obtained to assess these possibilities. A reevaluation for nongenital etiologies is also appropriate if there is any question regarding the location of the infection. If an abscess is identified, drainage will be necessary; however, it may often be performed by interventional radiology without requiring surgical drainage. When a patient has persistent fevers with resolution of her pain, there are two likely diagnoses. One is septic pelvic thrombophlebitis. This may occasionally be diagnosed by ultrasound (e.g., ovarian vein thrombosis). If a diagnosis of septic pelvic thrombophlebitis is made, prolonged therapy with antibiotics is usually adequate, as studies have failed to support the long held assumption that heparin accelerated recovery. An alternative explanation for prolonged febrile morbidity without tenderness is drug fever, and in that case, stopping the antibiotics will bring about resolution of the fever.

### Treatment of Abdominal and Vaginal Wound Infections

Wound infections are more commonly seen with c-sections than with vaginal lacerations. The most common presentation is of erythema and/or induration around the incision. The patient can have a fever, but this is not universal. Sometimes the incision will have opened with drainage of pus. Abdominal wound infections are generally caused by skin flora, and coverage should be considered accordingly (e.g., dicloxacillin, cephalexin). If a wound is fluctuant, it should be opened and drained. If there is necrotic tissue, debridement is necessary. When patients are admitted for wound infections, intravenous antibiotics are frequently given that offer coverage for skin flora (e.g., nafcillin). While wet-dry dressings may provide an appropriate initial treatment, they are appropriately but slowly being replaced by other "moisture-retentive" or "semi-occlusive" dressings involving hydrogels, hydrocolloids, calcium alginates, etc. These advanced dressings promote more rapid wound-healing at an overall lower total cost (19–22). Large open wounds may also benefit from negative pressure wound therapy.

When there is a vaginal laceration infection, a repair may appear to be failing or tearing out. The antibiotic coverage for infections of vaginal lacerations is often broader due to the range of possible bacteria (e.g., vibramicin and metronidazole, amoxicillin plus clavulanic acid, or sulfamethoxazole plus trimethoprim). If the examination finds a fluctuant mass, induration, substantial edema or cellulitis, a more aggressive course with inpatient therapy and broad-spectrum antibiotics may be necessary. While most patients show rapid improvement, spreading edema or erythema may indicate necrotizing fasciitis, and surgical exploration and debridement may be required. Rapidly progressing sepsis secondary to toxic shock syndrome or invasive group A streptococcal disease must be recognized rapidly (23,24). This condition is uncommon, but the risk of mortality is significant, so a high index of suspicion must be maintained. The CDC recommends high-dose parenteral penicillin and clindamycin for toxic shock syndrome or necrotizing fasciitis (25).

Because the timing to repair the dehiscence of a repaired laceration or episiotomy varies based on the condition of the tissue, patients should be referred to an obstetrician/gynecologist for consultation if they do not have one.

## MASTITIS

Mastitis is a frequent cause for women to seek medical care during the late postpartum. The incidence of mastitis is reported to be about 2.5%; however, the actual incidence is likely higher due to underreporting (26). Most infections are unilateral, but occasionally, it may affect both breasts. As with postpartum wound infections, the primary etiologic agents are maternal skin flora though infant nasal–oral flora may be the causative agent. The site of the infection is usually obvious upon breast observation. Erythema and tenderness with occasional induration are the hallmarks of this infection. Occasionally, an abscess can develop, and a fluctuant mass may be palpated. In the absence of an abscess, agents active against skin flora (e.g., dicloxacillin, cephelexin) are used. The mother should continue to breastfeed. Improvement is usually seen in the first 48 hours, although antibiotics are continued for 2 weeks. If an abscess is suspected, an obstetric or surgical consultation should be obtained for incision and drainage. The same antibiotics mentioned above are appropriate after an incision and drainage of an abscess. It is quite uncommon for mastitis to require admission for intravenous antibiotics.

## PYELONEPHRITIS

The incidence of pyelonephritis is higher during pregnancy due to the physiologic dilation of the urinary tract. This occurs secondary to the combination of pressure on the distal ureters from the gravid uterus and adjacent vasculature as well as a decrease in ureteral tone due to progestational effects. These factors result in urinary stasis with mild hydronephrosis and hydroureter (the "physiologic hydronephrosis of pregnancy"). Frequent vaginal examinations and possible bladder catheterizations may lead to an increased incidence of bacteriuria postpartum, with an increased risk of pyelonephritis. Women present with fever and costovertebral angle tenderness over the infected kidney. They will frequently report the other routine symptoms of a urinary tract infection including frequency, urgency, and dysuria. The most common etiology is *E. coli*; however, other organisms such as *Klebsiella, Enterobacter, Protues, Pseudomonas, Enterococcus,* and $\beta$-streptococcus are also seen. Because of the wide number of etiologic agents and the increased incidence of antibiotic resistance, it is important that a urine culture and sensitivity be obtained. In order to avoid contamination from the vaginal lochia, a catheter specimen is most appropriate. While pyelonephritis is usually treated as an outpatient in the nonpregnant state, pregnancy-associated pyelonephritis carries a significantly higher risk of urosepsis. Consequently, inpatient therapy with intravenous antibiotics is usually pursued. The initial choice for antibiotics is usually cefazolin or gentamicin, or both if the patient appears very ill and sepsis is suspected. Patients usually respond quickly with resolution of fever and costovertebral angle tenderness in 48 hours. Once the culture and sensitivity are available, the therapy may be altered as appropriate.

## PSYCHOLOGICAL ISSUES

The postpartum period is one that finds women at an increased risk for psychologic disorders. These may range from relatively mild disorders, such as the "baby blues" to more severe difficulties such as depression and psychosis. While these difficulties are often attributed to the "hormonal changes" women are undergoing at this time, the reasons are many and likely include such factors as a recognition of the incredible responsibility of raising an infant and the shift in focus of family members' and friends' attention from the pregnant mother-to-be to the newborn infant. Other risk factors include a family history of depression, being a single mother, or having marital/relationship difficulty and other socioeconomic stresses. It is critical to distinguish between the more severe and lesser conditions. As many as 40% of primiparous women have reported experiencing indifference to their infants when they first held them after birth (27). Several intrapartum factors were identified to be associated with this indifference including amniotomy, painful labor, and the dose of pethidine. This early maternal indifference resolved over the first few days after delivery. Even more common were the mild depression characterized as the "baby blues" or "postpartum blues." Over half of the women reported spells of tearfulness, insomnia, anxiety, depressed mood, headaches, confusion, fatigue, or other emotional distresses that lasted up to 2 weeks. For these milder conditions, reassurance and support from the medical team, family members, and friends are usually all that is necessary. When a mother has a past history of treatment for depression, anxiety, or similar conditions, treatment with selective serotonin reuptake inhibitors may be helpful. In many instances, women with a past history of postpartum psychological difficulty are started prophylactically on these medications. Referral to, or consultation with, a mental health care provider is always appropriate. When a woman presents with symptoms of major depression, consultation is mandatory, as this is a more severe disorder that hangs on much longer and is not likely to resolve quickly through enhanced family support. The symptoms to watch for are those seen in depression diagnosed outside of pregnancy: insomnia or hypersomnia, change in appetite or weight, feelings of worthlessness, inability to concentrate or make decisions, difficulty working, and thoughts of death or suicide. Women in this state may go beyond mere indifference and actually reject their infant. While some reports give an incidence of a major depressive disorder in up to 10% to 15% of postpartum women, this figure seems high in clinical experience (28). Because the symptoms are so oppressive and make life at home and work so difficult, these women almost always require medication and may be affected for up to 2 to 3 months.

The most serious condition, postpartum psychosis, is seen after only 0.2% of deliveries. Reported risk factors include nulliparity, not having an involved partner at the time of delivery, and delivery by cesarean section. A past history of bipolar disorder also carries an increased risk for psychosis, and a prior episode of postpartum psychosis carries a 15% risk of recurrence. Most episodes are affective (manic or depressive psychosis), while a minority are schizophrenia-like conditions. Psychiatric consultation is mandatory, and these patients are usually hospitalized. While the course of these conditions is usually measured in weeks, a controlled follow-up study found evidence that difficulties in the mother–child relationship may persist for as long as 4.5 years postpartum (29).

## SUMMARY

When a postpartum patient presents to the emergency department, it is vital that she is examined carefully and her concerns taken seriously without simply attributing symptoms to the "normal postpartum state." Some conditions are rapidly life-threatening, such as seizures, PPH, and PE, and treatments must be instituted rapidly. Other conditions, particularly infections may vary from inconvenience to potentially life-threatening, and an expeditious workup and initiation of appropriate therapy is critical. Some conditions such as pyelonephritis are managed differently during a pregnancy, and this must be taken into account. Postpartum psychological complaints should never be brushed aside and minimized. A careful evaluation to separate less serious psychological conditions that may be treated with reassurance and support, from more serious ones that need psychiatric consultation, is crucial to ensure that new mothers and their infants stay safe at a time when many women have mood fluctuations.

Finally, often the patient's midwife or obstetrician has information relating to the pregnancy or delivery that is very helpful, and they should be contacted. Consultation from that individual or the on-call obstetrician for the emergency department may be very useful to efficiently establish a diagnosis, institute treatment, and facilitate either discharge to home or admission to the hospital as is appropriate.

## References

1. Hofmeyr GJ, Walraven G, Gulmezoglu AM, Maholwana B, Alfirevic Z, Villar J. Misoprostol to treat postpartum haemorrhage: a systematic review. *BJOG.* 2005;112(5):547–553.
2. Blum J, Alfirevic Z, Walraven G, Weeks A, Winikoff B: Treatment of postpartum hemorrhage with misoprostol. *Int J Gynaecol Obstet.* 2007;99 (Suppl.2):S202–S205.
3. Hofmeyr GJ, Gulmezoglu AM. Misoprostol for the prevention and treatment of postpartum haemorrhage. *Best Pract Res Clin Obstet Gynaecol.* 2008;22(6):1025–1041.
4. Dabelea V, Schultze PM, McDuffie RS Jr. Intrauterine balloon tamponade in the management of postpartum hemorrhage. *Am J Perinatol.* 2007;24(6):359–364.
5. Nelson WL, O'Brien JM. The uterine sandwich for persistent uterine atony: combining the B-Lynch compression suture and an intrauterine Bakri balloon. *Am J Obstet Gynecol.* 2007;196(5):e9–e10.
6. Wells PS, Hirsh J, Anderson DR, et al. Comparison of the accuracy of impedance plethysmography and compression ultrasonography in outpatients with clinically suspected deep vein thrombosis: a two centre paired-design prospective trial. *Thromb Haemost.* 1995;74(6):1423–1427.
7. Douketis JD, Kearon C, Bates S, Duku EK, Ginsberg JS. Risk of fatal pulmonary embolism in patients with treated venous thromboembolism. *JAMA.* 1998;279(6): 458–462.
8. Koopman MM, Buller HR. Low-molecular-weight heparins in the treatment of venous thromboembolism. *Ann Intern Med.* 1998;128(12, pt 1):1037–1039.
9. Low-molecular-weight heparin in the treatment of patients with venous thromboembolism. The Columbus Investigators. *N Engl J Med.* 1997;337(10):657–662.
10. Kearon C, Kahn SR, Agnelli G, Goldhaber S, Raskob GE, Comerota AJ. Antithrombotic therapy for venous thromboembolic disease: American College of Chest Physicians Evidence-Based Clinical Practice Guidelines (8th Edition). *Chest.* 2008;133 (6 Suppl.):454S–545S.
11. Hyers TM, Agnelli G, Hull RD, et al. Antithrombotic therapy for venous thromboembolic disease. *Chest.* 1998;114(5 Suppl.):561S–578S.
12. Barritt DW, Jordan SC. Anticoagulant drugs in the treatment of pulmonary embolism. *Lancet.* 1960;1:1309–1312.
13. Oelsner G, Bider D, Goldenberg M, Admon D, Mashiach S. Long-term follow-up of the twisted ischemic adnexa managed by detorsion. *Fertil Steril.* 1993;60(6):976–979.
14. Zweizig S, Perron J, Grubb D, Mishell DR Jr. Conservative management of adnexal torsion. *Am J Obstet Gynecol.* 1993;168(6, pt 1):1791–1795.
15. Wager GP, Martin DH, Koutsky L, et al. Puerperal infectious morbidity: relationship to route of delivery and to antepartum *Chlamydia trachomatis* infection. *Am J Obstet Gynecol.* 1980;138(7, pt 2):1028–1033.

16. Sweet RL, Gibbs RS. Postpartum infection: infectious diseases of the female genital tract. 2nd Ed. Baltimore, MD: Williams & Wilkins; 1990:356–373.

17. Sokol ER, Casele H, Haney EI. Ultrasound examination of the postpartum uterus: what is normal? *J Matern Fetal Neonatal Med.* 2004;15(2):95–99.

18. Hoyme UB, Kiviat N, Eschenbach DA. Microbiology and treatment of late postpartum endometritis. *Obstet Gynecol.* 1986;68(2):226–232.

19. Alterescu V. The financial costs of inpatient pressure ulcers to an acute care facility. *Decubitus.* 1989;2(3):14–23.

20. Colwell JC, Foreman MD, Trotter JP. A comparison of the efficacy and cost-effectiveness of two methods of managing pressure ulcers. *Decubitus.* 1993;6(4):28–36.

21. Xakellis GC, Chrischilles EA. Hydrocolloid versus saline-gauze dressings in treating pressure ulcers: a cost-effectiveness analysis. *Arch Phys Med Rehabil.* 1992;73(5):463–469.

22. Bolton LL, van Rijswijk L, Shaffer FA. Quality wound care equals cost-effective wound care: a clinical model. *Adv Wound Care.* 1997;10(4):33–38.

23. Lurie S, Vaknine H, Izakson A, Levy T, Sadan O, Golan A. Group A Streptococcus causing a life-threatening postpartum necrotizing myometritis: a case report. *J Obstet Gynaecol Res.* 2008;34(4, pt 2):645–648.

24. Aronoff DM, Mulla ZD. Postpartum invasive group A streptococcal disease in the modern era. *Infect Dis Obstet Gynecol.* 2008;2008:796892.

25. Group A Streptococcal (GAS) Disease. Centers for Disease Control and Prevention; 2008. Available at: http://www.cdc.gov/ncidod/dbmd/diseaseinfo/groupastreptococcal_g.htm (updated 2008; cited 2009 March 7).

26. Marshall BR, Hepper JK, Zirbel CC. Sporadic puerperal mastitis: an infection that need not interrupt lactation. *JAMA.* 1975;233(13):1377–1379.

27. Robson KM, Kumar R. Delayed onset of maternal affection after childbirth. *Br J Psychiatry.* 1980;136:347–353.

28. O'Hara MW, Neunaber DJ, Zekoski EM. Prospective study of postpartum depression: prevalence, course, and predictive factors. *J Abnorm Psychol.* 1984;93(2):158–171.

29. Uddenberg N, Englesson I. Prognosis of post partum mental disturbance: a prospective study of primiparous women and their 4 1/2-year-old children. *Acta Psychiatr Scand.* 1978;58(3):201–212.

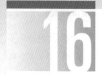

# Role of Imaging Modalities in Obstetric Emergencies

### Lama L. Tolaymat and Gwyn Grabner

Imaging has assumed a key role in the management of obstetric patients. Depending upon the patient population and clinical problem, a variety of imaging modalities are available for use, some more appropriate than others. Some women are exposed to x-rays before the diagnosis of pregnancy is known. Occasionally, x-ray procedures may be indicated during the pregnancy. To understand which modality to use for a specific concern, all imaging modalities must be reviewed with emphasis on the method of generating an image, common uses in pregnancy, and the associated risk with use. Table 16.1 summarizes the different modalities and the associated fetal exposure of radiation.

## RADIATION EXPOSURE IN PREGNANCY

There has been a growing concern about radiation exposure in the case of pregnant women who undergo radiological examinations. Lack of knowledge may result in unnecessary patient anxiety. Teratogenic effects have developed in animals exposed to large doses of radiation (up to 200 rad). The main effects of radiation on the human embryo and the fetus are prenatal death, growth restriction, congenital malformations, and mental retardation. Based on data from the atomic bomb survivors, it appears that the risk of central nervous system effects is greatest with exposures at 8 to 15 weeks of gestation (1,2). Prenatal doses from properly performed diagnostic procedures present no significant increased risk of prenatal death, malformation, or impairment of mental development over the background incidence of these entities. Rare consequences of prenatal radiation exposure include a slight increase in the incidence of childhood leukemia and, possibly, a very small change in the frequency of genetic mutations. Such exposure is not an indication of pregnancy termination. In 1977, the National Council on Radiation Protection and Measurement issued a report stating that "The risk [of abnormality] is considered to be negligible at 50 mGy [=5 rad] or less when compared to other risks of pregnancy, and the risk of malformation is significantly increased above control levels only at doses above 150 mGy [=15 rad]. Therefore, exposure of the fetus to radiation arising from diagnostic procedures would very rarely be the cause for terminating a pregnancy" (3). The accepted safe cumulative dose of ionizing radiation during pregnancy is **5 rad (0.05 Gy)**. The American College of Radiology established that "The interruption of pregnancy is rarely justified because of radiation risk to the embryo or fetus from a radiologic examination" (4). The most sensitive time period for central nervous system teratogenesis is between 10 and 17 weeks of gestation. Nonurgent radiologic testing should be avoided during this time.

### Risk Related to Gestational Age (5)
1. Fetal exposure prior to 2 weeks post-conception to 10 rad may lead to the death of the embryo.
2. Fetal exposure at 2 to 7 weeks post-conception to 5 to 50 rad leads to an increase in the risk of major malformations and growth restriction. An exposure to >50 rad leads to a substantial risk of malformations, growth restriction, and miscarriages.

Diagnostic Imaging Procedures and the Estimated Average Associated Fetal Exposure

| Study | Approximate Fetal Exposure |
|---|---|
| Dental x-ray | 0.006 mrad |
| Chest AP and lateral | 0.02–0.07 mrad |
| Hip x-ray | 200 mrad |
| IVP | ≥1 rad |
| Mammogram | 7–20 mrad |
| Head CT | <1 rad |
| Chest CT | <1 rad |
| CT pelvimetry | 250 mrad |
| Abdominal CT | 2.6 rad |
| Lumbar spine CT | 1 rad |
| Barium enema | 2–4 rad |
| Tc99m lung scan | 50 mrad |
| Xenon ventilation scan | 20 mrad |
| Tc99m HIDA scan | 150 mrad |

3. Fetal exposure 8 to 15 weeks post-conception to 5 to 50 rad leads to growth restriction, reduction in IQ, and 20% incidence of mental retardation. An exposure to >50 rad may result in a miscarriage.

4. Fetal exposure after 15 weeks post-conception to <50 rad may lead to noncancer health effects at exposures >50 rad.

## IMAGING MODALITIES

*x-Ray (plain films)*: Generally during pregnancy, the uterus is shielded for non-pelvic procedures. Plain films are useful in evaluating trauma, fractured bones, pneumonia, and urolithiasis in pregnant women.

*Fluoroscopy*: Most fluoroscopic examinations result in fetal exposure to millirads. Uses in pregnancy include cholelithiasis related pancreatitis and urolithiasis.

*Nuclear Medicine/angiography*: The most common nuclear medicine study performed during pregnancy is the ventilation–perfusion scan for suspected pulmonary embolism. Macroaggregated albumin labeled with Technetium Tc99m is used for the perfusion portion, and inhaled xenon gas is used for the ventilation portion. The radiation exposure to the fetus is usually 50 mrad (6). Radioactive iodine readily crosses the placenta and can adversely affect the fetal thyroid as early as 10 weeks, therefore, contraindicated in pregnancy. If a diagnostic scan of the thyroid is necessary during pregnancy, then using [123]I or Technetium Tc99m should be used (6).

*Computed Tomography (CT)*: The most common uses for CT during pregnancy include head CT to detect acute hemorrhage in eclamptic women or for the diagnosis of acute neurological catastrophe and spiral CT for evaluation of pulmonary embolism. Pelvimetry is used rarely, but when required, low-dose CT pelvimetry can be performed. Most radiopaque agents used with CT are derivatives of iodine and hence avoided in pregnancy.

*Ultrasound:* Since ultrasound does not involve any radiation, it is the preferred imaging modality in pregnant women. The International Society for Ultrasound in Obstetrics and Gynecology issued a safety statement that "routine clinical scanning of every woman during pregnancy using real-time B-mode imaging is not contraindicated" and "exposure time and acoustic output should be kept to the lowest levels" (7). Ultrasound is used in pregnancy to evaluate the fetus, the placenta, the adnexa, and the cervix. In addition, ultrasound may be used as an initial diagnostic tool to evaluate the kidneys when urolithiasis is suspected or in situations of abdominal trauma. It is the main modality used to evaluate vaginal bleeding any time during pregnancy.

*Magnetic Resonance Imaging (MRI):* Since MRI does not use any radiation, there is no known risk of using it in pregnant patients. In addition to the nonobstetric indications for MRI, it is used to evaluate fetal malformations specifically CNS (8) and for the evaluation and management of abdominal pregnancy (9). Most MRI machines have a patient weight limit of about 300 lbs, but this limit is usually higher for "open" MRI machines.

### General Principles to be Followed in Every Pregnant Patient

- Women should be counseled that x-ray exposure from a single diagnostic procedure (<5 rad) does not result in harmful fetal effects (10).
- Limit exposures to those that are essential for the diagnosis.
- Pelvic shielding should be used whenever possible.
- Fluoroscopy should be limited to short bursts as needed.
- Ultrasound and MRI should be considered instead of x-rays when appropriate, at least as an initial assessment tool (10).
- The use of radioactive isotopes of iodine is contraindicated in pregnancy.
- Radiopaque and paramagnetic contrast agents are unlikely to cause harm and may be of diagnostic benefit (10).

## OBSTETRIC EMERGENCIES AND IMAGING

The diagnosis of pregnancy requires a multifaceted approach using history and physical examination, hormonal assays, and endovaginal ultrasound. With the combination of early endovaginal ultrasound and beta subunit of human chorionic gonadotrophin (BhCG), we can reassure our patient of a normal progressing pregnancy versus failed early intrauterine pregnancy (miscarriage) or ectopic pregnancy. Readers may also wish to consult Chapter 3.

As early as 4.5 weeks after onset of last menstrual period, the first sign of pregnancy, gestational sac (Fig. 16.1), can be seen by endovaginal ultrasound. Normal gestational sac can be demonstrated when the hCG level is ≥1,800 mIU/mL (11). The second sign of pregnancy, the yolk sac, can be seen by endovaginal ultrasound at about 5.5 weeks. Its presence confirms that an intrauterine pregnancy is present (Fig. 16.2). The number of yolk sacs equals the number of amnions; accordingly, in twin gestations, the number of yolk sacs can be counted to determine if it is monoamniotic or diamniotic. The fetal pole is seen as a focal thickening on the yolk sac, hence the "diamond ring" sign. A distinct embryo will be identified adjacent to the yolk sac at 6 to 6.5 weeks with cardiac activity when the BhCG level is approximately 10,800 mIU/mL (11). A fetal pole of 5 mm is the discriminatory value for the presence of heart beat, although recent data

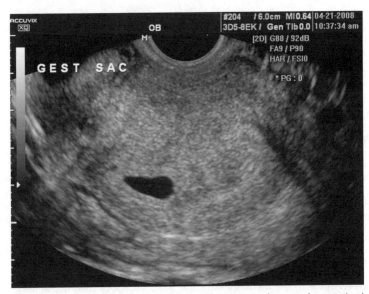

**FIGURE 16.1** Endovaginal image of an early intrauterine pregnancy demonstrating gestational sac.

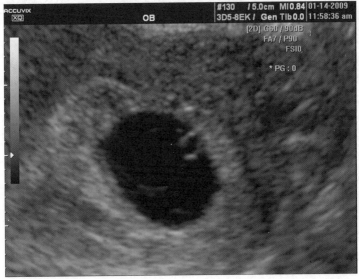

**FIGURE 16.2** Endovaginal image of an intrauterine gestational sac with a yolk sac visualized within it.

suggest that the cutoff should be lowered to 3 mm (12). Correlation of serum levels and endovaginal ultrasound findings are key when patients are being evaluated for pain or bleeding (13). It is important to keep in mind that these parameters depend largely on the operator's experience and the instrumentation used.

## VAGINAL BLEEDING IN PREGNANCY

Vaginal bleeding occurs in about 20% to 30% of all confirmed pregnancies in the first 20 weeks; about 50% of these end in spontaneous abortions (14). Disorders that commonly cause abnormal bleeding include ectopic (ruptured/unruptured) pregnancy, spontaneous abortion (to include complete, missed, inevitable, incomplete, blighted ovum, and threatened abortion), gestational trophoblastic disease, placenta previa/vasa previa, and placental abruption. Readers may also wish to consult Chapter 8.

### First Trimester Bleeding

*Implantation bleeding*: This term refers to a transient spotting associated with the normal implantation of the embryo into the uterine wall. Bleeding is usually minimal and is no cause for concern. Endovaginal ultrasound demonstrates a hypoechoic cleft in the decidua (endometrium thickened) near the sac.

*Threatened miscarriage/abortion*: This diagnosis refers to early pregnancies complicated by bleeding and/or cramping, while with endovaginal ultrasound, the fetal pole is visualized and fetal cardiac activity is present (Fig. 16.3). Contributing factors may include abnormal karyotype, infection, dehydration,

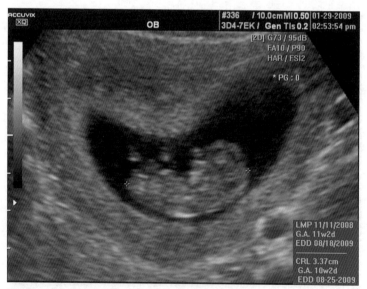

**FIGURE 16.3** Endovaginal image of a first trimester fetus. Measurement of the crown–rump length (CRL; calipers).

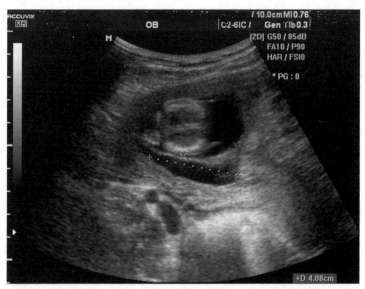

**FIGURE 16.4** Endovaginal image of a retroplacental hematoma (the hypoechoic region measured).

physical trauma, or use of drugs or medications. In many cases of threatened miscarriage, no contributing factors are identified. Occasionally, a retroplacental hematoma is seen (Fig. 16.4), and 25% of these pregnancies will miscarry, while without a hematoma, the risk of loss is 7% (15).

*Spontaneous (Complete) Abortion*: This term refers to heavy bleeding and cramping (in women with previously documented intrauterine pregnancy), and endovaginal ultrasound shows an empty endometrial cavity.

*Incomplete Abortion*: Partial expulsion of products of conception from the uterus with some retained products, usually clots and placental tissue. Sometimes the cervix appears to be open when inspected by speculum examination. Ultrasound may reveal the presence of tissue within the endometrial cavity.

*Blighted ovum (anembryonic)*: This terminology refers to pregnancies in the embryo that have failed to develop appropriately. The discriminatory criterion for anembryonic pregnancy by endovaginal ultrasound is a mean gestational sac diameter (MGSD) of >10 mm without a yolk sac or a MGSD >18 mm without a fetal pole. By transabdominal ultrasound, MGSD cutoffs of 20 mm without a yolk sac and 25 mm without embryo fetal pole are used (13). The accuracy of these parameters depends largely on the operator's experience and the instrumentation used.

*Ectopic pregnancy*: An ectopic pregnancy occurs when a fertilized ovum implants at a site other than the endometrial lining of the uterus. Diagnosis is often made by a pelvic examination and a combination of serum BhCG and endovaginal ultrasound. The sonographic identification of an intrauterine gestational sac with yolk sac essentially excludes an ectopic pregnancy. An intrauterine pregnancy should always be visualized at a BhCG level of

2,000 IU/L by endovaginal ultrasound and at a 6,500 IU/L by transabdominal ultrasound. An adnexal mass, in a patient with a BhCG level <2,000 IU/L, should not automatically be assumed to be an ectopic unless a sac with a yolk sac is seen within the mass. Most adnexal masses represent corpus luteum cysts associated with an early pregnancy. Although rare, a heterotopic pregnancy (an intrauterine pregnancy and an ectopic pregnancy present simultaneously) may be present. This underscores the importance of imaging the adnexa and ovaries when performing endovaginal ultrasound for women with early intrauterine pregnancies.

With ectopic pregnancy, the uterus is most commonly normal in appearance. However, fluid (known as a pseudosac) may be present in the endometrial cavity. As opposed to gestational sacs which are eccentrically located, a pseudosac is centrally located within the endometrial cavity. If an intrauterine fluid collection is identified, but no fetal pole or yolk sac is seen, the differentials include (a) an ectopic pregnancy with pseudosac, (b) an intrauterine pregnancy imaged too early for the development of the yolk sac, and (c) an abnormal intrauterine pregnancy. Such patients should be followed with serial assessments of serum BhCG levels and follow-up ultrasound when indicated (see chapter on ectopic pregnancy). Adnexal findings associated with ectopic pregnancy include tubal ring sign (Fig. 16.5), yolk sac/fetal pole with cardiac activity (Fig. 16.6), complex adnexal mass, simple adnexal cyst, and/or free fluid in the cul-de-sac (16).

***Molar pregnancy (gestational trophoblastic disease):*** Molar pregnancy refers to a rare condition in which the fetus and the amnion never form, and there is hydropic swelling of the chorionic villous stroma and absence of blood vessels within these villi. Ultrasound scans show absence of a fetus and a "Swiss Cheese" appearance within the placenta.

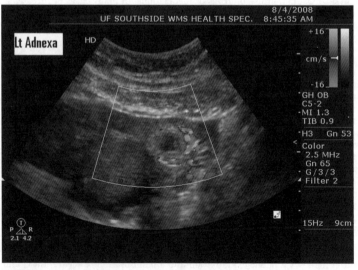

**FIGURE 16.5** Endovaginal image of the adnexa demonstrating the tubal ring (color flow) associated with an ectopic pregnancy.

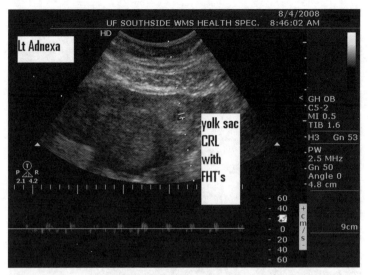

**FIGURE 16.6** Endovaginal image of an ectopic pregnancy with fetal cardiac activity present.

## BLEEDING IN THE SECOND AND THIRD TRIMESTER

Bleeding that occurs in the second and third trimesters (14 to 40 weeks) is abnormal and involves concerns different from bleeding in the first trimester.

*Cervical Incompetence:* Cervical incompetence represents a common cause of pregnancy failure in the second trimester, manifesting as *painless* dilatation of the cervix that leads to preterm delivery. The ultrasound signs that are suggestive of cervical incompetence in the second trimester include dilatation of the internal os also called funneling (Fig. 16.7), hourglassing of the membranes into the vagina, or short cervix (≤25 mm) in the absence of uterine contractions (17). Using endovaginal ultrasound, the cervical length (CL) is obtained by measuring the endocervical canal from the internal cervical os to the external os (Fig. 16.8). Endovaginal approach is a more accurate method since it does not have the distortion associated with the transabdominal approach. Because of the dynamic nature of the cervical canal and lower uterine segment throughout pregnancy, the normal length of a competent cervix falls within a wide range (0.5 to 5 cm) (17). Consequently, the sonographic assessment of the cervix requires attention to the temporal changes of the CL during every examination. Furthermore, the Valsalva maneuver or manual compression of the uterine fundus may corroborate the sonographic diagnosis of cervical incompetence. The sonographic determination of the residual closed length of the cervix may be used as a prognostic indicator of the risk of preterm labor progressing into preterm delivery. A cervical cerclage is a surgical procedure performed before 24 weeks that presents an option for women with cervical incompetence (18).

*Placenta previa:* This term refers to implantation of the placenta over or near the internal cervical os. It can be termed complete, partial, marginal or low-lying depending on its location relative to the internal os. Bleeding is usually bright red and painless. Since a pelvic digital examination is contraindicated in placenta previa, endovaginal ultrasound has been established as a safe assessment tool (19). Endovaginal ultrasound gives clear views of the cervical os and

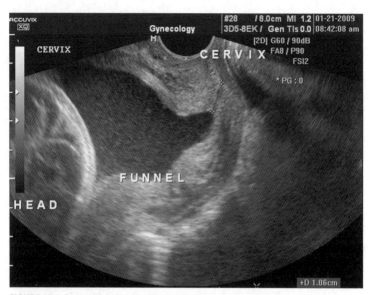

**FIGURE 16.7** Endovaginal ultrasound image of an incompetent cervix. Funneling indicates that the internal cervical os is dilated, allowing the amniotic sac to enter into the endocervical canal. Residual CL is measured with calipers.

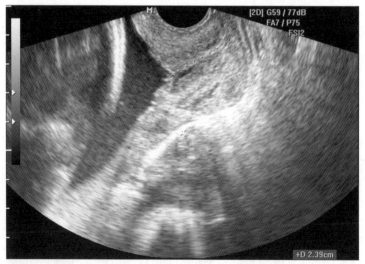

**FIGURE 16.8** Sagittal view of the maternal cervix with endovaginal ultrasound showing a normal endocervical canal. CL is measured from the internal os to the external os (calipers).

lower uterine segment, even at full term; therefore, it is used to improve the accuracy of diagnosis of placenta previa (Fig. 16.9).

***Vasa Previa:*** This term refers to an obstetric complication when fetal vessels traverse the fetal membranes over the internal cervical os. These vessels may be from either a velamentous insertion of the umbilical cord or may be joining an accessory placental lobe (succenturiate) to the main lobe of the placenta. If these fetal vessels rupture, the bleeding is from the fetoplacental circulation, and fetal exsanguination will rapidly occur, leading to fetal death. Vasa previa must be ruled out in all cases of bilobed, succenturiate, and low-lying placentas; pregnancies resulting from in vitro fertilization; and multiple pregnancies. Endovaginal ultrasound in combination with color Doppler is the most effective tool in antenatal diagnosis of vasa previa (20).

***Placental abruption:*** Abruption describes the condition which occurs when the placenta separates from the wall of the uterus prematurely and blood collects in that space between the two. On ultrasound examination, one may see a fluid collection of varying echogenicity based on the age of the hemorrhage with or without a connection to the placenta.

***Uterine Rupture:*** Uterine rupture may be associated with acute, potentially catastrophic complication which may result in maternal and perinatal mortality. It is defined as a full-thickness separation of the uterine wall and the overlying serosa. Uterine rupture is associated with clinically significant uterine bleeding; fetal distress; expulsion or protrusion of the fetus, placenta, or both into the abdominal cavity; and the need for prompt surgical intervention for delivery, uterine repair, or hysterectomy. Prior cesarean delivery is the most common risk factor. With complete wall disruption, protrusion of the amniotic sac beyond the uterus may be seen, as well as intraperitoneal or extraperitoneal hemorrhage.

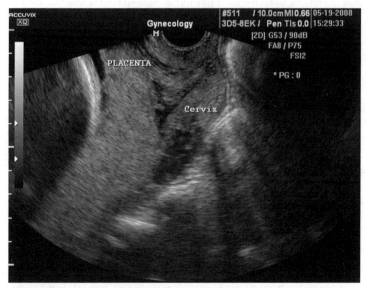

**FIGURE 16.9** Endovaginal image of the uterine cervix demonstrating a complete placenta previa (the placenta completely covers the internal os).

## TRAUMA IN PREGNANCY

Trauma and accidental injuries complicate 6% to 7% of all pregnancies (21) and are usually due to motor vehicle accidents, domestic abuse or assaults, and falls. Once fetal heart tones are confirmed, two patients exist and both require assessment and treatment. The anatomic and the physiologic changes of pregnancy make the trauma assessment more difficult. Readers may also wish to consult Chapter 4.

The cardinal principle in the management of trauma in pregnancy is that there can be no fetal survival without maternal survival, with the rare exception of the gravely injured mother late in pregnancy where urgent cesarean delivery may allow for fetal survival. With pregnancy, there is an increased risk of internal hemorrhage, and identification of bleeding is more difficult. Common adverse consequences to abdominal trauma in pregnancy include uterine contractions, preterm labor or delivery, and placental abruption. In many cases, external fetal monitoring and ultrasound may be adequate for assessment of the placenta, uterus, and fetal well-being. Obstetric and emergency department clinicians should recognize that even minor trauma in the pregnant woman can cause fetal demise (22).

From an imaging perspective, ultrasound is an excellent tool for initial evaluation of the trauma pregnant patient, but CT is the preferred modality when clinical or ultrasound findings suggest visceral injuries unaccompanied by intraperitoneal hemorrhage or injuries of the bones, chest, mediastinum, aorta, spine, retroperitoneum, bladder, and bowel. MRI is not a practical option for rapid evaluation of all these body parts in an unstable patient after trauma. Placental abruption typically appears on CT as a single avascular area of varying size that extends from the placental base to the placental surface. High attenuation in the nonplacental portion of the uterus indicates contusion, tear, or partial uterine disruption. Loss of amniotic fluid into the maternal peritoneum or free fetal parts in the maternal abdomen may indicate uterine rupture. But it may be difficult to determine if free intraperitoneal fluid is amniotic fluid or hemorrhage from a maternal visceral injury. In general, ultrasound may be sufficient for the initial imaging evaluation of a pregnant patient who has sustained trauma, but CT should be performed if a serious injury is suspected.

### References

1. Hall EJ. Scientific view of low-level radiation risks. *Radiographics.* 1991;11:509–518.
2. Schull WJ. The children of atomic bomb survivors: a synopsis. *J Radiol Prot.* 2003; 23:369–384.
3. National Council on Radiation Protection and Measurements. Medical radiation exposure of pregnant and potentially pregnant women. NCRP report no. 54. Bethesda, MD: *National Council on Radiation Protection and Measurement*; 1977.
4. American College of Radiology. A CoR 04–05 bylaws. Reston, VA: American College of Radiology, 2005.
5. Center for Disease Control Radiation Emergencies. Prenatal radiation exposure: a fact sheet for physicians. Available at: http://www.bt.cdc.gov/radiation/prenatal-physician.asp accessed March12, 2009.
6. Ginsberg JS, Hirsh J, Rainbow AJ, Coates G. Risks to the fetus of radiologic procedures used in the diagnosis of maternal venous thromboembolic disease. *Thromb Haemost.* 1989;61:189–196.
7. International Society for Ultrasound in Obstetrics and Gynecology. Safety statement, 2000 (confirmed 2002). *Ultrasound Obstet Gynecol.* 2000;16:594–596.
8. Malinger G, Ben-Sira L, Lev D, et al. Fetal brain imaging: a comparison between magnetic resonance imaging and dedicated neurosonography. *Ultrasound Obstet Gynecol.* 2004;23(4):333–340.
9. Bertrand G, Le Ray C, Simard-Emond L, Dubois J, Leduc L. Imaging in the management of abdominal pregnancy: a case report and review of the literature. *J Obstet Gynaecol Can.* 2009;31(1):57–62.

10. American College of Obstetricians and Gynecologists. Guidelines for diagnostic imaging during the pregnancy. *ACOG Committee Opinion.* Number 299, 2004.

11. Nyberg DA, Mack LA, Laing FC, et al. Early pregnancy complications: Endovaginal sonographic findings correlated with human chorionic gonadotropin levels. *Radiology.* 1988;167:619–622.

12. Abaid LN, As-Sanie S, Wolfe HM. Relationship between crown-rump length and early detection of cardiac activity. *J Reprod Med.* 2007;52:375–378.

13. Nyberg DA, Laing FC, Filly RA. Threatened abortion: sonographic distinction of normal and abnormal gestation sacs. *Radiology.* 1986;158:393–396.

14. Everett C. Incidence and outcome of bleeding before the 20th week of pregnancy: a prospective study from general practice. *Br Med J.* 1997;315:32–34.

15. Poulose T, Richardson R, Ewings P, Fox R. Probability of early pregnancy loss in women with vaginal bleeding and a singleton live fetus at ultrasound scan. *J Obstet Gynecol.* 2006;26(8):782–784.

16. Levine D. Ectopic pregnancy. *Radiology.* 2007;245(2):385–397.

17. Salomon LJ, Diaz-Garcia C, Bernard JP, Ville Y. Reference range for cervical length throughout pregnancy: non-parametric LMS-based model applied to a large sample. *Ultrasound Obstet Gynecol.* 2009; published on line by Wiley Interscience ahead of press.

18. Cunningham FG, Gant NF, Leveno KJ, Gilstrap LC III, Hauth JC, Wenstrom KD. General considerations and maternal evaluation. In: *Williams obstetrics.* 21st Ed. New York, NY: McGraw-Hill; 2001:1143–1158.

19. Timor-Tritsch IE, Yunis RA. Confirming the safety of transvaginal sonography in patients suspected of placenta previa. *Obstet Gynecol.* 1993;81(5):742–744.

20. Oyelese KO, Turner M, Lees C, Campbell S. Vasa previa: an avoidable obstetric tragedy. *Obstet Gynecol Survey.* 1999;54(2):138–145.

21. American College of Obstetricians and Gynecologists. Obstetric aspects of trauma management. *ACOG Educational Bulletin.* Number 251, 1998.

22. Weiss HB, Sauber-Schatz EK, Cook LJ. The epidemiology of pregnancy-associated emergency department injury visits and their impact on birth outcomes. *Accid Anal Prev.* 2008;40(3):1088–1095.

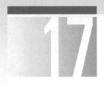

# Drug Therapy in Pregnancy

Thanh T. Hogan, Kristina E. Ward, Andrea L.
McKeever, William Renfro, and Linda Hastings

Ethical and legal limitations preclude drug studies in pregnant women, leaving the health care provider with little reliable information to base clinical decisions of drug use during pregnancy. As a result, some clinicians practice "therapeutic nihilism" where nothing is prescribed for the pregnant patient (1,2). However, avoiding medication use during pregnancy at all cost is not necessarily desirable. If left untreated, many conditions may jeopardize the health of the mother and/or the fetus. This chapter reviews the relative safety of common medications prescribed during pregnancy.

## FOOD AND DRUG ADMINISTRATION PREGNANCY CATEGORIES

During the 1960s and 1970s, the tragedy of thalidomide use, which resulted in thousands of babies being born with severe limb defects, heightened awareness of medication use in pregnant women.

In 1980, the Food and Drug Administration (FDA) required that the labeling of prescription drugs include information about the use in pregnancy. Five categories were established to indicate a drug's potential for causing birth defects. The category is assigned upon the drug's initial approval by the FDA. As a result, information available to categorize the drugs is usually limited human data and animal studies. This information can be found in the precautions section of the package insert. A description of the current categories is summarized in Table 17.1 (3).

This classification system was an important step for assisting the clinician in identifying potential teratogenic prescription drugs. However, the categories lack specific details to assist clinicians in prescribing to pregnant women and does not address timing of pregnancy, appropriate dosage of the drugs, or use during lactation. Additionally, health care professionals often mistakenly believe that there is a gradation of risk across the categories, assuming that a drug in category B is safer than one in category C which is safer than one in category D. However, by definition, category C drugs generally have the least data (Table 17.2) and can represent risks of unknown magnitude. A new labeling system has been under development at the FDA since 1977. However, the proposed regulation, which would provide more information on fertility, pregnancy, and breastfeeding, has not yet been finalized. In the meantime, health care professionals cannot assume relative safety for category C drugs. All available information must be carefully reviewed and the risks and benefits of each drug evaluated.

## TERATOGENESIS

Although initially designed to provide guidance, the current labeling system is often used to estimate teratogenic risk. Teratogenesis is defined as the dysgenesis of fetal organs as evidenced either structurally or functionally (e.g., brain functions) (4). Whether a given agent can induce congenital malformations in animals or humans is based on three fundamental principles of teratogenesis first described in 1959 (5). These include the particular dose of the substance, the susceptibility of the species, and the embryo's stage of development at the time of exposure.

**FDA Pregnancy Categories (3)**

Category A
Adequate, well-controlled studies in pregnant women have not shown an increased risk of fetal abnormalities.

Category B
Animal studies have revealed no evidence of harm to the fetus; however, there are no adequate and well-controlled studies in pregnant women.

**or**

Animal studies have shown an adverse effect, but adequate and well-controlled studies in pregnant women have failed to demonstrate a risk to the fetus.

Category C
Animal studies have shown an adverse effect and there are no adequate and well-controlled studies in pregnant women.

**or**

No animal studies have been conducted, and there are no adequate and well-controlled studies in pregnant women.

Category D
Studies, adequate, well-controlled, or observational, in pregnant women have demonstrated a risk to the fetus. However, the benefits of therapy may outweigh the potential risk.

Category X
Studies, adequate, well-controlled, or observational, in animals or pregnant women have demonstrated positive evidence of fetal abnormalities. The use of the product is contraindicated in women who are or may become pregnant.

 **Animal and Human Risk Exposure and Pregnancy Categories**

| Pregnancy Category | Animal Exposure | Human Exposure |
| --- | --- | --- |
| A | – | – |
| B | + | – |
|   | – | Unknown |
| C | + | Unknown |
|   | Unknown | Unknown |
| D (benefit may outweigh risk) | + | + |
| X (contraindicated) | + | + |

*Note*: –, no risk; +, known risk.

The timing of fetal exposure is the most important determinant of teratogenesis. There are four critical periods in human development in which drugs may adversely affect the fetus (6). Days 0 to 7 represent the preimplantation phase, in which fertilization and zygote formation occur. Exposure to teratogens during this period usually results either in death of the embryo or in replacement of damaged cells by undifferentiated cells that go on to develop normally. During organogenesis (days 14 to 60), the embryo is at its peak sensitivity to teratogens. Most morphologic congenital abnormalities are thought to be produced during this interval. As organogenesis ends, susceptibility to anatomic abnormalities declines. Minor structural malformation may still occur throughout histogenesis. Exposures during the fetal development period are associated with a much lower risk of major birth defects because most major organ systems are well developed by this time (7,8). Problems that do occur usually involve growth or functional deviations.

## PREGNANCY REGISTRIES

Beyond the current pregnancy categories, relevant clinical data on medications during pregnancy are found through a modest group of anecdotal case reports, case studies, observational studies, and retrospective chart reviews. Despite this lack of information about the effects of medications on the fetus, medication use during pregnancy appears to be increasing. A study conducted by the FDA in 1995 found that women under 35 years of age consumed on average three prescriptions during the course of their pregnancy (9). For those over 35 years of age, the number of prescriptions increased to five. A 2003 study estimates 80% of pregnant women taking some over-the-counter (OTC) or prescription medications (10). Known use of prescription and OTC medications in pregnant women, along with inadvertent exposures to medications during pregnancy (i.e., woman is unaware she is pregnant while taking a medication), provide another opportunity to collect relevant clinical data, through pregnancy registries.

A pregnancy registry is a surveillance study that enrolls pregnant women after they have been exposed to a medication and follows the women until the birth of the baby (11). Although regulations continue to be reviewed, pregnancy registries are currently voluntary with most administered through pharmaceutical companies and a few administered through specific organizations (i.e., hospitals, universities). Data from babies born to women taking a particular medication are compared to those born to women not taking the medicine. Patients may enroll directly to some but the majority require physician enrollment. A listing of available pregnancy registries is available on the FDA webpage.

To date, very few drugs are known to cause fetal harm (Table 17.3). Nonetheless, it is virtually impossible to prove drugs safe for use in pregnancy because no well-designed long-term studies can be ethically conducted. This leaves a huge void between known teratogenesis and known safety. Although this void is difficult to fill with our current labeling system and available literature, some clinically relevant conclusions can be reached (Table 17.4).

### Anti-infectives

Although penicillins and penicillin derivatives cross the placenta, they are considered safe for use in the nonallergic patient during pregnancy (12–14). A large study involving 3,546 fetal exposures to penicillin derivatives (primarily penicillin G) during the first trimester of pregnancy found no link to major or minor malformations (15). Other reports and the wide use of this class of drugs during pregnancy support this finding (14,16). Data on the newer penicillins (i.e., ticarcillin and piperacillin) are lacking. However, the FDA places each of these agents

| TABLE 17.3 | Medications Absolutely Contraindicated in Pregnancy (Category X) |

Acetretin

Androgens

Estrogens

Dihydroergotamine

Finasteride

Goserelin

HMG-CoA Reductase Inhibitors
 (Atorvastatin, Fluvastatin, Lovastatin, Pravastatin, Simvastatin)

Leuprolide

Megestrol

Progesterone

Ribavirin

Thalidomide

Warfarin

Yohimbine

in risk category B with the other penicillins. It is known that ticarcillin and piperacillin rapidly cross the placenta, but no reports of congenital defects with these agents have been located (14). Beta-lactamase inhibitors (i.e., clavulanate, sulbactam, tazobactam) are added to penicillin derivatives to broaden their spectrum of activity. Several studies have failed to find a teratogenic effect associated with exposure to clavulanate; however, the Michigan Medicaid Surveillance Study found a possible association with spina bifida (14,17–19). Limited data exist regarding sulbactam and tazobactam; however, available data suggest no evidence for concern (14,20).

The majority of *cephalosporins* readily cross the placenta and have pharmacokinetic parameters very similar to the penicillins. In the retrospective Michigan Medicaid Surveillance Study, increased numbers of birth defects were found for cefaclor, cephalexin, and cephradine, but not other cephalosporins (14,19). However, a large, population-based, case-control study assessing the incidence of birth defects with seven cephalosporins found no association (21). Generally, the cephalosporins are considered safe for use during pregnancy and are the preferred alternative in patients with nonanaphylactic penicillin sensitivity (14,20,21). Where it covers the appropriate microbial spectrum, erythromycin base should be used in penicillin-allergic patients demonstrating immediate-type sensitivity.

The *macrolide*, erythromycin, has been used during pregnancy with no known increased risk to the mother or the fetus (14,20). Although the drug crosses the placenta, plasma levels are low in the fetus (22). One salt of erythromycin, the estolate form, is considered contraindicated during pregnancy because of a reported 10% reversible incidence of hepatotoxicity (increases in serum aspartate

TABLE
17.4

Pregnancy Categories for Disease-Specific Medications

| Condition | FDA Pregnancy Category | Comments |
|-----------|------------------------|----------|
| **Acne** | | |
| Adapalene | C | No malformations seen in animal studies, but no well-controlled human trials available |
| Isotretinoin | X | Absolute contraindication, no safe dose, monthly pregnancy testing and two forms of contraception are required throughout therapy |
| Tazarotene | X | Absolute contraindication, negative pregnancy test should be obtained 2 weeks before therapy initiation |
| Tretinoin | C | Case reports of malformations with topical administration during the first trimester |
| **Anti-infectives** | | |
| Aminoglycosides | D | Streptomycin and kanamycin have been reported to cause congenital deafness. Serious side effects in the fetus have not been reported with other aminoglycosides |
| Azithromycin | B | No evidence of congenital defects |
| Cephalosporins | B | Less data than with penicillins, but generally considered safe in pregnancy |
| Daptomycin | B | Unknown risk to the fetus because of limited safety data |
| Erythromycin | B | The base is considered safe for use during pregnancy. No significant evidence of congenital defects reported. The estolate salt has been reported to cause hepatotoxicity in pregnant women |
| Linezolid | C | Unknown risk to the fetus because of limited safety data |
| Metronidazole | B | No compelling evidence of fetal harm. Recommended by CDC for treatment of trichomoniasis and bacterial vaginosis during pregnancy. Manufacturer lists first trimester use as a contraindication |
| Nitrofurantoin | B | Considered safe. Theoretically, could cause hemolytic anemia in newborn. Avoid in bacteremia, urosepsis, and pyelonephritis |
| Penicillins | B | Generally considered safe in pregnancy. Most safety experience with penicillin G |

| | | |
|---|---|---|
| Quinupristin/dalfopristin | C | Unknown risk to the fetus due to limited safety data |
| Quinolones | C | Avoid use during pregnancy. Have been associated with arthropathies in animals and children |
| Tetracyclines | D | Avoid if possible, especially during last half of pregnancy |
| Trimethoprim/Sulfamethoxazole | C | Trimethoprim inhibits folic acid synthesis. Sulfonamides can induce kernicterus in the newborn if used late in pregnancy |
| Vancomycin | C | Generally not thought to be teratogenic. Links to ototoxicity and nephrotoxicity not established |

**Analgesia**

| | | |
|---|---|---|
| Acetaminophen | B | Analgesic and antipyretic of choice in pregnancy |
| Aspirin | C | May produce adverse effects in the mother and the fetus. Can inhibit labor if used late in pregnancy. Avoid if possible |
| Codeine | C/D | High doses or long term use is not recommended. Likely to cause neonatal respiratory depression and withdrawal if used near term |
| Nonsteroidal anti-inflammatories | B/C/D | No association to date with congenital malformations. Can theoretically inhibit labor if used late in pregnancy. May cause constriction or closure of the ductus arteriosus if used near term |
| Hydromorphone | B/D | Not associated with congenital defects. High doses or long-term use is not recommended. Likely to cause neonatal respiratory depression and withdrawal if used near term |
| Fentanyl | C/D | Not associated with congenital defects. Likely to cause neonatal respiratory depression and withdrawal if used near term |
| Morphine | C/D | Not associated with congenital defects. High doses or long-term use is not recommended. Likely to cause neonatal respiratory depression and withdrawal if used near term |
| Oxycodone | B/D | Not associated with teratogenic effects. High doses or long-term use is not recommended. Likely to cause neonatal respiratory depression and withdrawal if used near term |

*(continued)*

TABLE
17.4

Pregnancy Categories for Disease-Specific Medications *(continued)*

| Condition | FDA Pregnancy Category | Comments |
|---|---|---|
| **Asthma** | | |
| $\beta$-Agonists | C | Safety differences between agents have not been identified. Oral/parenteral agents may delay delivery based on alternative indications (i.e., preterm labor) |
| Corticosteroids | C | Inhaled budesonide is preferred. ACOG does not mandate change from prior inhaled steroid agent despite category |
| Inhaled anticholinergics | B | No reports of teratogenicity in animals exposed to ipratropium, but few human investigations. No well-controlled studies in humans with tiotropium |
| Leukotriene receptor antagonists | B | No long-term data for this newer therapeutic class |
| Theophylline | C | Does not appear teratogenic. Drug clearance may be altered in pregnancy, monitor dose |
| **Coagulation** | | |
| Coumarin derivatives (warfarin) | X | Generally considered contraindicated. Risks include embryopathy, spontaneous abortion, stillbirth, prematurity, and hemorrhage |
| Heparin | C | Generally considered the agent of choice in pregnancy. Long-term therapy has been linked to maternal osteopenia |
| Low molecular weight heparins | B | Alternative therapy to UFH. Use of enoxaparin in pregnant women with a mechanical heart valve is controversial due to valvular clotting and deaths reported in clinical trial and post-marketing surveillance |
| Fondaparinux | B | Synthetic factor Xa inhibitor used in patients with heparin allergy or heparin |
| **Depression** | | |
| Monoamine oxidase inhibitors | C | Limited human data for pregnancy. Maybe increased risk for malformations; risk of use must be weighed against benefits |

| Drug | Category | Notes |
|---|---|---|
| Selective serotonin reuptake inhibitors (SSRIs) (*Paroxetine = D*) | C | Most experience with fluoxetine with no associated teratogenicity. Neonatal withdrawal syndrome has been estimated to occur in 30% of infants. Paroxetine use has been linked to cardiac malformations and PPHN |
| Tricyclic antidepressants (TCAs) *Imipramine = D* | C | This drug class may be associated with neonatal withdrawal (colic, cyanosis, tachypnea, and irritability). Animal trials and human case reports have documented congenital abnormalities with imipramine |
| Newer Antidepressants *Bupropion = B* *Duloxetine = C* *Mirtazapine = C* *Nefazodone = C* *Trazodone = C* *Venlafaxine = C* | B/C | Limited human data available for more recently approved agents. May consider for women refractory to other agents |
| **Diabetes** | | |
| Glyburide | C | One large prospective study has found that glyburide is as effective as insulin in women after the first trimester with gestational diabetes. Glyburide is a reasonable alternative to insulin in certain patients (e.g., fear of needles/injections) |
| Insulin (human), short-acting *Regular* *Aspart* *Lispro* *Glulisine* | Not available  B  B  B  C | Regular insulin is the agent of choice in pregnancy. Insulin aspart and lispro are alternatives for better postprandial glucose control. No human data available for glulisine |
| Insulin (human), long-acting *NPH* *Detemir* *Glargine* | C  C | NPH insulin is the basal insulin agent of choice in pregnancy. Limited pregnancy data available for insulin glargine and detemir (peak-less insulins); clinical implications of their increase in IGF-1 receptor affinity unknown |

*(continued)*

231

TABLE
17.4

Pregnancy Categories for Disease-Specific Medications *(continued)*

| Condition | FDA Pregnancy Category | Comments |
|---|---|---|
| Metformin | B | No morphological abnormalities observed in animals but some conflicting human data; results of one large clinical trial found metformin (with supplemental insulin) to be as effective and safe as insulin alone for gestational diabetes (after first trimester). PCOS clinical trials demonstrate safety. More research needed |
| **Gastrointestinal Reflux** | | |
| Aluminum-containing antacids | Not available | Use is controversial. Severe developmental retardation reported in a child after high-dose use during pregnancy; normal doses during pregnancy may be acceptable. Co-ingestion of acidic foods or beverages should be avoided due to potential for increased GI absorption of aluminum |
| Calcium/Magnesium-containing antacids | Not available | Generally considered first-line therapy for GERD in pregnancy; 10%–30% of calcium, 15%–30% of magnesium is absorbed |
| H$_2$ Receptor Antagonists | | |
| Cimetidine | B | Antiandrogenic effects observed in animals and nonpregnant humans; Limited data in humans suggest no association with increased risk of malformations |
| Ranitidine | B | Only H2RA with documented efficacy in pregnancy; available evidence suggests no congenital malformations or neonatal toxicity |
| Famotidine | B | Limited safety data in humans |
| Nizatidine | B | Caution recommended during pregnancy due to reports of abortions, low fetal weights, and fewer live fetuses in rabbits at doses significantly higher than recommended human doses |
| Magnesium trisilicates | Not available | Avoid long-term, high-dose use due to potential for fetal nephrolithiasis, hypotonia, respiratory distress, and cardiovascular effects |
| Proton Pump Inhibitors | | |
| Omeprazole | C | Reports regarding use in pregnancy are conflicting; use of safer alternatives preferred whenever possible (especially in the first trimester) |

| | | |
|---|---|---|
| Lansoprazole | B | Limited clinical experience available in humans. Use of safer alternatives preferred whenever possible (especially in the first trimester) |
| Rabeprazole | | |
| Pantoprazole | | |
| Esomeprazole | | |
| Metoclopromide | B | Available evidence suggests no congenital malformations or neonatal toxicity |
| Sodium bicarbonate | Not available | Avoid in pregnancy due to potential for maternal/fetal fluid overload and potential for metabolic alkalosis |
| Sucralfate | B | No data in animals, generally considered acceptable in pregnancy due to low absorption; Potential for fetal toxicity linked to aluminum content (1 g sucralfate = 207 mg aluminum) |
| **Hypertension** | | |
| Angiotensin-converting enzyme inhibitors (ACEIs) | D | Contraindicated in pregnancy. Can cause fetal toxicity and death |
| Angiotensin II receptor antagonists | D | Contraindicated. Similar to ACEIs |
| $\beta$-Blockers | C | Generally considered safe, but may be associated with fetal growth retardation |
| Calcium antagonists nifedipine | C | Limited data. No increase in major teratogenicity noted, but generally not used due to its association with cardiovascular events. Nifedipine use is controversial |
| Diuretics | B/C | Probably safe, but not first-line agents. Furosemide is embryotoxic. Thiazide diuretics considered safest in this class |
| Hydralazine | C | May be used as first or second line for acute hypertensive crisis, but second line after methyldopa for chronic treatment during pregnancy |
| Labetalol | C | May be used as first or second line for acute hypertensive crisis, but second line after methyldopa for chronic treatment during pregnancy. Should not be used in those with asthma or congestive heart failure |
| Methyldopa | B | Preferred agent for chronic hypertension during pregnancy. No adverse effects noted in long term follow-up study |

*(continued)*

TABLE

17.4

Pregnancy Categories for Disease-Specific Medications *(continued)*

| Condition | FDA Pregnancy Category | Comments |
|---|---|---|
| **Migraine/Headache** | | |
| Dihydroergotamine | X | Contraindicated. Has been linked to perinatal deaths and abnormalities |
| Ergotamine | X | Contraindicated. Has been linked to perinatal deaths and abnormalities |
| Sumatriptan | C | Not thought to be a human teratogen. Exposures, including those in the first trimester, linked to preterm labor and low birth weight infants |
| **Nausea and Vomiting** | | |
| Dimenhydrinate | B | Limited data available. Congenital defects were not found to be associated with dimenhydrinate |
| Diphenhydramine | B | Avoid near delivery |
| Doxylamine | A | Effective in combination with pyridoxine |
| Hydroxyzine | C | Given orally or IM. Possible congenital defects when given in first trimester |
| Meclizine | B | Several studies show safety in pregnancy |
| Metoclopramide | B | Enhances upper GI tract motility, increases lower esophageal sphincter tone, and in high doses, blocks serotonin in CTZ. EPS may be seen |
| Ondansetron | B | Blocks serotonin peripherally and in the CTZ |
| Promethazine | C | Safety data are conflicting. Use in labor is common, however, limited data regarding its use for NVP |
| Pyridoxine | A | Effective in combination with doxylamine |
| **Psychosis and Bipolar Disorder** | | |
| Benzodiazepines | C | Sedation and withdrawal seen in the neonate. Floppy infant syndrome (hypotonia, low Apgar scores, and neurological depression) |
| Low-potency antipsychotics | D (near term) | Tachycardia, GI dysfunction, sedation, and hypotension seen at birth and up to several days after |
| Chlorpromazine | C | delivery. Exposure during weeks 4–10 of gestation associated with increased risk of malformations. Chlorpromazine may cause insulin resistance in mother and respiratory |
| Thioridazine | | depression in the newborn exposed during the third trimester. Dose reduction near term can be considered to reduce risk of toxicity in infant |

| Drug | Category | Notes |
|---|---|---|
| **High-potency antipsychotics**<br>Fluphenazine<br>Perphenazine<br>Trifluoperazine<br>Thiothixine<br>Haloperidol | C | Extrapyramidal side effects (hyperactivity, tremor, hyperactive deep tendon reflexes, restlessness, abnormal movements, increased muscle tone, vigorous rooting or sucking, arching of back, and shrill crying) seen in newborn (especially if mother is given high doses). Exposure during weeks 4–10 of gestation associated with increased risk of malformations. Dose reduction near term can be considered to reduce risk of toxicity in the infant. Two case reports of limb reduction when haloperidol was administered in the first trimester; however, other studies have not confirmed this association |
| **Atypical Antipsychotics**<br>Clozapine | B | No defects seen in animals; one case report of intrauterine fetal death; accumulation of clozapine in neonate theoretically linked to floppy infant syndrome, neonatal seizures, gastrointestinal reflux disease, and agranulocytosis. Monitoring of white blood cells in newborns can be considered. Potential risk for gestational diabetes in mother |
| Olanzapine | C | Potential risk for gestational diabetes in mother; Limited data suggest olanzapine does not increase fetal teratogenic risk or rates of spontaneous abortion, however, more data are needed |
| Risperidone, Quetiapine, Ziprasidone | C | Data for these agents are limited or absent; ziprasidone is associated with developmental delays, possible teratogenic effects, and increased stillbirths in animals; however, limited human data are available |
| Lithium | D | Based on voluntary Register of Lithium Babies: higher rate of cardiovascular malformation (Ebstein's Anomaly); "floppy baby" syndrome (cyanosis and hypotonicity) common with exposure during labor; hypothyroidism and nephrogenic diabetes insipidus have been observed |
| **Seizure**<br>Carbamazepine | D | Estimated 1% risk of spina bifida; craniofacial defects, developmental delay (rate may be as high as 20%), may lessen effectiveness of contraceptives |
| Gabapentin | C | Gabapentin: No pattern of malformations reported to date, but often used with other agents, making causal determination difficult |

*(continued)*

**TABLE 17.4** Pregnancy Categories for Disease-Specific Medications *(continued)*

| Condition | FDA Pregnancy Category | Comments |
|---|---|---|
| Lamotrigine | C | Lamotrigine: may cause nervous system, heart, craniofacial, skeletal and urinary tract defects (Australian Birth Registry data) |
| Levetiracetam | C | Levetiracetam: no malformations or developmental delay reported in limited human evaluations |
| Oxcarbazepine | C | Oxcarbazepine: no major malformations reported to date; however, similar structure to carbamazepine which may cause neuronal tube defects; may lessen effectiveness of contraceptives |
| Phenobarbital | D | Congenital heart defects, facial clefts, dysmorphic features, fetal withdrawal syndrome, may lessen effectiveness of contraceptives |
| Phenytoin | D | Cleft palate, dysmorphic features, and craniofacial abnormalities; may lessen effectiveness of contraceptives |
| Primidone | D | Neonatal hemorrhagic syndrome, neural tube defects, may lessen effectiveness of contraceptives |
| Topiramate | C | Topiramate: developmental delay and teratogenicity in animal studies, may lessen effectiveness of contraceptives |
| Valproic Acid and salt derivatives | D | Doses >1,000 mg/d may heighten risk for spina bifida; other effects: dysmorphic features, developmental delay, cardiovascular and urogenital malformations |

**Herbal Products**

| | | |
|---|---|---|
| *Ginkgo biloba* | Not applicable | *Ginkgo* not recommended for use during pregnancy due to lack of standardization of products and need for further studies. No published evidence of major birth defects; however, more studies needed |
| Mugwort, Blue Cohash, Tansy, Black Cohosh, Scotch Broom, Goldenseal, Juniper Berry, Pennyroyal Oil, Rue, Mistletoe, and Chaste Berry | Not applicable | All are considered uterine stimulants or abortifacients and therefore contraindicated in pregnancy |
| Echinacea | Not applicable | Echinacea cannot be recommended for use during pregnancy, due to lack of standardization of products and need for further studies |
| St. John's wort | Not applicable | No studies regarding reproductive toxicity; animal studies suggest slight uterotonic activity. Due to lack of standardization of products and need for further studies, St. John's wort cannot be recommended for use during pregnancy |
| Ginger | Not applicable | Use could affect testosterone receptor binding in the fetus; use is controversial and not recommended |
| Ginseng | B | Associated with hypertension and hypoglycemia in the mother |

aminotransferase) occurring in the mother (14,20). Less evidence is available for clarithromycin and azithromycin. While teratogenic in animals, clarithromycin has, thus far, failed to demonstrate birth defects in small, epidemiologic studies of human pregnancy (14,23–25). Similar rates of major malformations and spontaneous abortions were observed with azithromycin and matched controls in a small study (26).

*Tetracyclines* are known to cause numerous potential problems to the mother and the fetus and should be avoided during pregnancy (14,20). Nearly all tetracyclines readily cross the placenta (14). Tetracycline is well-known to cause yellow-brown discoloration of the teeth after in utero exposure because of its ability to chelate calcium orthophosphate, which becomes incorporated into bones and teeth during calcification (14,20). Severe dysplasia of the teeth and inhibition of bone growth also have been demonstrated. These effects are more common when the drug is taken in the second and the third trimesters, when bone mineralization occurs (14,20). Tetracycline has also been reported to induce limb anomalies, inguinal hernia, and hypospadias (14). Potentially fatal maternal liver and renal toxicities, although rare, have been attributed to tetracycline (14,20).

*Sulfonamides* cross the placenta and accumulate in significant quantities in the fetus (14,20). Teratogenicity has been shown in some animal species, but a link to human malformations has not been demonstrated even in large trials (15,19). Sulfonamides should not be administered close to delivery as they can cause jaundice and kernicterus in the newborn through displacement of bilirubin from albumin-binding sites. Earlier in pregnancy, the placenta is capable of clearing the free unconjugated bilirubin; however, the clearing mechanism is no longer available at birth (14). Hemolysis may occur in the fetus or neonate because of relative deficiencies in glucose-6-phosphate dehydrogenase (G-6-PD) (14,20).

*Trimethoprim* used alone or in combination with sulfonamides should be avoided during pregnancy. The drug is a folic acid antagonist, a group of agents known to be potentially teratogenic. The Michigan Medicaid Surveillance Study and other retrospective reviews have suggested an increase in incidence of birth defects (cardiovascular and oral clefts) potentially up to twofold to threefold (14). Recent evidence suggests an association between trimethoprim and neural tube defects, congenital heart defects, and oral clefts (27–30).

*Nitrofurantoin* is not associated with an increased risk of birth defects in the neonate; however, administration of the drug close to delivery theoretically may cause hemolytic anemia in the newborn because of G-6-PD and glutathione deficiencies (14,19,20). Nitrofurantoin is popular for the treatment and prophylaxis of urinary tract infections in pregnancy but should not be used when bacteremia or urosepsis is suspected because of low therapeutic serum concentrations or in pyelonephritis because of inadequate tissue penetration (14,29,31).

*Metronidazole* crosses the placenta and appears in maternal and cord blood in equal amounts. Because the drug is mutagenic in bacteria and carcinogenic in rats, some recommend avoiding it in pregnancy (14). However, there are no good human data implicating metronidazole as a teratogen or a carcinogen. One human study reported 31 first-trimester exposures leading to four cases of birth defects (15). However, several more recent studies suggest that metronidazole does not adversely affect the fetus (32–35). Metronidazole has been recommended for the treatment of bacterial vaginosis and trichomoniasis (36). To date, the relative risk of metronidazole's use in pregnancy is unknown, and its use in pregnancy is controversial.

The *aminoglycosides* are frequently used to treat serious infections during pregnancy and have not caused fetal malformation (13,37). However, ototoxicity and deafness have been reported in infants exposed to *streptomycin* and *kanamycin* in utero (14,37). Gentamicin, amikacin, and tobramycin all cross the placenta and appear in the fetal circulation. Highest fetal concentrations are found in the kidneys and urine. Pharmacokinetics of aminoglycosides are usually significantly altered in pregnant women. Careful maternal serum level monitoring is required to limit fetal exposure yet assure therapeutic concentrations in the mother.

The *fluoroquinolones* distribute well to bone tissue and cartilage and have been associated with arthropathies in animals and in human children (14,31). However, some available data have failed to find this effect in the children of the women exposed to fluoroquinolones during pregnancy (20,38–40). Because of the availability of safer alternatives, fluoroquinolones should generally be avoided in pregnancy.

*Vancomycin* is not thought to be teratogenic (14). Vancomycin was present in significant amounts in the cord blood of a mother who received vancomycin (41). Ototoxicity and nephrotoxicity are potential problems, and a few cases have been reported; however, the relationship of these defects to vancomycin therapy has not been clearly established (14).

Limited data are available regarding the safety of *linezolid, daptomycin*, and *quinupristin/dalfopristin* in pregnant women. Linezolid has a low molecular weight; therefore, distribution across the placenta is likely. Animal studies have shown toxicity (i.e., total litter loss, decreased fetal weight, increased fusion of costal cartilage) at doses 6.5 times the expected human exposure and maternal toxicity (reduced body weight gain) at doses 0.64 times the expected human exposure (42). The manufacturer reports three cases of women found to be pregnant after linezolid study enrollment (two patients had spontaneous abortions and one delivered a healthy infant). Because of the unknown safety profile of *linezolid* in pregnancy, use should be considered only if the potential benefit to the patient outweighs the potential risks. In animals, *quinupristin/dalfopristin* was not teratogenic or embryotoxic or fetotoxic (14). No case reports of use in pregnant women are published. Two case reports of *daptomycin* use during the third trimester are published (43,44). In both reports, no adverse neonatal outcomes were reported.

## Analgesia

Although it crosses the placenta, acetaminophen has been widely used during pregnancy and is not teratogenic. Because acetaminophen does not affect platelet function or prostaglandin synthesis, short-term use of acetaminophen at therapeutic doses is considered the analgesic and antipyretic of choice in pregnant women (14,45,46). Aspirin is more controversial. The Collaborative Perinatal Project failed to associate 14,864 first-trimester fetal exposures to aspirin with malformations (15). Use in the first trimester has not been associated with birth defects, low birth weight, or still birth (47,48). However, aspirin can result in a narrowing of the ductus arteriosus when used in the third trimester (14). Women taking aspirin also run the risk of maternal and newborn bleeding through platelet inhibition, inhibition of uterine contractions, and prolonged labor through prostaglandin inhibition (47,49). Aspirin should be avoided, especially late in pregnancy.

The nonsteroidal anti-inflammatory drugs (NSAIDs) have not been linked with congenital malformations and have been used during pregnancy (47,50–53). Like aspirin, NSAIDs are prostaglandin inhibitors; therefore, they can prolong labor when used late in pregnancy and cause constriction or early closure of the ductus arteriosus (54,55). NSAIDs can cause oligohydramnios from decreased fetal urine output and renal dysfunction (47,51,56).

For severe pain, opioid analgesics have been used and are not associated with any major or minor malformations (14,15,57). Opioids may cause neonatal respiratory depression and withdrawal when used near delivery. Use for prolonged periods or in high doses at term is not recommended.

## Asthma

For most patients, the management of asthma is much the same during pregnancy as it is in the nonpregnant state. When left untreated, severe persistent asthma has the potential to lead to serious complications for both the mother and the child (58). In general, the inhalation route is preferred over oral or parenteral administration to limit localized absorption of the agent to the lungs.

Short-acting, beta-agonists, such as albuterol, are considered first-line therapy for patients with mild to moderate disease. There appears to be no safety differences between available inhaled beta-agonists; however, the use of the oral or parenteral route should be avoided because of limited safety data and the potential to delay delivery (terbutaline is used for tocolysis). Inhaled corticosteroids are a major component of asthma therapy for all patients, including those who may be pregnant. Budesonide is the preferred inhaled corticosteroid; however, the American College of Obstetricians and Gynecologists (ACOG) states that inhaled corticosteroids other than budesonide may be continued if symptoms were well-controlled prior to pregnancy (58).

Cromolyn is not known to be teratogenic (59,60). Nedocromil is not expected to be teratogenic (14). Both have minimal systemic absorption and associated adverse effects. The leukotriene receptor agonists zafirlukast and montelukast are not teratogenic in animals (14). However, there are limited safety data in humans. These agents may be considered alternative add-on controller medications in patients with moderate persistent asthma not stabilized on low-dose inhaled corticosteroids (58).

There are limited data for the use of ipratropium during pregnancy; however, animal models have shown no resulting fetal malformation during exposure (14). Compared to beta-agonists, ipratropium provides no significant benefit when safety data are considered, and as such, it is not considered first-line therapy during pregnancy (58,61). Theophylline does not appear to cause adverse fetal outcomes; however, use of theophylline in pregnancy should be undertaken with caution because theophylline pharmacokinetics change during pregnancy (60,62). Serum concentrations should be monitored frequently and doses adjusted accordingly.

Emergency management is the same as for nonpregnant patients because of the overwhelming benefits for the mother and the fetus and should consist of oxygen administration, use of nebulized beta-agonists and ipratropium, oral or intravenous corticosteroids, and intravenous agents when indicated (61).

## Coagulation

Thromboembolism is a serious complication of pregnancy occurring in 1 to 2 per 1,000 gestations and accounts for about 10% of deaths during gestation. About 65% of thromboembolic events occur during the antepartum period, and this risk continues with an incidence of 35% until about 6 weeks postpartum. Most emboli (80%) are venous in nature deep vein thrombosis (DVT) with the remaining 20% occurring as pulmonary emboli. Risk factors for venous thromboembolism (VTE) during normal pregnancy include increases in normal endogenous clotting factors, increased venous pooling, and compression of the iliac vein. Additive risk factors are age >35 years, prior history of VTE, obesity, genetic thrombophilia (factor V Leiden deficiency, antithrombin deficiency), preeclampsia, smoking, diabetes, anemia, Lupus, coronary disease, multiple gestation, hyperemesis, fluid/electrolyte imbalance, sickle cell disease, recent surgery, and prolonged immobility (63,64).

Based on the American College of Chest Physicians (ACCP), thromboembolism should be managed by using these comorbid factors (65,66):

1. Pregnant women with previous VTE prior to pregnancy require prophylactic unfractionated heparin (UFH) or low molecular weight heparin (LMWH) such as dalteparin, enoxaparin, or tinzaparin. Aspirin should be discontinued. Additionally, graduated elastic compression stockings (GECS) can be used as prophylaxis (67).
2. Women on warfarin for VTE who become pregnant should discontinue warfarin and begin treatment with UFH or LMWH in doses described below.
3. Women on anticoagulation for prosthetic heart valves should receive treatment with adjusted dose of UFH or LMWH.
4. Pregnant women with high-risk valves (older generation valve in the mitral position or history of thromboembolism) should consider therapy with oral anticoagulants instead of heparin.
5. Pregnant women with VTE during pregnancy should receive adjusted UFH as a bolus and then continuous infusion or UFH every 12 hours to achieve target activated partial thromboplastin time (PTT) values for at least 5 days and continue the same until delivery.
6. Pregnant women with prosthetic valves and high risk of VTE and/or preeclampsia should receive adjusted dose UFH or LMWH plus aspirin 75 to 100 mg per day.

The pharmacokinetics of heparin is altered in pregnancy to the point that significant increases in doses or frequency are required to keep aPTT values therapeutic. Therapeutic ranges for aPTT vary with the testing procedure run at different institutions (66,68). Women in labor should receive UFH instead of LMWH due to its longer duration and lack of a reversal agent (63). Protamine is the reversal agent for bleeding from heparin therapy. Approximately 1 mg of protamine reverses 100 units of heparin. In calculating the total dose of protamine required for reversal, only consider the amount of heparin given in the last several hours, as the duration of heparin is only 4 to 6 hours (64,66).

For women who develop adverse reactions to UFH or LMWH, the options are limited. Fondaparinux, a selective antifactor Xa, has limited and conflicting information in pregnancy but may be considered the treatment of choice if heparin products are not advised (allergy to heparin or heparin induced thrombocytopenia) (3,67,69,70).

Postpartum management should resume 12 hours after epidural or 24 hours after cesarean section. GECS devices should remain in place. If warfarin is indicated for continued treatment, it may be restarted 2 weeks after delivery and continued for 3 to 6 months after delivery (63,67).

## Depression

Recent data indicate that as many as 19% of women will have a major depressive episode at some point during pregnancy or the postpartum period (71). Untreated depression during pregnancy is associated with poor outcomes including low birth weight infants, preterm delivery, lower Apgar scores, poor prenatal care, and an increased risk of fetal abuse, neonaticide, or suicide (72,73). Treatment of maternal depression during pregnancy and the postpartum period is recommended, despite the potential risks to the fetus and the newborn (72,74). Selective serotonin reuptake inhibitors (SSRIs) have replaced tricyclic antidepressants (TCAs) as first-line treatment for depression in the general population (75). Of the SSRIs, fluoxetine has been the most commonly used and studied in pregnancy. Others are paroxetine, sertraline, citalopram, escitalopram, and fluvoxamine, as well as serotonin norepinephrine reuptake inhibitors (SNRIs) such as venlafaxine and duloxetine. The use of SSRI and SNRI drugs during gestation does not appear to be associated with an increased risk of major fetal anomalies (75,76).

Nevertheless, the safety of SSRIs is now in question with an emerging picture of neonatal problems such as neonatal behavioral syndrome, congenital heart disease, and persistent pulmonary hypertension (PPHN). Exposure to SSRIs in late pregnancy is associated with a threefold increased risk of neonatal behavioral syndrome, also termed neonatal abstinence syndrome (75,77). Signs and symptoms of this behavioral syndrome include jitteriness, poor muscle tone, tachycardia, hypoglycemia, hypothermia, respiratory distress, weak or absent cry, low Apgar scoring, and desaturation during feeding (75,77,78). This has been estimated to occur in approximately 30% of infants exposed to SSRIs in utero (75,77).

In December 2005, the FDA issued a public health advisory regarding the potential risk of ventricular septal defects (VSDs) in fetuses exposed to paroxetine in the first trimester (79). There are two reports from Glaxo-SmithKline based on a Swedish national registry and a U.S. insurance claims database that have raised concerns about a one-and-a-half- to twofold increased risk of congenital cardiac malformations (atrial and ventricular septal defects) associated with first-trimester paroxetine exposure (79). As a result, the manufacturer changed the pregnancy category rating from C to D. More recently, the cardiovascular teratogenic effect of SSRI use during the first trimester of pregnancy was examined in two large studies (73,80). These studies found no increase in cardiovascular defects associated with paroxetine use.

In July 2006, FDA issued another public health advisory regarding SSRI use in pregnancy and the potential risk of PPHN in newborns (81). One study that FDA cites found that PPHN was six times more likely in neonates whose mothers took an SSRI after the 20th week of pregnancy (82). A more recent study has found no evidence of an increase in the risk for PPHN associated with SSRI use (83).

The atypical antidepressants include bupropion, duloxetine, mirtazapine, nefazodone, and venlafaxine. Information on the use of these medications in pregnancy is limited (72).

### Diabetes

Diabetes during pregnancy has the potential to cause complications, such as macrosomia, hyperbilirubinemia, increased risk for cesarean delivery, and birth trauma to the fetus (84–87). The initial management of pregestational and gestational diabetes is diet and exercise. Drug therapy may be warranted if inadequate blood glucose control occurs. Based on the recommendations from the ACOG, the drug of choice for the treatment of pregestational and gestational diabetes is exogenous human insulin. Insulin does not cross the placenta unless bound to IgG antibody or forced through the placenta by high perfusion (e.g., fast infusion rate); therefore, fetal exposure is minimized (88). Traditionally, regular human insulin has been used to manage blood glucose levels with the addition of NPH human insulin (isophane suspension) as a longer acting basal source. Newer rapid acting insulins (e.g., insulin aspart and lispro) have been evaluated and appear to be safe for pregnant patients in place of regular insulin; these insulin analogs may be beneficial if better postprandial glucose control is desired. Limited pregnancy data are available for the newer peak-less, long-acting insulins (e.g., insulin glargine and detemir); the clinical implications of their increase in insulin-like growth factor-I (IGF-1) receptor affinity are unknown and warrant further evaluation before routine use in pregnancy.

Sulfonylureas stimulate insulin secretion from pancreatic islet $\beta$-cells to lower serum glucose levels (86,87,89). Animal and human models document placental transport of first-generation sulfonylureas (i.e., chlorpropamide, tolbutamide, tolazamide). Their low molecular weight (270 to 277) facilitates the placental transport and results in fetal hyperinsulinemia, which can be profound and prolonged; therefore, their use in pregnancy is contraindicated. Documentation of second-generation sulfonylurea's (i.e., glyburide, glipizide) use in pregnancy is primarily with glyburide (glibenclamide). Placental transport of glyburide in humans is minimal because of its significant plasma protein binding (95% to 99%) and relatively larger molecular weight (494). Results of a large randomized controlled study of 404 pregnant women post 11 weeks' gestation and diagnosed with gestational diabetes suggest glyburide is a clinically effective alternative to insulin; additionally, the incidence of complications (e.g., macrosomia) and adverse events (e.g., hypoglycemia, fetal anomalies) is similar between these therapies (90). A secondary analysis of the study population further substantiates the previously stated findings and concludes that glyburide and insulin are equally effective for all levels of gestational diabetes severity (91). Therefore, glyburide is a reasonable therapeutic alternative to insulin (e.g., patients fearful of injections) for the treatment of gestational diabetes.

Biguanides (i.e., phenformin, metformin) decrease serum glucose levels by reducing hepatic glucose production, decreasing intestinal glucose absorption, and increasing peripheral tissue glucose uptake and utilization (86,87,89). Phenformin, metformin's predecessor, was problematic because of its propensity to cause lactic acidosis in patients. Additionally, mouse embryo studies with phenformin documented fetal death and malformations (e.g., neural tube defect, craniofacial hypoplasia) at serum concentrations consistent with clinical use. Although metformin can cause lactic acidosis if used inappropriately (e.g., patients with severe renal insufficiency), it does not appear to be a major teratogen based on animal models. Animals exposed to metformin have experienced delayed closure of the neural tube; however, it has not translated into morphological abnormalities. One clinical trial comparing metformin, sulfonylureas, and insulin suggests that metformin may increase the occurrence of preeclampsia and perinatal death, but the investigators state these events could be attributed to other factors (e.g., obesity, metabolic syndrome) present in the metformin subjects (92). A more recent open-label study of 751 patients with gestational diabetes between 20 and 33 weeks' gestation demonstrates that metformin (with supplemental insulin if needed) is as effective and safe as insulin therapy alone; the composite endpoint of neonatal hypoglycemia, respiratory distress, need for phototherapy, birth trauma, 5-minute Apgar score <7, and prematurity did not differ between treatment groups (93). Metformin studies in pregnant patients with polycystic ovary syndrome (PCOS) further substantiate that metformin is not a human teratogen, as these patients continue metformin therapy into pregnancy postconception (89). However, more experience with metformin for the treatment of gestational diabetes is needed before routine use can be recommended (84).

Clinical pregnancy data for the remaining antidiabetic medication classes (e.g., meglitinides, thiazolidinediones, glucosidase inhibitors) predominately include published case reports (89). With limited clinical experience, the assessment of risk for these agents is difficult, thus restricting their use in pregnancy.

### Gastroesophageal Reflux Disease (94–96)

Gastroesophageal reflux effects 45% to 80% of pregnant women and is associated with maternal discomfort and complications (e.g., esophageal erosions). Non-pharmacologic interventions include avoidance of high-fat foods and caffeinated and carbonated beverages late in the day, elevating the head of the bed, and not smoking. Drug therapies for gastroesophageal reflux disease (GERD) include antacids, sucralfate, histamine-2 receptor blockers, prokinetic agents, and proton pump inhibitors.

Antacids are considered first-line agents in managing GERD symptoms, neutralizing gastric acid to prevent esophageal damage and discomfort. Calcium and magnesium containing antacids are preferred, whereas aluminum-based antacids are controversial due to aluminum's association with fetal neurological effects; however, systemic absorption of antacids is not significant. Likewise, magnesium trisilicate containing antacids (e.g., Gaviscon) should be avoided, as they have been associated with fetal complications such as nephrolithiasis, hypotonia, respiratory distress, and cardiovascular effects.

Like antacids, sucralfate is a first-line medication for GERD and is not generally systemically absorbed. It adheres to exposed mucosal lesions within the gastrointestinal tract until healing occurs and inhibits pepsin activity. Since sucralfate is an aluminum salt of a sulfated disaccharide (1 g sucralfate = 207 mg of aluminum), its use in pregnancy is controversial. Human fetal toxicity has not been reported, as findings of the Michigan Medicaid Surveillance Study of 229,101 pregnancies expected eight birth defects when only five were reported.

Histamine-2 receptor blockers are second tier therapeutic options, working to decrease gastric acid production. Of these agents, ranitidine is preferred, as available evidence suggests no congenital malformations or neonatal toxicity. Cimetidine's antiandrogen activity as well as its hepatotoxicity, as substantiated by a case report of hepatitis in a newborn, limits its clinical utility in pregnancy. Animal studies with nizatidine are conflicting. One rabbit pregnancy study involving nizatidine reports abortions, low fetal weights, and fewer live fetuses at doses significantly larger than human doses; however, other animal studies do not substantiate these findings. Famotidine is a pregnancy category B but limited human pregnancy data exist.

Metoclopramide is a prokinetic agent that increases lower esophageal sphincter (LES) tone and gastric motility. Animal studies do not demonstrate teratogenic effects, whereas human evidence conflicts. Of the 192 first-trimester pregnancy exposures documented in the Michigan Medicaid Surveillance Study, 10 cases (5.2%) of major birth defects occurred as compared to the eight expected; however, this does not establish a causal relationship between metoclopramide and birth defects.

Proton pump inhibitors block potassium–hydrogen–ATPase and inhibit the secretion of gastric acid. Limited safety data in pregnancy are available for proton pump inhibitors, limiting their use to severe and refractory cases. All of the proton pump inhibitors are classified as pregnancy category B, except omeprazole which is category C. Initial omeprazole animal studies demonstrated embryonic and fetal toxicity at clinical doses. Subsequent prospective human pregnancy studies suggest that omeprazole is not a teratogen. A 2002 metaanalysis evaluated all major malformations among the proton pump inhibitors, which revealed a nonsignificant relative risk of 1.18 (95% CI: 0.72 to 1.94; $p = 0.7$) despite maternal use in the first trimester. Judicious use of proton pump inhibitors and avoidance during the first trimester minimize these potential risks.

## Hypertension

Hypertension in pregnancy can lead to serious morbidity and mortality for the mother and fetus (97–101). Initial treatment options are lifestyle modifications such as restriction of activity, alcohol, tobacco products, and sodium intake. Close monitoring is essential to determine the response to interventions or the progression to severe hypertension (i.e., preeclampsia, eclampsia). If drug therapy is determined to be necessary, a few antihypertensive medications' use in pregnancy have been documented.

Methyldopa is the preferred oral agent based on long-term follow-up studies and supporting safety data (97–101). Its pharmacologic action arises from the drug's metabolism to alpha-methylnorepinephrine, which stimulates central inhibitory alpha-adrenergic receptors to lower arterial pressure; secondarily, methyldopa is believed to reduce plasma renin activity. Methyldopa is effective at controlling maternal blood pressure without adversely affecting uteroplacental or fetal blood flow. Additionally, a 7.5 year follow-up study found no adverse effects in children exposed to the drug in utero.

Labetalol has traditionally been reserved as a second-line therapy; however, prospective studies suggest similar efficacy and safety to methyldopa (97–101). Labetalol is a nonselective $\beta$-adrenergic blocker and a selective $\alpha_1$-adrenergic blocker; it reduces systemic vascular resistance and heart rate without decreasing peripheral, cerebral, coronary, or renal blood flow. Other ß-adrenergic blockers (e.g., metoprolol) may be acceptable alternatives for moderate hypertension with close monitoring of fetal effects if patient response is inadequate to first-line therapies. Use of atenolol in the first and the second trimesters has been associated with fetal growth retardation and is not recommended. Likewise, angiotensin-converting enzyme inhibitors (ACEIs) and angiotensin receptor blockers (ARBs) have been linked to fetal deaths and are contraindicated during pregnancy.

Historically, hydralazine has been the most commonly prescribed vasodilator for acute hypertension in pregnant women; however, a published meta-analysis suggests intravenous labetalol may be preferred over hydralazine for hypertensive emergencies (i.e., preeclampsia, eclampsia) (97–103). Results of the meta-analysis, including other anecdotal reports, reveal a higher incidence of adverse effects (e.g., placental abruption, increased caesarean sections, maternal oliguria, lower Apgar scores) with hydralazine. Therefore, practitioners are recommending labetolol as a first-line therapy and reserving hydralazine as a second-line therapy in acute, severe hypertension. Other agents for severe preeclampsia are available but fetal risk may be potentially greater. For example, esmolol is associated with fetal distress and bradycardia; thiazide diuretics may cause reduced placental perfusion.

## Migraines

Migraines and headache do not appear to negatively impact pregnancy outcomes. Studies of migraine in pregnancy have found no increased incidence of preterm labor, low birth weights, or congenital anomalies (104,105). On the other hand, pregnancy predisposes women to several potentially life-threatening conditions such as preeclampsia, stroke, and cerebral venous thrombosis which can present with headache. Therefore, careful diagnosis and treatment of headache during pregnancy are crucial.

Non-pharmacologic therapies such as relaxation, biofeedback, massage, and stress management have been shown to be highly effective in patients with recurring headaches (104–106). If drug therapy is necessary, acetaminophen is often recommended first. The NSAIDs, ibuprofen and naproxen, have a category B rating for use in the first trimester of pregnancy. NSAID use in the third trimester, however, is known to cause premature closure of the ductus arteriosus in utero resulting in fetal pulmonary hypertension. Therefore, NSAIDs carry a category D rating in the third trimester (104). Ergotamine and dihydroergotamine are rated category X and are contraindicated in pregnancy. These ergot alkaloids are known to cause vasospasm and a prolonged and marked increase in uterine tone. This, in turn, causes an impaired placental blood flow leading to spontaneous abortion and fetal distress.

The serotonin 5-HT$_1$ agonists (triptans) are very effective in the treatment of migraine headache in the general population and are considered relatively safe for the treatment of migraine in pregnancy (106,107). Current evidence from the sumatriptan and naratriptan registry in pregnancy suggests that sumatriptan does not carry a risk to either the fetus or the mother (107). Data regarding the other drugs in this class (zolmitriptan, naratriptan, almotriptan, eletriptan, frovatriptan, rizatriptan) are insufficient to draw the same conclusion.

## Nausea/Vomiting

Nausea and vomiting of pregnancy (NVP) is the most common complication of pregnancy affecting up to 85% of patients. The range of this condition includes a mild course of morning sickness to the rare (0.3% to 2.3%) but severe form of nausea–hyperemesis gravidarum (HG). Duration of symptoms may resolve by the 3rd month of pregnancy or may last until delivery (108,109). The exact etiology of NVP is not known but may involve rapid changes of hormones in the mother. In all forms/extent of NVP, protection of the mother and the fetus from the deleterious effects of nutrition depletion secondary to inadequate intake or excessive loss of nutrients is the most important goal of therapy. One example is neural tube defects secondary to folate deficiency. Pharmacologic measures should also demonstrate safety to the fetus as many agents pass the placenta and could affect normal fetal development, including teratogenicity.

Therapy of NVP includes many non-pharmacologic lifestyle interventions including avoidance of noxious smells or foods, smaller portions of tolerable foods eaten at shorter intervals, small feeding before arising in the morning, and avoidance of spicy or fatty foods. Pharmacologic therapy should be considered if these measures are not effective, other diseases causing nausea and vomiting are ruled out, or symptoms are severe (109).

Only two pharmacologic therapies for NVP are considered safe during pregnancy, the antihistamine, doxylamine, and pyridoxine or vitamin B$_6$. Prior to market withdrawal in 1983, these medications were available in the United States as a combination medication called Bendectin. Today, they are only available as single entities. These agents should be considered as first-line therapy as soon as other lifestyle interventions fail. Doses of doxylamine range from 12.5 to 25 mg twice daily or 12.5 mg twice a day with 25 mg at bedtime. Pyridoxine dose range from 10 to 25 mg three to four times daily (109,110). Higher doses have been studied, but they do not improve NVP and were associated with a higher hospitalization rates for rehydration (110). Preemptive antinausea medication has been reported to be more efficacious than therapy after symptoms of NVP (111). Other antihistamines such as dimenhydramine, diphenhydramine, and meclizine are considered as either replacement or additive for doxylamine. However, hydroxyzine, promethazine, and ranitidine should only be considered in more severe recalcitrant cases (109,112). Warnings of severe effects in children under 2 years of age were posted by the FDA in 2006 concerning the use of promethazine in infants

(113). Coupled with the fact that promethazine achieves similar fetal and maternal levels, there is some concern for the continued use of promethazine for NVP or HG.

Recently, newer therapies have emerged (109,114). Both metoclopramide and ondansetron are available as oral, intravenous, or continuous subcutaneous infusions. Oral therapy with either of these medications may be added to the doxylamine/pyridoxine regimen. Metoclopramide is a dopamine and serotonin antagonist that increases upper GI tract motility and blocks receptors in the chemoreceptor zone (CTZ). The CNS effects are associated with extrapyramidal symptoms (EPS) which may limit its use. Ondansetron works through antagonism of the 5-HT$_3$ receptor system, also blocking serotonin. Ondansetron works in the peripheral nerve receptors and also in the CTZ; however, there is no activity on peristalsis. Fatigue and headache are the most common side effects. More serious side effects, occur in <1% of patients, range from EPS/dystonia to cardiopulmonary arrest to seizures (115,116). The EPS/dystonia seen with ondansetron responds to intravenous benzodiazepines. The intravenous route for many of these agents is reserved for hospitalized patients. Recently, continuous subcutaneous infusions of metoclopramide and ondansetron have been utilized as home therapy.

### Psychosis/Bipolar Disorder

Women with bipolar disorder are at increased risk of relapse during pregnancy, and continued treatment with a mood-stabilizing drug can help reduce that risk. However, two of the most commonly used mood-stabilizing drugs, lithium and valproate, are known to increase the risk of congenital defects.

First-trimester exposure to lithium is associated with a small increased risk for all congenital malformations and in particular for cardiac anomalies (117). The most common lithium associated with malformation is Ebstein's anomaly. The risk for this cardiac malformation is 10 to 20 times greater than in the general population (118). Still, the absolute risk remains low at 1:1,000 to 1:2,000 (117,118).

The anticonvulsants, valproate and carbamazepine, may confer even greater risks of malformations than lithium (118). First-trimester exposure to valproate is associated with a 1% to 3.8% risk of neural tube defects, primarily spina bifida (119,120). Valproate exposure is also associated with craniofacial anomalies, microcephaly, and limb and cardiovascular anomalies (120). In utero exposure to valproate in any trimester has been associated with long term neurobehavioral effects in the children exposed (118,121). Malformations reported with carbamazepine include minor craniofacial defects, fingernail hyperplasia, cardiovascular and urinary tract anomalies, and cleft palate (121). It is unclear whether carbamazepine use increases risk of fetal neural tube defects or developmental delay (120).

Lamotrigine has been shown to be effective as a maintenance therapy for bipolar disorder in the general population (119). As monotherapy, lamotrigine has not been documented to cause teratogenic outcomes (118–121). To date, the number of reported exposures has been too small to fully assess the safety of lamotrigine's use in pregnancy.

Left untreated, schizophrenia in pregnancy has been linked to preterm birth, low birth weight infants, placental abnormalities, increased rates of congenital malformations, and a higher incidence of postnatal death (120). Typical antipsychotic agents (haloperidol, perphenazine, trifluoperazine, thioridazine, fluphenazine, and chlorpromazine) have been widely used for many years to treat schizophrenia in pregnancy. The available data suggest that the use of these agents confers a low risk in respect to teratogenic or toxic effects to the fetus

(120,122). There are limited data regarding the use of atypical antipsychotics in pregnancy.

## Seizure

Pregnancy with a comorbidity of seizure disorders can present a difficult management issue for the general obstetrician. Severe status epilepticus not only affects the mother, but can induce hypoxia or physical distress in the fetus. It is unclear if pregnancy alters seizure frequency in epileptic women as the literature reports opposing conclusions (123–125). Although the incidence of pregnancy with epilepsy is <1%, the use of traditional antiepileptic drugs (AEDs) is much higher, owing to the common use of AEDs for other disease states occurring during pregnancy (mood disorders, behavior disorders, etc.).

Of initial concern is that many AEDs reduce the effectiveness of systemic contraceptives, thereby increasing the chances of undesired pregnancy. Comprehensive family planning should be recommended to minimize unplanned pregnancy. Systemic oral contraceptives should contain at least 50 μg of estradiol, and patients should also consider secondary means of contraception, including barrier therapy (124). Well before a desired pregnancy, planning among the patient, neurologist, and the obstetrician should establish the safest AEDs for the patient.

Complete AED withdrawal (at least during the first trimester) has been advocated (126). However, this may not be possible. Single-drug therapy with the lowest effective dose during pregnancy should be the first goal as polytherapy increases adverse effects on the fetus. The rate of congenital malformations in women not taking AEDs is approximately 2%. Congenital malformations increase to 4% to 9% in those taking first-generation AEDs (phenobarbital, phenytoin, valproic acid, carbamazepine, and ethosuximide). These include intrauterine growth retardation, congenital malformations, cognitive disabilities, microcephaly, and fetal demise (124,125). Valproic acid appears to be the most associated with decreased neonatal cognition and physical malformations (124–126). Newer AEDs (lamtrogine, topirimate, gabapentin, oxcarbazepine, and levetiracetam) have shown teratogenicity in animals, but human data are incomplete at this point (127). Several major countries operate registries to track and report the effects of AEDs on pregnancy, but most differ in clinical data recorded, making interpretation between them impractical (127,128). Another confounding issue is keeping AED levels consistent from pre-pregnancy until delivery. First-generation AED levels decrease 40% to 70% by the third trimester (129). Lamotrigene, levetiracetam, and oxcarbazepine levels also decrease during pregnancy but information on other AEDs is lacking.

Seizures during labor are of particular concern for women with a generalized seizure disorder as this incidence increases sharply in women with partial disorders. During prolonged labor, oral AEDs may not be the preferred route as absorption can be erratic. Phenobarbital, phenytoin, fosphenytoin, valproic acid, and levetiracetam are alternatives available parenterally. Convulsive seizures occurring during labor should be treated aggressively with benzodiazepines. Measures to prevent hypoxia in the mother and the fetus and efforts to deliver the fetus should be instituted quickly (130).

High-dose folic acid supplementation (>4 mg per day) has been recommended for prevention of neural tube defects in women on phenytoin, carbamazepine, phenobarbital, and primidone (124). Additionally, vitamin K supplementation should be initiated for women on certain carbamazepine, phenytoin, phenobarbital, and ethosuximide. Dose of oral vitamin K is 10 mg daily beginning at 36 weeks' gestation and continued until delivery (130).

## References

1. Boothby LA, Doering PL. FDA labeling system for drugs in pregnancy. *Ann Pharmacother.* 2001;35:1485–1489.
2. Doering PL, Boothby LA, Cheok M. Review of pregnancy labeling of prescription drugs: is the current system adequate to inform of risks? *Am J Obstet Gynecol.* 2002; 187:333–339.
3. Meadows M. Pregnancy and the drug dilemma. FDA Consumer May-June 2001. Available at: URL:http://www.fda.gov/fdac/features/2001/301_preg.html
4. Koren G, Pastuszak A, Ito S. Drugs in pregnancy. *N Engl J Med.* 1998;338(16): 1128–1137.
5. Schardein JL. *Chemically Induced Birth Defects.* NewYork, NY: Marcel Dekker; 1985.
6. Moore KL. Causes of congenital malformations. In: *The Developing Human: Clinically Oriented Embryology.* 3rd Ed. Philadelphia, PA: WB Saunders; 1982.
7. Beely L. Adverse effects of drugs in the first trimester of pregnancy. *Clin Obstet Gynecol.* 1981;8:261.
8. Hayes DP. Teratogenesis: a review of the basic principles with a discussion of selected agents: Part I. *Drug Intel Clin Pharm.* 1981;15:544.
9. Henney JE. FDA/NICHD Conference. Clinical Pharmacology during pregnancy: addressing clinical needs through science. Available at: http://www.fda.gov/oc/ speeches/2000/nichdconference12–4.html (cited October 11, 2004).
10. Black RA, Hill A. Over-the counter medications in pregnancy. *Am Fam Physician.* 2003;67:2517–2524.
11. Information about pregnancy registries. US Food and Drug Administration. Available at: http://www.fda.gov/womens/registries/general.html (cited October 1, 2004).
12. Pacifici GM. Placental transfer of antibiotics administered to the mother: a review. *Int J Clin Pharmacol Ther.* 2006;44:57–63.
13. Nahum GG, Uhl K, Kennedy DL. Antibiotic use in pregnancy and lactation: what is and is not known about teratogenic and toxic risks. *Obstet Gynecol.* 2006;107: 1120–1138.
14. Briggs GG, Freeman RK, Yaffe SJ. *Drugs in Pregnancy and Lactation: A Reference Guide to Fetal and Neonatal Risk.* 8th Ed. Philadelphia, PA: Lippincott Williams & Wilkins; 2008.
15. Heinonen O, Slone D, Shapiro S. *Birth Defects and Drugs in Pregnancy.* Littleton, MA: Publishing Sciences Group; 1977.
16. Jepsen P, Skriver MV, Floyd A, et al. A population-based study of maternal use of amoxicillin and pregnancy outcome in Denmark. *Br J Clin Pharmacol.* 2003;55: 216–221.
17. Berkovitch M, Diav-Citrin O, Greenberg R, et al. First-trimester exposure to amoxycillin/clavulanic acid: a prospective, controlled study. *Br J Clin Pharmacol.* 2004; 58:298–302.
18. Czeizel AE, Rockenbauer M, Sorensen HT, Olsen J. Augmentin treatment during pregnancy and the prevalence of congenital abnormalities: a population-based case-control teratologic study. *Eur J Obstet Gynecol Reprod Biol.* 2001;97:188–192.
19. Macejko AM, Schaeffer AJ. Asymptomatic bacteriuria and symptomatic urinary tract infections during pregnancy. *Urol Clin North Am.* 2007;34:35–42.
20. Einarson A, Shuhaiber S, Koren G. Effects of antibacterials on the unborn child: what is known and how should this influence prescribing. *Paediatr Drugs.* 2001;3: 803–816.
21. Czeizel AE, Rockenbauer M, Sorensen HT, Olsen J. Use of cephalosporins during pregnancy and in the presence of congenital abnormalities: a population-based, case-control study. *Am J Obstet Gynecol.* 2001;184:1289–1296.
22. Philipson A, Sabath LD, Charles D. Transplacental passage of erythromycin and clindamycin. *N Engl J Med.* 1973;288:1219–1221.
23. Schick B HM, Librizzi R, Donnenfeld A. Pregnancy outcome following exposure to clarithromycin. Abstracts of the Ninth International Conference of the Organization

of Teratology Information Services, May 2–4, 1996, Salt Lake City, Utah. *Reprod Toxicol.* 1996;10:162. Abstract.

24. Einarson A, Phillips E, Mawji F, et al. A prospective controlled multicentre study of clarithromycin in pregnancy. *Am J Perinatol.* 1998;15:523–525.

25. Drinkard CR, Shatin D, Clouse J. Postmarketing surveillance of medications and pregnancy outcomes: clarithromycin and birth malformations. *Pharmacoepidemiol Drug Saf.* 2000;9:549–556.

26. Sarkar M, Woodland C, Koren G, Einarson AR. Pregnancy outcome following gestational exposure to azithromycin. *BMC Pregnancy Childbirth.* 2006;6:18 (DOI: 10.1186/1471–2393–6–18).

27. Shepard TH, Brent RL, Friedman JM, et al. Update on new developments in the study of human teratogens. *Teratology.* 2002;65:153–161.

28. Hernandez-Diaz S, Werler MM, Walker AM, Mitchell AA. Folic acid antagonists during pregnancy and the risk of birth defects. *N Engl J Med.* 2000;343:1608–1614.

29. Hernandez-Diaz S, Werler MM, Walker AM, Mitchell AA. Neural tube defects in relation to use of folic acid antagonists during pregnancy. *Am J Epidemiol.* 2001; 153:961–968.

30. Czeizel AE, Rockenbauer M, Sorensen HT, Olsen J. The teratogenic risk of trimethoprim-sulfonamides: a population based case-control study. *Reprod Toxicol.* 2001;15: 637–646.

31. Niebyl JR. Antibiotics and other anti-infective agents in pregnancy and lactation. *Am J Perinatol.* 2003;20:405–414.

32. Caro-Paton T, Carvajal A, Martin de Diego I, et al. Is metronidazole teratogenic? A meta-analysis. *Br J Clin Pharmacol.* 1997;44:179–182.

33. Czeizel AE, Rockenbauer M. A population based case-control teratologic study of oral metronidazole treatment during pregnancy. *Br J Obstet Gynecol.* 1998;105: 322–327.

34. Burtin P, Taddio A, Ariburnu O, Einarson TR, Koren G. Safety of metronidazole in pregnancy: a meta-analysis. *Am J Obstet Gynecol.* 1995;172(2, pt 1):525–529.

35. Piper JM, Mitchel EF, Ray WA. Prenatal use of metronidazole and birth defects: no association. *Obstet Gynecol.* 1993;82:348–352.

36. Workowski KA, Berman SM. Sexually transmitted diseases treatment guidelines, 2006. *MMWR Recomm Rep.* 2006;55(RR-11):1–94.

37. Czeizel AE, Rockenbauer M, Olsen J, Sorensen HT. A teratological study of aminoglycoside antibiotic treatment during pregnancy. *Scand J Infect Dis.* 2000;32:309–313.

38. Berkovitch M, Pastuszak A, Gazarian M, Lewis M, Koren G. Safety of the new quinolones in pregnancy. *Obstet Gynecol.* 1994;84:535–538.

39. Loebstein R, Addis A, Ho E, et al. Pregnancy outcome following gestational exposure to fluoroquinolones: a multicenter prospective controlled study. *Antimicrob Agents Chemother.* 1998;42:1336–1339.

40. Schaefer C, Amoura-Elefant E, Vial T, et al. Pregnancy outcome after prenatal quinolone exposure. Evaluation of a case registry of the European Network of Teratology Information Services (ENTIS). *Eur J Obstet Gynecol Repod Biol.* 1996;69: 83–89.

41. Bourget P, Fernandez H, Delouis C, Ribou F. Transplacental passage of vancomycin during the second trimester of pregnancy. *Obstet Gynecol.* 1991;78(5, pt 2):908–911.

42. Pfizer Pharmaceuticals, Inc. Linezolid use during pregnancy and breastfeeding (written communication). October 2004.

43. Shea K, Hilburger E, Baroco A, Oldfield E. Successful treatment of vancomycin-resistant Enterococcus faecium pyelonephritis with daptomycin during pregnancy. *Ann Pharmacother.* 2008;42:722–725.

44. Cunha BA, Hamid N, Kessler H, Parchuri S. Daptomycin cure after cefazolin treatment failure of Methicillin-sensitive Staphylococcus aureus (MSSA) tricuspid valve acute bacterial endocarditis from a peripherally inserted central catheter (PICC) line. *Heart Lung.* 2005;34:442–447.

45. Rebordosa C, Kogevinas M, Horvath-Puho E, et al. Acetaminophen use during pregnancy: effects on risk for congenital abnormalities. *Am J Obstet Gynecol.* 2008;198: 178. e1–7.

46. Czeizel AE, Dudas I, Puho E. Short-term paracetamol therapy during pregnancy and a lower rate of preterm birth. *Paediatr Perinat Epidemiol.* 2005;19(2):106–111.

47. Ostensen ME, Skomsvoll JF. Anti-inflammatory pharmacotherapy during pregnancy. *Expert Opin Pharmacother.* 2004;5:571–580.

48. Kozer E, Nikfar S, Costei A, et al. Aspirin consumption during the first trimester of pregnancy and congenital anomalies: a meta-analysis. *Am J Obstet Gynecol.* 2002; 187:1623–1630.

49. Kozer E, Costei AM, Boskovic R, et al. Effects of aspirin consumption during pregnancy on pregnancy outcomes: meta-analysis. *Birth Defects Res B Dev Reprod Toxicol.* 2003;68:70–84.

50. Ostensen M, Ramsey-Goldman R. Treatment of inflammatory rheumatic disorders in pregnancy: what are the safest treatment options? *Drug Saf.* 1998;19:389–410.

51. Chambers CD, Tutuncu ZN, Johnson D, Jones KL. Human pregnancy safety for agents used to treat rheumatoid arthritis: adequacy of available information and strategies for developing post-marketing data. *Arthritis Res Ther.* 2006;8:215 (DOI: 10.1186/ar977).

52. Tassinari MS, Cook JC, Hurtt ME. NSAIDs and developmental toxicity. *Birth Defects Res B Dev Reprod Toxicol.* 2003;68:3–4.

53. Nielsen GL, Sorensen HT, Larsen H, Pedersen L. Risk of adverse birth outcome and miscarriage in pregnant users of non-steroidal anti-inflammatory drugs: population based observational study and case-control study. *Br Med J.* 2001;322:266–270.

54. Loe SM, Sanchez-Ramos L, Kaunitz AM. Assessing the neonatal safety of indomethacin tocolysis: a systematic review with meta-analysis. *Obstet Gynecol.* 2005;106: 173–179.

55. Koren G, Florescu A, Costei AM, Boskovic R, Moretti ME. Nonsteroidal anti-inflammatory drugs during third trimester and the risk of premature closure of the ductus arteriosus: a meta-analysis. *Ann Pharmacother.* 2006;40:824–829.

56. Benini D, Fanos V, Cuzzolin L, Tato L. In utero exposure to nonsteroidal anti-inflammatory drugs: neonatal renal failure. *Pediatr Nephrol.* 2004;19:232–234.

57. Rathmell JP, Viscomi CM, Ashburn MA. Management of nonobstetric pain during pregnancy and lactation. *Anesth Analg.* 1997;85:1074–1087.

58. Dombrowski MP, Schatz M. ACOG practice bulletin: clinical management guidelines for obstetrician-gynecologists number 90, February 2008: asthma in pregnancy. *Obstet Gynecol.* 2008;111(2, pt 1):457–464.

59. Gilbert C, Mazzotta P, Loebstein R, Koren G. Fetal safety of drugs used in the treatment of allergic rhinitis: a critical review. *Drug Saf.* 2005;28:707–719.

60. Gluck JC, Gluck PA. Asthma controller therapy during pregnancy. *Am J Obstet Gynecol.* 2005;192:369–380.

61. Liccardi G, Cazzola M, Canonica GW, et al. General strategy for the management of bronchial asthma in pregnancy. *Respir Med.* 2003;97:778–789.

62. Chambers C. Safety of asthma and allergy medications in pregnancy. *Immunol Allergy Clin North Am.* 2006;26:13–28.

63. James A. Venous thromboembolism in pregnancy. *Arterioscler Thromb Vasc Biol.* 2009;29:326–331.

64. Weitz J. Prevention and treatment of venous thromboembolism during pregnancy, Proceedings from the Vascular Interventional Advances 06 meeting, Las Vegas, NV, USA September 26–29, 2006.

65. Bates S, Greer I, Pabinger I, Sofaer S, Hirsh J. Venous thromboembolism, thrombophilia, antithrombotic therapy, and pregnancy. *Chest.* 2008;133:844S–886S.

66. Hirsh J, Bauer K, Donati M, et al. Parenteral anticoagulants. *Chest.* 2008;133: 141S–159S.

67. Greer I. Thromboembolism and anticoagulant therapy in pregnancy. *Gend Med.* 2005;2(Suppl. A):S10–S17.

68. Patel J, Hunt B. Where do we go now with low molecular weight heparin use in obstetric care? *J Thromb Haemost.* 2008;6:1461–1467.

69. Bates S. Management of pregnant women with thrombophilia or a history of venous thromboembolism. *Hematology.* 2007;143–150.

70. Greer I, Hunt B. Low molecular weight heparin in pregnancy: current issues. *Br J Haematol.* 2004;128:593–601.

71. Gavin NI, Gaynes BN, Lohr KN, et al. Perinatal depression: a systematic review of prevalence and incidence. *Obstet Gynecol.* 2005;106:1071–1083.

72. Way CM. Safety of newer antidepressants in pregnancy. *Pharmacotherapy.* 2007; 27(4):546–552.

73. Belik J. Fetal and neonatal effects of maternal drug treatment for depression. *Semin Perinatol.* 2008;32:350–354.
74. Pearlstein T. Perinatal depression: treatment options and dilemmas. *J Psychiatry Neurosci.* 2008;33(4):302–318.
75. Davis RL, Rubanowice D, McPhillips H, et al. Risks of congenital malformations and perinatal events among infants exposed to antidepressant medications during pregnancy. *Pharmacoepidemiol Drug Saf.* 2007;16:1086–1094.
76. Andrade SE, Raebel MA, Brown J, et al. Use of antidepressant medications during pregnancy: a multi-site study. *Am J Obstet Gynecol.* 2008;198:194.e1–5.
77. Ter Horst PG, Jansman FG, Van Lingen RA, et al. Pharmacological aspects of neonatal antidepressant withdrawal. *Obstet Gynecol Survey.* 2008;63(4):267–279.
78. Food and Drug Administration. FDA public health advisory: paroxetine [electronic citation]. Available at: http://www.fda.gov/cder/drug/advisory/paroxetine200512.htm (accessed January 2009).
79. Einarson A, Pistelli A, DeSantis M, et al. Evaluation of the risk of congenital cardiovascular defects associated with use of paroxetine during pregnancy [published corrections appear in *Am J Psychiatry.* 2008;165(6):777 and 2008; 165(6):1208]. *Am J Psychiatry.* 2008;165(6):749–752.
80. Wichman CL, Moore KM, Lang TR, et al. Congenital heart disease associated with selective serotonin reuptake inhibitor use during pregnancy. *Mayo Clin Proc.* 2009; 84(1):23–27.
81. Food and Drug Administration. FDA public health advisory:treatment challenges of depression in pregnancy and the possibility of persistent pulmonary hypertension in newborns [electronic citation]. Available at: http://www.fda.gov/cder/drug/advisory/SSRI_PPHN200607.htm (accessed February 2009).
82. Chambers CD, Hernandez-Diaz S, Van Marter LJ, et al. Selective serotonin-reuptake inhibitors and risk of persistent pulmonary hypertension of the newborn. *N Engl J Med.* 2006;354(6):579–587.
83. Andrade SE, McPhillips H, Loren D, et al. Antidepressant use and risk of persistent pulmonary hypertension of the newborn. *Pharmacoepidemiol Drug Saf.* 2009; 18:246–252.
84. American College of Obstetricians and Gynecologists (ACOG) Practice Bulletin Number 30. Gestational diabetes. *Obstet Gynecol.* 2001;98:525–538.
85. Gabbe SG, Graves CR. Management of diabetes mellitus complicating pregnancy. *Obstet Gynecol.* 2003;102(4):857–868.
86. Homko CJ, Reece EA. Insulins and oral hypoglycemic agents in pregnancy. *J Matern Fetal Neonatal Med.* 2006;19(11):679–686.
87. Nicholson W, Bolen S, Witkop CT, et al. Benefits and risks of oral diabetes agents compared with insulin in women with gestational diabetes. *Obstet Gynecol.* 2009; 113(1):193–205.
88. Jovanovic L, Pettitt DJ. Treatment with insulin and its analogs in pregnancies complicated by diabetes. *Diabetes Care.* 2007;30:S220–S224.
89. Merlob P, Levitt O, Stahl B. Oral antihyperglycemic agents during pregnancy and lactation: a review. *Pediatr Drugs.* 2002;4(11):755–760.
90. Langer O, Conway DL, Berkus MD, et al. A comparison of glyburide and insulin in women with gestational diabetes mellitus. *N Engl J Med.* 2000;343:1134–1138.
91. Langer O, Yogev Y, Xenakis EM, et al. Insulin and glyburide therapy: dosage, severity level of gestational diabetes, and pregnancy outcome. *Am J Obstet Gynecol.* 2005;192:134–139.
92. Hellmuth E, Damm P, Mlsted-Pedersen L. Oral hypoglycemic agents in 118 diabetic pregnancies. *Diabet Med.* 2000;17:507–511.
93. Rowan JA, Hague WM, Gao W, et al. Metformin versus insulin for the treatment of gestational diabetes. *N Engl J Med.* 2008;358(19):2003–2015.
94. Richter JE. Review article: the management of heartburn in pregnancy. *Aliment Pharmacol Ther.* 2005;22:749–757.
95. Broussard CN, Richter JE. Treating gastro-esophageal reflux disease during pregnancy and lactation. *Drug Safety.* 1998;19(4):325–337.
96. Diav-Citrin O, Arnon J, Shechtman S, et al. The safety of proton pump inhibitors in pregnancy: a multicenter prospective controlled study. *Aliment Pharmacol Ther.* 2005;21:269–275.

97. Sibai BM. Chronic hypertension in pregnancy. *Am J Obstet Gynecol.* 2002;100(2): 369–377.
98. Montan S. Drugs used in hypertensive diseases in pregnancy. *Curr Opin Obstet Gynecol.* 2004;16:111–115.
99. Peters RM, Flack JM. Hypertensive disorders of pregnancy. *JOGNN.* 2004;33: 209–220.
100. National Institutes of Health (Joint National Committee on Prevention, Detection, and Treatment of High Blood Pressure). The seventh report of the Joint National Committee on Prevention, Detection, Evaluation, and Treatment of High Blood Pressure. (NIH Publication No. 04–5230). Washington, DC; 2004.
101. National Institutes of Health. Working group report on high blood pressure in pregnancy. (NIH Publication No. 00–3029). Washington, DC; 2000.
102. Magee LA, Cham C, Waterman EJ, Ohlsson A, Dadelszen PV. Hydralazine for treatment of severe hypertension in pregnancy: meta analysis. *Br Med J.* 2003;327: 955–965.
103. McCoy S, Baldwin K. Pharmacotherapeutic options for the treatment of preeclampsia. *Am J Health-Syst Pharm.* 2009;66:337–344.
104. Menon R, Bushnell C. Headache and pregnancy. *Neurologist.* 2008;14:108–119.
105. Soldin OP, Dahlin J, O'Mara DM. Triptans in pregnancy. *Ther Drug Monit.* 2008; 30(1):5–9.
106. Evans EW, Lorber KC. Use of 5-HT$_1$ agonists in pregnancy. *Ann Pharmacother.* 2008; 42:543–549.
107. Goadsby PJ, Goldberg J, Silberstein SD. Migraine in pregnancy. *Br Med J.* 2008; 336:1502–1504.
108. Tan P, Jacob R, Quek K, Omar S. Pregnancy outcome in hyperemesis gravidarum and the effect of laboratory clinical indicators of hyperemesis severity. *J Obstet Gynaecol Res.* 2006;33(4):457–464.
109. Sheehan P. Hyperemesis gravidarum. *Aust Fam Physician.* 2007;36(9):699–701.
110. Atanackovic G, Navioz Y, Moretti M, Koren G. The safety of higher than standard dose of doxylamine-pyridoxine for nausea and vomiting of pregnancy. *J Clin Pharmacol.* 2001;51:842–845.
111. Koren G, Maltepe C. Pre-emptive therapy for severe nausea and vomiting of pregnancy and hyperemesis gravidarum. *J Obstet Gynaecol.* 2004;24(5):530–533.
112. AGOG Issues Guidance on Treatment of Morning Sickness During Pregnancy, The American College of Obstetricians and Gynecologists news release. March 29, 2004.
113. Anon FDA. Alert for Promethazine HCL, U.S. Food and Drug Administration Bulletin, April 25, 2006.
114. Reichmann J, Kirkbride M. Nausea and vomiting of pregnancy-cost effective pharmacologic treatments. *Manag Care.* 2008;17:41–45.
115. Spiegel J, Kang V, Kunze L, Hess P. Ondansetron-induced extrapyramidal symptoms during cesarean section. *Int J Obstet Anesth.* 2005;6:368–369.
116. Pasricha Pankaj J. Treatment of disorders of bowel motility and water flux and Antiemetics agents used in biliary and pancreatic disease. In: Brunton LL, Lazo JS, Parker KL. *Goodman & Gilman's the Pharmacological Basis of Therapeutics.* 11th Ed. Available at: http://www.accessmedicine.com/content.aspx?aID=946551
117. Giles JJ, Bannigan JG. Teratogenic and developmental effects of lithium. *Curr Pharm Des.* 2006;12:1531–1541.
118. Frieder A, Dunlop AL, Culpepper L, Bernstein P. The clinical content of preconception care: women with psychiatric conditions. *Am J Obstet Gynecol.* 2008;199 (6 Suppl. 2):S328–S332.
119. Yonkers KA, Wisner KL, Stowe Z, et al. Management of bipolar disorder during pregnancy and the postpartum period. *Am J Psychiatry.* 2004;161(4):608–620.
120. Use of psychiatric medications during pregnancy and lactation. ACOG Practice Bulletin No. 92. American College of Obstetricians and Gynecologists. *Obstet Gynecol.* 2008;111:1001–1020.
121. Dodd S, Berk M. The safety of medications for the treatment of bipolar disorder during pregnancy and the puerperium. *Curr Drug Saf.* 2006;1:25–33.
122. Reis M, Kallen B. Maternal use of antipsychotics in early pregnancy and delivery outcome. *J Clin Psychopharmacol.* 2008;28(3):279–288.

123. Battino D, Tomson T. Management of epilepsy during pregnancy. *Drugs.* 2007; 67(18):2727–2746.
124. Pennell P. Antiepileptic drugs during pregnancy: what is known and which AEDs seem to be safest? *Epilepsia.* 2008;49(Suppl. 9):43–55.
125. Uziel D, Rozental R. Neurologic birth defects after prenatal exposure to antiepileptic drugs. *Epilepsia.* 2008;49(Suppl. 9):35–42.
126. Harden C, Sethi N. Epliptic disorders in pregnancy: an overview. *Curr Opin Obstet Gynecol.* 2008;20:557–562.
127. Karceski S. Epilepsy and pregnancy, are seizure medications safe? *Neurology.* 2008;71:e32–33.
128. Meador K, Pennell P, Harden C, et al. Pregnancy registries in epilepsy, a consensus statement on health outcomes. *Neurology.* 2008;71:1109–1117.
129. Yerby M, Kaplan P, Tran T. Risks and management of pregnancy in women with epilepsy. *Clev Clin J Med.* 2004;71(Suppl. 2):S25–S37.
130. Pennell P. Pregnancy in women who have epilepsy. *Neurol Clin.* 2004;22:799–820.

# 18 Complications of Medical and Surgical Abortion

Rosanne L. Botha, Paula H. Bednarek, Andrew M. Kaunitz, and Alison B. Edelman

## EPIDEMIOLOGY AND HISTORY OF ABORTION IN THE UNITED STATES

Abortion is one of the most common medical procedures for women aged 15 to 44 years in the United States (1,2). Each year, almost half of all pregnancies among American women are unintended, and about half of these unplanned pregnancies end in abortion. If current rates continue, it is estimated that 35% of all reproductive-age women in America will have had an abortion by the time they reach the age of 45 (3). In 2005, approximately 1.2 million abortions were performed in the United States, with nearly 90% performed in the first trimester (before 12 weeks) (3). Both medical and surgical abortions are low-risk procedures when performed early in gestation, and in a safe, legal setting. Fewer than 0.3% of abortion patients experience a complication that requires hospitalization (4). The risk of death from abortion is 1 in 100,000 or less while the risk of a woman dying from giving birth is 10 times higher (5–7).

Abortion has not always been so safe. Before its legalization in the United States in 1973, many women died or had serious complications following procedures by untrained practitioners with suboptimal techniques in unsanitary conditions or after attempts to self-induce abortion using knitting needles or wire coat hangers. These practices resulted in sepsis, thrombosis of the pelvic vasculature, disseminated intravascular coagulation (DIC), and death. In countries where abortion is still illegal, unsafe abortion remains a leading cause of maternal death (8).

## SURGICAL ABORTION

Over 90% of surgical abortions are performed in outpatient settings, using either electric or manual (handheld syringe) vacuum aspiration (9). Perioperative antibiotics are routinely provided to patients. Women typically experience cramping and bleeding similar to a period for a few days to several weeks following the procedure. Regular menses usually returns in 4 to 6 weeks postprocedure.

## MEDICAL ABORTION

In the United States, medical abortion is offered at gestational ages 9 weeks or less using 200 mg of oral mifepristone followed by 800 µg of misoprostol vaginally or buccally 6 to 48 hours later (10). Misoprostol-alone regimens have lower rates of successful complete abortion but are still utilized by some women to self-induce abortion or in countries where mifepristone is not available (10). Patients are asked to return for an ultrasound approximately 2 weeks after their medical abortion to confirm that the procedure is complete. During the actual abortion, bleeding can be heavy and cramping may require narcotic analgesia. Both symptoms are expected to last for several hours while passing the pregnancy but usually improve within 24 hours (11). Nausea, vomiting, and diarrhea are known side effects of misoprostol and are also frequently reported (12). Symptoms of recovery following a medical abortion are similar to those with surgical abortion.

## MANAGING SPECIFIC COMPLICATIONS OF ABORTION

Although first trimester medical and surgical abortions are safe with low rates of major complications, these are common procedures, and therefore it is not unusual for women with abortion complications to present for emergent care. Physicians in such settings may encounter complications such as bleeding, infection, retained products of conception, continuing pregnancy, or ectopic pregnancy. Gynecologic consultation or referral is appropriate for these patients.

### Hemorrhage

Hemorrhage associated with an abortion may indicate retained pregnancy tissue; placental abnormalities (such as placenta accreta); cervical laceration; DIC; or uterine perforation, atony, or rupture. Following an abortion, patients typically have 1 to 2 weeks of bleeding that does not substantially decrease hemoglobin levels (13). For patients with ongoing heavy bleeding, suction evacuation is recommended. If the bleeding has decreased on its own and the patient is clinically stable, expectant management or medical management with misoprostol (800 μg buccally or vaginally) or methylergonovine (0.2 mg intramuscularly) may be considered as well.

The need for transfusion following induced abortion is rare and only seen in 0.2% of both medical and surgical cases (11,14,15). Transfusion should be considered in patients according to standard criteria used in other clinical situations, but suction evacuation is the mainstay of treating excessive vaginal bleeding.

If there is evidence of intra-abdominal free fluid on ultrasound, then uterine perforation or ruptured ectopic pregnancy should be considered in the differential diagnosis, and further surgical intervention may be necessary.

### Infection

Endometritis occurs in <1% of cases of induced abortion (16). Antibiotic guidelines for treating pelvic inflammatory disease (PID) are applicable to postabortion infections (17). If retained products of conception are suspected in the setting of infection, prompt resuctioning after initiating antibiotics is usually necessary to prevent the worsening infection or sepsis.

**Clostridium sordellii** *Toxic Shock Syndrome with Medical Abortion*: Since the FDA approved mifepristone for use in 2000, six women have died as a result of toxic shock secondary to a rare infection of the uterus with *Clostridium sordellii* following medical abortion (18,19). Fatal infections have also occurred following surgical abortions, miscarriages, and childbirth and in cases unrelated to pregnancy. Given the large number of uncomplicated medical abortions that have occurred, risk of death from medical abortion remains low at 1 per 100,000 cases (20).

Sepsis due to *Clostridium sordellii* is atypical in presentation. Patients may only describe general malaise and flu-like symptoms, without fever or significant findings on pelvic examination. Tachycardia and hypotension are later findings. In the laboratory workup, a dramatic leukocytosis with left shift and hemoconcentration is seen, but blood cultures are usually not revealing. **Urgent endometrial biopsy with Gram stain can establish the diagnosis** (20).

Treatment should include aggressive surgical debridement, often including a hysterectomy, and parenteral antibiotic therapy with anaerobic coverage.

*Infection Related to Illegal Abortion*: Women who have obtained an illegal abortion tend to present to emergency settings later than women with complications of legal abortion, and therefore they often have more severe consequences (21). Delayed care for infections related to unsanitary instruments, caustic substances, or retained tissue means that these infections can be more severe and associated with pelvic abscesses and septic shock.

### Retained Tissue

*Hematometra* (blood clots accumulating in the uterus) occurs in 0.2% to 1.0% of abortions (22). Typically, patients experience severe and progressive lower abdominal cramping immediately following or within 24 hours of the abortion with often lighter than normal postprocedure vaginal bleeding. Pelvic examination reveals a distended and tender uterus. Prompt suction aspiration of the uterus should be performed. Although no published data support this recommendation, it is standard practice for US clinicians to administer methylergonovine 0.2 mg intramuscularly followed by a scheduled 0.2 mg oral dose three times daily for 24 to 48 hours in patients free of hypertension to decrease the risk of reaccumulation of intrauterine blood clots.

*Retained products of conception*, including fetal or placental tissue, may result in infection, bleeding, or both and occur in approximately 1% of surgical abortion patients (23). Typically, within 1 to 2 weeks of the abortion, the patient experiences cramping and heavy bleeding, which may be accompanied by fever. With medical abortion, most patients expel the pregnancy within 4 to 8 hours after the misoprostol dose, but 5% to 8% of patients will have evidence of retained pregnancy tissue on the follow-up ultrasound at 2 weeks (24).

Depending upon the clinical presentation and patient preference, treatment for retained products of conception can be via surgical evacuation or misoprostol 800 μg buccally or vaginally to help induce uterine contractions to expel the tissue. Surgical evacuation is the safest option if the patient has severe pain, signs of infection, or ongoing heavy bleeding.

*Continuing pregnancy* following abortion results either from a failure to abort an intrauterine pregnancy or because of a previously undiagnosed ectopic pregnancy. Performance of the abortion at <6 weeks' gestational age, in the presence of a uterine anomaly or a uterine cavity distorted by fibroids, increases the risk of failure in surgical abortions (25). Although most US abortion clinics confirm the presence of an intrauterine pregnancy via ultrasound prior to an abortion, a pseudogestational sac associated with an early ectopic pregnancy may be mistaken for an early intrauterine pregnancy. Another rare phenomenon called heterotopic pregnancy refers to simultaneous intrauterine and ectopic pregnancies and may complicate abortion care. As more women conceive using assisted reproductive technologies, including in vitro fertilization, heterotopic pregnancies are becoming more common. In women presenting for emergent care following an abortion, a pelvic ultrasound can evaluate for evidence of retained tissue or signs of ectopic pregnancy, such as an adnexal mass or intra-abdominal free fluid.

Occasionally, when a pregnancy continues following an attempted abortion, a patient may decide to continue the pregnancy. Misoprostol is a known teratogen, but mifepristone alone has unknown risks to the pregnancy (26–28). There is less concern about the teratogenicity of medications used in surgical abortion, but instrumentation of the uterine cavity may increase the risk of infection or other complications for an ongoing pregnancy. Patients who are considering continuing a pregnancy following a failed abortion should be counseled about these risks.

| | Possible complications of surgical and medical abortion |

| Surgical Abortion | Medical Abortion |
| --- | --- |
| Hemorrhage | Hemorrhage |
| Incomplete abortion | Incomplete abortion |
| Uterine or pelvic infection | Uterine or pelvic infection |
| Ongoing intrauterine pregnancy, requiring a second procedure | Ongoing intrauterine pregnancy (failure of the medications to stop the pregnancy from progressing), requiring a surgical abortion for completion |
| Misdiagnosed/unrecognized ectopic pregnancy | Misdiagnosed/unrecognized ectopic pregnancy |
| Hematometra (blood clots accumulating in the uterus) | |
| Uterine perforation | |
| Cervical laceration | |

### Abortion in the Second Trimester

Cervical dilation and/or softening can be accomplished with mechanical osmotic dilators (e.g., laminaria) and/or misoprostol 1 to 2 days prior to a second trimester abortion. Occasionally following this cervical preparation, patients can develop heavy bleeding or symptoms of labor and may present to the emergency department prior to their scheduled abortion. In this setting, delivery of the fetus may occur with or without the delivery of the placenta. Retained placenta in this situation usually requires urgent surgical evacuation of the uterus to minimize bleeding.

## CONTRACEPTION FOLLOWING ABORTION

Ovulation can occur as early as 2 to 3 weeks following first trimester abortion (29), so it is recommended to start birth control as soon as possible after an abortion is completed. Immediate initiation of contraception including the insertion of an intrauterine device (IUD) or subdermal implant during the same visit as a surgical abortion is a safe and effective practice that is becoming more common in the United States. Patients who have an IUD in place following their abortion may suffer the same complications as other abortion patients, but pain, irregular or heavy bleeding, and infection are unlikely to be specifically caused by the IUD. For this reason, it is not usually necessary or helpful to remove the IUD while these complications are being evaluated and treated. An IUD does not need to be removed in the setting of endometritis unless the patient does not show clinical improvement with the use of antibiotics (30,31).

## SUMMARY

Although an induced abortion is safe, the fact that this procedure is common means that women presenting with complications will be encountered in the emergency department. The recommendations described in this chapter will help clinicians provide timely, appropriate, and effective treatment for women experiencing these complications (Table 18.1).

## References

1. Owings MF, Kozak LJ. Ambulatory and inpatient procedures in the United States, 1996. *Vital Health Stat.* 1998;13(139):1–119.
2. Judge DE. Reported voluntary abortions: numbers inch downward. *J Watch Women Health.* 2009;14;11–12.
3. Finer LB, Henshaw SK. Disparities in rates of unintended pregnancy in the United States, 1994 and 2001. *Perspect Sex Reprod Health.* 2006;38(2):90–96.
4. Henshaw SK. Unintended pregnancy and abortion: a public health perspective. In: Paul M, et al., ed. *A Clinician's Guide to Medical and Surgical Abortion.* New York, NY: Churchill Livingstone; 1999:11–22.
5. Grimes DA. Risks of mifepristone abortion in context. *Contraception.* 2005;71(3):161.
6. Bartlett L, Berg C, Shulman H, et al. Risk factors for legal induced abortion-related mortality in the United States. *Obstet Gynecol.* 2004;103(4):729–737.
7. Christiansen LR, Collins KA. Pregnancy-associated deaths: a 15-year retrospective study and overall review of maternal pathophysiology. *Am J Forensic Med Pathol.* 2006;27(1):11–19.
8. van Lerberghe W, ed. *The World Health Report 2005: Make Every Mother and Child Count.* Geneva, Switzerland: WHO; 2005.
9. Cates W Jr, et al. Legalized abortion: effect on national trends of maternal and abortion-related mortality (1940 through 1976). *Am J Obstet Gynecol.* 1978;132(2):211–214.
10. Grimes DA. Medical abortion in early pregnancy: a review of the evidence. *Obstet Gynecol.* 1997;89(5, pt 1):790–796.
11. Spitz IM, et al. Early pregnancy termination with mifepristone and misoprostol in the United States. *N Engl J Med.* 1998;338(18):1241–1247.
12. Schaff EA, et al. Low-dose mifepristone 200 mg and vaginal misoprostol for abortion. *Contraception.* 1999;59(1):1–6.
13. Thonneau P, et al. A comparative analysis of fall in haemoglobin following abortions conducted by mifepristone (600 mg) and vacuum aspiration. *Hum Reprod.* 1995;10(6):1512–1515.
14. Haskell WM. Surgical abortion after the first trimester. In: Paul M, et al., ed. *A Clinician's Guide to Medical and Surgical Abortion.* New York, NY: Churchill Livingstone; 1999:123–138.
15. Tietze C. *Induced Abortion: A Worldwide Review.* New York, NY: Guttmacher Institute; 1996.
16. Shannon C, et al. Ectopic pregnancy and medical abortion. *Obstet Gynecol.* 2004;104(1):161–167.
17. Workowski KA, Berman SM. Sexually transmitted diseases treatment guidelines, 2006. *MMWR Recomm Rep.* 2006;55(RR-11):1–94.
18. *Clostridium sordellii* toxic shock syndrome after medical abortion with mifepristone and intravaginal misoprostol—United States and Canada, 2001–2005. *MMWR Morb Mortal Wkly Rep.* 2005;54(29):724.
19. Cohen AL, et al. Toxic shock associated with *Clostridium sordellii* and Clostridium perfringens after medical and spontaneous abortion. *Obstet Gynecol.* 2007;110(5):1027–1033.
20. Fischer M, et al. Fatal toxic shock syndrome associated with *Clostridium sordellii* after medical abortion. *N Engl J Med.* 2005;353(22):2352–2360.
21. Stubblefield PG, Grimes DA. Septic abortion. *N Engl J Med.* 1994;331(5):310–314.
22. Kaunitz AM. First trimester abortion technology. In: Corson S, ed. *Fertility Control.* Boston, MA: Little, Brown and Company; 1985:63.
23. Grimes DA, Cates W Jr. Complications from legally-induced abortion: a review. *Obstet Gynecol Surv.* 1979;34(3):177–191.
24. Guest J, et al. Randomised controlled trial comparing the efficacy of same-day administration of mifepristone and misoprostol for termination of pregnancy with the standard 36 to 48 hour protocol. *BJOG.* 2007;114(2):207–215.

25. Kaunitz AM, et al. Abortions that fail. *Obstet Gynecol.* 1985;66(4):533–537.
26. Gary MM, Harrison DJ. Analysis of severe adverse events related to the use of mifepristone as an abortifacient. *Ann Pharmacother.* 2006;40(2):191–197.
27. Sitruk-Ware R, Davey A, Sakiz E. Fetal malformation and failed medical termination of pregnancy. *Lancet.* 1998;352(9124):323.
28. Orioli IM, Castilla EE. Epidemiological assessment of misoprostol teratogenicity. *BJOG.* 2000;107(4):519–523.
29. Vorherr H. Contraception after abortion and post partum: an evaluation of risks and benefits of oral contraceptives with emphasis on the relation of female sex hormones to thromboembolism and genital and breast cancer. *Am J Obstet Gynecol.* 1973;117(7):1002–1025.
30. Rinehart W. *WHO Updates Medical Eligibility Criteria for Contraceptives.* Baltimore, MD: Johns Hopkins University; 2004.
31. World Health Organization. Improving access to quality care in family planning. 3rd Ed. *Medical Eligibility Criteria for Contraceptive Use.* Geneva, Switzerland: World Health Organization (WHO); 2003.

# 19

# Sexually Transmitted Diseases

**Shireen Madani Sims**

## PELVIC INFLAMMATORY DISEASE

Any discussion of gynecologic infectious emergencies should begin with a review of pelvic inflammatory disease (PID). Approximately one million cases of PID per year result in 160,000 hospitalizations, and more than 100,000 surgical procedures annually (1). Aside from the personal, physical, and emotional distress associated with PID, the financial cost to the individual and to society is staggering. In the United States, the total cost associated with PID and its sequelae in 2006 was estimated at $4.2 billion (1).

It is important for the clinician to recognize certain risk factors that may be associated with an increased risk of PID. A major risk factor is age. Young women are at greater risk of acquiring PID as a consequence of the greater prevalence of sexually transmitted diseases, a lower prevalence of protective chlamydial antibodies, larger zones of cervical ectopy, and a greater penetrability of cervical mucus (2). Sexually active adolescents are three times more likely to be given the diagnosis of PID than women who are 25 to 29 years old (1). Multiple sexual partners, a high frequency of sexual intercourse, and a high rate of new partner acquisition within the previous 30 days all appear to increase the acquisition risk of PID (3). The perception of the role of an intrauterine device (IUD) and the risk of PID is undergoing review. The primary risk centers around the time of insertion (4). It is presumed to be secondary to the introduction of vaginal and cervical pathogens into the endometrium during IUD insertion. However, even in areas with high prevalence of STDs, the use of an IUD appears to only minimally increase the risk of PID (4,5). Other factors that appear to be associated with an increased risk of PID include douching, smoking, and proximity to menses. It has been observed that symptoms develop significantly more often in women with chlamydial or gonococcal salpingitis within 7 days of menses than at other times during the cycle (6).

Although *Neisseria gonorrhoeae* and *Chlamydia trachomatis* are considered to be the primary pathogens in PID, other organisms are also isolated from tubal and peritoneal fluids. These organisms include aerobes (*Streptococcus* species, *Escherichia coli*, and *Haemophilus influenzae*) and anaerobes (*Bacteroides bivius, Bacteroides fragilis, Peptostreptococcus*, and *Peptococcus*) (7). Other organisms that have been isolated but whose significance is still indeterminate include *Mycoplasma* and *Actinomycosis*. Finally, tuberculosis is a remote consideration in patients at risk (particularly in underdeveloped countries and immunosuppressed patients). Although PID may be caused by a single agent, infection is frequently polymicrobial. The polymicrobial nature of PID may result when more than one primary pathogen infects the oviductal epithelium or it may result from damage created by a single primary pathogen, resulting in altered host immune defense mechanisms and secondary infections by other bacteria. These secondary invading organisms may be normal inhabitants of the upper vagina that become pathogenic upon contact with damaged tubal epithelium.

PID has always posed a diagnostic dilemma for the examining physician. Mild disease may be misdiagnosed as cystitis or gastroenteritis. Severe disease may be misdiagnosed as ovarian torsion, diverticulitis, or, most commonly, appendicitis. Frequently, this diagnostic dilemma results from the lack of sensitivity and specificity of the patient's complaints, physical findings, and laboratory evaluation. Therefore, the index of suspicion for the clinical diagnosis of PID should be high. The CDC has recommended a minimal set of criteria for empiric treatment in order to reduce missed or delayed diagnosis (8,9). It may be appropriate to overtreat as undertreatment may cause significant damage to the oviducts, resulting in chronic pelvic pain, infertility, or a future ectopic pregnancy. When no other cause can be identified, empiric treatment should be started in women with pelvic pain and at least one of the following: (a) cervical motion tenderness or uterine/adnexal tenderness; (b) oral temperature >101°F (>38.3°C); (c) peripheral leukocytosis or left shift; (d) abnormal cervical or vaginal mucopurulent discharge; (e) presence of white blood cells (WBCs) on saline microscopy of vaginal secretions; (f) elevated erythrocyte sedimentation rate; and (g) elevated C-reactive protein. Patients with pelvic pain and any of the following are considered confirmed cases: (a) endometrial biopsy with histopathologic evidence of endometritis; (b) laparoscopy findings consistent with PID; (c) laboratory evidence of cervical infection with *N. gonorrhoeae* or *C. trachomatis*; and (d) imaging studies demonstrating thickened, fluid-filled oviducts with or without free fluid or tubo-ovarian complex.

The use of ultrasonography and computed tomography (CT) scanning may be useful in examining the patient with severe rebound tenderness in whom an adequate pelvic examination is impossible to perform. Ultrasonography may demonstrate echogenic fluid in the pelvis consistent with pus (Fig. 19.1). CT scanning may demonstrate abscess formation with fluid and air collection (Fig. 19.2).

When significant uncertainty exists concerning the diagnosis, the "gold standard" has been the performance of a diagnostic laparoscopy. One major study of patients with signs and symptoms of PID undergoing a laparoscopic examination demonstrated that in 65% of the patients, the correct preoperative diagnosis had been made, 23% had normal pelvic anatomy, and 12% had other pathology (appendicitis or endometriosis) (10).

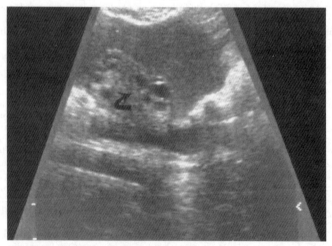

**FIGURE 19.1** Transvaginal probe demonstrating ovary with follicles (*arrow*) surrounded by echogenic fluid (pus).

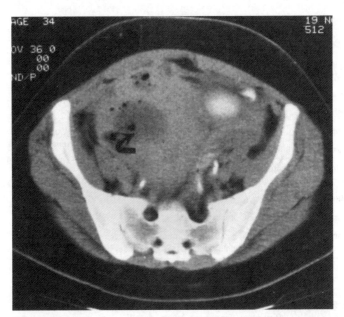

**FIGURE 19.2** CT scan demonstrating tubo-ovarian abscess with fluid collection and gas (*arrow*).

The decision to admit the patient to the hospital for further evaluation or treatment should be based on certain well-established criteria. These include the following: (a) significant peritoneal signs or rebound tenderness, (b) presence of an IUD, (c) pregnancy, (d) an adnexal mass consistent with a tubo-ovarian abscess (on pelvic examination or diagnostic imaging), (e) gastrointestinal symptoms precluding appropriate outpatient therapy or suggestive of bowel pathology, (f) failed outpatient therapy, (g) nulliparity, and (h) an uncertain diagnosis. Patients with an uncertain diagnosis require further evaluation and institution of therapy. The decision to perform laparoscopy to delineate the disease process may be based on the patient's severity of symptoms on admission or on her response to antibiotic therapy. If the decision is to initiate treatment with antibiotics and no resolution of symptoms occurs in 24 to 48 hours, or if symptoms increase in severity during this time frame, a laparoscopy should be considered. Treatment regimens for PID are outlined in Tables 19.1 and 19.2. Appropriate follow-up ensures compliance and resolution of symptoms in patients undergoing the outpatient regimen.

Ruptured tubo-ovarian abscess or leaking tubo-ovarian abscess may present as a serious threat to life. Mortality rate associated with a ruptured tubo-ovarian abscess ranges from 10% to 15%. Appropriate diagnosis and therapy are necessary. When a tubo-ovarian abscess ruptures, endotoxin is released into the systemic circulation. The lipid A portion of the lipopolysaccharide results in the release of numerous factors or mediators: $\beta$-endorphins, bradykinin, activators of the complement and coagulation cascades, plasminogen, and histamine. Decreased systemic resistance, a low pulmonary artery occlusive pressure, and increased cardiac output are noted in the initial stage of shock. As shock progresses, systemic vascular

**Inpatient Treatment Options for PID**

| Regimen A | Regimen B |
|---|---|
| Cefoxitin IV, 2 g q 6 hr | Clindamycin IV, 900 mg q 8 hr |
| **or** | |
| Cefotetan IV, 2 g q 12 hr | **plus** |
| **plus** | Gentamicin loading dose IV or IM (2 mg/kg), followed by a maintenance dose (1.5 mg/kg) q 8 hr |
| Doxycycline, 100 mg q 12 hr orally or IV | |

**Alternative Parchterol Regimens**
Ampicillin/Sulbactam IV, 3 g q 6 hr

**plus**

Doxycycline, 100 mg q 12 hr orally or IV

Continue the regimen for at least 48 hr after clinical improvement. Following hospital discharge, continue doxycycline, 100 mg orally twice a day for 10–14 d.

*Note*: IV, intravenously; IM, intramuscularly.

**Outpatient Treatment Options for PID**

**Option 1**
Ceftriaxone, 250 mg IM

**plus**
Doxycycline, 100 mg orally for 14 d

**with or without**
Metronidazole, 500 mg orally b.i.d. for 14 d

**Option 2**
Cefoxitin, 2 g IM[a]

**plus**
Doxycycline, 100 mg orally b.i.d. for 14 d

**with or without**
Metronidazole, 500 mg orally b.i.d. for 14 d

*Note*: b.i.d., twice daily; IM, intramuscularly.
[a]Plus, probenecid, 1 g orally, concurrently.

resistance increases and cardiac output decreases. Microvascular hypoperfusion resulting from microembolization from fibrin degradation products and precapillary sphincteric dilatation resulting from hypoxia result in arterial venous shunting and loss of effective intravascular volume. Myocardial depression results in a diminution of effective cardiac output. Inadequate perfusion of vital organs results in renal dysfunction and accentuated acidosis. It is imperative that the managing physician recognize the presence of septic shock and respond appropriately. The hypotensive, tachycardic patient with abdominal findings suggestive of diffuse peritonitis, secondary to a ruptured tubo-ovarian abscess, should be managed aggressively with fluid resuscitation. Large volumes of crystalloid should be administered intravenously through two large-bore catheters. If there is a failure to correct hypotension with fluid administration, intravenous sympathomimetic amines should be initiated. Dopamine is the primary agent to be considered. Administered at a dose of 1 to 3 µg/kg per minute, dopamine has minor inotropic and chronotropic effects on the heart, with concomitant dilatation of mesenteric, cerebral, coronary, and renal arteries (11,12). At dosages between 4 and 10 µg/kg per minute, there is a further increase in cardiac output and an increased heart rate. The decision to initiate invasive monitoring for fluid resuscitation should be based on the patient's response to crystalloid administration and urine output. If blood pressure fails to respond to intravascular volume repletion and sympathomimetic amines and if urine output is not appropriate (>30 mL per hour), then pulmonary capillary wedge pressure monitoring should be considered to prevent the development of adult respiratory distress syndrome. Broad-spectrum antibiotic therapy should be initiated promptly to cover the polymicrobial gamut of pelvic pathogens. Preparation should be made for emergency admission to the hospital and laparotomy to remove the ruptured abscess and irrigate the peritoneal cavity. Blood should be sent for type and cross-match, coagulation panel, electrolytes, and blood gases. It is imperative that the physician managing the patient in septic shock from a ruptured tubo-ovarian abscess understand that this is a surgical disease, and pharmacologic intervention is supportive and preparatory to laparotomy.

## GONORRHEA

*Neisseria gonorrhea* requires emergency care in two situations: (a) when it is associated with acute PID and (b) when it is the cause of a disseminated gonococcal infection.

Only 1% to 2% of patients with gonorrhea develop disseminated gonococcal infections. Women appear to be more commonly affected by this presentation than men. This may be explained by the relative lack of symptoms in women harboring *N. gonorrhea* in the lower reproductive tract, specifically the cervix. With a breakdown in host immune defense, gonococcemia may occur. With the invasion of the bloodstream, symptoms include fever, chills, and arthralgias. Gonococcal dermatitis–arthritis syndrome develops within 2 to 3 weeks of the primary genital infection. Cutaneous manifestations usually consist of fewer than 25 lesions, usually on the distal extremities and in various stages of development. Lesions begin as pinpoint erythematous macules, which progress to papules, vesicular pustules, or hemorrhagic bullae. Advanced lesions contain a necrotic-appearing center surrounded by an erythematous halo. Rarely are cultures of cutaneous lesions positive for *N. gonorrhea*; however, immunofluorescent tissue stains may be of assistance in demonstrating organisms. Blood, urethral, cervical, pharyngeal, and rectal cultures may be of assistance in defining the etiology of the rash. A high index of suspicion is imperative (13).

With dissemination, the patient may have an acutely inflamed septic joint. Disseminated gonococcal disease is the most common cause of septic arthritis in patients younger than 30 years of age. The arthritis may be monoarticular or oligoarticular. Joints most commonly affected are the knees, elbows, ankles, wrists, and small joints of the hands and feet (14). The knee is the most commonly involved joint from which the gonococcus is recovered, but this may reflect the relative ease with which this joint is aspirated. The fluid withdrawn from the involved joint usually contains polymorphonuclear neutrophils, but a Gram stain for Gram-negative intracellular diplococci is positive only 10% to 30% of the time. Cultures likewise are positive in approximately 20% to 30% of cases. Once again, it is imperative that appropriate cultures be obtained from blood, urethral, pharyngeal, rectal, and cervical sites.

With the dissemination of the gonococcus to the heart, endocarditis may develop. Patients may have fever, chills, arthralgias, malaise, fatigue, dyspnea, and chest pain. Most patients have a murmur, and evidence of embolization may be present (conjunctival petechia, Osler's nodes, and splinter hemorrhages). Occasionally, splenomegaly and arthritis may be noted. Depending on the degree of cardiac compromise, congestive heart failure may be manifested by rales, ascites, edema, or a gallop rhythm on auscultation of the heart. The chest x-ray film may demonstrate cardiomegaly as a manifestation of congestive heart failure. The electrocardiogram may demonstrate left ventricular hypertrophy, bundle branch block, or intraventricular conduction delay. Usually, blood cultures are positive for *N. gonorrhea*. Echocardiography is useful in determining whether vegetations exist on the heart valves. The most common involvement is of the aortic and mitral valves. Without treatment, the endocarditis is almost always fatal.

Rarely, *N. gonorrhea* may disseminate to the meninges and cause manifestations of meningitis. Fever and nuchal rigidity in a patient complaining of headache, general malaise, and arthralgias should prompt a lumbar puncture to evaluate for organisms. As with synovial fluid, Gram stain and cultures may be negative, and therefore it is imperative to perform appropriate blood, cervical, urethral, rectal, and pharyngeal cultures for *Neisseria*.

Hospitalization is recommended for patients with disseminated gonococcal infection. Endocarditis and meningitis should be ruled out. Ongoing CDC investigation demonstrates that fluoroquinolone-resistant gonorrhea is now widespread in the United States. Therefore, this class of antibiotic is no longer recommended for treatment. When bacteremia and arthritis are present, the recommended therapy is ceftriaxone, 1 g intravenously (IV) daily for 7 to 10 days. Meningitis should be treated with ceftriaxone, 1 to 2 g IV every 12 hours for at least 10 days. Endocarditis should be treated with ceftriaxone, 1 to 2 g IV every 12 hours for at least 4 weeks. Depending on the severity of the valvular involvement with vegetations, cardiac surgery with valvular replacement may be necessary. Consultation with the appropriate specialist should be obtained early (15,16).

## ACQUIRED IMMUNODEFICIENCY SYNDROME

Even though the decade of the 1980s began with human immunodeficiency virus (HIV) as a male-specific entity, this virus is clearly not gender specific. The estimated number of new infections in the United States in 2006 was 56,300. Women account for 25% of patients living with HIV, with a prevalence of 278,400 in 2006 (17). The gynecologist cannot avoid the potential for exposure to patients infected with HIV, whether or not the patient's infectivity status is known.

HIV is an RNA retrovirus, which uses reverse transcriptase to transcribe DNA from RNA. It targets the CD4 molecule on the surface of the T4 lymphocyte. After being incorporated into the T4 lymphocyte and using reverse transcriptase to transcribe DNA, the virus is integrated into the host genome and the production of viral RNA begins. T4 cells are comprised of inducer and helper cells. Inducer cells stimulate the maturation of T lymphocytes from precursor cells, and T4 helper cells help cytotoxic T cells destroy foreign cells. T4 cells constitute approximately 60% to 80% of the circulating T-cell population. As a result of the infection and depletion of T4 lymphocytes by the invading HIV, the B cells cannot produce antibodies to HIV or other microorganisms. The cytotoxic response is depressed. There is a decreased secretion of interleukin-2, and T4 cells are incapable of antigen recognition. Not only does HIV attack the T helper cells but also the virus may attack macrophages and other target cells, resulting in direct infection of bowel, nervous tissue, heart, and lung (18). It is well recognized that the infected host may transmit HIV to susceptible individuals through blood or body fluids, including vaginal secretions, semen, peritoneal fluid, and amniotic fluid (19). Once individuals are infected with HIV, seroconversion may not occur for a mean of 18 months, with a range of 3 to 42 months (20). The mean latency period from seroconversion to AIDS is usually 10 to 11 years. Once AIDS develops, death is inevitable. As the disease progresses in the female patient, a number of opportunistic infections may result in infections that prompt the need for emergent therapy.

Because AIDS is a sexually transmitted disease, the AIDS patient is prone to acquisition of other sexually transmitted diseases, and it is important to keep this in mind when evaluating them. For example, an AIDS patient with signs and symptoms of PID may not demonstrate leukocytosis. For this reason, strong consideration should be given to admitting the AIDS patient with signs and symptoms of PID for intravenous antibiotic therapy. Currently, there appears to be no basis to provide treatment regimens other than those currently recommended by the Centers for Disease Control for acute PID (9).

The observant physician should be alert to clinical manifestations of AIDS in any patient seen in an emergency setting. Such manifestations include enlarged lymph nodes, night sweats, fevers, oral candidiasis, chronic cough, paresthesias, nausea, vomiting, diarrhea, weight loss, and skin ulcerations.

The primary pulmonary emergency in the patient with AIDS is *Pneumocystis jiroveci* (formerly *Pneumocystis carinii*) pneumonia. This most common of the opportunistic infections in patients with AIDS poses the greatest risk to those who have CD4 T-lymphocyte counts of <200. Patients may have shortness of breath and appear septic. Physical examination demonstrates diminished breath sounds and dullness to percussion. Chest x-ray study shows diffuse bilateral interstitial pneumonia (Fig. 19.3). Blood gases may show a diminished $PO_2$ and acidosis. If the presumptive diagnosis is *P. jiroveci* pneumonia with evidence of pulmonary compromise, the patient should be admitted for trimethoprim–sulfamethoxazole therapy. The medication may be given orally or intravenously as trimethoprim, 15 to 20 mg/kg per day, and sulfamethoxazole, 75 to 100 mg/kg per day, in three or four doses for 21 days (21). Adjunctive glucocorticoids should be given to patients with a room air $PAO_2$ ≤70 mm Hg or alveolar–arterial oxygen gradient ≥35 mm Hg (22).

Tuberculosis is becoming an increasing concern in AIDS patients and should be considered in any pulmonary emergency in a seropositive or at-risk individual. Typical symptoms include cough, fever, night sweats, and weight loss. Purified protein derivative (PPD) testing should be considered in at-risk patients unless there is a known history of tuberculosis or a prior positive PPD. A reaction of 5 mm in an immunocompromised person suggests exposure to tuberculosis, and chest x-ray study and sputum stains should be obtained for confirmation (23). Standard therapy consists of isoniazid, rifampin, pyrazinamide, and ethambutol. Other considerations in patients with pulmonary symptoms include community-acquired bacterial and viral pneumonias and fungal pneumonias (cryptococcosis, coccidiomycosis, and histoplasmosis).

AIDS patients may present with abdominal manifestations. The female AIDS patient with an acute abdomen is a diagnostic dilemma. The differential may include PID or primary bowel involvement by HIV or an opportunistic infection. Right upper quadrant pain associated with either jaundice or abnormal liver function tests may suggest cytomegalovirus (CMV) or cryptosporidia organisms and a resultant cholangitis. The differential diagnosis also includes liver abscess, hepatitis, CMV infection of the intestinal tract, HIV enteritis and colitis, neoplasms, and perforations (23).

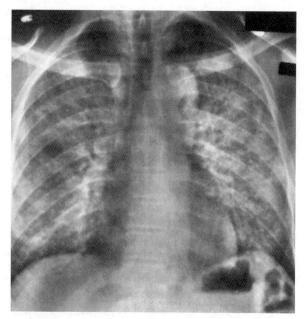

**FIGURE 19.3** Extensive, bilateral pulmonary infiltrates in a patient with *P. jiroveci* pneumonia complicating acquired immunodeficiency syndrome.

CMV colitis patients may have lower quadrant pain, weight loss, diarrhea, hematochezia, and fever. If perforation has occurred, the patient may have symptoms and signs of peritonitis. Surgical intervention is imperative. In the patient with symptoms suggestive of colonic involvement without impending perforation, CT scanning demonstrates marked bowel thickening typically involving the terminal ileum and right colon. Colonoscopic examination reveals erythema, submucosal hemorrhages, and ulcerations. CMV vasculitis on biopsy is diagnostic (24). Prompt admission with the initiation of therapy with ganciclovir at 5 mg/kg IV every 12 hours for 14 to 21 days is warranted (21).

Disabling vulvar symptoms may cause the AIDS patient to seek emergency care. The differential should include candidiasis, chancroid, HSV, or a primary HIV ulceration of the vulva (24) (Fig. 19.4).

Other crises that may prompt the HIV patient to request emergency care usually involve the central nervous system or the eye. Disorientation, headache, seizures, hallucinations, and altered motor activity should prompt CT scanning of the cranium to rule out an intracranial mass. The presence of a mass raises the diagnostic possibility of toxoplasmosis or non-Hodgkin's lymphoma. Appropriate studies for immunoglobulin G antibody against *Toxoplasma gondii* should be obtained. A diagnosis of toxoplasmosis should prompt therapy with pyrimethamine and sulfadiazine (23). Other diagnostic possibilities in the AIDS patient with central nervous system symptoms include meningitis, which may be bacterial (*H. influenzae, Mycobacterium tuberculosis,* and *Listeria monocytogenes*), and cryptococcal or viral (CMV and varicella) causes. With the elevation in the incidence of syphilis seen in AIDS patients, neurosyphilis should be considered in patients with central nervous

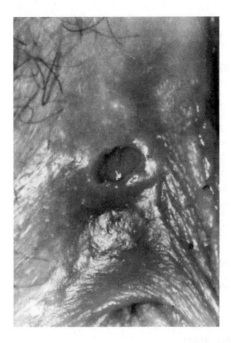

**FIGURE 19.4** Vulvar ulceration in a patient with acquired immunodeficiency syndrome. Cultures and biopsies were negative for all pathogens, resulting in the diagnosis of HIV ulceration.

system symptoms. Parenteral therapy for this condition is warranted and consists of aqueous penicillin G, 12 million units per day IV for 10 days, or procaine penicillin, 2.4 million units intramuscularly per day for 10 days, plus probenecid, 500 mg by mouth twice a day for 10 days (22).

If the AIDS patient has visual changes (e.g., blurred vision or loss of visual fields), CMV retinitis should be suspected. Fundoscopic examination may reveal multifocal white or yellow patches with or without hemorrhage. Therapy should be initiated with ganciclovir, 5 mg/kg IV every 12 hours for 14 to 21 days (22).

With the increasing incidence of seropositivity in the female patient population, it is imperative that the gynecologist practice defensive medicine. If a health care professional makes transcutaneous contact with HIV-infected blood, there is an approximately 1-in-300 chance of seroconversion (25). Gynecologists should take every reasonable precaution to prevent transcutaneous needle exposure to infected blood. Eye protection and double gloves should be worn. Needles should be handled with instruments and not fingers. Body fluids, drapes, catheters, and needles should be handled and disposed of with care and according to preestablished guidelines. These protective medical practices should apply to contact with all patients, whether or not serum status is known.

## SYPHILIS

*Treponema pallidum* was responsible for epidemic outbreaks of syphilis in the 15th and 16th centuries in Europe. Widespread prevalence of the disease was observed until the availability of penicillin after World War II. In 1943, 575,000 cases were reported in the United States (26). In 2000, the rate was the lowest since reporting began in 1941. However, a disturbing trend emerged, with the rate of syphilis increasing steadily between 2000 and 2007, with 40,920 cases reported in 2007 (27).

*T. pallidum* is a delicate, spiral-shaped organism, which is spread by sexual contact. After inoculation, the average incubation period is 3 weeks, with a range of 9 to 90 days. The initial lesion of syphilis, known as the primary lesion or chancre, is usually found in the genital region, although extragenital chancre may occur on the lip or finger (Fig. 19.5). The chancre is a firm, well-circumscribed painless ulceration with a clean base. If superinfection is present, the ulceration may be painful. Regional painless lymphadenopathy is also observed. The chancre may persist for 3 to 8 weeks and then heal spontaneously; however, the lymphadenopathy may persist for longer durations. Without therapy, within weeks to months, the stage of secondary syphilis is entered. Approximately 50% of patients demonstrate signs and symptoms during this stage, which may consist of low-grade fever, meningismus, arthralgia, nocturnal bone pain, coryza, and malaise. The painless chancre of primary syphilis may go unobserved, especially if it is located on the cervix, and therefore women often do not seek evaluation until they have entered this stage. Skin lesions in this stage of the disease may be annular, maculopapular, papular, or macular. The most common skin lesion is the maculopapular syphilid, which occurs in approximately 70% of cases and consists of distinctive brownish or coppery macules and papules on the palms and soles (Fig. 19.6). Another characteristic lesion of secondary syphilis is condyloma latum, which is often confused with condyloma acuminata

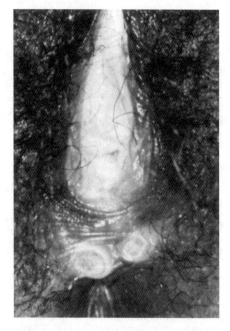

**FIGURE 19.5** Primary chancres.

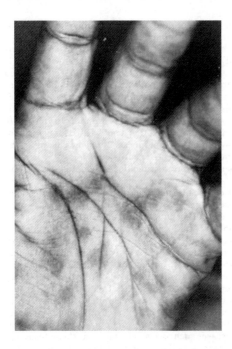

**FIGURE 19.6** Maculopapular secondary syphilis.

induced by human papillomavirus. This lesion is broad based, moist, and grayish white in coloration. It is highly contagious and may also be found in other warm moist regions of the body, such as the inner thighs, the axilla, and underneath the breasts. Dark-field examination, serologic testing, or biopsy may confirm the diagnosis.

If the *Treponema* organisms induce osteomyelitis that spreads to the periosteum, patients may complain of bone pain, which classically is nocturnal and exaggerated by heat, frequently being relieved by movement of the involved bone (28). The skull, clavicle, tibia, and radius are the most commonly involved bones in patients with periostitis as a manifestation of secondary syphilis. This bone pain may precede or follow the mucocutaneous manifestations of secondary syphilis and may be the only manifestation of secondary syphilis.

The liver may be involved in secondary syphilis, and patients may complain of abdominal pain and upper quadrant discomfort. Approximately 50% of patients with secondary syphilis may have liver function abnormalities, and 1% to 12% may demonstrate jaundice. Most cases of hepatic dysfunction, during the course of early syphilis, are a result of inflammation of the liver by the spirochetes. It has been suggested that rectal inoculation with *T. pallidum* results in direct portal venous inoculation and a higher incidence of hepatic involvement (29).

Ocular involvement in secondary syphilis may result in a patient seeking care for visual disturbances. The pathogenesis of syphilitic episcleritis and scleritis is related to lymphocytic infiltration and subsequent vasculitis. Patients may have a painful, reddened eye. Iritis presenting as pain, photophobia, and dimness of vision may be noted, and adhesions of the iris to the anterior lens may produce a fixed pupil. This is not to be confused with the Argyll Robertson pupil, which is also seen as a component of symptomatic neurosyphilis and presents as a small irregular pupil that reacts to accommodation but not to light (30).

The central nervous system is commonly involved in early syphilis, affecting at least 50% of patients (31). Although central nervous system involvement is frequent, symptomatic neurosyphilis develops in fewer than 10% of untreated patients. Patients with symptomatic neurosyphilis may have cranial nerve palsies, paresthesias, weakness, sensory loss in extremities and trunk, progressive mental deterioration, convulsions, ataxia, areflexia, bladder and eye disturbances, optic atrophy, coma, and death. These manifestations of syphilis are typically seen in late syphilis, particularly in patients not treated for primary or secondary syphilis. Patients with these symptoms should be evaluated for the possibility of untreated or suboptimally treated neurosyphilis.

The evaluation of a patient with the aforementioned symptoms suggestive of syphilis is well established. The lesions should be examined for spirochetes. Obvious care should be exercised, because mucocutaneous lesions are infectious. Serology is likewise helpful, but because primary syphilis manifests as a chancre, initial serology may be positive in 70% of patients and negative serologic examination in the absence of the ability to perform a dark-field examination does not exclude the diagnosis of primary syphilis. Antibodies against cardiolipin, known as reaginic or nontreponema antibodies (VDRL [Venereal Disease Research Laboratory] and RPR [Rapid Plasma Reagin]), are quantitative measurements and serum titers usually reflect disease activity. The specific treponemal antibody test, the fluorescent treponemal antibody absorbed test (FTA-ABS), is very sensitive and specific and usually remains reactive indefinitely without regard to treatment status. This test is useful in ruling out false-positive, nontreponemal tests, which may be caused by pregnancy, recent immunizations, sarcoidosis, hepatitis, and autoimmune diseases such as systemic lupus erythematosus. For the patient with a lesion of primary syphilis, the initial screen should include a dark-field examination of the chancre, qualitative and quantitative nontreponemal assays (VDRL or RPR), and a specific treponemal assay (the FTA-ABS). The differential diagnosis of such a lesion includes HSV, chancroid, and HIV. Appropriate cultures for *Haemophilus ducreyi* and HSV should be obtained if suspected, and HIV testing should be considered. Syphilis is the great masquerader, and even though it may be highly likely that secondary syphilis will be suspected in patients with maculopapular diffuse eruptions involving the palms and soles, the diagnosis must also be entertained in patients with right upper quadrant pain, bone pain, ocular symptoms, and neurologic symptoms. The most consistently observed laboratory abnormality in syphilitic hepatitis is a marked elevation in alkaline phosphatase. The differential diagnosis should include viral hepatitis, cholecystitis, and Fitz Hugh–Curtis syndrome. In addition to the liver function tests, studies should be obtained for hepatitis B and treponemal and nontreponemal serologies. Patients with bone pain may demonstrate tenderness on physical examination while the involved bone is palpated. In the absence of obvious mucocutaneous lesions of secondary syphilis for dark-field studies, the VDRL and FTA-ABS should be obtained. The erythrocyte sedimentation rate may be elevated. Radiographs may show no radiologic changes. Bone scanning may show increased uptake in the involved bones suggestive of inflammation. Patients with syphilitic scleritis typically have positive nontreponemal and treponemal serologies. Other causes for the inflammation should be evaluated with assays for rheumatoid factor and antinuclear antibody.

Lumbar puncture is recommended to rule out neurosyphilis in all patients with syphilis of more than 1 year's duration or in patients with clinical symptoms of meningitis or focal neurologic findings. The issue of whether all patients should have a lumbar puncture remains unanswered; however, it has been observed that patients with concurrent HIV infection and positive central nervous system serology have a higher failure rate on standard treatment with the usually recommended dose of 2.4 million units of benzathine penicillin as a single-dose therapy for primary syphilis. Until the optimum therapy for HIV- testing for HIV in all patients with syphilis. Lumbar puncture should be strongly considered in patients who are HIV positive and seropositive for syphilis before the initiation of therapy (32).

Therapy for early syphilis (primary syphilis, secondary syphilis, and latent syphilis of <1 year's duration) consists of 2.4 million units of benzathine penicillin given intramuscularly on one occasion. An alternative therapy for the patient who is allergic to penicillin and who is not pregnant would be 100 mg of doxycycline twice a day for 14 days or, alternatively, tetracycline, 500 mg orally four times a day for 14 days (32). The treatment for late syphilis, defined as syphilis existing for more than 1 year, or cardiovascular syphilis consists of 2.4 million units of benzathine penicillin intramuscularly given weekly for 3 weeks. Patients with neurosyphilis should receive penicillin G, 3 million to 4 million units IV every 4 hours for 10 to 14 days. This implies admission to the hospital for receipt of therapy. An alternative approach is procaine penicillin G, 2.4 million units intramuscularly daily, plus probenecid, 500 mg four times a day orally, both for 10 to 14 days (33). As mentioned previously, patients with syphilis who are HIV positive and have asymptomatic central nervous system involvement may not respond to a single-dose benzathine penicillin therapy. If examination of the cerebral spinal fluid demonstrates that the patient has neurosyphilis, then more aggressive therapy is warranted, with appropriate serologic follow-up testing. If cerebrospinal fluid testing demonstrates no evidence of neurosyphilis, current recommendations do not dictate therapy more intensive than the currently recommended single-dose therapy for early syphilis. However, it is imperative that regular serologic testing be obtained to confirm that the initially positive VDRL has converted to negative. Relapse in the HIV-positive patient may be more common and should be carefully monitored for reinstitution of therapy.

All patients who have received therapy for syphilis should be monitored with VDRLs or RPRs drawn at 3-month intervals to document the conversion to seronegativity, implying successful therapy. As many as 95% of patients with seropositive primary syphilis and 55% of patients with seronegative primary syphilis demonstrate the Jarisch–Herxheimer reaction after therapy for syphilis is administered. Clinical manifestations include fever, chills, diaphoresis, malaise, myalgia, arthralgia, headache, anorexia, nausea, vomiting, and skin eruptions (34). The pathogenesis of the reaction is poorly understood but appears to be related to circulating immune complexes, complement activation, plasma kinins, and possibly endogenous opioids.

Because Jarisch–Herxheimer reaction is self-limited, it may be managed with bed rest and anti-inflammatory agents.

## HERPES SIMPLEX VIRUS INFECTIONS

From the mid-1970s through the mid-1980s, genital infections with HSV dominated both the professional and the lay press. As concern mounted in the 1980s over the increasing prevalence of HIV and AIDS, public education concerning safe sexual practices dominated national educational efforts. As a result, it appears that "safe sex" practices have resulted in a diminution of the number of patients with herpetic genital infections.

HSV is a member of the same viral family as varicella zoster, CMV, and Epstein–Barr. The double-stranded DNA virus has two primary serotypes: HSV I and HSV II. Both serotypes infect cells by incorporating their DNA into the host cellular DNA and proceeding to either remain in the latent phase or initiate the production of viral DNA, with the release of infectious viral particles and destruction of the host cell. HSV II infections are most commonly seen in the genital region, although type I infections may result as a consequence of orogenital spread. Herpetic infections are to be considered sexually transmitted and they require direct contact for transmission.

Manifestations of infection with HSV typically occur after an incubation period of 3 to 7 days (35). Initial symptoms may consist of vulvar pruritus, burning, or pain. Within 1 to 3 days, a vesicular eruption develops. Vesicles may rupture, with resultant widespread multicentric painful ulcerations. Systemic manifestations include fever, malaise, and headaches. Approximately 30% of patients develop nuchal rigidity, photophobia, or fever, all suggestive of viral meningitis. Because of the involvement of the autonomic nervous system with the virus, bladder dysfunction may be noted and patients may complain of urinary retention. In addition to lesions on the vulva, vagina, and cervix, extragenital lesions may be noted on the chest, buttocks, thighs, and fingers and are consistent with autoinoculation. If lesions are noted in multiple extragenital sites, then the possibility of disseminated mucocutaneous HSV must be entertained. Usually when this condition is diagnosed, one is dealing with an immunocompromised patient, and progression to disseminated visceral infection runs a fulminant course and terminates in death. Rarely has disseminated mucocutaneous HSV II virus been noted in nonimmunocompromised patients (36). Primary lesions of HSV usually persist for 2 to 6 weeks, after which healing occurs without scarring.

Even though patients may be seen for emergent care for recurrent herpetic lesions, the most frequent request for evaluation and treatment is from patients who are experiencing their first episode of primary herpes. The local pain from the vulvar ulcerations, the systemic symptoms of fever and headache, or the painful bladder spasms from urinary retention will, separately or together, prompt urgent gynecologic evaluation. The diagnosis is usually made based on visual inspection. The vesicles or the subsequent ulcerations are classic in appearance and are typically quite painful. Even though they may be unifocal, they are most frequently multifocal and can be differentiated from the painless unifocal lesion of syphilis. Although suspicion of the diagnosis is by physical examination, it can be confirmed only by culturing for the virus. The stage of the disease has a direct impact on the recovery of the virus by culture. Recovery rates from lesions of primary herpes are 100% for vesicular lesions, 89% for pustular lesions, and 82% for ulcerative lesions. Crusted lesions have an approximately 25% recovery rate (37). Serologic studies are not particularly helpful in the patient experiencing a primary episode of herpes. Even though titers rise after an acute infection, the gold standard is the viral culture.

Therapy for primary HSV involving the genitalia is based on the clinical status of the patient. Typically, treatment is on an outpatient basis, with acyclovir, 200 mg orally five times daily for 7 to 10 days. Many physicians use 400 mg orally three times daily as a more effective and convenient form of oral therapy (38). Other options include famciclovir, 250 mg orally three times a day for 7 to 10 days, and valacyclovir, 1 g orally twice daily for 7 to 10 days. Patients experiencing urinary retention require insertion of a catheter until symptoms subside and bladder function returns to normal. The decision to hospitalize a patient for intravenous acyclovir therapy is based on the severity of systemic symptoms. The patient with severe meningeal signs, the patient unable to tolerate oral medication, and the patient with disseminated mucocutaneous HSV need to be hospitalized. Acyclovir should be administered intravenously at 5 mg/kg every 8 hours for 5 to 7 days (38). In AIDS patients with severe herpes genitalis, strong consideration should be given to hospitalization for intravenous therapy (39).

Certainly, patients with nonprimary first-episode herpes or patients with recurrent herpes may have significant discomfort from their disease; however, attacks are less likely to be associated with severe systemic symptoms or urinary retention. Patients with nonprimary first-episode herpes have circulating antibodies from a prior herpes infection that usually limit the manifestations of the disease. The same can be said for patients who have episodes of recurrent herpes virus infections. The diagnosis is suspected after observing the genital lesion, which is typically ulcerative when first seen by the physician. The patient may have noted the erythematous papule developing into a painful vesicle, usually within the first day of a recurrent infection. With progression, the vesicle ruptures and ulceration forms. Viruses are recoverable from the lesion between the first and the fourth days of recurrence. Recovery rates are lower with each stage of the disease than in primary infections. Treatment of recurrent genital herpes with acyclovir, 200 mg orally five times a day for 5 days, has been shown to reduce viral shedding by 1 day and shorten the duration of the episode by 1 to 2 days (40). It is imperative that therapy for recurrence be initiated early in the course of the disease or the ameliorative effect is lost.

## CHANCROID

Chancroid is a relatively infrequent disease in the United States, accounting for 33 cases in 2006 (41). The disease is caused by *H. ducreyi*, a Gram-negative facultative anaerobic bacillus. After an incubation period of 4 to 7 days, a chancre appears, which rapidly erodes to form an ulcer approximately 48 hours after its initial appearance. The ulcer is extremely tender, with irregular undermined edges. The base of the ulcer is necrotic, whereas the syphilitic chancre is clean, without evidence of necrosis. Multiple lesions develop in 33% of patients, and contiguous lesions may coalesce into giant ulcers. Lesions in women are most common on the fourchette, the labia, the vestibule, and the clitoris. Without treatment, extensive ulceration and massive edema of the vulva and perineum may be observed. Inguinal lymphadenopathy develops in half of patients, and these may develop into a bubo with rupture and adjacent ulceration.

The diagnosis of chancroid is suspected when the characteristic lesion is noted. Gram stain from the base of the ulcer shows Gram-negative coccobacillary forms in chains. Special culture media (gonococcal agar base and Mueller Hinton agar base) can be used to culture for the organism. Strong consideration should be given to HIV testing, because there is an increased rate of chancroid infection among patients with HIV.

The recommended regimen for the treatment of chancroid is either azithromycin, 1 g orally once, or ceftriaxone, 250 mg intramuscularly once. Other regimens include ciprofloxacin, 500 mg orally twice a day for 3 days, or erythromycin, 500 mg orally four times a day for 7 days (42). With successful treatment, ulcers will improve within 3 days symptomatically and within 7 days objectively. If no clinical improvement is observed by 7 days, the clinician should determine whether the prescribed medication was taken and rule out coinfection with another sexually transmitted disease such as syphilis or herpes, in addition to ruling out infection with HIV. A final consideration would be antibiotic resistance, and appropriate susceptibilities should be determined.

## *References*

1. www2a.cdc/gov/std. Last accessed 6/09.
2. Cates W, Rolfs RT, Aral SO. Sexually transmitted diseases, pelvic inflammatory disease, and infertility: an epidemiologic update. *Epidemiol Rev.* 1990;12:199–220.
3. Washington EA, Aral SO, Wolner-Hanssen P, et al. Assessing risk for pelvic inflammatory disease and its sequelae. *JAMA.* 1991;266:2581–2586.

4. Meirik O. Intrauterine devices—upper and lower genital tract infections. *Contraception.* 2007;75:S41–S47.
5. Shelton JD. Risk of clinical pelvic inflammatory disease attributable to an intrauterine device. *Lancet.* 2001;357:443.
6. Sweet EL, Blankfort-Doyle M, Robbie MO, et al. The occurrence of chlamydial and gonococcal salpingitis during the menstrual cycle. *JAMA.* 1986;255:2062–2064.
7. Rice PA, Schachter J. Pathogenesis of pelvic inflammatory disease: diagnostic and prognostic value of routine laparoscopy. *Am J Obstet Gynecol.* 1969;105(7):1088–1098.
8. Kahn JG, Walker CK, Washington E, et al. Diagnosing pelvic inflammatory disease. *JAMA.* 1991;266:2594–2604.
9. Workowski KA, Berman SM. Sexually transmitted diseases treatment guidelines, 2006. *MMWR Recomm Rep.* 2006;55(RR-11):1–94.
10. Jacobson L, Swastrom L. Objectivized diagnosis of acute pelvic inflammatory disease: diagnosis and prognostic value of routine laparoscopy. *Am J Obstet Gynecol.* 1969;105:1088–1098.
11. Drugs for sexually transmitted infections. *Med Lett.* 1999;41(1062):85–90.
12. Septic shock: Where are we now? *Emerg Med Rep.* 1991;33:856.
13. Buntin DM, Rosen T, Lesher JL, et al. Sexually transmitted diseases: bacterial infections. *J Am Acad Dermatol.* 1991;25(2) 287–299.
14. Dallabetta G, Hook E. Gonococcal infections. *Infect Dis Clin North Am.* 1987;1:25–54.
15. Wall TC, Peyton RB, Corey GR, et al. Gonococcal endocarditis: a new look at an old disease. *Medicine.* 1989;68:375–380.
16. Update to CDC's sexually transmitted diseases treatment guidelines, 2006: fluoroquinolones no longer recommended for treatment of gonococcal infections. *Morbid Mortal Wkly Rep.* 2007;56(14):332–336.
17. Hall HL, Song R, Rhodes P, et al. Estimation of HIV incidence in the United States. *JAMA.* 2008;300(5):520–529.
18. Levy JA. Changing concepts in HIV infection: challenges for the 1990's. *AIDS.* 1990;4:1051.
19. US Department of Health and Human Services, Public Health Services, Centers for Disease Control. Acquired immunodeficiency syndrome United States, 1989. *Morbid Mortal Wkly Rep.* 1990;39(5):81.
20. Wolinsky SM, Rinaldo CR, Kowk S, et al. Human immunodeficiency virus type 1 (HIV-1) infection in a median of 18 months before a diagnostic Western blot: evidence from a cohort of homosexual men. *Ann Intern Med.* 1989;111:961.
21. Drugs for AIDS and associated infections. *Med Lett.* 1995;37:(959):87–94.
22. Briel M, Bucher HC, Furrer H. Adjunctive corticosteroids for *Pneumocystis jiroveci* pneumonia in patients with HIV-infection. *Cochrane Database Syst Rev.* 2006 Jul;3:CD006150.
23. Dwyer B. HIV in the 2nd decade: clinical manifestations and emergency management. *Emerg Med Rep.* 1991;12:22.
24. Covino JM, McCormach WM. Vulvar ulcer of unknown etiology in a human immunodeficiency virus-infected woman: response to treatment with zidovudine. *Am J Obstet Gynecol.* 1990;163:1.
25. Henderson DK, Fahey BJ, Willy M, et al. Risk for occupational transmission of human immunodeficiency virus type I (HIV-1) associated with clinical exposures. *Ann Intern Med.* 1990;113:740.
26. CDC. *Sexually Transmitted Disease Statistics—1987.* Atlanta, GA: Centers for Disease Control; 1988:136;988.
27. CDC. *Sexually Transmitted Disease Surveillance-2007.* Atlanta, GA: Centers for Disease Control.
28. Meier JL, Mollet E. Acute periostitis in early acquired syphilis simulating shin splints in a jogger. *Am J Sports Med.* 1986;14(4):327–328.
29. Sclossberg D. Syphilitic hepatitis: a case report and review of the literature. *Am J Gastroenterol.* 1987;82(6):552–553.
30. Wilhelmus K, Yokoyama C. Syphilitic episcleritis and scleritis. *Am J Ophthalmol.* 1987;104:595–597.
31. Zenker RN, Rofs RT. Treatment of syphilis, 1989. *Rev Infect Dis.* 1990;12:5590–5609.

32. Lukehart SA, Hook EW, Baker-Zander SA, et al. Invasion of the central nervous system by *Treponema pallidum*: implications for diagnosis and treatment. *Ann Intern Med*. 1988;109:855–862.

33. Centers for Disease Control and Prevention. 2006 Guidelines for Treatment of Sexually Transmitted Diseases. *Morbid Mortal Wkly Rep*. 2006;55:22.

34. Rosen T, Rubin H, Ellner K, et al. Vesicular Jarisch–Herxheimer reaction. *Arch Dermatol*. 1989;125:77–81.

35. Landy HJ, Grossman JH. Herpes simplex virus: sexually transmitted diseases. *Obstet Gynecol Clin North Am*. 1989;16(3):495–515.

36. Gutmann D, Beard BA, Collinge ML, et al. Nonfatal disseminated mucocutaneous herpes simplex type 2 infection in a healthy woman. *Obstet Gynecol*. 1988;72:506–507.

37. Webb D, Fife K. Genital herpes simplex virus infections: sexually transmitted diseases. *Infect Dis Clin North Am*. 1987;(1):1:97–122.

38. Drugs for sexually transmitted infections. *Med Lett*. 1999;41(1062):85–90.

39. Kroon S. Genital herpes—When and how to treat. *Semin Dermatol*. 1990;9(2):133–140.

40. Stone K, Whittington W. Treatment of genital herpes. *Rev Infect Dis*. 1990;12(6):610–619.

41. Centers for Disease Control and PRevention, Division of SExually Transmitted Diseases. Sexually Transmitted Diseases Surveillance, Other Sexually Transmitted Diseases, 2006 National Report. Available at: http://www.cdc.gov/std/stats/other.htm. Accessed May 7, 2008.

42. Centers for Disease Control and Prevention. 2006 Guidelines for Treatment of Sexually Transmitted Diseases. *Morbid Mortal Wkly Rep*. 2006;55:15.

# 20

# Vulvar and Vaginal Diseases

## Guy I. Benrubi

Vaginitis is the most common reason for visits to the offices of obstetrics and gynecology physicians as well as constitutes a very large component of visits to primary care providers. Vulvovaginal discomfort does not usually create in a patient a sense of urgency, therefore, most of these patients are not going to present either to emergency departments or to urgent care centers or call physician offices for emergency consultations. However, with the effects of the Great Recession in the United States and with the increasing loss by patients of coverage for health care, there has been an increase in the number of patients presenting with these symptoms to urgent settings. Therefore, this chapter will briefly discuss some of the overall aspects of care of patients presenting with these conditions as well as the most common causes for these symptoms.

In the medical literature, the three most common causes identified as creating vulvovaginal discomfort are bacterial vaginosis, candidiasis, and trichomoniasis (1). Though these three conditions have been so described for quite a long time, currently, the most common cause of vulvovaginal discomfort in the United States is mucosal atrophy secondary to insufficient estrogen (2). This particular diagnosis will be seen increasingly in the next few years as the population of women in this country ages. Additionally, the result of the publication of the Women's Health Initiative in 2002 lead to a 70% decline in the use of hormone replacement therapy in US postmenopausal women.

In approaching this problem, it should be understood that the term "itis" in vaginitis is probably a misnomer. "Itis" refers to inflammation. Very frequently, what is causing the symptoms in the patient's vulvovaginal area is not an inflammation but a colonization or an abnormality in the bacterial flora of the vagina. Another concept that should be understood is that a lot of the symptoms are not arising in the vagina but in the vulva. The vulva in addition to being part of the urogenital system is also part of the integumentary system. Vulva is skin and any condition which can arise in the skin can also arise on the vulva.

One of the most common presentations of vulvovaginal atrophy due to estrogen deficiency is urethral meatal irritation, which the patient interprets as a urinary tract infection. Frequently, when these patients arrive at the care area, urine culture and urinalysis are negative. Other symptoms of estrogen lack are nonspecific sense of irritation as well as occasionally mild burning and some dyspareunia both intromissional as well as post coital. In the emergent setting, the patient should be reassured and a determination should be made as to whether the patient wants to be placed on systemic hormone replacement therapy or to be on localized therapy. There are multiple options for localized therapy (3–5). Estradiol vaginal tablets (Vagifem®) can be inserted vaginally twice weekly and can deliver $50 \mu g$ of estradiol per week. Another option is an estradiol vaginal ring (Estring®) which is inserted in the vagina and stays in place for 90 days and delivers $52 \mu g$ of estradiol each week. Other options are to use estradiol creams with an applicator which allows the patient to use a small amount on a weekly basis.

Bacterial vaginosis is the term that is now used to describe a whole host of conditions that have had multiple other names prior to 1984 when the current term was adopted. It is important to note that "vaginosis" implies a colonization and not an inflammatory process. Vaginosis is a condition where the normal lactobacillus bacteria in the vagina have decreased in number and the vagina becomes colonized with anaerobic bacteria. These bacteria come from the rectum. This is due to proximity and not hygiene deficiency. The patient presents with a complaint of a profuse smooth vanilla yogurt-like discharge as well as possibly a "fishy" odor which is most profound after partner ejaculation during intercourse. On examination, the most notable aspect will be the profuse white discharge which is frequently found in the introitus even before a speculum is inserted. On wet prep, the diagnostic sign will be the clue cells which are squamous cells covered by anaerobic bacteria clinging to their surface. The presence of clue cells in conjunction with a profuse smooth white discharge is diagnostic 99% of the time for bacterial vaginosis. The other important sign is that there is no evidence of inflammation, that is, no redness of the vaginal or vulvar tissues and no white blood cells in the wet prep. This condition is treated efficaciously with metronidazole or clindamycin. These medications can be given systemically or topically (6). A high incidence of this disease is seen in lesbian couples. This may be due to the use of sexual toys. If the patient keeps reappearing in the urgent care area and the patient does not go to her primary physician, a discussion should be carried out with her as to sexual practices. Although this is not, strictly speaking, a sexually transmitted disease, it is a disease which may be impacted by the patient's type of sexual practice.

The next frequently seen etiology for vulvovaginal discomfort is a yeast infection. Most yeast infections in this country are candida albicans. There are some that are candida tropicalis, and also there is an increasing incidence of candida glabrata. Most yeast infections at the time the patient presents to the physician are not inflammatory in nature but are colonizations of the vagina with yeast. If the patient has delayed care, then a yeast infection may in fact become inflammatory. The patient will frequently describe, in addition to a discharge, a pruritic sensation. This pruritus is secondary to an IgA reaction on the tissues and is similar to a contact dermatitis or an allergic dermatitis. On wet prep, the squamous cells will appear normal. There may be some white blood cells, and the diagnostic sign would be yeast forms, either budding yeast forms or mycelial forms. One frequent cause of a yeast infection is the use of antibiotics by the patient prior to the start of the yeast colonization problem (7). The antibiotics knock out the lactobacilli, and this results in an overgrowth of yeast. These infections are invariably treated with azoles whether it is fluconazole, butoconazole, terconazole, etc (8). Therapy can be either oral or by insertion of vaginal ovules or cream depending on the preference of the patient.

Trichomoniasis is the true inflammatory infection of the vagina. Once the patient contracts a vaginal trichomonal infection, the infection will spread to the draining lymph nodes in the obturator as well as the hypogastric area of the pelvis. The patient therefore will present not only with a discharge but also with pelvic pain because of the lymphatic involvement. The diagnosis is made by looking at a wet prep which shows not only a profuse number of white blood cells but also the trichomonads which are swimming against Brownian motion. Once the diagnosis is made, the patient is most efficaciously treated with metronidazole. This should be given systemically not topically because the metronidazole must get into the pelvic lymph nodes; otherwise, the infection will recur (9,10). One of the problems that trichomoniasis presents is that the patient's partner also needs to be treated, and the partner must be referred to the appropriate physician for the appropriate therapy.

The above are the most common conditions which would necessitate a patient to seek care in an urgent or semi-urgent manner. There is a whole host of other conditions of the vagina that one must consider which may cause symptoms but in fact are not applicable to treatment in the urgent care area. These include inflammatory conditions such as desquamative inflammatory vaginitis, lichen planus, lichen sclerosus, vulvar hypertrophy, as well as vulvar intraepithelial neoplasia. The reader is referred to the appropriate literature and texts for these conditions as it would be unlikely that the urgent care physician would have to provide definitive therapy. The physician, however, must be aware that these conditions occur because if the patient presents with symptoms and none of the four conditions described above are obvious, then the patient must be told about other possibilities and must be referred for appropriate care.

### References

1. Schorge JO, Schaffer JI, Halvorson LM, et al. *Williams Gynecology.* New York, NY: The McGraw-Hill Companies, Inc.; 2008.
2. Mehta A, Bachmann G. Vulvovaginal complaints. *Clin Obstet Gynecol.* 2008;51:549–555.
3. Bachmann G, Lobo RA, Gut R, et al. Efficacy of low-dose estradiol vaginal tablets in the treatment of atrophic vaginitis: a randomized controlled trial. *Obstet Gynecol.* 2008;111:67–76.
4. Chollet JA, Carter G, Meyn LA, et al. Efficacy and safety of vaginal estriol and progesterone in postmenopausal women with atrophic vaginitis. *Menopause.* 2009 April [Epub ahead of print].
5. Bachmann G, Bouchard C, Hoppe D, et al. Efficacy and safety of low-dose regimens of conjugated estrogens cream administered vaginally. *Menopause.* 2009 June [Epub ahead of print].
6. Livengood CH. Bacterial vaginosis: an overview. *Rev Obstet Gynecol.* 2009;2:28–37.
7. McClelland RS, Richardson BA, Hassan WM, et al. Prospective study of vaginal bacterial flora and other risk factors for vulvovaginal candidiasis. *J Infect Dis.* 2009; 199:1883–1890.
8. Mills EJ, Perri D, Cooper C, et al. Antifungal treatment for invasive candida infections: A mixed treatment comparison meta-analysis. *Ann Clin Microbiol Antimicrob.* 2009; 8:23.
9. Peixoto F, Camargos A, Duarte G, Linhares I, Bahamondes L, Petracco A. Efficacy and tolerance of metronidazole and miconazole nitrate in treatment of vaginitis. *Int J Gynaecol Obstet.* 2008;102:287–292.
10. Huppert JS. Trichomoniasis in teens: an update. *Curr Opin Obstet Gynecol.* 2009 May [Epub ahead of print].

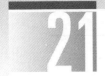

# Menorrhagia and Abnormal Vaginal Bleeding

## Deborah S. Lyon

Most gynecology textbooks begin a discussion of abnormal vaginal bleeding by first carefully outlining the endocrinology of normal bleeding and then detailing various pathologic conditions that can lead to menorrhagia. In addition, most texts clearly distinguish pregnancy-related bleeding from other vaginal bleeding problems and (depending on whether it is an obstetric or a gynecologic text) concentrate on only one of those categories.

For the emergency department (ED) physician, however, the proper focus is the patient and the chief complaint. This is one of many processes in which the initial focus should be stabilization and appropriate categorization (i.e., obstetric, gynecologic, or gastrointestinal) with later emphasis on more precise diagnosis and pathology-specific therapy.

## INITIAL EVALUATION AND STABILIZATION

Vaginal bleeding is a common ED complaint and may represent anything from a catastrophic, life-threatening hemorrhage to a normal menstrual period in an anxious patient. An algorithm for patient assessment is presented in Fig. 21.1. To begin an assessment of the severity of the bleeding, the most helpful starting point is the patient's vital signs. Of particular importance is the pulse rate, because many young patients demonstrate a hyperdynamic pulse well before blood pressure is affected. Some patients can tolerate remarkable anemia with relatively unchanged vital signs, but this generally occurs when bleeding is of a chronic nature. Acute bleeding episodes of hemodynamic consequence manifest themselves in vital signs before blood counts, and these should be the foundation of the initial assessment. If the vital signs point to an acute and profound process, the patient should be managed as a trauma patient, with large-bore intravenous lines, fluid resuscitation, and rapid transfusion.

The patient's history is extremely important. Even though patients tend to exaggerate blood loss, semiquantitative evaluations such as pad counts and days of bleeding can be helpful in determining whether a vaginal bleeding episode is of clinical consequence. Of special concern is a patient whose stated history suggests less blood loss than her vital signs or her complete blood count (CBC) does; these patients may have a known problem, such as uterine leiomyomata, with a second hidden problem, such as gastrointestinal bleeding. Alternatively, the patient with an impressive history but normal vital signs may, in fact, be well compensated, and the CBC may be a better diagnostic tool.

While collecting the vaginal bleeding history, particularly if the report does not seem to accurately reflect the clinical picture, information that might elucidate other sources of bleeding should be sought. This might include gastrointestinal symptoms, hematuria, a history of liver disease or chronic illness, and a family history of blood dyscrasia.

## EXAMINATION OF A PATIENT WITH VAGINAL BLEEDING

Many women are reluctant to be examined when they are actively bleeding, although in the case of an ED visit, this is less often a problem. Nonetheless, it is helpful to explain to the patient what you hope to accomplish by performing a

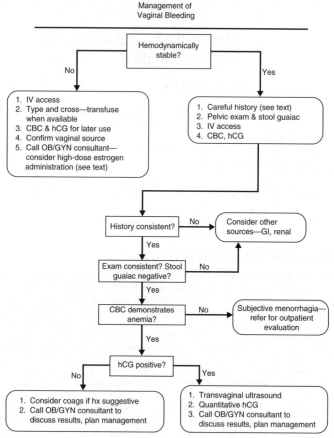

Management of
Vaginal Bleeding

Hemodynamically
stable?

No

Yes

1. IV access
2. Type and cross—transfuse
   when available
3. CBC & hCG for later use
4. Confirm vaginal source
5. Call OB/GYN consultant—
   consider high-dose estrogen
   administration (see text)

1. Careful history (see text)
2. Pelvic exam & stool guaiac
3. IV access
4. CBC, hCG

History consistent?    No    Consider other
                             sources—GI, renal

Yes

Exam consistent? Stool    No
guaiac negative?

Yes

CBC demonstrates    No    Subjective menorrhagia—
anemia?                   refer for outpatient
                          evaluation

Yes

hCG positive?

No    Yes

1. Consider coags if hx suggestive
2. Call OB/GYN consultant to
   discuss results, plan management

1. Transvaginal ultrasound
2. Quantitative hCG
3. Call OB/GYN consultant to
   discuss results, plan management

**FIGURE 21.1** Menorrhagia and abnormal vaginal bleeding.

pelvic examination. This includes confirming the source of the bleeding, evaluating for areas of active bleeding, inspecting for anatomic abnormalities such as cervical lesions or large leiomyomata uteri, and evaluating for abdominal tenderness. In addition, a Hemoccult test should always be performed on a stool sample obtained with a fresh glove to avoid possible cross-contamination from the vagina.

Conventional medical practice places the performance of an examination before obtaining laboratory tests. It is helpful, however, to know the results of a urine pregnancy test before examining the patient, because it may focus the physical examination on a more narrow, differential diagnosis.

A detailed examination is important. Abdominal tenderness should be noted. Even in the absence of pregnancy or trauma, intra-abdominal bleeding is possible (as in the case of a ruptured corpus luteum cyst or diverticulum). Active bleeding should be recorded, as should a quantification of the amount of blood in the vault. Point sources of bleeding should be sought. The cervix should be carefully inspected for lesions as well as possible extruding products of conception. A bimanual pelvic examination should make a faithful attempt to identify the uterine size, recognizing that operator inexperience and patient body habitus may limit the utility of this step. Examiners who are not comfortable with the convention of sizing in comparison to weeks of pregnancy may use fruit (orange, grapefruit, honeydew, and watermelon) or sports equipment (golf ball, tennis ball, baseball, and basketball) to describe findings. Adnexal masses should be sought; although if ectopic pregnancy is on the differential diagnosis list, a vigorous adnexal examination is discouraged. Finally, a thorough rectal examination should be performed, with attention to palpable lesions, as well as Hemoccult testing.

## ANCILLARY TESTING TO EVALUATE VAGINAL BLEEDING

Two laboratory tests are critical in the evaluation and management of vaginal bleeding: a CBC and a qualitative human chorionic gonadotropin (hCG) measurement. A quantitative hCG test is not necessary to establish the diagnosis of pregnancy, because most commercial qualitative kits are sensitive to 25 IU. Most ectopic pregnancies do not become symptomatic until the hCG level reaches four-digit numbers, so a negative qualitative hCG makes ectopic pregnancy unlikely. Little diagnostic refinement and much delay result from conducting a quantitative test. There is a place for the quantitative test but not in the initial evaluation.

The CBC is useful in differentiating patients who are hemodynamically compromised from those who are well but concerned. Experienced gynecologists may be surprised when, in the course of an outpatient evaluation of vaginal bleeding, they encounter a hemoglobin of 5 or 6. These numbers occur in patients whose menorrhagia is long-standing and who are relatively well compensated but, nevertheless, require prompt therapy. By the same token, it is common for a woman to be seen in the ED with menorrhagia as her chief complaint, yet her hemoglobin is 12 or 13. In the event of an impressively acute history and an examination compatible with profound acute loss, this hemoglobin may be thought of as spurious, because blood loss takes time to be reflected in the blood count. If the history and examination are less impressive, however, the patient may be assumed to be stable. It is important in this setting to validate the patient's concern, which may be legitimate in light of her past experience, while still providing her the reassurance she needs to pursue a more problem-specific outpatient evaluation.

The hCG serves a much more direct purpose. As mentioned earlier, many texts consider vaginal bleeding exclusively within the context of a positive or a negative hCG. A positive hCG demands a relatively immediate diagnosis, because therapy may be immediately necessary and will be tailored to the diagnosis.

If the hCG is positive for pregnancy, the likelihood is that either the pregnancy is intrauterine and threatening to abort or it is ectopically located. Physical examination may make this distinction, because incomplete spontaneous abortions often are seen with an open os and with tissue extruding. If physical examination is unrevealing, the next step in the workup is to identify the gestational age with reasonable assurance. This can sometimes be accomplished if the patient can confidently establish the date of her last menstrual period; often, laboratory testing is required. It is in this setting that a quantitative hCG is useful. Although not an accurate measure of gestational age per se, this test provides information regarding the quantity of hormone being produced, which is an indirect measure of fetal age as well as viability. The primary value of this test in the acute setting is in the context of the *discriminatory zone*. This is a level above which a pregnancy, if intrauterine, can confidently be expected to be of such mass and development that it will be apparent on ultrasound. For most institutions with transvaginal ultrasound capability, this number ranges from 1,500 to 2,500 IU (see Chapter 3). If the facility has only transabdominal ultrasound capability, the range jumps to approximately 6,500 IU, and many ectopic pregnancies will have already ruptured by that level. Thus, the ability to detect ectopic pregnancies early and to manage them optimally is dependent on the presence of both quantitative hCG and transvaginal ultrasound capability.

A full bladder is not required for a transvaginal probe scan. This is helpful, because many patients find it difficult to fill their bladders sufficiently to form a good acoustic window for a first-trimester scan. However, when necessary, the bladder can be filled by administering intravenous fluids or placing a transurethral catheter that fills it retrograde.

Having emphasized the importance of technology in discriminating between intrauterine and extrauterine pregnancies, it should be repeated that this distinction can often be made on clinical grounds alone. Thus, the physical examination should always precede the ordering of a quantitative hCG or transvaginal probe ultrasound.

## MANAGEMENT OF VAGINAL BLEEDING WITH A POSITIVE PREGNANCY TEST

Pregnancies with a quantitative hCG below the discriminatory zone must be evaluated strictly on clinical criteria. Certainly, an acute abdomen or a hemodynamically significant bleed must be addressed. On the other hand, a less significant bleed may be managed by observation and repeat quantitative hCG testing in 48 to 72 hours. This follow-up is best done by on obstetric care provider, and transfer of care may be arranged by telephone from the ED. It is important from a liability perspective that the ED provider documents explaining the differential diagnosis to the patient, along with the importance of keeping follow-up evaluation appointments. If the patient is stable, management of ectopic pregnancy may be conservative (methotrexate): otherwise, management should be surgical. Management of a spontaneous abortion may include dilation and curettage versus expectant management with close follow-up (Chapters 3 and 8).

## MANAGEMENT OF VAGINAL BLEEDING WITH A NEGATIVE PREGNANCY TEST

If the pregnancy test is negative, follow-up is determined by the patient's clinical condition. In terms of additional testing, a coagulation profile may be considered if the patient has a history or stigmata of liver disease, has a family history of blood dyscrasia, or is an adolescent just beginning menstruation (a time when many bleeding disorders are diagnosed). It is probably not cost effective in other settings. A patient with profound hemodynamic changes, a very low hemoglobin, or brisk bleeding is best managed by admission, whereas a less acute blood loss may easily be managed by prompt outpatient evaluation.

Acute bleeding in the nonpregnant patient is managed by liberal use of intravenous fluid replacement and blood products. Products other than packed red cells should be reserved for use in accordance with institutional protocols rather than by a preset formula. Appropriate indications for replacement of platelets or cryoprecipitate might be a diagnosed dyscrasia, need for immediate surgery, or ongoing bleeding not responding to other medical management (listed below).

There have been many proposed interventions to stop uterine bleeding in the nonpregnant patient. The most common of these is high-dose estrogen, either intravenously or orally (1–3). Estrogen increases coagulation factors V and IX, increases platelet aggregation, and decreases capillary permeability. In addition, estrogen promotes rapid growth of the endometrium, thereby stabilizing bleeding at denuded surfaces. Older literature emphasized the use of intravenous preparations of up to 25 mg every 6 hours. More recent review shows lower and oral doses to be equally efficacious, and intravenous administration is largely limited to patients not tolerating oral intake or for whom oral estrogens induce profound nausea. Even though the possibility of an underlying estrogen-sensitive neoplasia is of concern, achieving hemodynamic stability takes priority. Once bleeding has been stopped, endometrial biopsy can be performed if indicated.

Oral estrogen use is less standardized than intravenous, and many regimens exist for its use. At our institution, we prescribe a 35-$\mu$g pill and instruct the patient to take four pills per day for 4 days, three pills per day for 3 days, two pills per day for 2 days, and then finish the remaining pack at one pill per day. The patient must be specifically instructed to discard the placebo pills in the first pack of pills. This tapered dose is intended to allow endometrial and hemodynamic restoration before estrogen withdrawal leads to another bleeding episode. It is highly effective in treating the acute bleeding episode. It is then up to the gynecologic provider to begin evaluation of the source of the bleeding and its optimal control.

Massive bleeding generally occurs in the setting of a cervical or endometrial malignancy, a prolapsing or necrosing fibroid, or a recent intervention such as curettage of an infected uterus. In any case, when the several hours necessary to achieve control through use of estrogen does not appear to be a viable option, four emergent options are available. The first is packing, either of the vagina, if bleeding is primarily cervical, or of the uterine cavity, if bleeding is coming from the uterus. Packing should be done with the goal of putting pressure on every bleeding point, so attention should be given to completely reaching all crevices with the packing material. This may be either ordinary laparotomy sponges or balloons such as a Foley catheter or ablation balloon. Various hemostatic agents have been used in association with the packing. One report from Jamaica described soaking the packing with formaldehyde (4), although at our institution we have used Monsel solution. This is readily available wherever colposcopy is performed and does not have the exposure risks associated with formaldehyde.

The second option is emergent endometrial ablation. This requires an anatomically intact cervical canal, so it cannot be used in cases of bulky tumor or prolapsing fibroid. Ablation can be done fairly quickly and has become quite routine as a management option for more indolent bleeding problems, but a case report has been published showing efficacy in the emergency setting (5), and there is some evidence of durable benefit even in cases of natural or iatrogenic (overanticoagulation) coagulopathies(6).

The third option, transported from more routine menorrhagia management into emergent management, is uterine artery embolization. This is not available at many institutions, and even where interventional radiology capabilities are present, the radiologist must be willing to respond emergently. This limits the utility of embolization. When used, however, it can be extremely successful and may also be employed even in the face of common dyscrasias such as disseminated intravascular coagulopathy and von Willebrand's disease. Response is quite rapid, and in experienced hands, the complication rate is relatively low. In the one retrospective series of embolizations, fertility appeared to be spared despite occlusion of both uterine arteries (7), although pregnancy is not recommended due to case reports of growth restriction and other vasculopathy-related complications of pregnancies subsequent to uterine artery embolization (8).

Finally, emergent hysterectomy may be required. Packing will usually provide enough time to call in appropriate surgical support and transport the patient to the operating theater. Except in the immediate postpartum period, the requirement for a truly emergent hysterectomy is relatively uncommon.

In summary, management of vaginal bleeding is as follows:

Assess vital signs
Take a thorough history
Perform a rapid qualitative hCG test
Perform a thorough physical examination with stool guaiac
Obtain a CBC and, if indicated, coagulation studies
If indicated, order a quantitative hCG and transvaginal ultrasound
Control bleeding, if necessary, via fluid resuscitation, transfusion, surgical intervention (dilation and curettage for incomplete abortion and laparoscopy or laparotomy for intra-abdominal hemorrhage), mechanical tamponade, and pharmaceutical management.

## LONG-TERM MANAGEMENT GOALS IN MENORRHAGIA

Control of heavy vaginal bleeding is readily achieved in the acute setting by use of the aforementioned steps. In the patient who is not pregnant and who does not have a vaginal or cervical laceration (the true menorrhagia patient), bleeding tends to recur unless long-term management goals are established. Although these are frequently undertaken in the gynecologist's office, the possible outcomes and goals are of interest to the ED physician for two reasons. First, it is important to know what potential options the patient may have, so that she may be appropriately counseled. There should be no need for the frustrated patient in the gynecologist's office saying, "But the emergency doctor told me I needed a hysterectomy," when the gynecologist has simply prescribed an increase in the patient's thyroid medication dose. Second, there may be a relatively high rate of return to the ED in some populations, particularly in urban indigent care centers (9). Thus, the ED physician becomes de facto part of the patient's continuity care team. Understanding the therapeutic plan provides considerable assistance in dealing with recidivism.

Management of menorrhagia depends on its source. There are four common areas of possible dysfunction leading to menorrhagia (Table 21.1). Thinking in terms of these compartments allows an orderly workup and management of the patient's bleeding.

### Cytologic/Architectural Bleeding

Bleeding of cytologic/architectural origin includes cervical and uterine cancers, as well as endometritis, leiomyomata, and polyps. Diagnostic evaluation mandated for all menorrhagia patients starts with a Papanicolaou smear and endometrial biopsy. If there are any suspicious lesions on the cervix, they should be biopsied as part of the initial evaluation. Cervical cytology is designed as a screening tool and carries a relatively high false-negative rate (10), so it should not replace visual inspection and biopsy of abnormal-appearing areas. Large leiomyomata should be appreciable on bimanual examination, but significant menorrhagia may result from relatively small fibroids if they are submucous. Thus, a sonohysterogram may be helpful. This involves cannulating the cervix and injecting sterile saline into the uterine cavity while performing ultrasound. An acoustic window is developed by the sterile saline, which clearly demonstrates intracavitary lesions. These may then be managed via hysteroscopic resection versus hysterectomy, depending on the size of the lesion and the childbearing wishes of the patient. Uterine artery embolization has become a well-accepted alternative

| TABLE 21.1 | Causes of Menorrhagia |
|---|---|

**Architectural/Cytologic**
  Cervical cancer
  Endometrial cancer/hyperplasia
  Endometritis
  Leiomyomata
  Polyp
  Cervical trauma

**Endocrine**
  Polycystic ovarian syndrome
  Excessive exogenous estrogen use
  Excessive endogenous estrogen production or storage (ovarian tumor and obesity)
  Hypothyroidism
  Hyperthyroidism
  Hyperprolactinemia
  Hypothalamic—major changes in weight or exercise status, perimenopause

**Systemic**
  Hemophilia
  von Willebrand's disease
  Thrombocytopenia (idiopathic or autoimmune)
  Leukemia
  Pancytopenia (immunosuppression, chemotherapy, and bone marrow suppression)
  Anticoagulation (iatrogenic)

**Idiopathic Menorrhagia**

to surgery in many instances and is an ideal option for patients with increased surgical risks. Its primary drawback, as noted above, is the requirement for a skilled interventional radiologist, which may not be possible in all areas. Malignancies must be staged, and management may include surgery or radiation.

### Endocrine Bleeding

Bleeding of endocrine origin includes polycystic ovarian syndrome and hypothalamic/pituitary disorders. Menorrhagia is typically associated with estrogen excess, whereas estrogen deficiency may cause amenorrhea or irregular spotting. This explains why many patients on depot medroxyprogesterone for contraception spot irregularly (progestins stabilize estrogen exposure and, at high doses, may be considered relatively antiestrogenic). Hypothalamic/pituitary disorders most often fall into the hypoestrogenic category, so that anorectics, athletes, and patients with prolactinomas rarely have menorrhagia. Polycystic ovarian syndrome, on the other hand, is a relatively hyperestrogenic state. These patients often have very irregular periods and may only bleed once or twice a year, but those periods may be of profound hemodynamic consequence. Although the chain of endocrine events behind this syndrome is complex, the critical issue in this context is the loss of cyclic hormonal surges and suppressions in the face of normal or supranormal amounts of estrogen. The regular withdrawal bleeding that should be induced by an appropriate pattern of hormone secretion is lost, but estrogen continues to stimulate endometrial cell proliferation. Thus, a very thick endometrium is developed, which eventually outgrows its blood supply, causing sloughing and menorrhagia.

Endocrine bleeding is often a diagnosis of exclusion, presumed to be the source of menorrhagia when no architectural/cytologic abnormality is identified. Two blood tests are important, however, to make specific diagnoses. These are prolactin and thyroid-stimulating hormone levels. Hypothyroidism and hyperthyroidism can cause menorrhagia by influencing the feedback loop to the hypothalamus, driving follicle-stimulating hormone and luteinizing hormone levels up. Prolactin may be artifactually elevated in this case, so thyroid disease should always be sought and treated before evaluation for a prolactinoma. Hyperprolactinemia in the absence of thyroid disease is fairly common in women of reproductive age and is often treatable by simple means, so testing for it should not be overlooked.

Virtually all sources of endocrine bleeding problems are managed similarly in the patient not desiring immediate pregnancy. The use of oral contraceptives suppresses and eliminates the need for regular signals from the hypothalamic–pituitary–ovarian axis and provides regular hormonal stimulation and withdrawal, so that an orderly bleeding pattern can be developed. Most patients with exclusively endocrine-mediated bleeding problems are able to establish a normal bleeding pattern on an oral contraceptive regimen without the need for surgical intervention, and it is currently a standard of care in the gynecologic community to attempt medical management of bleeding before undertaking surgical management. Medical management may also be attempted if the patient has fibroids, because it is not uncommon for a patient to have both architectural and endocrine abnormalities. Upon correction of the endocrine abnormalities, the architectural distortion may become clinically irrelevant (11).

An exception to the rule of oral contraceptive use is in the case of the patient with high prolactin levels (12). These patients may have pituitary macroadenomas, and further imaging is indicated to rule out extrinsic compression of the sella turcica or optic chiasm. A more specific treatment such as bromocriptine may be indicated instead of or in addition to oral contraceptives in these patients. A second category of patients who should not receive oral contraceptives is those for whom they are relatively contraindicated (13). This includes patients with a history of prior deep venous thrombosis, severe hepatic disease, or cerebrovascular accident, as well as obese women, hypertensives, and smokers older than 35 years (because estrogen, age, and each of these are multiplicative risk factors for thrombogenesis). For these patients, menorrhagia can be effectively controlled with depot medroxyprogesterone, but there is a high likelihood of persistent spotting. Long-term use of high-dose progestins has also been associated with early onset of osteopenia, so the benefits of medical therapy must be weighed against its risks. Recent evidence supports use of local progestin therapy in the form of the levonorgestrel-releasing intrauterine system (Mirena®) for excellent long-term control of abnormal uterine bleeding with minimal side effects and a high degree of patient satisfaction (14,15).

## SYSTEMIC CAUSES OF BLEEDING

The third category of menorrhagia sources is systemic. The most obvious are the bleeding dyscrasias. Congenital bleeding disorders may be diagnosed in a young teenager who is seen for a life-threatening hemorrhage from her first period. Many of these patients are proven to have von Willebrand's disease (relatively common) or a variant of hemophilia (extremely uncommon). It is rare to diagnose congenital coagulopathies in older patients, but secondary coagulopathies from liver disease or bone marrow suppression should not be overlooked if the patient's history is suggestive. Appropriate diagnosis depends on a high index of suspicion, because clotting function testing is not recommended routinely. A special subset of this category is the iatrogenic menorrhagia caused by anticoagulation therapy. It is not unusual for a patient on warfarin therapy to have very heavy bleeding, particularly if she becomes overanticoagulated. The best management for this type of bleeding is to hold one or more doses of warfarin and adjust the desired therapeutic window downward. It is rare for coagulopathies to require surgical intervention. The primary mechanism of hemostasis in menstruation is mechanical (constriction of the myometrial muscle) rather than hematologic. Menstrual bleeding in these patients is often a nuisance but not of profound hemodynamic consequence. This is particularly important to remember, because these patients are obviously suboptimal operative candidates as well.

## IDIOPATHIC MENORRHAGIA

The fourth category of menorrhagia is idiopathic. This is a diagnosis of exclusion made when architectural abnormalities are ruled out and the patient fails to resume a normal bleeding pattern when exposed to three or more cycles of oral contraceptive management. These patients may have very high endogenous levels of estrogen or simply endometrial receptors that are exquisitely sensitive to estrogen. This is an uncommon category, and most patients who complain of persistent menorrhagia after exclusion of the aforementioned diagnoses are found to have a normal hemoglobin. Thus, it is the perception of the patient that her menstruation is excessive, but objectively, she is maintaining adequate hematopoiesis. These patients can be demanding; nevertheless, a policy of nonintervention is in the physician's best interest, because any untoward outcome from therapy is likely to be weighed against the therapeutic benefit of the therapy. The ED physician should keep in mind that repetitive somatic complaints, particularly gynecologic ones, have been associated with a history of or current domestic violence in some studies (16–18). Sensitively offered questions on this topic may allow appropriate diagnosis and referral.

If the objective findings support the patient's claim of menorrhagia, she may be offered endometrial ablation versus hysterectomy. Endometrial ablation may also be appropriate for the patient with endocrine problems discussed earlier but should be undertaken with caution in that category, because ablation does not destroy all the endometrial glands, and the continued hyperestrogenic state may increase the patient's risk of subsequent endometrial carcinoma. Ablation should only be undertaken in women who have no further childbearing desires, and its long-term success rate (measured as no further need for intervention) is approximately 60% to 85%, with typical short-term satisfaction rates in the range of 90% to 95% (19). Levonorgestrel-releasing intrauterine systems may be a highly satisfactory choice in the setting of iatrogenic menorrhagia as well (14,15).

## SUMMARY

In summary, menorrhagia may be due to any of several causes, which should be sought and treated specifically. Even though removal of the endometrium via hysterectomy ultimately solves all cases of uterine bleeding, this treatment is imprecise at best and carries a significant risk of iatrogenic morbidity. With a little patience and a small armamentarium of tests, the physician can confidently establish a diagnosis and undertake specific treatment. Surgical management should be reserved for the patient who will clearly not respond well to more conservative management. This includes the patient with significant anatomic distortion or high-grade cytologic derangements, the patient who has failed medical management, and the patient whose compliance with medical management is poor enough that she is repetitively exposed to major hemodynamic insults.

## References

1. DeVore GR, Odell O, Kase N. Use of intravenous Premarin in the treatment of dysfunctional uterine bleeding: a double-blind randomized control study. *Obstet Gynecol.* 1982;59:285–291.
2. Bayer SR, DeCherney AH. Clinical manifestations and treatment of dysfunctional uterine bleeding. *JAMA.* 1993;269:1823–1828.
3. Chuong CJ, Brenner PF. Management of abnormal uterine bleeding. *Am J Obstet Gynecol.* 1996;175:787–792.
4. Fletcher H, Wharfe G, Mitchell S, Simon T. Treatment of intractable vaginal bleeding with formaldehyde soaked packs. *J Obstet Gynecol.* 2002;22(5):570.
5. Nichols CM, Gill EJ. Thermal balloon endometrial ablation for management of acute uterine hemorrhage. *Obstet Gynecol.* 2002;100:1092–1094.
6. El-Nashar SA, Hopkins MR, Feitoza SS, et.al. Global endometrial ablation for menorrhagia in women with bleeding disorders. *Obstet Gynecol.* 2007;109:1381–1387.
7. Ornan D, White R, Pollak J, Tal M. Pelvic embolization for intractable postpartum hemorrhage: long-term follow-up and implications for fertility. *Obstet Gynecol.* 2003; 102:904.
8. Usadi RS, Marshburn PB. The impact of uterine artery embolization on fertility and pregnancy outcome. *Curr Opin Obstet Gynecol.* 2007;19(3):279–283.
9. Lyon DS, Ballard L, Jones JL. A retrospective review of inpatients with menometrorrhagia: etiologies, treatments, and outcomes. *South Med J.* 2000;93(6):571–574.
10. DiSaia PJ, Creasman WT, eds. *Clinical Gynecologic Oncology.* 5th Ed. St. Louis, MO: Mosby; 1997.
11. ACOG Practice Bulletin No. 96. Alternatives to hysterectomy in the management of leiomyomas. August 2008.
12. Speroff L, Glass RH, Kase NG, eds. *Clinical Gynecologic Endocrinology and Infertility.* 5th Ed. Philadelphia, PA: Williams & Wilkins; 1994.
13. ACOG Practice Bulletin No. 73. Use of hormonal contraception in women with coexisting medical conditions. June 2006.
14. Rauramo I, Elo I, Istre O. Long-term treatment of menorrhagia with levonorgestrel intrauterine system versus endometrial resection. *Obstet Gynecol.* 2004;104: 1314–1321.
15. Busfield RA, Farquhar CM, Sowter MC, et.al. A randomised trial comparing the levonorgestrel intrauterine system and thermal balloon ablation for heavy menstrual bleeding. *BJOG.* 2006;113:257–263.
16. Fillingim RB, Wilkinson CS, Powell T. Self-reported abuse history and pain complaints among young adults. *Clin J Pain.* 1999;15(2):85–91.
17. Jamieson DJ, Steege JF. The association of sexual abuse with pelvic pain complaints in a primary care population. *Am J Obstet Gynecol.* 1997;177(6):1408–1412.
18. Reiter RC, Shakerin LR, Gainbone JC, et al. Correlation between sexual abuse and somatization in women with somatic and nonsomatic chronic pelvic pain. *Am J Obstet Gynecol.* 1991;165(1):104–109.
19. Feitoza SS, Gebhart JB, Gostout BS, Wilson TO, Cliby WA. Efficacy of thermal balloon ablation in patients with abnormal uterine bleeding. *Am J Obstet Gynecol.* 2003; 189:453.

# Pelvic Mass

### Karl H.S. Smith

A pelvic mass in a female must always be considered in the context of other parameters. Is the woman symptomatic with abdominal pain and swelling, or has her mass been detected incidentally by an imaging study performed for another reason? What is her age, menstrual and pregnancy history? What has she been using for contraception? Has she had previous pelvic infection or surgery? Has she had any recent pain with sexual intercourse or change in urinary or bowel habits? The answer to each of these questions may have a bearing on determining the ultimate cause of a pelvic mass and lead a clinician through a logical and efficient process of evaluation.

## ASYMPTOMATIC PELVIC MASSES

In the 21st century in the United States, the plethora of imaging studies has made the incidental finding of a pelvic mass common. Abdominal and pelvic computerized tomograms (CT scans), sonograms, magnetic resonance imaging (MRI), and positron emission test (PET) scans are being performed with much more frequency than in the past. In 2006, it was estimated that over 60 million CT scans were performed in the United States (1). Sometimes these procedures are performed for nonspecific abdominal complaints or to evaluate urologic, intestinal, or orthopedic problems. Sometimes these tests are performed to further evaluate a known problem such as cancer. There is an increase in the performance of these imaging studies in asymptomatic women as part of a general executive health screening (2). Small asymptomatic cystic ovarian masses assessed on vaginal ultrasound to be <5 cm diameter without septae or nodularity within (simple cysts) may be followed with repeat vaginal sonography in several months time (3). Generally, asymptomatic masses that do not grow are considered benign. In reproductive age women not using hormonal contraception, a functional ovarian cyst (including hemorrhagic corpora lutea and dominant follicles) would be a common finding. Such cystic masses can sometimes be associated with uterine changes indicating an early pregnancy. In such cases, a pregnancy test is indicated. An adnexal mass imaged in a reproductive age woman with a positive pregnancy test and absence of an intrauterine gestational sac could be the first evidence of an early ectopic pregnancy. Management of ectopic pregnancy is covered in Chapter 3 of this book.

For the premenarchal female, an asymptomatic pelvic mass could represent a congenital anomaly involving the upper genital tract, urinary tract, vagina, or colon and rectum. Prior to the availability of sophisticated imaging studies such as sonography and CT scans, a pelvic kidney was commonly misdiagnosed as an ovarian mass. Although the finding of an asymptomatic pelvic mass in a premenarchal girl is not a medical emergency, further evaluation is appropriate. Some of the more common premenarchal conditions that could present as a pelvic mass in an infant or adolescent are as follows: hematocolpos from an imperforate hymen, uterine anomalies, ovarian germ cell or stromal neoplasia, and rarely, endometriomas or abscesses (4,5). Other information obtained by history and general physical examination will be helpful in determining an appropriate differential diagnosis. For example, the presence of precocious puberty with premature breast and pubic hair development or premature menarche may lead to the discovery of an ovarian stromal neoplasm. It is always prudent to consider simple problems such as urinary retention with a full bladder or constipation with a dilated colon or rectum as the cause of a so-called "asymptomatic pelvic mass" in a female child. Further elucidation is beyond the scope of this chapter. The reader is referred to well-documented previous works (6–8).

In reproductive-age women with an intact uterus, the most common asymptomatic pelvic mass after a functional ovarian cyst or early pregnancy is uterine leiomyoma. This occurs in 20% to 30% of women over 30 years of age (9) and is found in up to 75% of hysterectomy specimen (10). Leiomyoma is often discovered on routine screening pelvic examinations. Women with leiomyoma may have unrecognized symptoms of heavy menstrual periods and pelvic fullness with urinary frequency and/or constipation. The presence of uterine leiomyoma does not represent a medical emergency unless it is causing severe symptoms such as pain or uterine bleeding significant enough to cause acute anemia with decreased intravascular volume. A very large or rapidly growing leiomyoma may cause ureteral obstruction or hydronephrosis. The development of uterine leiomyosarcoma is a feared sequela of uterine leiomyoma. Fortunately, this is a rare condition that occurs in <1% of women with suspected leiomyoma (11). Occasionally, a pelvic mass that is thought to represent a leiomyoma is later determined to be an ovarian mass. If normal ovaries cannot be clearly identified in a women with a pelvic mass suspected to represent leiomyoma, additional studies including combined abdominal/vaginal ultrasound or MR of the pelvis should be considered.

The most feared pelvic mass is ovarian cancer. This is an insidious condition with a peak incidence among women in their mid 50s. Like uterine leiomyoma, women with ovarian cancer may experience abdominal fullness, swelling, or early satiety. As women go through menopause and stop menstruating, uterine leiomyoma tend to get smaller, but ovarian masses may continue to grow. Fortunately, most ovarian neoplasms are benign with cystic teratomas being the most common (12). Like leiomyoma, benign ovarian tumors may reach great size, distorting the abdominal contour while causing little in the way of symptoms.

Ovarian masses that are detected during routine prenatal sonograms are particularly challenging. Ovarian masses are detected in approximately 6% of pregnancies during routine obstetrical sonography (13,14). Most of these resolve representing physiologic cysts of pregnancy. Those that persist may cause the same complications seen in nonpregnant women (e.g., torsion, rupture, or hemorrhage), but these events are uncommon. Approximately 2% of ovarian masses detected during pregnancy will prove to be malignant and most of these are stage 1 (15). In the past, persistent adnexal masses in pregnancy were managed surgically in the second trimester between 14 and 20 weeks' gestation. Masses detected later were managed by elective cesarean delivery at term followed by surgical management of the ovarian mass. Within the past decade, there has been a trend toward a more conservative management with careful sonographic monitoring allowing vaginal delivery and then management of the mass weeks to months after delivery (15–18).

As previously noted, ovarian cancer is the most dreaded cancer of the female reproductive tract because of its insidious and lethal nature. In 2008, it was estimated that 21,650 women in the United States would develop this cancer and 15,520 would die (19). With serous ovarian cancer, the most common type of malignant ovarian epithelial cancer, the ovarian neoplasia may grow as an ovarian mass, spread by direct extension to the peritoneal cavity or other structures in the abdomen and pelvis or development of ascites causing subtle symptoms of bloating and indigestion. These symptoms can be misinterpreted as a primary gastrointestinal (GI) problem. It is not uncommon for a woman to present with ovarian cancer claiming to have no "gynecologic symptoms," yet she has seen an internist or gastroenterologist for intestinal "problems." It is not uncommon to have a woman undergo an upper and a lower GI imaging or endoscopy prior to having a pelvic examination or a pelvic sonogram. According to Goff et al. (20), early symptoms associated with the subsequent diagnosis of ovarian cancer consisted of pelvic or abdominal pain, urinary urgency or frequency, increased abdominal size or bloating, and difficulty eating or feeling full.

Common causes of asymptomatic nonovarian pelvic masses in premenopausal women are abnormalities of the fallopian tubes such as hydrosalpinx and paraovarian cysts. These conditions can often be diagnosed by transvaginal ultrasound, and in most cases, expectant management is appropriate. Other less common conditions of the ovary that can present as an asymptomatic pelvic mass are polycystic ovaries, hyperstimulated ovaries, and, occasionally, an ovarian abscess. These conditions will usually be associated with other suggestive findings in the history and the physical examination leading the clinician to make an appropriate diagnosis. Unfortunately, a final diagnosis sometimes cannot be made without surgery such as a diagnostic laparoscopy.

## SYMPTOMATIC PELVIC MASS

While asymptomatic pelvic masses are concerning, they rarely present as a medical emergency. Symptomatic pelvic masses are of greater concern because they may represent a serious or even life-threatening situation. One of the most common symptomatic conditions in a reproductive age female is abdominal pain due to ovulation or a ruptured corpus luteum. Rupture of a cyst, though painful, is usually self-limiting and not life threatening. The diagnosis is usually one of the exclusions, and in cases of severe, unrelenting pain, confirmation may require surgical intervention by laparoscopy.

The most serious symptomatic condition in a reproductive age female is an ectopic pregnancy. Despite advances in imaging technology in the 21st century, ectopic pregnancies are still misdiagnosed resulting in serious and sometimes fatal consequences. The importance of obtaining a pregnancy test in a reproductive age women with abdominal pain and menstrual irregularity cannot be over emphasized (see Chapter 3).

After ectopic pregnancy, the most serious symptomatic pelvic mass is a tuboovarian abscess. This usually occurs in a setting of pelvic inflammatory disease as discussed in Chapter 19 of this book. These masses will usually resolve with medical management but will occasionally require surgical intervention.

The next most serious symptomatic pelvic mass is the torsed adnexa. Adnexal torsion has been found to account for about 3% of surgical emergencies in women (21). Adnexal enlargement on sonography in the presence of abdominal pain and a negative pregnancy test should point to ovarian torsion in the differential diagnosis. These findings indicate the need to consider surgical intervention by laparoscopy or laparotomy (see Chapter 23).

The differential diagnosis of a pelvic mass with abdominal pain must also include endometrioma, appendicitis, and colonic diverticulitis. Endometriosis may be associated with a history of progressive dysmenorrhea leading to the presenting episode. Sonographic features of the ovary are also distinctive with the hemorrhagic ovarian cyst and endometrioma showing a ground-glass appearance and sometimes a fluid and solid interface within the ovarian mass where blood has clotted and layered. An ovarian abscess may have nonspecific solid and cystic sonographic features that could be confused with an ovarian malignancy. A pelvic infection often occurs after a menstrual period and may be associated with cervical motion tenderness, fever, and elevated white blood count (WBC). These same findings may be present in a woman with a diverticular abscess. In this case, a history of progressively worsening constipation may be significant and may lead to the diagnosis. Often, a sonogram will not be sufficient to establish a diagnosis, and additional imaging studies such as a CT scan with oral, intravenous (IV), and rectal contrast may need to be considered. If pain persists and the WBC rises, surgical evaluation by laparoscopy may need to be considered.

A uterine disorder is the most common cause of a symptomatic midline pelvic mass. After pregnancy, symptomatic uterine leiomyoma are most common. Rapidly growing or cystically degenerated leiomyoma is a common cause of midline mass with pain. Adenomyosis often occurs in the presence of uterine leiomyoma leading to heavy menstrual bleeding and pelvic pain. The timing of the pain is critical. If the uterus is infected due to pelvic inflammatory disease or endomyometritis, the picture may be confusing. Imaging studies such as pelvic sonograms and CT scans become critical. In this setting, endometrial biopsy may also help determine if an infection is present. WBC will usually be elevated in the presence of infection. Uterine cancer (endometrial or myometrial) or cervical cancer may rarely present as a painful midline pelvic mass. This will usually occur in a perimenopausal woman and be associated with abnormal bleeding. Pelvic examination and pelvic sonography are useful in establishing a diagnosis of uterine cancer; however, a final diagnosis cannot be established without histological evaluation of tissue from the endometrium or the cervix.

In women who have undergone a hysterectomy, the diagnosis of a midline symptomatic pelvic mass can be more challenging. Recent history of surgery such as a hysterectomy should lead to a differential that might include a hematoma or an abscess. With a more remote history of hysterectomy (over 6 months), the differential could include an ovarian or tubal mass in the cul-de-sac, endometrioma, inclusion cyst of the vaginal cuff, or malignancy of the bladder, colon, or rectum. Once again, simple problems such as cystitis with urinary retention and chronic constipation with fecal impaction must be considered. These conditions can usually be established by taking a careful history.

Rarely, symptomatic pelvic masses include metastatic disease to the ovary from cancers of the breast, colon, stomach, small intestine, kidneys, or lymphoma. The ovarian mass may be the first sign of cancer. Cancers metastatic to the ovary tend to be bilateral and solid; however, cystic lesions have been reported (22). A history of breast, GI, renal, or hematologic malignancy should raise suspicion of a metastatic process.

## UNUSUAL SITUATIONS PRESENTING AS A PELVIC MASS

The most common causes of pelvic mass have been described. To complete a discussion of the differential diagnosis of a pelvic mass, other diagnoses must be considered. These include neoplasic masses caused by retroperitoneal sarcomas, lymphomas, and retroperitoneal cysts. Pelvic inclusion cysts, which are not neoplastic, can occur in women who have undergone multiple intra-abdominal and/or pelvic surgeries. Radiated bowel can become agglutinated, forming a mass that is hard to distinguish from a neoplastic process on examination. Also, fluid-filled spaces may occur between loops of intestine simulating a cystic mass. Past history of pelvic surgery with lymph node dissection and a pelvic sidewall cyst could indicate the presence of a lymphocyst. Careful review of imaging studies will usually allow for a correct diagnosis. However, sometimes the correct diagnosis cannot be made until surgery. As noted previously, in the presence of abdominal pain, fever, and elevated WBC, it is sometimes hard to distinguish a

| TABLE 22.1 | Differential Diagnosis of Pelvic Masses |

| Gynecologic | Nongynecologic |
|---|---|
| **Uterus—benign** | Distended bladder |
| Pregnancy | Feces (impaction) |
| Leiomyoma | Pelvic kidney |
| Congenital anomalies | Urachal cyst |
|  | Urinoma |
| **Uterus—malignant** | Diverticular abscess |
| Cervical carcinoma | Appendiceal abscess |
| Endometrial carcinoma | Lymphoma |
| Sarcoma | Lymphocyst |
|  | Anterior sacral teratoma |
| **Ovary—benign** | Retroperitoneal fibrosis |
| Cystadenoma | Metastatic cancer |
| Follicle cyst | GI tumor |
| Sclerocystic ovary | Abdominal wall hematoma |
| Corpus luteum cyst | Abdominal wall radiation fibrosis |
| Endometriotic cyst |  |
| Germinal inclusion cyst |  |
| Theca-lutein cyst |  |
| Benign cystic teratoma (dermoid) |  |
| Ovarian hyperstimulation syndrome (OHSS) |  |
| **Ovary—malignant** |  |
| Epithelia carcinoma |  |
| Germ cell tumor |  |
| Gonadal stromal tumor |  |
| Metastatic cancer to ovary |  |
| **Fallopian tube** |  |
| Ectopic pregnancy |  |
| Hydrosalpinx |  |
| Paratubal cyst |  |
| Carcinoma |  |

right-sided ovarian abscess from a diverticular abscess or a left-side mass from a diverticular abscess. Other causes of pelvic cysts are listed in Table 22.1.

## METHODS OF EVALUATING A MASS

As mentioned earlier, asymptomatic masses are often detected by CT or MRI performed for another reason. For example, a pelvic or abdominal CT or MRI may be ordered to evaluate back pain and a pelvic mass will be discovered. Unfortunately, if only a pelvic CT or MRI is ordered, lower lung fields, diaphragm, liver, stomach, spleen, pancreas, omentum, much of the intestinal tract, and kidneys with upper ureters may not be visible. Sometimes, with very large masses, only the lower aspect of the mass will be seen. These are all sites that may be impacted by a primary ovarian cancer. An abdominal CT or MRI on the other hand often stops at the level of vertebral body L5 or S1 and misses important pelvic structures such as the uterus, bladder, rectosigmoid colon, and bony pelvis. If a complete survey of the abdomen and the pelvis is to be conducted, imaging of both the abdomen and the pelvis should be ordered when evaluating nonspecific symptoms. For general surveillance of the abdominal and pelvic organs, a CT scan is a better study than an MRI because imaging with the MRI occurs at a slower speed and results in more intestinal or respiratory motion and artifact. The MRI is better for evaluating bony structures. When ordering a CT, it is also prudent to use both oral and IV contrasts. This will allow intestinal and urologic structures to be more easily distinguished from vascular structures and muscles. IV contrast should generally be avoided in patients with a serum creatinine of 1.5 mg/dL to prevent contrast induced nephropathy.

If a mass is detected on pelvic examination and requires further characterization, a pelvic and abdominal sonogram may be more useful than a CT. The sonogram will allow for better characterization of the internal features of an ovarian mass such as septations or papillary features. As previously noted, ovarian masses that are simple (i.e., those containing no internal echoes such as septations, papillary features, or fluid layering) and 5 cm in diameter or less are rarely neoplasic (3). For large pelvic masses, sonographic evaluation of the kidneys and ureters can exclude hydronephrosis or hydroureter. An abdominal ultrasound will also allow ascites or free peritoneal blood to be identified. This is the strategy of the focused assessment with sonography for trauma (FAST scan) used by emergency department physicians and general surgeons in evaluating someone with pelvic trauma (23). Finding free fluid in the pelvis or abdomen following trauma warrants an emergency paracentesis. It is always prudent in the evaluation of a woman of menstrual age to consider a pregnancy condition as a source of hemoperitoneum, emphasizing the importance of performing a screening urine pregnancy test in this situation.

## MANAGEMENT OF PATIENTS WITH A MASS

Asymptomatic masses may usually be managed in an orderly fashion by referring the patient to a gynecologic surgeon and preparing for surgery. However, in a symptomatic patient, some urgency will ensue (Fig. 22.1). In patients with worrisome vital signs such as tachycardia and hypotension, IV hydration should be initiated and blood should be made ready in the blood bank (type and crossmatch). Basic laboratory tests should include a complete blood count (CBC) and basic metabolic profile (BMP) that includes serum electrolytes, glucose, blood urea nitrogen (BUN), and creatinine. If there is any concern about bleeding or liver disease, a coagulation screen consisting or prothrombin time (PT) and partial thromboplastin time (PTT) should be ordered. As noted previously, a urine pregnancy test is warranted in reproductive age women. The patient should be kept from eating or drinking as this can result in anesthetic complications. Depending on the status of the patient and time constraints, simple x-rays of the chest and the abdomen should be obtained (obstructive series). These tests will allow the gynecologic or general surgical consultant to rapidly take a patient to surgery if indicated. Air under the diaphragm suggests a perforated viscous and intestinal obstruction indicating the need for nasogastric tube placement. Both findings warrant consideration for more urgent surgical intervention.

In situations where the need for surgery is not emergent, additional procedures such as a bowel prep or thoracentesis for a pleural effusion might be considered. For patients with large pelvic masses, there is a possibility of respiratory compromise. In the presence of pleural effusion or marked abdominal distension due to ascites or a very large abdominal mass, arterial blood gases should be considered. Finally, attention should be directed to managing comorbid conditions such as diabetes, hypertension, or chronic obstructive pulmonary disease.

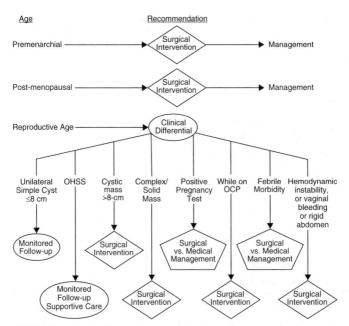

**FIGURE 22.1** Algorithm for symptomatic ovarian mass.

The gynecologic or general surgeon who decides to take a patient to surgery must determine the timing (emergent or urgent) and the best approach to surgery (laparoscopic versus open) and then the best type of incision. These decisions should be discussed with the patient. It is important for the surgeon to ask the patient about her future desires for fertility and to determine any limits on surgery. For example, a woman <40 years of age may wish to preserve her uterus for future fertility if possible. This issue becomes critical in situations where both ovaries are involved in a process such as infection, endometriosis, or cancer. Some patient would want the uterus removed if both ovaries were removed, while others would want the uterus preserved. Bilateral ovarian masses have a greater incidence of malignancy (24). Patients should be informed that sometimes the best solution to a particular situation cannot be determined prior to surgery. It should be determined if a patient desires conservative surgery even at the risk of requiring additional surgery in the future. Finally, it is important for the surgeon to explain that unforeseen circumstances may occur that necessitate surgery to the intestinal or urinary tract. This is especially important if there is a possibility that bowel resection or colostomy is necessary.

## SUMMARY

The diagnosis and management of a pelvic mass require taking a careful history of recent and past events, a thorough physical examination including a pelvic examination, and a selection of appropriate laboratory tests and imaging studies. The differential diagnosis should be discussed with the patient and her support system (family and/or friends) to determine the best course of treatment based on the most likely diagnosis, severity of symptoms, and desire for future fertility. Once a treatment plan is established, the plan should be implemented with efficiency and safety while maintaining communication with the patient and her family.

## References

1. Brenner DJ, Hall EJ. Computed tomography—an increasing source of radiation exposure. *N Engl J Med*. 2007;357:2277–2284.
2. Beinfeld MT, Wittenberg E, Gazelle GS. Cost-effectiveness of whole-body CT screening. *Radiology*. 2005;234:415–422.
3. Van Nagell JR, Depriest PD, Ueland FR, et al. Ovarian cancer screening with annual transvaginal sonography. *Cancer*. 2007;109:1887–1896.
4. Emans DP. Office evaluation of the child and adolescent. In: Emans SJH, Goldstein DP, eds. *Pediatric & Adolescent Gynecology*. 3rd Ed. Boston, Toronto, London: Little, Brown and Company; 1990.
5. Muram D. Developmental abnormalities. In: Copeland LJ, ed. *Textbook of Gynecology*. Philadelphia, PA: W.B. Saunders; 2000.
6. Emans SJH, Goldstein DP, eds. Ovarian masses. In: *Pediatric & Adolescent Gynecology*. 3rd Ed. Boston, Toronto, London: Little, Brown and Company; 1990.
7. Sanfiliippo JS. Pediatric and adolescent gynecology. In: Copeland LJ, ed. *Textbook of Gynecology*. Philadelphia, PA: W.B. Saunders; 2000.
8. BekiesiÅska-Figatowska M, Jurkiewicz E, Iwanowska B, et al. Magnetic resonance imaging as a diagnostic tool in case of ovarian masses in girls and young women. *Med Sci Monit*. 2007;13(Suppl. 1):116–120.
9. Zaloudek C, Hendrickson M. Mesenchymal tumors of the uterus. In: Kurman RJ, ed. *Blaustein's Pathology of the Female Genital Tract*. 5th Ed. New York, NY: Springer-Verlag; 2002.
10. Cramer SF, Patel A. The frequency of uterine leiomyomas. *Am J Clin Pathol*. 1990; 94(4):435–438.
11. Parker WH, Fu YS, Bereek JS. Uterine sarcoma in patients operated on for presumed leiomyoma and rapidly growing leiomyoma. *Obstet Gynecol*. 1994;83:414–417.
12. Koonings PP, Campbell K, Mishell DR Jr, Grimes DA. Relative frequency of primary ovarian neoplasms: a 10-year review. *Obstet Gynecol*. 1989;74(6):921–926.
13. Bernhard LM, Klebba PK, Gray DL, et al. Predictors of persistence of adnexal masses in pregnancy. *Obstet Gynecol*. 1999;93:585–589.
14. Condous G, Khalid A, Okaro E, et al. Should we be examining the ovaries in pregnancy? Prevalence and natural history of adnexal pathology detected at first-trimester sonography. *Ultrasound Obstet Gynecol*. 2004;24:62–66.
15. Leiserowitz GS, Xing G, Cress R, et al. Adnexal masses in pregnancy: how often are they malignant? *Gynecol Oncol*. 2006 May;101(2):315–321.
16. Schmeler KM, Mayo-Smith WW, Peipert JF, et al. Adnexal masses in pregnancy: surgery compared with observation. *Obstet Gynecol*. 2005;105:1098–1103.
17. Zanetta G, Mariani E, Lissoni A, et al. A prospective study of the role of ultrasound in the management of adnexal masses in pregnancy. *BJOG*. 2003;110(6):578–583.
18. Giuntoli RL, Vang RS, Bristow RE. Evaluation and management of adnexal masses during pregnancy. *Clin Obstet Gynecol*. 2006;49(3):492–505.
19. Jemal A, Siegel R, Ward E, et al. Cancer statistics, 2008. *CA Cancer J Clin*. 2008;58;71–96.
20. Goff BA, Mandel LS, Drescher CW, et al. Development of an ovarian cancer symptom index: possibilities for earlier detection. *Cancer*. 2007 109(2):221–227.
21. Hibbard LT. Adnexal torsion. *Am J Obstet Gynecol*. 1985;152:456.
22. Young RH, Scully RE. Metastatic tumors of the ovary. In: Kurman RJ, ed. *Blaustein's Pathology of the Female Genital Tract*. 5th Ed. New York, NY: Springer-Verlag; 2002.
23. Von Kuenssberg Jehle D, Stiller G, Wagner D. Sensitivity in detecting free intraperitoneal fluid with the pelvic views of the FAST exam. *Am J Emerg Med*. 2003;21(6): 476–478.
24. Koonings PP, Grimes DA, Campbell K, Sommerville M. Bilateral ovarian neoplasms and the risk of malignancy. *Am J Obstet Gynecol*. 1990;162(1):167–169.

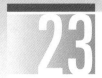

# Torsion of Ovary

## Mehdi Parva and Charles J. Dunton

Causes of acute abdominal pain unique to women include pelvic inflammatory disease, ectopic pregnancy, endometrioma, rupture or hemorrhage of a corpus luteum cyst, and torsion of adnexal structures (1). Although uncommon, adnexal torsion is not rare and comprises approximately 3% of surgical emergencies in women (2). Diagnosis of this condition is challenging. Prompt diagnosis may allow for preservation of the adnexal structures and fertility.

## ETIOLOGY

Torsion of the adnexa is caused by rotation of the ovary or the adnexa about the ovarian pedicle, resulting in arterial, venous, or lymphatic obstruction (Fig. 23.1). Initially, the venous and lymphatic obstruction without arterial obstruction produces edema and enlargement of the ovary. If arterial obstruction occurs, the organs may become necrotic and gangrenous. This in turn may lead to peritonitis and intestinal obstruction. In some cases, the twisted adnexa may be absorbed, leading to unilateral absence of the adnexa. Torsion of the fallopian tube alone is rare and has been associated with hydrosalpinx, neoplasms of the tube, and previous tubal ligation (2–5) (Fig. 23.2). Torsion of the adnexa is increased in ovarian hyperstimulation syndrome (OHSS) caused by menotropin therapy for infertility (6–8).

Pregnancy has been associated with an increased risk of adnexal torsion (9,10). If an adnexal mass is associated with a pregnancy, a recent review found that the most frequent complication was torsion (11). This may be due to the repositioning of the ovaries by the enlarging uterus. Torsion is most likely in the first trimester (10,12).

Torsion of the adnexa may involve the ovary, the fallopian tube, or both structures together. In most cases, an ovarian neoplasm is involved (9). Nonetheless, in up to 18% of cases, the torsion may involve normal tubes and ovaries. In keeping with the age of the patient population, the neoplasms are usually benign (Table 23.1). The most common neoplasm is the dermoid cyst. Paraovarian cysts have the highest relative risk of torsion (9,13).

It is unusual for malignant neoplasm to present with symptoms of torsion. A review of 10 years' experience at the Women's Hospital, Los Angeles County, showed only two cases of malignant neoplasms undergoing torsion. In comparison, the relative risk for a benign neoplasm to undergo torsion was 12.9% (95% CI, 10.2 to 15.9) (14,15). However, if a postmenopausal woman presents with torsion, clinicians should consider the possibility of malignancy. In series with a high percentage of malignancy reported with torsion, most patients were postmenopausal (13,16). Postmenopausal patients also had a delayed diagnosis compared to younger patients (13).

Torsion of a normal ovary may present as a massive ovarian edema. This tumor-like condition presents with significant ovarian enlargement and pathologically shows only edema of a normal ovary (17).

## CLINICAL FEATURES

The clinical diagnosis of adnexal torsion is often difficult. It occurs mainly in young women and less frequently in children and postmenopausal females. Pain,

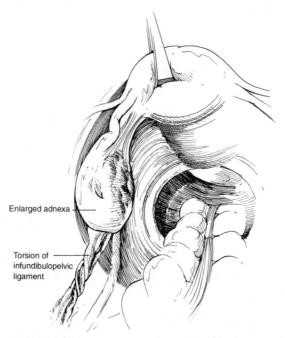

**FIGURE 23.1** Torsion of infundibulopelvic ligament.

Enlarged adnexa

Torsion of
infundibulopelvic
ligament

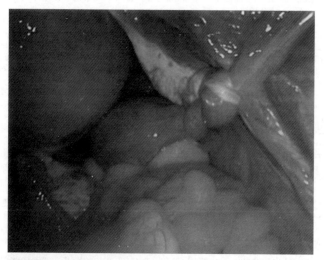

**FIGURE 23.2** Torsion of the adnexa.

TABLE
23.1 Pathology of Torsed Adnexes

| Pathologic Diagnosis | Number |
|---|---|
| Dermoid cyst | 38 |
| Serous adenoma | 12 |
| Serous carcinoma | 2 |
| Mucious adenoma | 6 |
| Fibroadenoma | 4 |
| Fibroma/thecoma | 1 |
| Struma ovarii | 1 |
| Hemangioma | 24 |
| Paraovarian cyst | 7 |
| Corpus luteum | 8 |
| Serous cyst | 6 |
| Endometrioma | 2 |
| Total | 101 |

*Source*: With permission from Lomano JM, Trelford JD, Ullery JC. Torsion of the uterine adnexa causing an acute abdomen. Obstet Gynecol. 1970;Vol.no. 35, issue.no. 2.

low-grade temperature, moderate leukocytosis, and nausea and vomiting (70%) are present in most cases. The pain associated with torsion may be unilateral or bilateral (25%) and either intermittent or constant. The pain may be acute, in onset, and may be associated with a vigorous activity or a change in position. The pain may be out of proportion to other findings. Later in the course, if necrosis occurs, high fever and marked leukocytosis may be seen (17–20) (Table 23.2). Symptoms may be present for a number of days prior to the patient seeking medical attention, and physician delay prior to surgical treatment is not uncommon. Reviews showed that the median onset of pain was 1 day, but the range was 0 to 210 days, with a median of 7 to 8 days (18).

Abdominal examination may show initial rigidity, spasm, tenderness, and unilateral pain on deep palpation. On pelvic examination, unilateral adnexal tenderness and a palpable mass are usually present. The torsion is more likely to involve the right adnexal (3:2), perhaps because of the proximity of the sigmoid colon to the left adnexa, resulting in less space in which the torsion can occur (21). Half of the patients may have radiation to the back, flank, or groin. One third of patients may exhibit only mild abdominal tenderness and some have no pelvic tenderness (18).

In Bouguizane et al. (22), a review of 135 cases of adnexal torsion, only 57.8% of patients were diagnosed accurately at the first clinical examination. Incorrect preoperative diagnoses in patients subsequently having torsion include adnexal mass, appendicitis, myoma, ectopic pregnancy, abscess, and ruptured viscus (23). Torsion must be considered in the differential diagnosis of abdominal pain, especially when a palpable pelvic mass is present.

If no palpable mass is present, ultrasonography may prove helpful in the diagnosis (17,24). Ultrasonography has been shown to demonstrate a mass in all patients

| TABLE 23.2 | Symptoms Associated With Adnexal Torsion in 44 Patients |

| Symptom | Percentage of Patients |
| --- | :---: |
| Pain | 100 |
| Nausea or vomiting | 66 |
| Abdominal fullness | 16 |
| Menstrual dysfunction | 9 |
| Diarrhea | 7 |
| Dysuria | 7 |
| Constipation | 5 |
| Rectal pressure | 2 |
| Syncope | 2 |
| Gradual onset of pain | 59 |
| Sudden onset of pain | 41 |

*Source*: With permission from Lomano JM, Trelford JD, Ullery JC. Torsion of the uterine adnexa causing an acute abdomen. Obstet Gynecol. 1970;Vol.no. 35, issue.no. 2.

with torsion. However, the ultrasonic appearance of the masses was nonspecific (17). The use of Doppler flow examination has recently been shown to be helpful in the diagnosis and management of ovarian torsion. Doppler ultrasound is able to identify the twisted vascular pedicle in the majority of cases (24,25). If normal arterial and venous flow can be demonstrated, untwisting of the pedicle is possible. If no blood flow is seen, this is generally associated with necrotic adnexa (17). However, more recent studies of Doppler ultrasound have shown that normal flow does not exclude the diagnosis of ovarian torsion (17,26). In fact, in one case report, up to 60% of confirmed ovarian torsions had normal flow (27). Approximately 20% of patients with an adnexal torsion will have a concomitant intrauterine pregnancy. Ultrasound can demonstrate the location of the pregnancy and aid in differentiation of torsion with intrauterine pregnancy from an ectopic gestation.

Magnetic resonance imaging (MRI) and computed tomography (CT) scanning have been described in a small number of patients. CT and MRI findings are generally nonspecific unless edema or hemorrhagic findings are present. MRI findings of large areas of high signal intensity on both $T_1$- and $T_2$-weighted images are associated with passive congestion of the torsed mass. The common CT and MRI features of adnexal torsion include thickening of the twisted fallopian tube, smooth thickening of the wall of the cystic ovarian mass, ascites, and uterine deviation to the side of torsion (28–30).

## DIFFERENTIAL DIAGNOSIS

The diagnosis of torsion of the adnexa must be considered in women with abdominal pain. The differential diagnoses include ectopic pregnancy, appendicitis, pelvic inflammatory disease, adnexal mass without torsion, endometrioma, degeneration of a myoma, renal calculi, urinary tract infection, and ruptured functional cyst (1,19).

Ectopic pregnancy without an acute abdomen is diagnosed by serial β-human chorionic gonadotropin (β-hCG) testing along with appropriate use of ultrasound when the quantitative β-hCG level reaches the discriminatory zone. Although intrauterine pregnancy is associated with torsion of the adnexa, ultrasound and β-hCG testing should be used to differentiate an intrauterine pregnancy with torsion from an ectopic gestation. In the event of an unstable patient, emergency laparotomy is indicated with either diagnosis (Chapter 3).

In appendicitis, the symptoms of midline abdominal pain with migration to the right lower quadrant and negative pelvic findings other than tenderness on rectal examination differentiate this entity from torsion. In addition, the nausea and vomiting seen in torsion generally occur rapidly after the onset of pain, rather than gradually, as in acute appendicitis.

Pelvic inflammatory disease is usually characterized by bilateral pain and tenderness. Temperature elevation and leukocytosis may be more marked. Pertinent history—such as episodes of pelvic inflammatory disease, intrauterine device use, and multiple or new sexual partners—points to pelvic inflammatory disease.

Patients who have an adnexal mass without torsion generally present without pain. Those who have a ruptured functional cyst may present at the midpoint of the menstrual cycle (Mittelschmerz) or just prior to the next expected period. Symptoms of nausea and vomiting are less frequent. In cases where there is no hemorrhage, symptoms are less severe than those seen with adnexal torsion and resolve over 48 hours.

Renal calculi usually present with flank pain and hematuria. There is also lack of a palpable pelvic mass. Degeneration of a myoma, especially if pedunculated, may require laparoscopy to confirm the diagnosis. A history of chronic pelvic pain will usually accompany endometriosis. Fever, acute pain, and increased leukocyte count are not seen with endometriomas unless there is a rupture. In cases of rupture, an acute abdomen may be seen necessitating operative intervention.

In all cases of acute pain, an empty bladder is necessary to ensure that urinary retention is not the cause of the pain. It will also allow for a more complete and accurate pelvic examination.

A high index of suspicion for torsion in cases of abdominal pain with a palpable or ultrasonically detected pelvic mass is necessary. Combined with laparoscopy in equivocal cases, early diagnosis and prompt treatment of this condition are possible.

Serum concentrations of interleukin-6 have been reported to be elevated in ovarian torsion in 75% of cases (six of eight) (31). Ovarian torsion has also been reported along with cases of inguinal hernia (32).

## TREATMENT

Treatment for adnexal torsion is surgical and depends on the condition of the ovary at the time of surgery. In most series, treatment has consisted of removal of the affected adnexa because of fear of embolism from thrombosed ovarian veins or necrosis of the ovary and the tube. In these cases, it is wise to expose the ureter to determine its location prior to ligating the ovarian blood supply, as the tenting of the peritoneum by the torsion may cause the ureter to be in or adjacent to the twisted pedicle.

Laparoscopic management of ovarian torsion has become the standard of care. If the ovary is not necrotic and fertility is important, it may be untwisted and stabilized by suturing it to the posterior wall of the uterus or by shortening the ovarian ligament. Observation is important to determine viability. Long-term follow-up has demonstrated that normal ovarian function is present in the great majority of cases. Follow-up ultrasounds have demonstrated normal follicular function in 95% of cases. Two important facto rs that may influence a successful conservative management of adnexal torsion are the surgeon's experience and the time interval from the beginning of abdominal pain (36 hours) to definitive treatment (33–38). Since torsion is usually associated with neoplasms of the ovary, the ovary should be carefully inspected and cystectomy carried out if necessary. If there is suspicion of a malignancy, unilateral adnexectomy should be performed. Appropriate surgical staging should be carried out if a frozen section shows malignancy (2).

Laparoscopic oophoropexy has been described to prevent recurrent ovarian torsion. This may be performed if the surgeon feels that the risk of recurrent torsion is high based on physical findings or if it represents the remaining ovary in premenopausal women (36).

Ovarian torsion has been described in postmenopausal women on tamoxifen therapy (39).

## SPECIAL CONSIDERATIONS

Torsion of the ovary is associated with OHSS caused by the hMG (Pergonal) use for ovulation induction. This syndrome is characterized by high estrogen secretion, enlargement of the ovaries, abdominal discomfort, and nausea and vomiting. In severe cases, clinical manifestations may include ascites, pleural effusions, electrolyte imbalance, oliguria, and shock. Torsion of the ovary was present in 7.4% of cases of OHSS in one series. It was more common (16%) in patients who were pregnant and had OHSS (40). A review of assisted reproductive technologies demonstrated nine cases of ovarian torsion in 10,583 cycles. However, 3 of 104 patients with OHSS demonstrated torsion. All cases were treated conservatively (41). Recent reports of treatment of these patients by the untwisting of the ovarian pedicle even when the ovary appears necrotic have demonstrated no complications. Normal subsequent ovarian function has been demonstrated by ultrasound in these patients. Continuation of pregnancy without problems was also demonstrated. Although the number of patients treated in this manner is still small, this option should be considered for these patients, in whom fertility is such an important issue. This method of treatment may not be applicable to patients who do not have OHSS (38,40).

The diagnosis of ovarian torsion must be considered in children presenting with abdominal pain. In children, the adnexal torsion may present as an abdominal mass. The diagnosis in children is especially important. Kokoska et al. (42) reported on 51 children with ovarian torsion. At their institution, all 51 underwent salpingo-oophorectomy. Earlier diagnosis may allow for conservative treatment (36). This entity has been reported in the infant as well (43).

## CONCLUSIONS

Torsion of the adnexal structures must be considered in women of all ages presenting with abdominal pain. The incidence is highest in the reproductive-age group. A palpable or an ultrasonically detected pelvic mass along with pain should alert the clinician to consider this diagnosis. Because of the difficulty of clinical diagnosis, the more frequent use of laparoscopy may lead to early treatment and preservation of fertility.

## References

1. Silen W. *Cope's Early Diagnosis of the Acute Abdomen*. 21st Ed. New York, NY: Oxford Press; 2005:208.
2. Oelsner G, Shashar D. Adnexal torsion. *Clin Obstet Gynecol*. 2006;49(3):459–463.
3. Orazi C, Inserra A, Lucchetti M, et al. Isolated tubal torsion: a rare cause of pelvic pain at menarche. Sonographic and MR findings. *Pediatr Radiol*. 2006;36(12):1316–1318.
4. Antoniou N, Varras M, Akrivis C, et al. Isolated torsion of the fallopian tube: a case report and review of the literature. *Clin Exp Obstet Gynecol*. 2004;31(3):235–238.
5. Krissi H, Shalev J, Bar-Hava I, et al. Fallopian tube torsion: laparoscopic evaluation and treatment of a rare gynecological entity. *J Am Board Fam Pract*. 2001;14(4):274–277.
6. Gorkemli H, Camus M, Clasen K. Adnexal torsion after gonadotrophin ovulation induction for IVF or ICSI and its conservative treatment. *Arch Gynecol Obstet*. 2002;267(1):4–6.
7. Robson S, Kerin JF. Acute adnexal torsion before oocyte retrieval in an in vitro fertilization cycle. *Fertil Steril*. 2000;73(3):650–651.
8. Zhu W, Li X, Chen X, et al. Conservative management of adnexal torsion via transvaginal ultrasound guided ovarian cyst aspiration in patients with ovarian hyperstimulation. *Fertil Steril*. 2008;89(1):229, e1–3.
9. McWilliams GD, Hill MJ, Dietrich CS III. Gynecologic emergencies. *Surg Clin North Am*. 2008;88(2):265–283, vi.
10. Whitecar MP, Turner S, Higby MK. Adnexal masses in pregnancy: a review of 130 cases undergoing surgical management. *Am J Obstet Gynecol*. 1999;181(1):19–24.
11. Kumari I, Kaur S, Mohan H, et al. Adnexal masses in pregnancy: a 5-year review. *Aust N Z J Obstet Gynaecol*. 2006;46(1):52–54.
12. Chittacharoen A, Wangpusayavisut A, O-Prasertsawat P. Adnexal masses in pregnancy. *J Med Assoc Thai*. 2005;88(Suppl. 2):S37–S40.
13. Eitan R, Galoyan N, Zuckerman B, et al. The risk of malignancy in post-menopausal women presenting with adnexal torsion. *Gynecol Oncol*. 2007;106(1):211–214.
14. Sommerville M, Grimes D, Koonings P, et al. Ovarian neoplasms and the risk of adnexal torsion. *Am J Obstet Gynecol*. 1991;164(2):577–578.
15. Koonings PP, Grimes DA. Adnexal torsion in postmenopausal women. *Obstet Gynecol*. 1989;73(1):11–12.
16. Lee RA, Welch JS. Torsion of the uterine adnexa. *Am J Obstet Gynecol*. 1967;97(7):974–977.
17. Chang HC, Bhatt S, Dogra VS. Pearls and pitfalls in diagnosis of ovarian torsion. *Radiographics*. 2008;28(5):1355–1368.
18. Houry D, Abbott JT. Ovarian torsion: a fifteen-year review. *Ann Emerg Med*. 2001;38(2):156–159.
19. Marx J. *Rosen's Emergency Medicine: Concepts and Clinical Practice*. 6th Ed. St. Louis, MO: Mosby; 2006.
20. Lomano JM, Trelford JD, Ullery JC. Torsion of the uterine adnexa causing an acute abdomen. *Obstet Gynecol*. 1970;35(2):221–225.
21. Weitzman VN, DiLuigi AJ, Maier DB, et al. Prevention of recurrent adnexal torsion. *Fertil Steril*. 2008; 90(5):2018el–3.
22. Bouguizane S, Bibi H, Farhat Y, et al. Adnexal torsion: a report of 135 cases. *J Gynecol Obstet Biol Reprod (Paris)*. 2003;32(6):535–540.
23. Hiller N, Appelbaum L, Simanovsky N, et al. CT features of adnexal torsion. *AJR Am J Roentgenol*. 2007;189(1):124–129.
24. Moore C, Meyers AB, Capotasto J, et al. Prevalence of abnormal CT findings in patients with proven ovarian torsion and a proposed triage schema. *Emerg Radiol*. 2009;16(2):115–120.
25. Chang YJ, Yan DC, Kong MS, et al. Adnexal torsion in children. *Pediatr Emerg Care*. 2008;24(8):534–537.
26. Albayram F, Hamper UM. Ovarian and adnexal torsion: spectrum of sonographic findings with pathologic correlation. *J Ultrasound Med*. 2001;20(10):1083–1089.
27. Pena JE, Ufberg D, Cooney N, et al. Usefulness of Doppler sonography in the diagnosis of ovarian torsion. *Fertil Steril*. 2000;73(5):1047–1050.
28. Kimura I, Togashi K, Kawakami S, et al. Ovarian torsion: CT and MR imaging appearances. *Radiology*. 1994;190(2):337–341.
29. Singh A, Danrad R, Hahn PF, et al. MR imaging of the acute abdomen and pelvis: acute appendicitis and beyond. *Radiographics*. 2007;27(5):1419–1431.

30. Minutoli F, Blandino A, Gaeta M, et al. Twisted ovarian fibroma with high signal intensity on T1-weighted MR image: a new sign of torsion of ovarian tumors? *Eur Radiol.* 2001;11(7):1151–1154.
31. Cohen SB, Wattiez A, Stockheim D, et al. The accuracy of serum interleukin-6 and tumour necrosis factor as markers for ovarian torsion. *Hum Reprod.* 2001;16(10): 2195–2197.
32. Merriman TE, Auldist AW. Ovarian torsion in inguinal hernias. *Pediatr Surg Int.* 2000;16(5–6):383–385.
33. Oelsner G, Bider D, Goldenberg M, et al. Long-term follow-up of the twisted ischemic adnexa managed by detorsion. *Fertil Steril.* 1993;60(6):976–979.
34. Dane B, Dane C, Kiray M, et al. Sonographic findings in adnexal torsion: a report of 34 cases. *Arch Gynecol Obstet.* 2008.
35. Rody A, Jackisch C, Klockenbusch W, et al. The conservative management of adnexal torsion—a case-report and review of the literature. *Eur J Obstet Gynecol Reprod Biol.* 2002;101(1):83–86.
36. Rousseau V, Massicot R, Darwish A, et al. Emergency management and conservative surgery of ovarian torsion in children: a report of 40 cases. *J Pediatr Adolesc Gynecol.* 2008;21(4):201–206.
37. Aziz D, Davis V, Allen L, et al. Ovarian torsion in children: is oophorectomy necessary? *J Pediatr Surg.* 2004;39(5):750–753.
38. Eckler K, Laufer MR, Perlman SE. Conservative management of bilateral asynchronous adnexal torsion with necrosis in a prepubescent girl. *J Pediatr Surg.* 2000;35(8):1248–1251.
39. Barbieri RL, Ferracci AL, Droesch JN, et al. Ovarian torsion in a premenopausal woman treated with tamoxifen for breast cancer. *Fertil Steril.* 1993;59(2):459–460.
40. Delvigne A, Rozenberg S. Review of clinical course and treatment of ovarian hyperstimulation syndrome (OHSS). *Hum Reprod Update.* 2003;9(1):77–96.
41. Mashiach S, Bider D, Moran O, et al. Adnexal torsion of hyperstimulated ovaries in pregnancies after gonadotropin therapy. *Fertil Steril.* 1990;53(1):76–80.
42. Kokoska ER, Keller MS, Weber TR. Acute ovarian torsion in children. *Am J Surg.* 2000;180(6):462–465.
43. Fitzhugh VA, Shaikh JR, Heller DS. Adnexal torsion leading to death of an infant. *J Pediatr Adolesc Gynecol.* 2008;21(5):295–297.

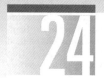

# Oncologic Emergencies

## Sarah Adams and Stephen C. Rubin

The American Cancer Society reports that approximately 78,500 new invasive cancers of the female reproductive tract were diagnosed in the United States in 2008 (1). With the increasing age of the population and an increased prevalence of human papillomavirus infection, the number of women that develop gynecologic cancers is expected to rise (2). Some women learn that they have a gynecologic cancer during a visit to the emergency department with symptoms such as vaginal bleeding, pain, or intestinal obstruction. Women diagnosed with cancer may also require emergent medical care due to postoperative complications or symptoms resulting from chemotherapy, radiotherapy, or recurrent disease. This chapter reviews the most frequent symptoms experienced by women with gynecologic cancers that require emergency medical care.

## VAGINAL BLEEDING

Endometrial cancer and cervical cancer, as well as less common malignancies such as sarcomas, gestational trophoblastic disease, and advanced vulvar cancer, may present with vaginal bleeding (3). As with any patient, initial evaluation of a woman presenting with vaginal bleeding should determine whether she is hemodynamically stable based on blood pressure and pulse, and patients who appear syncopal should be resuscitated appropriately. As part of this initial evaluation, a pregnancy test should be performed for all women of reproductive age. Once the patient is stable, the cause of vaginal bleeding can be determined by its pattern and findings on physical examination.

### Cervical cancer

Vaginal bleeding caused by cervical cancer is usually painless and often occurs between menses or postcoitally. Given the success of cervical cancer screening in the United States, most patients presenting with advanced cervical cancer may have a history of poor health maintenance without regular Pap smears or a history of abnormal Pap smears or other pelvic infections. Because cervical cancer is not hereditary, family history is noncontributory; however, tobacco use is associated with a higher rate of transformation of intraepithelial neoplastic cervical lesions to carcinoma (3).

On physical examination, it is important to visualize the cervix with a speculum prior to performing a bimanual examination so that any bleeding resulting from manipulation of the cervix will not compromise the speculum examination. After gently inserting the speculum, any clots in the vaginal vault can be evacuated and the source of bleeding can be determined. Advanced cervical cancer may present with a large fungating tumor or with ulceration of the cervix or the upper vagina. Biopsy of the cervix to confirm the diagnosis may be performed at this time or deferred until a planned examination under anesthesia to avoid causing further bleeding. Small areas of bleeding may be treated with Monsel solution or silver nitrite. Brisk bleeding may require tamponade with vaginal packing and admission to a gynecologic oncology service. If the bleeding is unremitting, the patient may need hypogastric artery ligation, embolization, or high-dose radiation therapy (4). Following the speculum examination, a bimanual examination will reveal the size and the extent of the disease, including the presence of parametrial spread, or the involvement of the rectum or the bladder. Laboratory studies should include a pregnancy test and a complete blood count as well as a chemistry panel to check for evidence of renal dysfunction which might suggest obstruction of the distal collecting system. If the bleeding is not severe, the patient can be discharged once appropriate referral and prompt follow-up by a qualified gynecologic oncologist has been arranged.

### Endometrial Cancer

Vaginal bleeding caused by endometrial or other corpus cancers is usually not as severe as that caused by cervical cancer. The majority of patients with endometrial cancer are postmenopausal, with a mean age of 60 years (3). Essential points of the history in older patients include use of unopposed exogenous estrogens and obesity. In younger women, obesity, nulliparity, infertility, and a family history of endometrial, colon, or ovarian cancer are associated with the development of endometrial cancer. Although vaginal bleeding is the most common presenting complaint for this disease, it is seldom of sufficient magnitude to cause an emergency department visit, unless the patient lacks a primary physician.

In most cases, it will not be possible to make a definitive diagnosis of endometrial cancer during an emergency department visit, although postmenopausal women presenting with vaginal bleeding are considered to have endometrial cancer until proven otherwise. The differential diagnosis is much broader in a premenopausal woman and may include such benign causes as anovulatory bleeding, fibroids, complications from pregnancy, and infection.

On speculum examination, the bleeding will be from the cervical os. A pelvic examination will determine whether the uterus is enlarged and whether there is any extrauterine spread of the tumor. The bleeding is seldom life threatening, and most patients can be discharged from the emergency department as long as adequate provisions are made for prompt referral to a qualified gynecologist.

### Gestational Trophoblastic Disease

Women with gestational trophoblastic neoplasia most commonly present with vaginal bleeding (5). This disease is seen at early or late reproductive ages and affects 1 in 1,200 pregnancies in the United States. Patients may report recurrent vaginal bleeding and an absence of fetal movements.

On examination, the uterine size is often greater than expected for gestational age. Bleeding will be seen from the cervical os on speculum examination, and occasionally, vesicular material also may be seen extruding through the os (3). The definitive diagnosis is made by ultrasonography, which shows a distinctive multiechogenic pattern. The patient with gestational trophoblastic neoplasia should be admitted after a prompt obstetric consultation.

### Vulvar Cancer

Bleeding caused by vulvar cancer is rare (6). Women presenting with bleeding usually have an advanced vulvar lesion. Patients with advanced diseases and bleeding should be admitted to initiate treatment.

## THROMBOEMBOLISM

Patients with gynecologic malignancy have a high risk of thromboembolic disease due to an acquired coagulopathy due to the cancer combined with compression and venous stasis caused by large pelvic tumors (7). This risk is increased in the postoperative period and should be considered for women presenting with asymmetric edema or shortness of breath. Women with deep venous thrombosis usually present with unilateral lower extremity edema, which may be difficult to differentiate from lymphedema resulting from lymphadenectomy. Venous Doppler ultrasound is required to identify clots, and evaluation should include the upper thigh if possible.

Pulmonary embolus is a dangerous complication of pelvic surgery and malignancy and should be suspected in patients reporting shortness of breath or pleuritic chest pain. Conversely, patients presenting with a pulmonary embolus should undergo evaluation for malignancy as a possible etiology of their coagulopathy. Women with pulmonary clots are likely to be tachycardic and hypoxic. Lung examination is often unremarkable, but decreased breath sounds or dullness to percussion may be evident if the thrombus is accompanied by pleural effusion. Lab values such as d-dimer may assist with the diagnosis, but a helical CT will be most sensitive in confirming the present of a clot. If the patient cannot tolerate IV dye for the CT scan, a ventilation–perfusion study can be performed. Patients with new venous thrombosis or pulmonary embolism are usually admitted to initiate anticoagulation.

## POSTOPERATIVE WOUND COMPLICATIONS

### Wound Infections

Common postoperative infections include superficial wound cellulitis, infected hematomas, abscesses, and infections of the vaginal cuff after hysterectomy. Cellulitis presents with warmth and erythema around the incision, but the skin should be dry and intact. The patient can be treated with antibiotics as an outpatient and should follow-up with her surgeon to ensure that the infection has cleared. Infected hematomas or seromas often result in fluctuance, erythema, and discharge from the incision site and should be drained if possible. This can be done by probing the wound gently or by removing some of the staples over the area of fluctuance to evacuate clots or fluid collections. Gentle probing should also determine whether the underlying fascia is intact. Cultures of the wound often show polymicrobial infection but may be helpful in directing treatment if antibiotic resistant organisms are found. If a large defect remains, it can be packed with moist gauze twice daily until it closes. Signs of necrotizing fasciitis (skin discoloration, skin necrosis, and crepitus) require prompt consultation for surgical debridement (8).

### Wound Dehiscence

Wound dehiscence usually occurs 5 to 7 days after surgery but may present after staple removal 10 days to 2 weeks postoperatively. If the wound is healthy, without discharge or signs of infection, and if the defect is small, the patient can be managed with debridement and dressing changes. Larger defects may benefit from a wound vac or closed suction system. In either case, the patient's surgeon should be consulted.

### Evisceration

Evisceration, with fascial separation, may present as an incisional mass or bulge with valsalva, and patients may report pain or nausea which can be sudden in onset or related to exertion or coughing. Risk factors for evisceration include a history of prior hernia, steroid use, immunosuppression, poorly controlled diabetes, obesity, infection, chronic cough, and tobacco use (9). Evaluation of the wound will reveal a fascial defect and sometimes bowel herniation. If the bowel is exposed, the wound should be covered with sterile, moist towels, and arrangements made for the patient to be taken to the operating room for fascial closure.

## Vaginal Cuff Cellulitis

The other common postoperative infections in patients with gynecologic malignancies are vaginal cuff cellulitis and cuff abscess. Vaginal cuff cellulitis occurs in 8% of those who receive antibiotic prophylaxis before a hysterectomy (8). The most common cause is a mixed infection of anaerobes endogenous to the vagina and Gram-negative aerobic bacteria. Women with cuff cellulitis may present with purulent discharge, persistent vaginal bleeding, and fever. On examination, the cuff will be erythematous and friable. Most patients are treated with oral antibiotics, but women who are acutely febrile or who have evidence of an abscess should be admitted for treatment and possible drainage of the pelvic collection in the operating room.

## Vaginal Cuff Dehiscence

Vaginal cuff dehiscence is a rare complication following hysterectomy that requires prompt medical attention. Risk factors include early resumption of intercourse postoperatively, increased intra-abdominal pressure, smoking, history of prior surgery or radiation, connective tissue disease, and steroid use (10). Patients may present with vaginal pain or pressure or with protrusion of bowel into the vaginal vault. The diagnosis can be confirmed with a sterile speculum examination and requires an immediate gynecologic consult for surgical management.

## GASTROINTESTINAL COMPLICATIONS

### Bowel Obstruction

Because ovarian cancer metastasizes to the serosal surfaces of the bowel, bowel obstruction is a common problem for patients with advanced or recurrent disease and is the presenting symptom for approximately 5% of patients (11). Bowel obstruction may also occur postoperatively as a consequence of adhesion formation or bowel stricture. Women with bowel obstruction present with persistent nausea and vomiting or anorexia, often have abdominal pain and distention, and may report an absence of flatus or bowel movements. They are typically dehydrated and may be tachycardic or mildly hypotensive as a result. Tympany, distention, and tenderness may be evident on abdominal examination, and radiographic studies will show air-fluid levels and bowel distention. It is critical to note overdistention of the large bowel as a diameter >10 cm is associated with a high risk of perforation and requires prompt surgical decompression (12). Women with a bowel obstruction usually require admission for hydration and bowel rest or surgery. Placement of a nasogastric tube to drain the stomach and decompress the bowel will alleviate some of their symptoms and may hasten recovery.

### Bowel Perforation

Less commonly, patients may present with bowel perforation resulting from obstruction or from tumor infiltration of the bowel wall. In addition to women with massive dilation of the bowel, patients with recurrent cancer and a history of prior obstruction or those treated with anti-angiogenic chemotherapies, such as bevacizumab, are at increased risk of bowel perforation. In some cases, the symptoms may be unexpectedly subtle, but most patients with bowel injury will have abdominal pain that can be severe. This may be accompanied by fever, tachycardia, and abdominal rigidity resulting from acute peritonitis. A CT scan with gastrografin may be helpful to confirm the diagnosis but should not delay surgical intervention. These patients should be resuscitated with IV fluid and given broad-spectrum antibiotics. Consultation with a gynecologic oncologist or surgeon should be obtained immediately.

## Gastrointestinal Fistulas

Women with gynecologic malignancies may develop gastrointestinal fistulas as a consequence of tumor infiltration of the bowel or as a complication of surgery or treatment with radiation or chemotherapy. Fistulas developing in the postoperative period can result from an unrecognized enterotomy at the time of surgery, from erosion of a foreign body such as an intraperitoneal drain or from infection and wound breakdown. In patients treated with radiation or antiangiogenic chemothearpy, fistulas result from devascularization and breakdown of the affected tissue. Patients with enterocutaneous fistulas may present with discharge from a prior incision site from surgery or a percutaneous drain site. Subcutaneous fluid collections may yield feculent material, and local necrosis or an overlying cellulitis with erythema, warmth, or tenderness may be evident. Enterovaginal or rectovaginal communications cause persistent vaginal discharge which can be caustic small bowel contents or feculent material if the distal intestinal tract is involved. It is often difficult to localize the fistulous tract due to patient discomfort, especially in patients who have vaginal stenosis from prior irradiation, but a gentle speculum examination may be helpful to confirm the diagnosis. CT fistulograms can also be performed to document the location of the fistulous tract for treatment planning. Women with a new fistula, or with evidence of infection from a chronic fistula, should be admitted for workup and management.

## Bowel Prolapse

Many women with ovarian cancer or other gynecologic malignancies require colostomy or ileostomy to achieve optimal surgical results or to manage a bowel obstruction from recurrent disease. Colostomy complications, including stenosis of the stoma, peristomal hernia, wound infection, and prolapse, occur in approximately 30% of patients (13). Women may present with complaints of a mass at the site of the stoma or prolapse of the bowel through the stoma which can be associated with bleeding or tenderness. Peristomal herniation of bowel requires admission for prompt surgical correction. Mucosal prolapse of the stoma can be reduced by gentle digital pressure, but it should be done expeditiously to prevent infection or edema. In either case, consultation should be requested from a gynecologic oncologist or a surgeon for management, and the exposed bowel should be kept moist and protected with gauze.

## UROLOGIC COMPLICATIONS

### Ureteral Obstruction

Ureteral obstruction can be caused by compression from a large pelvic tumor or by stricture from radiation treatment or postoperative adhesions, or it may result directly from an intraoperative injury. Women with ureteral obstruction often present with nonspecific flank pain, occasionally radiating to the pelvis and the groin. The onset may be gradual and is often associated with concurrent urinary infection or even urosepsis. In cases of bilateral obstruction, anemia and azotemia may result. The diagnosis can be made using intravenous pyelography, computed tomography, renal nuclear scanning, or renal ultrasonography showing hydronephrosis. Management depends on the severity of the obstruction, but antibiotics should be administered after specimens for blood and urine cultures have been obtained. Postoperative patients should be admitted for surgical consultation and repair, and women with renal compromise or urosepsis will also require hospitalization for treatment. Stable patients with insidious signs of ureteral obstruction may be discharged once arrangements are made for follow-up care.

## Urologic Fistulas

Urinary fistulas may develop following radical surgery or radiation or as a result of extensive tumor involvement of the lower pelvis, most commonly in patients with cervical or vaginal cancer. Postoperative fistulas occur from 7 to 21 days after surgery and are most common in patients undergoing radical hysterectomy requiring extensive ureterolysis and pelvic dissection (14). The incidence of fistula formation after radical hysterectomy is approximately 1%, but this rate is three times higher in patients treated with adjuvant radiation therapy (14). Ureteral fistulas caused by radiation therapy typically develop 6 to 12 months after completion of treatment. In patients with advanced cervical or vaginal tumors, large fistulas may develop from erosion of the tumor into the base of the bladder or the urethra.

Symptoms of ureteral fistulas include urinary incontinence, frequency, dysuria, hematuria, and watery vaginal discharge. Fistulas can be diagnosed either by directly observing urine in the vagina or by injecting indigo carmine intravenously and placing a tampon in the vagina. Most do not require emergent hospital admission, but patients should be referred to a gynecologic oncologist for management and repair.

## Urinary Conduit Complications

Urinary conduits may be constructed using a segment of ileum or colon as a reservoir and conduit. Complications include blockage of the ureteroconduit anastomotic site, with ureteral obstruction and possibly urosepsis; conduit necrosis; stomal necrosis; and electrolyte imbalance owing to absorption of chloride in an overly long conduit, resulting in hyperchloremic acidosis (15,16). Management in the emergency department is supportive. Admission considerations depend on the patient's overall electrolyte balance, the presence of urinary obstruction, and the patient's ability to return for follow-up care. Intravenous pyelography or ultrasonography usually defines the problem. If urinary obstruction has resulted in urosepsis, emergency percutaneous nephrostomy may be necessary (17). Appropriate consultation with the gynecologic oncologist should be obtained.

## NEUROLOGIC DEFICITS

The differential diagnosis for patients presenting with a change in mental status is broad and in patients with a history of malignancy, includes infection, cerebrovascular accident, and metastatic disease. The most common etiology is infection, particularly in elderly patients, which requires a thorough workup including imaging studies and cultures of blood, urine, and possibly spinal fluid. Patients undergoing chemothearpy may be neutropenic and unable to mount an inflammatory response with fever or leukocytosis. In patients in whom infection is suspected, admission and empiric treatment with broad-spectrum antibiotics is advised.

As discussed above, patients with gynecologic malignancies are also coagulopathic and, consequently, are at risk for both hemorrhagic and embolic strokes. Women presenting with neurologic deficits and a history of prior clot or patients who are currently anticoagulated with warfarin or heparin should have imaging studies performed to rule out an intracranial bleed.

Although relatively uncommon except in very advanced disease, metastasis to the brain is possible in women with ovarian, endometrial, uterine, or cervical cancers. Depending on the location of the lesion, patients with intracranial masses may present with headache, changes in mental status, vertigo, seizure, or neurologic deficits. CT or MRI scans may show a distinct mass, or lumbar puncture may reveal evidence of meningeal carcinomatosis with high opening pressure, elevated protein or white blood cell count, low glucose, and positive cytology. Patients with acute neurologic changes, or evidence of spinal cord compression, should have a neurosurgery consultation for operative decompression or steroid treatment to decrease swelling and inflammation.

## COMPLICATIONS OF RADIATION THERAPY

### Radiation Enteritis
Radiation therapy is used for the primary treatment of advanced cervical cancer, as well as uterine cancers, vulvar cancer, and locally recurrent ovarian cancer. An early complication during or immediately following treatment with radiothearpy is radiation proctitis or enteritis with diarrhea (18). Patients with severe diarrhea may become dehydrated and present to the emergency department for evaluation and resuscitation. These women can usually be treated with diphenoxylate (Lomotil) and fluid resuscitation, without admission. In some cases, rectal bleeding may result from radiation proctitis. Cort enemas (hydrocortisone) and a low-residue diet can be recommended for mild bleeding, but bleeding heavy enough to require fluid resuscitation or transfusion also requires consultation to a gynecologic or surgical service. In severe cases that do not respond to medical management, angiographic embolization or colostomy may be required.

### Hemorrhagic Cystitis
Hemorrhagic cystitis can be caused by radiation therapy or some types of chemotherapy. Bleeding can be managed in the emergency department with bladder irrigation using a three-way catheter. If the bleeding is not severe once any clots are removed from the bladder, the patient may be discharged with follow-up care. In severe hemorrhage, the patient will need to be admitted for more aggressive management and both urologic and gynecologic consultations are necessary.

## COMPLICATIONS OF CHEMOTHERAPY

### Nausea and Vomiting
The most commonly used drugs in gynecologic oncology are cisplatin, carboplatin, and paclitaxel. Complications caused by cisplatin and carboplatin, which are administered as a bolus, include nausea and vomiting, which may be unremitting despite the use of prophylactic antiemetics (19). Symptoms are most severe on the day of treatment and, occasionally, may require emergent medical attention in the days following instillation. Once fluid and electrolyte statuses are assured, the patient can often be managed with additional antiemetic medications and rarely will need to be admitted for hydration.

### Hypersensitivity Reactions
Paclitaxel (Taxol) is used for induction chemotherapy for women with ovarian cancer and uterine cancers. The most severe toxicity associated with taxol is an immediate hypersensitivity reaction, which can require transfer to the emergency room during infusion. Patients may become acutely hypertensive or hypotensive and flushed. They may experience shortness of breath or chest pain and can become hypoxic. Taxol can also cause cardiac toxicity manifested by sinus bradycardia (30%), bradyarrhythmia with AV blockade, and short-lived ventricular tachycardia (20). Although most of these side effects are noted while the patient is receiving chemotherapy, they can occasionally occur after discharge, particularly if the patient is given a 3-hour taxol infusion. Most patients recover quickly following treatment with steroids, antihistamines, fluids, and supportive care, but severe cases may require respiratory support.

## Bone Marrow Suppression

Many chemotherapeutic drugs, including taxol and platinum compounds, can cause bone marrow suppression with neutropenia, anemia, and thrombocytopenia. It is unusual for these patients to be seen in the emergency department; however, women presenting with fever or evidence of infection and an absolute neutrophil counts <500 should be admitted for empiric broad-spectrum antibiotic therapy. Rarely, patients with anemia or severe thrombocytopenia will require admission for transfusion of platelets and packed red cells.

## SUMMARY

Women with gynecologic cancers are susceptible to medical complications from their tumor burden as well as from surgery, chemotherapy, or radiation therapy that may require emergent medical attention. It is important to consider effects and toxicities of these interventions when evaluating patients with a history of malignancy in the emergency department and to consult with a gynecologic oncologist to assist with diagnosis and management to ensure that these women receive the care they need.

## COMMON PITFALLS

- In the presence of vaginal bleeding in a patient of reproductive age, pregnancy should be ruled out.
- If the cecum is dilated to 10 cm from large bowel obstruction, prompt decompression is mandatory.
- Necrotizing fasciitis requires prompt surgical debridement and admission.
- If any amount of ureteral obstruction is diagnosed, urosepsis must be ruled out before the patient is discharged from the ED.
- Febrile neutropenic patients must be admitted.

## *References*

1. www.cancer.org.
2. Guijon F. Sexually transmitted disease and cervical neoplasia. *Curr Opin Obstet Gynecol.* 1990;2:857.
3. Disaia P, Creasman W. *Clinical Gynecologic Oncology.* 5th Ed. St. Louis, MO: Mosby; 1997.
4. Dehaeck C. Transcatheter embolization of pelvic vessels to stop intractable hemorrhage. *Gynecol Oncol.* 1986;24:9.
5. Kohorn EI. What we know about low-level hCG: definition, classification and management. *J Reprod Med.* 2004;49:433.
6. Morley G. Cancer of the vulva: a review. *Cancer.* 1981;48:597.
7. Wang X, Fu S, Freedman RS, Kavanagh JJ. Venous thromboembolism syndrome in gynecologic cancer. *Int J Gynecol Cancer.* 2006;16(S1):458–71.
8. Nichols D. *Reoperative Gynecologic Surgery.* St. Louis, MO: Mosby Year Book; 1991.
9. Molpus KL. Intestinal tract in gynecologic surgery. *Telinde's Operative Gynecology* 9th Ed. Philadelphia PA: Lippincott Williams & Wilkins; 2003.
10. Croak AJ, Gebhart JB, Klingele CJ, Schroeder G, Lee RA, Podratz KC. Characteristics of patients with vaginal rupture and evisceration. *Obstet Gynecol.* 2004;103(3): 572–576
11. Rubin S, Sutton G. *Ovarian Cancer.* New York, NY: McGraw–Hill; 1993
12. Schwartz S. *Principles of Surgery.* 6th Ed. New York, NY: McGraw–Hill; 1994:1213.
13. Kretschiner P. *The Intestinal Stoma.* Philadelphia, PA: WB Saunders; 1978.
14. Delgado G, Smith J. *Management of Complications in Gynecologic Oncology.* New York, NY: John Wiley and Sons; 1982.
15. Chamberlain D, Hopkins M, Roberts J, et al. The effects of early removal of indwelling urinary catheter after radical hysterectomy. *Gynecol Oncol.* 1991;43:98.
16. Hancock K, Copeland L, Gershenson D. Urinary conduits in gynecologic oncology. *Obstet Gynecol.* 1986;67:680.

17. Dudley B, Gershenson D, Kavanaugh J, et al. Percutaneous nephrostomy catheter use in gynecologic malignancy: M. D. Anderson Hospital experience. *Gynecol Oncol.* 1986;24:273.

18. Beer W, Fan A, Halsted C. Clinical and nutritional implications of radiation enteritis. *Am J Clin Nutr.* 1985;41:85.

19. Benrubi G, Norvell M, Nuss R, et al. The use of methyiprednisolone and metoclopramide in control of emesis in patients receiving cis-platinum. *Gynecol Oncol.* 1985; 21:306.

20. McGuire W, Hopkins W, Brady M, et al. Cyclophosphamide and cisplatin compared with pacitaxel and cisplatin in patients with stage III and stage IV ovarian cancer. *N Engl J Med.* 1996;334:1–6.

# Postoperative Complications and Postoperative Emergencies

**Brent E. Seibel**

Emergencies following gynecologic surgery may present as immediate, early, and late occurring events that require proper diagnosis and management by the gynecologic surgeon and/or emergency physician. In this chapter, postoperative complications are discussed as they pertain to the gynecologic or obstetric patient after abdominal, vaginal, and minimally invasive procedures. This chapter is divided into potential problems encountered after surgery, including wound complications, urinary tract injuries, gastrointestinal complications, infectious complications, and other postoperative emergencies that are more specific to gynecologic procedures and therefore possibly less familiar to the emergency physician. Complications such as pneumonia, pyelonephritis, deep vein thrombosis, pulmonary embolus, and other conditions that may be encountered postoperatively, but are not unique to this setting, are not emphasized.

## WOUND COMPLICATIONS

The most common wound complications associated with gynecologic surgery include hematoma, seroma, infection, fascial dehiscence, and hernia. Risk factors include obesity, diabetes, immunosuppression, cardiovascular disease, smoking, cancer, malnutrition, previous surgery or radiation, and infection. Surgical factors include contamination, devitalization of tissues, the presence of foreign bodies, prolonged operating time, extensive wound dissection, and the presence of dead space in the surgical wound. Strategies for the prevention of wound complications obviously address these issues when possible and include prophylactic antibiotics when appropriate, proper surgical preparation and sterile technique, avoiding excessive dissection or devitalization of tissues, and closure of subcutaneous spaces when appropriate. A 2004 metaanalysis by Chelmow et al. (1) reviewed six studies addressing subcutaneous fat closure during c-section and found a 34% decrease in the risk of wound disruption when the subcutaneous fat thickness is >2 cm. In a randomized trial of abdominal hysterectomy patients, subcutaneous closure, when this layer was >2.5 cm, was associated with a significantly lower incidence of wound disruption (2). The type of incision is dictated by the requirements of the specific surgery, prior surgical scars, and body habitus of the patient. Incisions utilized in obstetrics and gynecologic procedures include longitudinal or median, transverse, infraumbilical, and those associated with laparoscopy. Although infection, hematoma, seroma, dehiscence, and hernia can be seen with any type of incision, wound dehiscence and hernia occur at a higher rate following vertical midline incisions (3).

### Hematoma and Seroma

Over 1.2 million cesarean section deliveries and nearly 600,000 hysterectomies, two of the most common obstetric and gynecologic procedures, were performed in the United States during 2005 (4). The estimated incidence of wound infections ranges from 3% to 15% for cesareans and 3% to 8% for abdominal hysterectomies. An additional 3% to 14% of cesareans are complicated by wound seroma and hematoma (5). Practicing physicians must therefore be familiar with the recognition and management of these conditions. Hematomas are collections of blood that accumulate in the subcutaneous tissues due to failure of primary hemostasis or a bleeding diathesis. Similarly, collections of serum are responsible for seromas. They both usually occur in the immediate or early postoperative period but may not present until much later with swelling, pain, drainage, and even incisional separation. Seromas may not pose a serious threat to patients but the sudden release of copious amounts of serosanguinous drainage can create significant anxiety often prompting them to seek care in the emergency department. In these circumstances, the truly emergent condition of fascial dehiscence must be ruled out. Seromas and hematomas also are associated with increased risk of wound infection.

Hematoma and seroma can usually be identified by inspection, palpation, and partially opening or probing the wound. Ultrasonography can be used to differentiate subcutaneous fluid collections from subfascial or bladder-flap hematomas. Small and asymptomatic seromas and hematomas may simply be observed. If staples are present over the fluctuant or draining area, they should be removed. The remaining staples should be left in place until the nature and extent of the defect are known. Incisions secured with subcuticular sutures may need to be opened to adequately drain and assess the wound. Cultures should be obtained if an infection is suspected. After opening part or all of the wound, copious irrigation may be required to debride tissues or express clotted blood. Digital palpation or sterile swab is then used to check the fascial layer as the integrity of the fascia must be established.

Treatment options include secondary closure of the uninfected wound, either immediate or delayed, versus wound care and healing by secondary intention. Secondary closure in this setting has been found to be successful in over 80% of patients and significantly reduces healing time over secondary intention without risks of serious complications (5–7).

Total hysterectomy by any route and vaginal repair procedures can result in postoperative hematomas above the vaginal cuff or at the site of vaginal closure. These patients may present with vaginal bleeding or complaints of pain and pressure as well as anemia. Fever and leukocytosis may be observed in the presence of infection. If a mass is not observed or palpated on examination, pelvic ultrasound or computed tomography (CT) scan may help identify a pelvic hematoma. If no systemic infection is evident, the hematoma may be allowed to gradually resolve over time. Opening the vaginal repair or vaginal cuff and evacuating the clot in the emergency department or operating room may be necessary. CT-directed drainage of a pelvic hematoma can sometimes be achieved.

Laparoscopic procedures can result in significant hematomas of the abdominal wall even though trocar incisions appear small. In a review of the Finnish National Registry, 1,165 laparoscopic hysterectomies were associated with a vascular injury rate of 1.2% (8). Large vessel injuries are typically recognized intraoperatively, whereas superficial vessels and inferior epigastric injuries may not present themselves until after the patient has been discharged home from outpatient surgery. Patients may present with pain, induration, ecchymosis, and occasionally bleeding from the trocar site. Hemotomas can be large with discoloration of the anterior abdomen and can radiate around to the flank or back. CT or ultrasound can be used to determine the extent of the hematoma. Such hematomas may result in anemia which may require transfusion. These hematomas are usually self-limited and eventually resolve with observation but surgery may be required if bleeding persists or infection develops. Embolization of the inferior epigastric artery was recently described when other interventions failed to control hemorrhage of a lateral accessory trocar site (9).

## Surgical Site Infections

Surgical site infections are classified by the CDC as superficial incisional (involving only the skin or subcutaneous tissue of the incision), deep incisional (involving fascia and/or muscular layers), and organ/space. They occur in 2% to 5% of patients undergoing inpatient surgery in the United States, resulting in approximately 500,000 infections each year (10). Many gynecologic procedures and all cesarean sections are classified as "clean contaminated" procedures as the genitourinary tract is entered, thus increasing the risk of wound infection. Infections usually present late in the first postoperative week with erythema and either subcutaneous pockets of exudate (if the epithelium is intact) or frank sero-sanguinous or seropurulent drainage from an open incision. *Staphylococcus aureus* is common but enteric or vaginal flora is also commonly involved. Wound cultures should be obtained initially due to the increasing rate of methicillin-resistant Staphylococcus aureus (MRSA). Fascial integrity must be established as described above. The wound should be adequately opened for drainage and debridement performed as indicated followed by dressing changes or wound vacuum. Hospitalization and antibiotics may be required in cases of extensive involvement or sepsis, diabetes, obesity, immunosuppression, and suspected MRSA or when adequate outpatient wound care is not possible.

Necrotizing fasciitis represents a life-threatening soft-tissue infection primarily involving the superficial fascia. It is characterized by skin discoloration, skin and subcutaneous necrosis, crepitus, and sometimes hypesthesia as cutaneous nerves become ischemic. Systemic toxicity and multiorgan involvement can occur quickly. Wong et al. reviewed 89 consecutive patients over a 5-year span with necrotizing fasciitis and reported the following: polymicrobial synergistic infection was the most common cause with streptococci and enterobacteriaceae being the most common isolates. Group-A streptococcus was the most common cause of monomicrobial necrotizing fasciitis. The most common associated comorbidity was diabetes mellitus followed by advanced age. These factors and a delay in surgery of >24 hours adversely affected the outcome. Multivariate analysis showed that only a delay in surgery of >24 hours was correlated with increased mortality. Similarly, Bilton et al. reviewed 68 cases of necrotizing fasciitis, finding that the major predictor of favorable outcome was prompt aggressive surgical debridement (11,12). When such a treatment was delayed, mortality occurred in more than one third of cases, compared with <5% with prompt aggressive surgical debridement (11,12). To summarize, when necrotizing fasciitis is suspected, prompt diagnosis, aggressive surgical debridement, supportive care, and broad-spectrum antibiotics appear to be the keys to avoiding overwhelming sepsis and death.

## Fascial Dehiscence and Hernia

Dehiscence describes the separation of any of the layers of the abdominal wall, but the term is commonly used when partial or complete fascial disruption occurs. This separation may be associated with evisceration where small bowel and abdominal contents herniate through the defect. When the fascial layer does not heal properly, evisceration may occur in the early postoperative period, while such failure of healing may present later as an incisional hernia.

Fascial dehiscence as a complication of pelvic laparotomy performed for hysterectomy and other gynecologic surgeries occurs at a rate of 0.3% to 0.7%. Dehiscence occurs more frequently in midline incisions as opposed to transverse incisions (13). Age, underlying medical disease, obesity, infection, and malignancy increase the risk. Dehiscence tends to occur during the first 1 to 2 weeks of postoperative period and can present with the skin layer either open or intact. The most common associated complaint is serosanguinous discharge from the wound. The patient may also describe an associated sudden tearing or popping sensation brought on by coughing, lifting, or Valsalva maneuver. The fascia must be evaluated in such situations digitally or by probing with a sterile Q-tip. Imaging studies such as ultrasound, MRI, or CT scan may reveal the disrupted fascia with herniated abdominal contents when the skin is intact or the examination is inconclusive. Wound dehiscence should be considered a surgical emergency as it is associated with a mortality rate of up to 10%.

Initial treatment involves protecting the wound with a large moist sterile dressing and arranging for prompt surgical debridement and fascial closure in the operating room. The patient must be medically stabilized, cultures obtained, and broad-spectrum antibiotics initiated as wound infection or sepsis is often present. If the fascia cannot be reapproximated without tension, incorporating a synthetic fascial graft into the repair may be necessary. Skin and subcutaneous layers are typically left open for wound care and healing by secondary intention. Secondary closure may be an option once the wound appears adequately healthy.

Incisional hernia implies that superficial layers and peritoneum have healed but a facial defect is present. Hernias can be expected in nearly 1% of uncomplicated surgeries, in 10% when wound infection has occurred, and in 30% of patients with fascial repair after dehiscence (14). Once again, the incidence is higher with midline incisions but ventral hernias have been described in essentially all incisions employed in gynecologic surgery. Most incisional hernias present within the first 2 years following surgery with over 50% occurring within the first 6 months. Patients typically complain of a bulge beneath the surgical scar which may or may not be associated with discomfort and often exacerbated by straining or Valsalva maneuver.

If the contents of the hernia become entrapped in the fascial defect, incarceration with strangulation or obstruction can occur. Pain, peritoneal signs, and symptoms of bowel obstruction differentiate this patient from the easily reduced hernia and require stabilization and emergent surgical repair.

Minimally invasive procedures can also result in symptomatic hernias despite the relatively small incisions utilized. Reported incisional bowel herniation rates after laparoscopy range from 0.02% to 0.17% and are related to larger trocar size, multiple ancillary ports, tissue extraction, and longer operative times (15–17). In spite of recommendations to close the fascia on all trocar sites 10 mm and larger, 18% of the hernias cited in the AAGL (American Academy of Gynecologic Laparoscopists) survey cited above occurred despite fascial closure. Any laparoscopic patient with unusual pain at the incision site, the presence of a bulge, nausea, and vomiting, or symptoms of bowel obstruction must be evaluated for port site herniation and potential infarction of herniated omentum or bowel.

## Vaginal Cuff Dehiscence

Unique to gynecologic surgery is the potential for postoperative vaginal cuff dehiscence and vaginal evisceration. Although vaginal evisceration can be associated with vaginal trauma, spontaneous rupture of a large enterocele, or large uterine perforation with suction curettage, it should be suspected in the symptomatic posthysterectomy patient. An extensive review of the literature by Ramirez and Klemer in 2002 (18) found that although a rare event, with only 59 patients reported, vaginal evisceration represents a surgical emergency. Of those cases reported, 37 (63%) occurred following vaginal hysterectomy, 19 (32%) after abdominal hysterectomy, and 3 (5%) after laparoscopic hysterectomy. Small bowel was the most common organ to eviscerate. The most common presenting symptoms among these cases of vaginal evisceration were vaginal bleeding, pelvic pain, or a protruding mass. In postmenopausal women, vaginal evisceration was associated with increased intra-abdominal pressure. In premenopausal women, however, it was most often preceded by sexual intercourse. Some suggest an increased risk of cuff dehiscence following total laparoscopic hysterectomy with the use of thermal energy for colpotomy or inadequate laparoscopic cuff closure postulated as factors. One series of over 7,000 assorted hysterectomies over a 6-year span encountered 10 cuff dehiscences, 6 of which included bowel evisceration. Most (80%) were complications of total laparoscopic hysterectomies with the remaining two (one in each) associated with total abdominal hysterectomy (TAH) and transvaginal hysterectomy (TVH). The median time from surgery to dehiscence was 11 weeks. In each of these 10 cases, repair was accomplished vaginally (19).

## UROLOGIC EMERGENCIES

The incidence of surgical injuries to the ureter and bladder during gynecologic procedures is dependent upon several factors including the type and route of the procedure, anatomic distortions by adhesions or diseases, skill level of the performing surgeon, and the lack of intraoperative recognition of the injury. Reported rates of injury to the bladder during gynecologic operations range from 0.2% to 1.8% and for ureteral injuries from 0.03% to 1.5% (20). Actual figures are uncertain as many injuries go unrecognized. Ibeanu et al. (20) described their experience with cystoscopy during 839 hysterectomies for benign disease and found a total incidence of urinary tract injury of 4.3%, with bladder and ureteral injury rates of 2.9% and 1.8%, respectively. Cystoscopy detected 97.4% of injuries compared to only a 25.6% detection rate by visual inspection, suggesting an increased role for intraoperative cystoscopy. The most common types of ureteral injuries were transections and kinking, which occurred 80% of the time at the level of the uterine artery and ureter junction. With potentially undetected injuries and often rapid hospital discharge after many gynecologic procedures, the diagnosis and treatment of postoperative urologic conditions often fall upon the emergency physician.

### Urinary Retention
Although most postoperative patients have passed a voiding trial prior to catheter removal and hospital discharge, some may develop difficulty voiding and suffer urinary retention. Women who undergo incontinence procedures and difficult or radical hysterectomies are at increased risk for postoperative urinary retention. These patients describe the limited ability or inability to void with progressive pain and suprapubic mass. This condition can be diagnosed and easily treated by catheterization, either indwelling or intermittent self-catheterization. If presentation or diagnosis is delayed, the patient may develop an associated infection and require antibiotic treatment. Most cases of retention resolve over time but some cases persist, requiring chronic catheterization or the removal of anti-incontinence mesh.

### Bladder Injuries
Incidental injuries to the bladder can occur during any type of gynecologic procedure, including abdominal, vaginal, laparoscopic, hysteroscopic, or cesarean section. The incidence of bladder injuries associated with hysterectomy appears to be higher now than the 0.2% to 1% reported in the older literature, with increases observed when additional procedures for prolapse or incontinence are added and in the presence of prior surgeries. In a series of 257 hysterectomies done between 1986 and 1988, Gambone et al. (21) reported a rate of 2.3% for inadvertent bladder injury with two thirds of those occurring in patients with prior

c-section. Obvious bladder defects, bloody urine, or carbon dioxide gas in the urine collection bag during laparoscopy may lead to intraoperative recognition and repair. Injuries may also go undetected and present later with intraperitoneal urine collection or urine loss through various fistulas. Thermal intraoperative injury may also present days later even though the bladder appeared intact at the time of surgery.

Vesicoperitoneal fistula results in decreased urine output and the accumulation of intraperitoneal urine which can result in a peritonitis associated with pain, fever, and decreased bowel function. This can make differentiating this type of fistula from a bowel injury difficult. A CT urogram can reveal the bladder defect, but cystoscopy and retrograde evaluation of the ureters may be necessary to confirm the location of the defect. Although prolonged catheterization alone may result in spontaneous healing of small bladder injuries, surgical repair is often required.

Vesicovaginal fistulas can be seen after hysterectomies, prolapse repairs, and incontinence procedures. Vesicouterine fistulas have been reported after c-section and hysteroscopies (22,23). In both instances, patients present with continuous urine loss in spite of bladder catheterization. Differentiation from ureterovaginal fistula may be difficult and again could require CT urogram, cystoscopy, and hysteroscopy.

## Ureteral Injuries

Ureteral injury is a relatively rare but well-known complication of gynecologic surgery as the path of the ureter lies in close proximity to critical anatomic structures such as the infundibulopelvic ligament, uterine artery, and anterior vagina. Ureteral ligations, angulation or kinking, and transection can occur acutely whereas strictures from scarring, devascularization, and thermal injury may appear later. As stated previously, the actual incidence of injuries associated with gynecologic surgery is difficult to pinpoint as many injuries go undetected at the time of surgery and the risk is highly dependent on the technical difficulty of the procedure. The Collaborative Review of Sterilization (CREST) study published by Dicker (24) in 1982 reported a 0.2% ureteral injury rate for 1,851 elective hysterectomies. In comparison, Daly and Higgins (25) reported a significantly higher rate of 1.4% in 1,093 patients undergoing major gynecologic surgeries which included reoperative procedures involving the ovaries, malignancies, and emergency cases. Twelve injuries occurred at the pelvic brim and four others occurred elsewhere in the pelvis. Risk factors included previous surgical procedures in the pelvis, endometriosis, ovarian neoplasm, pelvic adhesions, distorted anatomic features of the pelvis, and repair of the bladder.

Symptomatic ureteral obstruction presents with ipsilateral flank pain or tenderness due to the distention of the collection system or renal capsule and occasionally radiates to the groin or labia with lower obstructions. Fever can indicate an associated pyelonephritis. Urine output is usually normal unless bilateral injuries have occurred. If no infection is present, urinalysis may also be normal. The plasma creatinine concentration also is usually normal or only slightly elevated with a unilateral injury. Only in rare cases does unilateral obstruction lead to anuria and acute renal failure when vascular or ureteral spasm is thought to result in loss of function in the nonobstructed kidney (26). Asymptomatic obstruction can be an incidental finding months or years later during a workup for an unrelated condition, making it too late for intervention to salvage the renal function.

Bladder catheterization should be the initial step in the patient with symptoms of obstruction in the postoperative period as urinary retention may be involved. Renal ultrasonography can usually detect hydronephrosis and hydroureter, but a false-positive rate of up to 25% can be seen when minimal criteria for obstruction are used (27). A CT urogram or an intravenous pyelogram (IVP) has the advantage of low false-positive rates and is more likely to identify the level of obstruction. In some instances where hydronephrosis is present but ureteral obstruction is questionable, a diuretic renogram involving the administration of furosemide prior to a radionuclide renal scan can be performed. However, cystourethroscopy with retrograde ureteropyelography has the advantage of both diagnosing a partial obstruction and attempting retrograde ureteral stent placement. If successfully placed, stents are left in place for several months to be removed later. If unsuccessful with retrograde stents, percutaneous nephrostomy should be performed allowing an attempt at antegrade stent placement.

Surgical management of ureteral injuries depends on the type and location of the injury. Obstructing or kinking sutures should be removed and, in the case of minor injury, stents placed. Major injuries, thermal injuries, or complete transections require excision of the damaged ureteral segment and definitive repair. Most distal ureteral injuries can be repaired by ureteroneocystostomy, but those near or above the pelvic brim require ureteroureterostomy (28).

Postoperative genitourinary fistulas generally present with continuous transvaginal urinary leakage developing anytime up to several weeks after surgery. Vaginal examination alone may yield evidence of the urethrovaginal, vesicovaginal, or ureterovaginal fistula, but transurethral instillation of an indigo carmine–colored solution can be helpful. Direct visualization of the blue dye or staining of a vaginal tampon suggests vaginal or urethral leakage. Blue staining of the tampon after intravenous indigo carmine or orange staining after oral pyridium suggests a ureterovaginal fistula. A CT urogram, cystourethroscopy, and retrograde studies can confirm the site of injury and document renal function. Prolonged catheterization of the bladder may allow for spontaneous healing of an early, small vesicovaginal fistula as may successful stenting of ureterovaginal defects, but surgical repair is often required.

## GASTROINTESTINAL EMERGENCIES

Postoperative nausea and vomiting related to medical or anesthetic factors typically are evident in the immediate period after surgery and are usually managed prior to patient discharge. The use of general anesthesia and opioid analgesics increase the risk of ileus. When patients present with nausea and vomiting following gynecologic surgery, distinguishing ileus from bowel obstruction represents a critical, and sometimes challenging, task for the clinician.

### Postoperative Ileus

A dynamic or paralytic ileus potentially occurs to some degree with any surgical procedure or intra-abdominal inflammation, but delay in return to normal function beyond the typical 24 to 48 hours for uncomplicated procedures defines postoperative ileus. Factors that delay the recovery of bowel motility include the extent of bowel manipulation, length of the procedure, intraoperative bowel injury, peritonitis, intraperitoneal hemorrhage, and electrolyte imbalances such as hypokalemia, hyponatremia, and hypomagnesemia. The possibility of unrecognized bowel injury or inadequate repair of a recognized injury should always be entertained when return of normal bowel function is delayed. This is particularly important when delayed postoperative ileus develops in a patient that was recovering normally. The aforementioned CREST study reported an incidence of paralytic ileus of 2.2% with abdominal hysterectomy and 0.2% for vaginal procedures (24).

Patients typically present with abdominal discomfort, lack of flatus or bowel movements, and abdominal distention accompanied by nausea and sometimes vomiting. Differentiating ileus from bowel obstruction or an injury is crucial and can be difficult. Ileus typically is not associated with fever, leukocytosis, localized tenderness, or peritoneal signs. Bowel sounds are absent and the distended abdomen may be tympanitic and usually nontender. Initial laboratory studies should include a complete blood count and serum electrolytes. The plain abdominal radiographs or "KUB" show multiple dilated loops of small bowel with gas visible throughout including the colon and rectum. Differential air-fluid levels are usually absent and their presence is suggestive but not always diagnostic of small bowel obstruction (SBO). CT with oral contrast can be utilized when differentiating between ileus and obstruction is difficult. Megibow et al. (29) reported the overall sensitivity of CT was 94%, specificity was 96%, and accuracy was 95% for cases of obstruction. In addition, CT imaging correctly predicted the cause of obstruction in 47 of 64 cases [73%].

The treatment of postoperative ileus involves bowel rest, intravenous fluids, and electrolyte management. If vomiting or significant abdominal distention persists, the patient may benefit from nasogastric tube decompression. Limiting the use of opioids is also suggested.

## Postoperative Bowel Obstruction

Although postoperative adhesions occur in over 60% of women undergoing a major gynecologic surgery, they usually do not result in significant complications but are implicated as a common contributing factor in SBO. The incidence of adhesion-related intestinal obstruction after gynecologic surgery for benign conditions without hysterectomy is approximately 0.3%. This increases to 2% or 3% among patients who undergo hysterectomy, and up to 5% if a radical hysterectomy is performed (30). Patients may present days or weeks after surgery, but symptoms can also occur years after the procedure. In one series of SBO attributed to adhesions, 50% were related to a benign abdominal hysterectomy (31). Hernia represents the next most common cause of SBO followed by tumors, intussusception, volvulus, and Crohn's disease. As the small bowel dilates and compromises blood flow, necrosis, strangulation, and sepsis can result.

Intermittent or crampy abdominal pain and abdominal distention with nausea, vomiting, and the absence of flatus are symptoms of bowel obstruction. Peristalsis of the obstructed bowel proximal to the obstruction can result in the characteristic high-pitched tinkling bowel sounds. Laboratory findings suggest hypovolemia and hemoconcentration as significant blood and fluid are sequestered in the bowel resulting in the air-fluid levels seen on plain radiographs of the abdomen. Leukocytosis is particularly concerning and may indicate strangulation and necrosis.

Treatment may require surgical intervention, but the patient should be stabilized, metabolic abnormalities corrected, and broad-spectrum antibiotics initiated when possible. Decompression by nasogastric tube, stabilization, and observation may be adequate treatment in many instances, but most series suggest that a majority of patients ultimately require surgery.

Obstruction of the large intestine is rare and usually involves cecal or sigmoid volvulus. The patient may not present with the symptoms of dehydration and vomiting as seen in SBO. Careful colonoscopy may be employed to correct the condition but surgery may also be required.

## Laparoscopic Bowel Injury

Bowel injury during laparoscopy may result from the insertion of the Veress needle, placement of primary and secondary trocars, inadvertent thermal injury, and direct trauma during manipulation or dissection. These injuries can pose serious consequences, as up to 25% of all laparoscopic entry complications are not recognized until the postoperative period (32). Combined data show that diagnostic and minor operative laparoscopies in gynecology are associated with a 0.08% risk of bowel injury, and in major operative laparoscopy, the risk increases to 0.33%. Up to 15% of these injuries are not diagnosed during laparoscopy, and one of five cases of delayed diagnosis results in death (33).

The key to avoiding delayed diagnosis is maintaining a high degree of suspicion in any laparoscopy patient that displays abnormal pain, increasing pain, peritoneal signs, or a general failure to thrive. One must consider bowel perforation, incarcerated hernia, bladder, or ureteral injuries in such patients and employ close observation. Symptoms from penetrating trauma or lacerations usually present in the early postoperative period. Small injuries that temporarily seal, or thermal injury followed by bowel necrosis, may not be apparent for 4 to 5 days. Ileus after laparoscopic surgery is not normal and warrants evaluation.

The initial treatment, laboratory, and imaging studies are the same as those discussed above for laparotomy cases. The presence of free air on upright abdominal radiographs does not indicate a ruptured viscus as 40% of patients will have >2 cm of free air imaged between the hepatic surface and the diaphragm at 24 hours postlaparoscopy (34). Failure of free air to decrease, or increasing intra-abdominal air, must be presumed to represent a ruptured viscous. In general, if a patient reports pain, fever, tachycardia, and abdominal distention, the assumption must be intraperitoneal injury until proven otherwise. Unnecessary delays in surgical intervention can be catastrophic.

## POSTOPERATIVE INFECTIONS

Routine administration of perioperative prophylactic antibiotics has reduced the incidence of postoperative infections. Nonetheless, postoperative infections still constitute the most common type of postoperative complication. In a review of 10,110 hysterectomies of all types, infections were the most common complication with incidences of 10.5%, 13.0%, and 9.0% in the abdominal, vaginal, and laparoscopic groups, respectively (35). The highest infection rate of 7.3% was urinary tract infections in the vaginal hysterectomy group, which is similar to the 7.0% rate in abdominal hysterectomies from the CREST study. As discussed earlier, wound infections among abdominal hysterectomy are also common, reaching an incidence of 3.1% in this series. Vaginal site infections occurred in 0.2%, 1.8%, and 1.4% of the abdominal, vaginal, and laparoscopic procedures, respectively.

It is important to remember that low-grade fever alone within the first 48 hours of surgery is not always indicative of infection but often reflects cytokine release from tissue trauma. Rates of unexplained fever range from 1.9% to 30%; this wide range reflects a lack of consistency in criteria among studies. Extensive fever workup should be reserved for high-risk patients such as those with malignancy, bowel injury or resection, high or prolonged fever, and increased white blood cell count.

### Pelvic Cellulitis and Abscess

Patients presenting several days to a week after gynecologic surgery with persistent fever, pelvic pain, vaginal cuff induration, and purulent discharge should be evaluated for pelvic cellulitis and abscess. Occasionally, peritoneal signs or ileus is also present. The diagnosis is somewhat subjective, but speculum examination typically reveals a purulent discharge from an indurated and tender vaginal cuff. If pelvic examination and ultrasound or CT scan shows a pelvic fluid collection, this usually represents a cuff abscess or an infected hematoma. The cause is usually a mixed infection of endogenous vaginal bacteria including anaerobes and occasionally Gram-negative aerobic bacteria. Once the diagnosis is made, broad-spectrum antibiotics should be initiated.

If an abscess or infected hematoma is identified and antibiotics alone are ineffective, drainage is indicated. If an abscess or infected hematoma is located in proximity to the vaginal cuff, transvaginal drainage in the operating room can be accomplished. CT-guided percutaneous drainage can be attempted when the abscess cannot be reached via the vaginal cuff. Occasionally, surgical drainage or evacuation of an abscess or hematoma must be performed via laparotomy or laparoscopy.

## Septic Pelvic Thrombophlebitis
Septic pelvic thrombophlebitis should be considered in the postoperative female patient with continued fever in spite of adequate broad-spectrum antibiotic therapy. Iliofemoral vein involvement may be accompanied by radiating pain toward the leg while ovarian vein thrombus contributes to unilateral pelvic or low back pain. Pulmonary embolus can occur from the pelvic thrombus. Fortunately, pulmonary embolus is a rare occurrence after gynecologic procedures. Pulmonary embolus is more common after vaginal delivery and cesarean section with reported incidences of 1:9,000 and 1:800, respectively (36). In the past, the diagnosis was implied when the patient responded to heparin therapy, but CT scan or MRI will confirm the diagnosis.

In many cases, simply continuing or changing antibiotic coverage will result in patient improvement as was shown by Brown et al. (36) where women given heparin in addition to antimicrobial therapy for septic pelvic thrombophlebitis did not have better outcomes than did those for whom antimicrobial therapy alone was continued. The other option is to add therapeutic heparin to the broad-spectrum antibiotic regimen until the patient is afebrile and clinically well for 48 hours, after which the anticoagulant can be discontinued.

## OTHER GYNECOLOGIC POSTOPERATIVE EMERGENCIES
Serious complications can be seen after relatively minor gynecologic procedures such as uterine dilatation and evacuation, operative hysteroscopy, and uterine artery embolization (UAE). Since these are outpatient procedures, the patient may present first to the emergency room seeking care.

### Uterine Perforation
Cervical dilatation and curettage, uterine evacuation, and hysteroscopy all can result in uterine perforation, which can be associated with bleeding, infection, and bladder or bowel injury. Endometritis, pelvic inflammatory disease or abscess, and sepsis require broad-spectrum antibiotic treatment and stabilization. Operative hysteroscopy and global endometrial ablation techniques add the potential of thermal energy injuries to the bowel. Patients presenting with atypical pain, fever, or peritoneal symptoms should be aggressively evaluated and managed.

### Uterine Artery Embolization
UAE is becoming a common minimally invasive alternative to myomectomy and hysterectomy in the treatment of symptomatic uterine leiomyomata. Performed by the interventional radiologist, this procedure can be associated with rare but serious conditions including pain, infection, fibroid expulsion, catheter site hematoma, and sequelae from inadvertent embolization of other structures. Ischemia from inadvertent embolization can affect the bowel, bladder, nerve, muscle, and skin as well as ovarian function. Postembolization syndrome commonly occurs

following UAE and consists of low-grade fever, malaise, nausea, and leukocytosis. Pain is the most common cause for hospital readmission (37).

Hysterectomy may be necessary after UAE as was reported in a 2003 multi-center prospective trial following 555 patients. By 3 months, eight women (1.5%) underwent complication-related hysterectomy [39]. Indications for hysterectomies were infections [2], postembolization pain [4], vaginal bleeding [1], and prolapsed leiomyoma [1] (38). Ischemic uterine rupture, sepsis, and even death have been reported following UAE (39).

### Retained Foreign Objects

In an attempt to identify risk factors for retained foreign bodies, authors from a 2003 study reviewed 10 hospitals over 15 years and found 54 patients with a total of 61 retained foreign objects. Over two thirds were sponges and 31% were instruments. Statistically significant risk factors for the retention of a foreign body were emergency surgery, unplanned change in the operation, and increased body mass index (40).

In the event of an incorrect count, plain radiographs of the entire abdomen and pelvis must be performed and reviewed before the patient leaves the operating room. This does not benefit the situations, however, when sponge, needle, and instrument counts are reported to be correct and the object remains in the patient undetected.

Retained foreign objects are ideally managed by prompt removal but occasionally remain asymptomatic until they are discovered during unrelated radiologic studies or present with symptoms much later. Removal of retained laparotomy pads or sponges can be difficult due to extensive adhesions. Retained instruments must be removed as they may cause pain and risk perforation injury. Small needles arguably pose little risk and may not require removal, but larger ones may result in injury.

## SUMMARY

As with all surgical procedures, gynecologic surgeries entail the risk of postoperative complications. Obstetricians, gynecologists, and emergency department physicians who are cognizant of the spectrum of possible complications, and appropriate management strategies, can improve outcomes for women experiencing these complications.

### References

1. Chelmow D, Rodriguez EJ, Sabatini MM. Suture closure of subcutaneous fat and wound disruption after cesarean delivery: a meta-analysis. *Obstet Gynecol.* 2004; 103:974–980.
2. Kore S, Vyavaharker M, Akolekar R, et al. Comparison of closure of subcutaneous tissue versus non-closure in relation to wound disruption after abdominal hysterectomy in obese patients. *J Postgrad Med.* 2000;46:26–28.
3. Bucknal TE, Cox PJ, Ellis H. Burst abdomen and incisional hernia: a prospectice study of 1129 major laparotomies. *Br Med J (Clin Res Ed).* 1982;284:931–933.
4. DeFrances CJ, Cullen KA, Kozak LJ. National Hospital Discharge Survey: 2005 annual summary with detailed diagnosis and procedure data. National Center for Health Statistics. *Vital Health Stat 13.* 2007;165:1–209.
5. Wechter ME, Pearlman MD, Hartman KE. Reclosure of the disrupted laparotomy wound: a systematic review. *Obstet Gynecol.* 2005;106:376–383.
6. Dodson MK, Magann EF, Meeks GR. A randomized comparison of secondary closure and secondary intention in patients with superficial wound dehiscence. *Obstet Gynecol.* 1992;80:321–324.
7. Walters MD, Dombroski RA, Davidson SA, et al. Reclosure of disrupted abdominal incisions. *Obstet Gynecol.* 1990;76:597–602.

8. Harki-Siren P, Sjoberg J, Makinen J, et al. Finnish national register of laparoscopic hysterectomies: a review of complications of 1165 operations. *Am J Obstet Gynecol.* 1997;176:118–122.

9. Lavery S, Porter S, Trew G, et al. Use of inferior epigastric artery embolization to arrest bleeding at operative laparoscopy. *Fertil Steril.* 2006;86:719.e13–719.e14.

10. Anderson DJ, Kaye KS, Classen D, et al. Strategies to prevent surgical site infections in acute care hospitals. *Infect Control Hosp Epidemiol.* 2008;29:s51–s61.

11. Wong CH, Chang HC, Pasupathy S, et al. Necrotizing fasciitis: clinical presentation, microbiology, and determinants of mortality. *J Bone Joint Surg Am.* 2003;85:1454–1460.

12. Bilton BD, Zibari GB, McMillan RW, et al. Aggressive surgical management of necrotizing fasciitis serves to decrease mortality: a retrospective study. *Am Surg.* 1998;64(5):397–400.

13. Harris JW. Early complications of abdominal and vaginal hysterectomy. *Obstet Gynecol Surv.* 1995;50(11):795–805.

14. Ellis H, Gajraj H, George CD. Incisional hernias: when do they occur? *Br J Surg.* 1983;70:290–291.

15. Montz FJ, Holschneder CH, Munro MG. Incisional hernia following laparoscopy: a survey of the American Association of Gynecologic Laparoscopists. *Obstet Gynecol.* 1994;84:881–884.

16. Kadar N, Reich H, Liu CY, et al. Incisional hernias after major laparoscopic procedures. *Am J Obstet Gynecol.* 1993;168:1493–1495.

17. Jansen FW, Kapiteyn K, Trimbos-Kemper T, et al. Complications of laparoscopy: a prospective multicentre observational study. *Br J Obstet Gynaecol.* 1997;104:595–600.

18. Ramirez PT, Klemer DP. Vaginal evisceration after hysterectomy: a literature review. *Obstet Gynecol Surv.* 2002;57(7):462–467.

19. Hur HC, Guido RS, Mansuria SM, et al. Incidence and patient characteristics of vaginal cuff dehiscence after different modes of hysterectomies. *J Minim Invasive Gynecol.* 2007;14(3):311–317.

20. Ibeanu OA, Chesson RR, Echols KT, et al. Urinary tract injury during hysterectomy based on universal cystoscopy. *Obstet Gynecol.* 2009;113:6–10.

21. Gambone JC, Reiter RC, Lench JB. Quality assurance indicators and short-term outcome of hysterectomy. *Obstet Gynecol.* 1990;76:841–844.

22. Mokrzycki ML, Hampton BS. Vesicouterine fistula presenting with urinary incontinence after primary cesarean section: a case report. *J Reprod Med.* 2007;52(12):1107–1108.

23. De Iaco P, Golfieri R, Ghi T, et al. Uterine fistula induced by hysteroscopic resection of an embolized migrated fibroid: a rare complication after embolization of uterine fibroids. *Fertil Steril.* 2001;75:818–820.

24. Dicker RC, Grenspan JR, Strauss LT, et al. Complications of abdominal and vaginal hysterectomy among women of reproductive age in the United States. *Am J Obstet Gynecol.* 1982;144:841–848.

25. Daly JW, Higgins KA. Injury to the ureter during gynecologic surgical procedures. *Surg Gynecol Obstet.* 1988;176:19–22.

26. Maletz R, Berman D, Peelle K, et al. Reflex anuria and uremia from unilateral ureteral obstruction. *Am J Kidney Dis.* 1993; 22:870.

27. Webb JA. Regular review: ultrasonography in the diagnosis of urinary tract obstruction. *Br Med J.* 1990;301:944.

28. Hurt GH. Gynecologic injury to the ureters, bladder, and urethra. In: Walters MD, Karram MM, eds. *Urogynecology and Resconstructive Pelvic Surgery.* 2nd Ed. St. Louis, MO: Mosby; 1999:377–386.

29. Megibow AJ, Balthazar EJ, Cho KC, et al. Bowel obstruction: evaluation with CT. *Radiology.* 1991;180:313–318.

30. Monk BJ, Berman ML, Montz FJ. Adhesions after extensive gynecologic surgery: clinical significance, etiology, and prevention. *Am J Obstet Gynecol.* 1994;170:1396–1403.

31. Al-Sunaidi M, Tulandi T. Adhesion-related bowel obstruction after hysterectomy for benign conditions. *Obstet Gynecol.* 2006;108:1162.

32. Magrina JF. Complications of laparoscopic surgery. *Clin Obstet Gynecol.* 2002;202(45):469–480.

33. Brosens I, Gordon A, Campo R, et al. Bowel injury in gynecologic laparoscopy. *J Am Assoc Gynecol Laparosc.* 2003;10:9–13.
34. Farooqui MO, Bazzoli JM. Significance of radiologic evidence of free air following laparoscopy. *J Reprod Med.* 1976;16:119.
35. Makinen J, Johansson J, Tomas C, et al. Morbidity of 10110 hysterectomies by type of approach. *Hum Reprod.* 2001;16:1473–1478.
36. Brown CE, Stettler RW, Twickler D, et al. Puerperal septic pelvic thrombophlebitis: incidence and response to heparin therapy. *Am J Obstet Gynecol.* 1999;181:143–148.
37. Wong JJ, Roberts AC. Pre-op work-up and post-op care of uterine fibroid embolization. In: Golzarian J, Sun S, Sharafuddin M, et al. eds. *Vascular Embolotherapy: A Comprehensive Approach.* Germany: Springer-Verlag; 2006:125–139.
38. Pron GP, Mocarski E, Cohen M, et al. Hysterectomy for complications after uterine artery embolization for leiomyoma: results of a Canadian multicenter trial. *J Am Asoc Gynecol Laparosc.* 2003;10:99–106.
39. De Blok S, de Vries C, Prinssen HM, et al. Fatal sepis after uterine artery embolization with microspheres. *J Vasc Interv Radiol.* 2003;14:779–783.
40. Gawande AA, Studdert DM, Orav EJ, et al. Risk factors for retained instruments and sponges after surgery. *N Engl J Med.* 2003; 348:229–235.

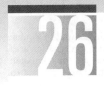

# 26 Emergency Evaluation and Treatment of the Sexual Assault Victim

## James L. Jones

Sexual assault or rape is a common violent crime in the United States. According to the National Crime Victimization Survey, there were 260,940 rapes and sexual assaults in the United States in 2006 (1).

Accurate statistics are difficult to obtain because sexual assault is a common crime and not often reported to authorities. The Rape, Abuse and Incest National Network statistics for 2001 show that 38.6% of rape was not reported to the police (2). Most rape victims who know their assailant are less likely to report the crime when the perpetrator is an acquaintance. These factors make sexual assault the most underreported crime in the United States.

Since the 1970s, rape crisis centers have been developed in urban areas of the United States to deal with the particular problems of the sexual assault victims. Rape crisis centers often provide training for physicians and nurses in performing sexual assault examinations. These centers also provide continuity of care and counseling that is difficult to obtain in many other settings. The multidisciplinary approach used by many centers underscores the importance of the psychological aspects of sexual assault. In addition to meeting the acute medical needs of the patient, the medical staff is responsible for advocating for the immediate and long-term emotional needs of the victim as well.

Many physicians are uncomfortable performing sexual assault examinations. Sexual assault examinations are performed by nurse examiners in many states (3,4). The most important considerations in determining who should perform a sexual assault examination are experience and interest, as well as local statutes related to medical care. The forensic aspects of the examination require strict attention to detail and experience in performing sexual assault examinations. The psychological aspects of sexual assault demand that the examiner be compassionate, patient, and understanding. A list of the responsibilities of the examiner in caring for a victim, as described by Kobernick et al. (5), follows:

1. Prompt treatment of physical injuries
2. Collection of legal evidence
3. Careful physical examination
4. Documentation of pertinent history
5. Prevention of pregnancy
6. Prevention of sexually transmitted disease
7. Psychological support and arrangement for follow-up counseling

The physician or examiner should be familiar with all these aspects of care of sexual assault victims.

Five to ten percent of adult sexual assault victims are men. It is important to realize that male victims deserve the same respect and treatment considerations as female victims.

## TRIAGE

Upon arrival at the emergency department, the victim should not wait in a public area but should be quickly and discreetly escorted to a private examination area. An assessment of the extent of the victim's injuries should be made on admission. Critically injured victims should be treated without delay in an urgent care area. The forensic examination should be performed only after the victim is stabilized. If the victim has to be taken to the operating room, specimens can often be safely collected during an operative procedure. Fortunately, sexual assault victims are not usually severely injured. An unpublished review of 100 consecutive assaults reported to the Sexual Assault Recovery Center at Shands Hospital, Jacksonville, Florida, found that only two patients required hospitalization for injuries sustained during an assault. One patient was bleeding heavily from a labial laceration and required an examination under anesthesia; the other was a victim of a severe beating. A study by Hicks of rape victims presenting to a Miami emergency room also found that <1% of all victims require hospitalization (6).

The victim should be instructed not to wash, use the toilet, eat, or drink until the examination is completed. If friends or family members are present, they may remain with the victim if she wishes. If the victim is alone, a nurse or rape crisis counselor should stay with her. The victim should not be left alone.

Loss of control is an important psychological factor in rape; it is important to help the victim reestablish control over her surroundings. It is important that the victim be reassured as to her safety. The examiner should carefully explain the procedures that will be performed. At the Sexual Assault Recovery Center at Shands Hospital, the victim is given a folder containing information about each step of the examination. A list of tests that have been ordered is included along with the expected completion date. The victim should be informed that she may refuse any part of the examination. Consents for the examination and the release of the information to the police should be reviewed carefully and signed. Whether the victim intends to report the crime should be immaterial; she is still entitled to medical care.

## FORENSIC MEDICINE

Many physicians find the medicolegal aspects of sexual assault intimidating. The examining physician must be familiar with the specific guidelines issued by the prosecuting attorney for sexual assault examination (7). Prepackaged rape kits are also available that should fulfill a particular state's guidelines for collecting evidence. Common medical practices, such as using the newer rapid DNA probe technologies for detection of *Neisseria gonorrhoeae* and *Chlamydia trachomatis*, may not be admissible in some courts and cannot replace a traditional culture in making a diagnosis. As newer technologies are introduced, state guidelines change, and the hospital's protocol should be updated.

The most important aspect of a forensic examination is adequate and careful documentation. Notes must be legible. Physicians may be called to testify years after the assault, and they must be able to rely solely on notes taken during the examination. It is equally important that physicians not make remarks that may be misinterpreted at a later date or in court. This can be avoided if physicians realize that their role is not to determine whether the victim has been raped but to determine whether the examination is consistent with sexual assault. Physicians should avoid conclusive statements that are not supported by facts or their experience. Remarks concerning the victim's behavior should not be entered into the record unless they are purely descriptive. Coping mechanisms produce a wide spectrum of responses to rape, thus physicians may encounter behavior that seems incongruent with a history of assault. Therefore, statements such as the victim's behavior is inconsistent with sexual assault are inappropriate. The patient's affect can be described instead.

Physicians should also understand the concept of "chain of custody." Courts will not consider evidence admissible if a direct line of custody cannot be established between the examiner and the court. As the evidence is gathered, it is placed into separate envelopes, sealed, and initialed. All specimens must be clearly labeled with the victim's name, the date, the examiner's name, and the source of the specimen. Clothing is placed in paper bags. Glass slides should be placed in carriers with rigid sides. The bags, envelopes, and carriers should be sealed with plastic tape and the examiner's initials written across the tape or the seal. This should be done in such a fashion that if the container were opened, the tampering would be obvious. The evidence should then be placed in a large paper bag or envelope and sealed. The evidence is then either handed directly to a police officer or placed in a locked cabinet. A receipt should be obtained for the evidence when it is transferred to the police. Breaking the chain of custody, by faulty handling or record keeping, may make the entire examination inadmissible in court.

## OBTAINING A MEDICAL HISTORY

The purpose of obtaining a history in a sexual assault case is to record as soon as possible the events that have occurred and to guide the physician during the examination. If the patient is an adult and a good historian, the physician may eliminate some parts of the exam and tests, such as obtaining rectal or oral cultures when only vaginal penetration has occurred. In the absence of an adequate history, the physician should perform an encompassing physical examination. If the physician records remarks made directly by the victim, these should be placed in quotations; otherwise, the remarks are assumed to be paraphrased.

The history should include the following:

1. Medical and surgical history: This should include allergies and medications.
2. Gynecologic history: The examiner should emphasize last coitus, menstrual history, current method of contraception, history of sexually transmitted disease, history of pelvic inflammatory disease, tampon use, and douching practices.
3. Obstetric history: Methods of delivery, gravidity, and parity.
4. Location, date, and time of assault.
5. Description of assault: The victim should be asked to describe the assault in her own words. The examiner should ask the victim to include the number of assailants, whether force was used, the presence of weapons, and what type of assault occurred. If the patient does not volunteer enough information, it is appropriate to ask, for example, "Did he put his penis in your vagina?"

## PHYSICAL EXAMINATION OF THE ADULT

It is particularly important to inform the patient again of exactly what the examination involves and to reassure her that the examination will not be painful. The examiner should collect as much of the victim's clothing as feasible, particularly the panties. The victim should remove the clothing herself, preferably over a clean paper or cloth sheet to catch any debris. If it is necessary to cut the victim's clothing to remove it, torn or stained areas should be left intact.

The victim should then be carefully examined, paying close attention to lacerations, bruises, and foreign material (Fig. 26.1). Any foreign material should be carefully removed, placed in an envelope, and identified as to the location of origin. Bruises, bite marks, and lacerations should be carefully described and diagrammed. Lacerations should be inspected carefully, particularly if a sharp object was used in the assault, to rule out a deep, penetrating injury. Photographs may be helpful if they effectively demonstrate an injury but should be taken by a

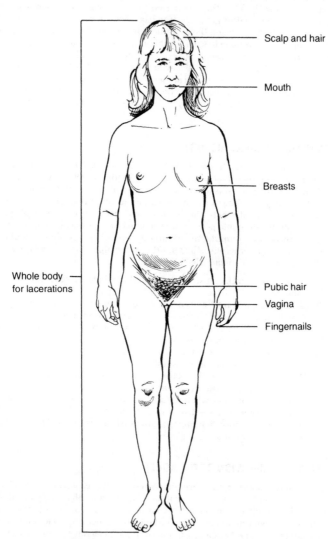

Scalp and hair

Mouth

Breasts

Whole body
for lacerations

Pubic hair

Vagina

Fingernails

**FIGURE 26.1** Examination of the sexual assault victim.

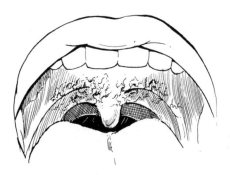

**FIGURE 26.2** Fellatio syndrome: ecchymoses of the palate.

police or a medical photographer. Photographs can actually harm a case if they do not add significant graphic detail. The photograph should be labeled with an indelible marker or by other permanent means of identification.

A tongue blade or a moist, cotton-tipped applicator should be used to collect any suspicious stains or deposits on the skin. Since semen fluoresces a bright yellow-green, deposits can often be identified with a Woods light. The head hair should be combed with a new comb over a paper towel, carefully collecting foreign material. Loose pubic hair should be collected in a similar fashion.

The oral cavity should be carefully examined with a tongue blade. Victims will often bite themselves during a sexual assault, producing small abrasions in the buccal mucosa. Fellatio may also cause small submucosal hemorrhages, which are usually seen at the junction of the hard and the soft palates (Fig. 26.2) (8). If there is a history of fellatio, the oral cavity, especially the areas between the gum and the lips, should be swabbed with a cotton-tipped applicator and glass slides should be prepared. When obtaining specimens for determination of the presence of sperm, two slides should be made. One goes directly to the forensic laboratory; the other is used immediately as a wet mount. The specimens should be made with several swabs. After the slides are prepared, the swabs are allowed to air-dry before placing them in an envelope. The presence of sperm as noted by the examiner should be recorded in the chart, and a separate notation should be made as to whether the sperm are motile. Pharyngeal cultures should be taken for *N. gonorrhoeae*. A saliva specimen is obtained from the victim for blood antigen determination. A small square of filter paper is placed in the victim's mouth, and the victim is encouraged to saturate it with saliva. It is important that no one handles the filter paper except the victim. If there is a history of fellatio, the victim should rinse her mouth out with water and wait 5 minutes before preparing the specimen.

The fingernails should be inspected for foreign material under the nails. If any foreign material is present, including dirt, it should be collected over a paper towel with a blunt wooden probe. Scrapings from each hand should be submitted separately.

The victim is then asked to lie on the examination table in the dorsal lithotomy position, so that a pelvic examination can be performed. The labia, posterior fourchette, and vestibule are carefully inspected under adequate lighting. Bruises, lacerations, and tender areas are carefully explored, diagrammed, and photographed, if necessary. Wood's light should again be employed to highlight semen deposits. In younger victims, the posterior fourchette is very susceptible to injury, which appears as fine lacerations. In cases of chronic sexual abuse, the examiner should look for scarring in the posterior fourchette and the posterior vestibule.

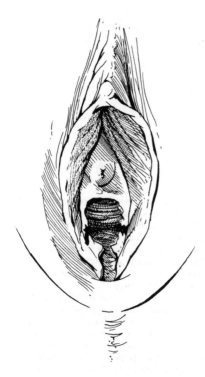

**FIGURE 26.3** Laceration of hymenal ring and posterior fourchette.

Physical findings suggestive of vaginal penetration are present in approximately 50% of sexual assault victims, but only 2% show clinical evidence of significant genital trauma (9). Injuries are typically minor and appear as small abrasions and lacerations. The examiner should describe any visible lesions and diagram their locations. The most commonly injured sites are the posterior aspect of the introitus, the hymen, labia minora, and the posterior fourchette (Fig. 26.3) (8). In a study of 311 rape victims by Slaughter et al. (10), 76% of the victims had an average of 3.1 sites of injury. Victims with nongenital injury are more likely to have genital trauma. In the absence of gross laceration, two techniques can be employed to highlight microlacerations: colposcopy and toluidine blue staining. The colposcope is a medium-powered binocular microscope with an internal light source that is commonly used to visualize the cervix (9). In a study of 18 volunteers examined within 6 hours after coitus, Norvell et al. (11) showed that microlacerations of the introitus and the vagina could be identified in 61%. Toluidine blue staining can also be used in the absence of gross lesions to highlight microlacerations (12). The stain should be applied directly to the perineum and then carefully wiped off using lubrication jelly on a gauze. Toluidine blue is a nuclear stain, so normal keratinized skin will not stain. Microlacerations show up as finely stained blue lines.

The buttocks are then gently separated and the anus is inspected for evidence of small fissures, lacerations, and scarring. Hemoccult should be obtained for evidence of occult rectal bleeding. If there is a history of anal penetration, the physician should look for evidence of rectal bleeding. Unexplained rectal bleeding should alert the physician to the possibility of bowel perforation. Proctoscopy or flexible sigmoidoscopy is then indicated.

Anal swabs should be taken and glass slides prepared. Sperm may be recovered from the rectum, but the yield is usually significantly lower than that from the vagina or the cervix (13).

A speculum moistened with warm water (do not use lubricant) can then be gently inserted in the vagina. The cervix is visualized for any evidence of trauma. Microlacerations on the cervix resulting from sexual trauma can be visualized with the aid of the colposcope (9). A specimen should be taken from the external os, and two glass slides should be prepared. Samples are also taken from the vaginal pool. Whether the sperm are motile should be noted. Sperm may remain motile in the vaginal pool for 12 hours. Sperm survival in the cervical os is considerably longer; motile sperm can be recovered from the cervix for up to 7 days (14). Cultures for gonorrhea and *Chlamydia* should be taken. As noted earlier, most courts will not accept direct antigen tests for determination of gonorrhea. At Shands Hospital in Jacksonville, Florida, the sensitivity and the specificity of the BD Probe Tec (15) assay are 100% and 100% for both *N. gonorrhoeae* and *C. trachomatis*.

Two vaginal swabs are obtained for antigen determination. Blood group antigens are secreted into body fluids by approximately 80% of the population (16). Although it cannot identify a specific assailant, this technique is useful to exclude or include someone from a list of suspects.

Vaginal swabs are also obtained for analysis of the prostatic antigen, p30, and acid phosphatase. Finding these seminal factors can establish penile penetration in the absence of sperm.

Additional swabs, usually six to eight, also can be obtained from the vaginal pool for DNA profiling. DNA profiling depends on the diversity of repetitive regions of DNA, variable number tandem repeat (VNTR) for forensic analysis. These regions are targeted with specific primers, amplified using PCR and separated with either capillary or gel electrophoresis. First described in 1985, there are a number of analytical techniques including short tandem repeat (STR), Y-STR, and mitochondrial DNA testing in common use. STR is primarily used for forensic analysis. In the United States, the FBI has designated 13 STR loci for analysis and maintains the CODIS, Combined DNA Index System, database. Unlike fingerprint analysis, DNA profiling cannot identify a specific individual. It can, however, indicate the probability that an individual is involved to greater than one in a trillion.

The vaginal walls are then inspected for lacerations. This is most easily accomplished while slowly withdrawing the speculum. In very young or postmenopausal patients, who have poorly estrogenized vaginal mucosa, lacerations of the vaginal sidewalls are more common. Laceration of the cul-de-sac or the posterior vaginal fornix can also be seen, particularly if a foreign object is inserted into the vagina. Injury from insertion of a foreign object can also cause perforation of the cul-de-sac and bowel injury. If a penetrating injury is suspected, a laparotomy should be performed to rule out injury to the bowel.

## EXAMINATION OF THE CHILD

A discussion of sexual abuse in children must begin with the physician's legal requirement for reporting of cases. In all states, a physician having a reason to suspect child sexual abuse must report to a designated agency. Agencies that receive reports vary in different states and localities, and it is essential that the physician learns these requirements before performing any examination.

The services of a multidisciplinary assessment team, if available, can be of great assistance in evaluating the child and the total family situation.

Examinations for alleged sexual abuse in children usually do not result from allegations of acute rape (17). More commonly, the allegation is of incest, fondling, molestation, or exploitation. This being the case, serious questions must be raised as to whether an emergent examination is required or whether the child should be referred to a team for a total evaluation. In the unusual case where there may be forensic collection considerations, the protocol for obtaining specimens should be similar to that used in adult patients. The expected yield from collection of evidence in child victims, however, is quite different in children than in adults. In the study done at Children's Hospital of Philadelphia, Christian et al. (18) found that forensic evidence, when present, was found on clothes or bedclothes, not on the prepubertal child. Chronic or recurrent sexual abuse in children is usually manifested by subtle physical signs and is likely to be accompanied by behavioral or developmental signs or symptoms. For this reason, the child sexual assault examination must be carried out in the context of a total pediatric health assessment and by an examiner skilled in assessing for the specific manifestations of child sexual abuse (19). After a history has been taken by the examiner or by a trained interviewer, the examiner should decide the extent of the examinations necessary, decide the cultures and specimens to be collected, and incorporate an explanation for the child, who should know that the examination is not painful or more intrusive than necessary. The examiner should be understanding and patient but should not play games with the child to gain cooperation. This is a common ploy of abusers.

Children should never be examined against their will. If examination is absolutely necessary for medical reasons, the examination should be performed under anesthesia. Genital examinations in children should be carried out in the modified dorsal lithotomy (frog-leg) and/or knee–chest position. Children are often uncomfortable in the knee–chest position, but it may offer visualization up to the cervix without instrumentation. Uncooperative or frightened children often do quite well in their mother's lap on an examining table (Fig. 26.4). Stirrups may be used in older children but are usually unnecessary and frightening in younger children. The use of a colposcope in the examination offers a light source, magnification, and photographic documentation and greatly simplifies evaluation and documentation (20).

Findings associated with child sexual abuse have been more clearly delineated in recent years. In addition, there is a greatly enhanced understanding of normal anatomic variations based on recent studies (21–27). Most of the physical findings seen with sexual abuse are indicators of genital trauma and must be coupled with the history to raise a serious question of abuse. Some findings or combinations of findings, however, are so compelling as to be reasonably diagnostic of abuse. In our experience with a highly selected referral population, 65% of examinations result in no finding, 30% have findings consistent with sexual abuse, and 5% have findings considered diagnostic of sexual abuse. It is useful to remember that a normal examination is often seen with any kind of allegation. Many times the offender has confessed to specific sexual acts and there is no physical finding. A physical examination alone can never rule out the possibility of sexual abuse (28,29).

The genital examination is best performed by using labial traction, in which the labia majora are grasped between the thumbs and the index fingers and are gently lifted laterally and toward the examiner, or labial separation, where the thumbs of the examiner are placed on the labia majora and mild lateral pressure is applied. The latter is more comfortable, whereas the former usually offers better direct visualization of the edges of the hymen. Digital or speculum examinations are rarely advisable or necessary except in sexually active older children.

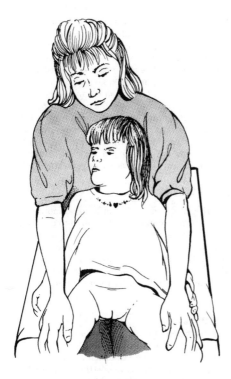

**FIGURE 26.4** Position of a child on the mother's legs for examination.

Many of the findings associated with genital trauma focus on changes in the hymen. A clear understanding of normal variants is essential. The hymen can normally be circular (annular), semilunar (crescentic, with attachments at about 2 o'clock and 10 o'clock), cribiform, or septate. In unusual circumstances, the hymen may be imperforate, which has medical implications but no implications for sexual abuse. Congenital absence of the hymen has never been reported (30). In the first few months of life, the hymen is still estrogenized from maternal influences and becomes estrogenized again in early puberty. Estrogenization produces an appearance of hypertrophy, redundancy, and white, pearl-like mucosa. It often is more difficult to assess for scars with these changes.

Findings statistically diagnostic of penetrating trauma or sexual abuse are

- Fresh lacerations of the anus or posterior fourchette
- Acute laceration or healed complete transection of the hymen
- Bruising of the hymen
- Absence of a part of the hymen
- Scars on the anus, posterior fourchette, penis, or scrotum
- Pregnancy (31–34).

Documentation issues are even more important in children than in adults, as the time between the examination and the possible testimony is even longer. Photographs are the method of choice for accurate documentation of findings, but detailed diagrams of body findings and specific genital findings may suffice. Laboratory support may be very useful in supporting the diagnosis of child sexual abuse. Cultures for *N. gonorrhoeae* should routinely be done in all postpubertal cases where genital contact by the abuser is possible. Cultures in prepubertal children are indicated only if there are signs of infection. Since positive cultures from sites other than the primary contact are common, cultures should be obtained from vaginal, rectal, and oropharyngeal sites. A positive result from culture makes sexual contact a certainty if the patient is not a newborn. Cultures for *C. trachomatis* and herpes, types 1 and 2, may be indicated under certain clinical conditions. The presence of genital warts on gross inspection or *Trichomonas vaginalis* in wet preparations is usually considered a strong indicator of sexual abuse in children. However, condylomata can be acquired either through autoinoculation or perinatal transmission (35). Human immunodeficiency virus (HIV) antibody testing and serologic testing for syphilis are not routinely done unless more specific indicators are present (19,36).

## TREATMENT OF SEXUAL ASSAULT VICTIMS

Most physical injuries sustained during rape or sexual assaults are minor. Minor cuts, abrasions, and bruises on the external genitalia will respond to cold compresses and sitz baths. Vaginal sidewall lacerations often do not require repair unless they are deep. Deep lacerations are best repaired under anesthesia, where the extent of the lesion can be more fully appreciated. As noted earlier, penetrating injuries to the cul-de-sac also require examination under anesthesia and possible exploratory laparotomy. Patients assaulted with foreign objects should also receive tetanus prophylaxis.

### Prevention of Sexually Transmitted Disease

The risks of acquiring a sexually transmitted disease from a single act of sexual assault are difficult to determine. The risks depend on the prevalence of the disease in the local community and on the nature of the assault. Infections detected within 24 hours of the assault most likely represent a preexisting condition (37). In a small study of 109 sexual assault victims who returned for follow-up, Jenny et al. (38) found that the risks of acquiring *N. gonorrhoeae* and *C. trachomatis* from a single act of sexual assault were 4% and 2%, respectively. The baseline prevalence of these infections in assault victims is higher: 6% for *N. gonorrhea* and 10% for *Chlamydia*. The prevalence of syphilis in rape victims has been reported in several studies to be <3% (38). The risk of acquiring HIV from a single act of unprotected vaginal intercourse has been estimated as between 0.1% and 0.2%. The risk of transmission of HIV from penile–anal penetration is somewhat higher, between 0.1% and 3.0% (36).

Sexual assault may result in an increased risk of the transmission of HIV since transmission of the virus is facilitated if the normal barriers that intact vaginal and vulvar mucosa provide are broken down.

Many sexual assault centers provide prophylactic antibiotics at the time of the sexual assault examination. Although the risk of acquiring a sexually transmitted disease from a single assault is low, treatment at the time of the initial examination is safe and effective and avoids treatment failure due to poor follow-up. Lack of adequate follow-up is a significant challenge in treating sexual assault victims. At Shands Hospital, Jacksonville, Florida, only 20% of victims return for follow-up counseling or testing. In the study by Jenny et al. (38), cited previously, follow-up was accomplished in only 53%.

The treatment should cover the most common pathogens, gonorrhea, *Chlamydia*, and incubating syphilis. The Centers for Disease Control (CDC) recommendations for treatment of common sexually transmitted diseases are outlined in Table 26.1 (36). Selection of prophylaxis should also be determined by

**TABLE 26.1** CDC 2006 Guidelines for Treatment of Sexually Transmitted Diseases

| Disease | Treatment |
| --- | --- |
| **Chlamydia** | |
| Recommended regimens | Azithromycin, 1 g orally in a single dose, OR Doxycycline, 100 mg twice a day for 7 d |
| Alternative regimens | Erythromycin base, 500 mg orally four times a day for 7 days, OR Erythromycin ethylsuccinate, 800 mg orally four times a day for 7 d |
| **Gonococcal infections** | |
| Recommended regimens | Cefixime, 400 mg orally in a single dose, OR Ceftriaxone, 125 mg IM in a single dose, OR |
| Alternative regimens | Spectinomycin, 2 g IM in a single dose, OR Ceftizoxime, 500 mg IM, OR Cefotaxime, 500 mg IM, OR Cefotetan, 1 g IM |
| **Syphilis** | |
| Recommended regimen | Benzathine penicillin G, 2.4 million units IM once |
| Alternative regimens | Doxycycline, 100 mg orally twice a day for 2 weeks, OR Tetracycline, 500 mg orally four times a day for 2 weeks |
| **Trichomoniasis** | |
| Recommended regimen | Metronidazole, 2 g orally in a single dose |
| Alternative regimen | Metronidazole, 500 mg twice a day for 7 d |

*Note:* CDC, Centers for Disease Control; IM intramuscularly.
*Source:* Ref. 36.

local sensitivity studies. It should be noted that the CDC no longer recommends the use of fluroquinolones for the treatment of gonorrhea due to antibiotic resistance (39).

Antibiotics that can be given as a single dose are preferred. The risk that young children will acquire *N. gonorrhoeae* or *Chlamydia* from sexual assault is low. Prophylaxis is not recommended unless the assailant is known to be infected, and treatment with antibiotics is withheld until diagnostic tests are completed. Treatment of *N. gonorrhoeae* and *C. trachomatis* in children is adjusted to body weight (36).

### Postexposure Prophylaxis for Sexually Transmitted Viruses

The management of patients exposed to HIV, human papillomavirus (HPV), herpes simplex virus, and hepatitis continues to evolve. Postexposure prophylaxis (PEP) for health care workers exposed to hepatitis and HIV has become standard practice. It has been estimated that the use of zidovudine has led to an 81% reduction in the transmission of HIV to health care workers after a needle stick (40). PEP is unavailable for HPV and not routinely offered for herpes simplex.

Prophylactic treatment of sexual assault victims for HIV is more controversial. The medications are expensive and funding issues may present obstacles to treatment. Complicating the decision process is the low follow-up rate of rape victims. PEP for HIV is effective but there are significant possible side effects, some so severe as to lead to discontinuance of the medications. Serial laboratory studies such as liver function tests and complete blood counts should be obtained. Close follow-up with psychological support is essential but may be difficult to obtain. Patients requesting such prophylaxis must be carefully counseled prior to initiating treatment.

While the risk of acquiring HIV after a sexual assault is low, approximately 5 per 10,000 exposures, sexual assault victims should be offered prophylaxis for HIV (41).

Such guidelines are based on the familiar Public Health Service guidelines for management of health care workers exposed to HIV (42). When there is a significant risk of exposure to HIV, a course of highly active antiretroviral therapy, HAART, should be initiated as soon as possible. These medications must be initiated within 72 hours of the assault, otherwise, HAART is not recommended. The CDC recommends a 4-week regimen of two drugs, such as zidovudine and lamivudine, for most HIV exposures (42). At this time, there are insufficient clinical data to suggest a specific antiviral regime. A protease inhibitor such as indinavir is added if the exposure involves an increased risk of transmission of the virus or if resistance to one of the drugs used for PEP is suspected. Oral, rectal, or vaginal penetration by the assailant's penis should be considered a high-risk exposure. The CDC recommendations for management of patients after a sexual exposure are listed in Table 26.2.

Unfortunately, there are no clear-cut guidelines for health care workers regarding counseling of sexual assault victims. It is important to remember that clinical data support only the use of zidovudine. Additional drugs were added based on the experience gathered in treating HIV-infected patients. As this field of medicine is rapidly evolving, patients should be referred to physicians who are expert in the use of these medications and the management of HIV.

If the assailant was known, attempts should be made to determine if he is a carrier of hepatitis B. If the victim requests, she should be offered prophylaxis with hepatitis B immunoglobulin. Prophylactic treatment for hepatitis B is usually not offered to rape victims unless the assailant is a known carrier or the victim requests it.

| TABLE 26.2 | Basic and Expanded PEP Regimens |
|---|---|

**Basic regimen**
4 weeks of both zidovudine, 600 mg PO every day in divided doses (i.e., 300 mg b.i.d.), and lamivudine, 150 mg PO b.i.d.

**High-risk exposure**
Basic regimen plus either

- Indinavir, 800 mg PO q 8 hr
  OR
- Nelfinavir, 750 mg PO t.i.d.
  OR
- Abacavir, 300 mg b.i.d.
  OR
- Efavirenz, 600 mg daily at bedtime

It is important that these medications be started immediately.

*Note*: PO, by mouth; b.i.d., twice daily; t.i.d., three times per day.
*Source*: Ref. 36.

It is also important that the victim understands that sexually transmitted viruses are chronic infections. HPV-related cervical dysplasia may surface years after an exposure, and it is important that the victim understands that yearly Pap smears are essential. Follow-up testing for HIV and hepatitis B may also be indicated.

### Prevention of Pregnancy

The risk of pregnancy after an unprotected act of intercourse ranges from 0% to 26%, depending on the timing of the victim's cycle. If the victim is at risk for pregnancy and the examination occurs within 72 hours of the assault, postcoital (emergency) hormonal birth control should be offered.

While a number of hormonal preparations have been used to prevent pregnancy, a progestin-only formulation, Plan B, is widely used and approved by the US Food and Drug Administration for emergency contraception (43). This method is somewhat more effective than a regime based on the Yuzpe method and is associated with less nausea. However, the original method of Yuzpe is very effective and widely available (44). This technique uses high-dose ethinyl estradiol and norgestrel/levonorgestrel to prevent pregnancy. A commercially available product, Preven, is marketed as an emergency contraceptive based on the Yuzpe technique. The principal mechanism of action is to prevent fertilization. A study of the effectiveness of the Yuzpe method of emergency contraception estimates that the technique reduces the risk of pregnancy by 75.4% (45). One hundred micrograms of ethinyl estradiol and either 1.0 mg of norgestrel or 0.5 mg of levonorgestrel is given orally within 72 hours of the assault; this is repeated 12 hours later. Any combination of birth control pills that provides the equivalent amount of ethinyl estradiol and norgestrel may be used. The pregnancy rate with this regime is approximately 1.6% (43). The ACOG Practice Bulletin on Emergency Contraception (December 2005) outlines 21 separate regimens which may be used for emergency contraception in addition to Plan B (46). The most common side effect of these regimens is nausea and vomiting, which may be treated with antiemetics.

Insertion of a copper-bearing intrauterine device (IUD) within 5 days of conception is also an effective means of preventing implantation (46). In patients in whom hormonal therapy is counterindicated, the copper IUD is a reasonable option. As there are no studies regarding the efficacy of progesterone secreting IUDs in such settings, these devices should not be used.

It should be remembered that postcoital hormonal or IUD birth control is considered by some to be a form of abortion. The mechanism of action of these techniques should be carefully explained to the victim so she can make an informed decision. In addition, a sensitive pregnancy test should be obtained before any treatment is initiated.

### Psychological Support and Counseling

The most significant medical problem that the rape victim presents with is a psychological one. Rape trauma syndrome was initially described by Burgess and Holmstrom in 1974 (47). The syndrome is composed of two phases, an acute phase and a long-term reorganization phase.

The response to sexual assault seen in the acute phase is described as either controlled or expressive. Expressive behaviors, demonstrated by 75% of victims, include anger, grief, and anxiety. Twenty-five percent of victims respond in a controlled fashion and internalize their emotions. Such controlled behavior has led some examiners to conclude that the victim has not been assaulted because her behavior is different from what is expected.

Somatization is a common feature of the acute phase. Victims may complain of a wide variety of somatic manifestations of the sexual assault, including sleep disturbances, muscle tension, headaches, and gastrointestinal problems. The acute phase typically lasts from 3 to 6 months (48).

The long-term reorganization phase may last for years. The clinical signs include depression, sexual dysfunction, substance abuse, and low self-esteem (48). Felitti (49) found a significant increase in morbid obesity in victims of child abuse. Chronic pelvic pain is also strongly associated with a history of sexual abuse. When dealing with patients who present with complaints of depression, sexual dysfunction, or chronic pain, one should rule out sexual abuse as an underlying factor. Physicians commonly treat sexual assault victims, but they are not always aware of it.

## CONCLUSION

Sexual assault is a major social and medical problem in the United States. Treatment of sexual assault victims presents a unique challenge to the physician. The examination should only be performed by professionals who have both the technical skills to perform and interpret the physical examination and the compassion and understanding to deliver medical care to victims.

Acknowledgement: The author is indebted to Dr Jay M. Whitworth (deceased) who was an invaluable resource in the writing of this chapter.

### References

1. Bureau of Justice Statistics. *Criminal Victimization, 2006*. Washington, DC: U.S. Department of Justice; 2008.
2. The Rape, Abuse and Incest National Network. Available at: www.rainn.org.
3. Antognoli-Toland P. Comprehensive program for examination of sexual assault victims by nurses: a hospital-based project in Texas. *J Emerg Nurs*. 1985;11(3):132.
4. Houmes BV, Fagan MM, Quintana NM. Establishing a Sexual Assault Nurse Examiner (SANE) program in the emergency department. *J Emerg Med*. 2003;25(1):111–121.

5. Kobernick ME, Seiferts S, Sanders AB, et al. Emergency department management of the sexual assault victim. *J Emerg Med.* 1985;2:205.
6. Hicks DJ. Rape: sexual assault. *Am J Obstet Gynecol.* 1980;137(8):931.
7. Office of the Attorney General. *Protocol for Sexual Assault Examinations.* FL: Office of the Attorney General; 2002.
8. Geist RF. Sexually related trauma. *Emerg Med Clin North Am.* 1988;6(3):439.
9. Slaughter L, Brown C. Cervical findings in rape victims. *J Obstet Gynecol.* 1991; 164(2):528.
10. Slaughter L, Brown CR., Crowley S, et al. Patterns of genital injury in female sexual assault victims. *Am J Obstet Gynecol.* 1997;176:609–616.
11. Norvell MK, Benrubi GI, Thompson RJ. Investigation of microtrauma after sexual intercourse. *J Reprod Med.* 1984;29(4):269–271.
12. Lauber AA, Souma ML. Use of toluidine blue for documentation of traumatic intercourse. *Obstet Gynecol.* 1982;60(5):644.
13. Tucker S. Claire E, Ledray LE, et al. Sexual assault evidence collection. *Wis Med J.* 1990;89(7):407.
14. Soules MR, Pollard AA, Brown KM, et al. The forensic laboratory evaluation of evidence in alleged rape. *Am J Obstet Gynecol.* 1978;130(2):142.
15. BD Probe Tec. Sparks, MD: Becton, Dickinson & Co.
16. Cabaniss ML, Scott SE, Copeland L. Gathering evidence for rape cases. *Contemp Obstet Gynecol.* 1985;25(3):160.
17. American Academy of Pediatrics, Committee on adolescence: rape and the adolescent. *Pediatrics.* 1988;81:595.
18. Christian C, Lavele J, DeJong A, Loiselle J, Brenner L, Joffe M. Forensic evidence findings in prepubertal victims of sexual assault. *Pediatrics.* 2000;106(1):100–104.
19. American Academy of Pediatrics, Committee on Child Abuse and Neglect. Guidelines for the evaluation of sexual abuse of children. *Pediatrics.* 1999;103:186–191.
20. McCann J. The use of culposcope in childhood sexual abuse examinations. *Pediatr Clin North Am.* 1990;37(4):863.
21. Heger AH, Ticson L, Guerra L, et al. Appearance of the genitalia in girls selected for non-abuse: review of hymenal morphology and non-specific findings. *J Pediatr Adolesc Gynecol.* 2002;15:27–35.
22. Heger A, Emans SJ, Muram D, eds. *Evaluation of the Sexually Abused Child. A Medical Textbook and Photographic Atlas.* 2nd Ed. New York, NY: Oxford University Press; 2000.
23. Berenson A, Heger A, Andrews S. Appearance of the hymen in newborns. *Pediatrics.* 1991;87:458–465.
24. McCann J, Wells R, Simon M, Voris J. Genital findings in prepubertal girls selected for non-abuse: a descriptive study. *Pediatrics.* 1990;86:428–439.
25. Berenson AB, Heger AH, Hayes JM, et al. Appearance of the hymen in prepubertal girls. *Pediatrics.* 1992;89:387–394.
26. Berenson AB, Grady JJ. A longitudinal study of hymenal development from 3 to 9 years of age. *J Pediatr.* 2002;140:600–607.
27. Berenson AB, Chacko MR, Wiemann CM, Mishaw CO, Friedrich WN, Grady JJ. A case-control study of anatomic changes resulting from sexual abuse. *Am J Obstet Gynecol.* 2000;182:820–834.
28. Muram D. Child sexual abuse: relationship between sexual acts and genital findings. *Child Abuse Negl.* 1989;13:211.
29. DeJong A, Rose M. Legal proof of child sexual abuse in the absence of physical evidence. *Pediatrics.* 1991;88(3):506.
30. Jenny C, Kuhns ML, Arakawa F, et al. Hymens in female infants. *Pediatrics.* 1987; 80(3):399.
31. McCann J, Voris J, Simon M. Genital injuries resulting from sexual abuse, a longitudinal study. *Pediatrics.* 1992;89:307–317.
32. McCann J, Voris J. Perianal injuries resulting from sexual abuse: a longitudinal study. *Pediatrics.* 1993;91:390–397.
33. Heppenstall-Heger A, McConnell G, Ticson L, et al. Healing patterns in anogenital injuries: a longitudinal study of injuries associated with sexual abuse, accidental injuries, or genital surgery in the preadolescent child. *Pediatrics.* 2003;112: 829–837.

34. Heger A, Ticson L, Velasquez O, Bernier R. Children referred for possible sexual abuse: medical findings in 2384 children. *Child Abuse Negl.* 2002;26:645–659.
35. Wynne JM, Hobbs CJ. Anogenital warts in prepubertal children; sexual abuse or not? *Int J Std AIDS.* 1993;4(5):271–279.
36. Update to CDC's Sexually Transmitted Diseases Treatment Guidelines, 2006: Fluoroquinolones No Longer Recommended for Treatment of Gonococcal Infections. *MMWR Morb Mortal Wkly Rep.* 2007;56(14):332–336.
37. Schwarcz SK, Whittington WL. Sexual assault and sexually transmitted diseases: detection and management in adults and children. *Rev Infect Dis.* 1990;12(Suppl. 6): S680–S690.
38. Jenny C, Hooten TM, Bowers A, et al. Sexually transmitted diseases in victims of rape. *N Engl J Med.* 1990;322(11):713.
39. Mastro TD, deVincenzi I. Probabilities of sexual HIV-1 transmission. *AIDS.* 1996; 10(Suppl A):S75–S82.
40. Management of possible sexual, injecting-drug-use, or other non-occupational exposure to HIV, including considerations related to antiretroviral therapy. *MMWR Morb Mortal Wkly Rep.* 1998;47(RR-17):1–137.
41. Antiretroviral Postexposure Prophylaxis After Sexual, Injection-Drug Use, or Other Nonoccupational Exposure to HIV in the United States. *MMWR Morb Mortal Wkly Rep.* 2005;54(RR02):1–20.
42. Updated U.S. Public Health Service Guidelines for the Management of Occupational Exposures to HBV, HCV, and HIV and Recommendations for Postexposure Prophylaxis. *MMWR Morbid Mortal Wkly Rep.* 2001;50(RR11):1–42.
43. Grimes D. Progestin-only emergency contraception. *Contracept Rep.* 1999;10(5): 8–10.
44. Yuzpe A, Smith P, Rademakeer A. A multi-center clinical investigation employing ethinyl estradiol combined with dl norgestrel as a postcoital contraceptive agent. *Fertil Steril.* 1982;37(509):580.
45. Trussel J, Rodriiguex G, Ellertson C. New estimates of the effectiveness of the Yuzpe regime for emergency contraception. *Contraception.* 1998;57(6):363–369.
46. ACOG. *Emergency Contraception. ACOG Practice Bulletin #69*, Washington, DC: American College of Obstetricians and Gynecologists; 2005.
47. Burgess AW, Holmstrom LL. Rape trauma syndrome. *Am J Psychiatry.* 1974; 131(9):981.
48. Gise LH, Paddison P. Rape, sexual abuse, and its victims. *Psychiatr Clin North Am.* 1988;11(4):629.
49. Felitti VJ. Long term medical consequences of incest, rape and molestation. *South Med J.* 1991;84(3):329.

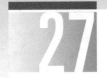

# Gynecologic Traumas

**Tracey Maurer**

Gynecologic trauma can result from a variety of situations. Included in this discussion are sexually related trauma, trauma associated with women's sports or leisure activities, and trauma that occurs from pelvic fractures.

## SEXUALLY RELATED TRAUMA

A substantial body of literature addresses trauma from rape, as well as trauma occurring during consensual coitus (1–10). The major forms of sexually related trauma dealt with in the literature result from unexpected trauma occurring between consenting adults. Even though sexual abuse and its related trauma may be seen in emergency departments (EDs), abused women without life-threatening injuries or hemorrhage are generally evaluated in a well-controlled setting established for rape victims (1–3) (Chapter 26). Nevertheless, the gyneco-logic injuries that can occur during consensual and forced coitus are similar.

Women who are seen for emergency evaluation associated with sexually related trauma not only are in pain but also harbor feelings of embarrassment and anguish. In such a setting, compassion is as important as diagnostic acumen.

Trauma resulting from oral–genital sex can present in many ways. One finding seen in the oral cavity is referred to as fellatio syndrome. Erythema, pete-chia, purpura, and ecchymoses of the soft palate are seen (4). These are due to hemorrhage, possibly from repetitive negative pressure in the oral cavity, com-bined with the action of the tensor and levator veli palatini muscles, or solely from thrusting against the highly vascular soft palate (4). The lesions are pain-less, nonulcerative, and nonblanching (4). A history of fellatio can deter an exten-sive diagnostic workup, but a differential diagnosis includes paroxysmal coughing, sneezing, vomiting, infection, tumors, blood dyscrasias, and capillary fragility (4). Cunnilingus syndrome results from oral–genital sex in which the tongue is used on the partner's genital areas (4). The findings are pain of the ven-tral surfaces of the tongue and throat with abrasions and ulcerations of the lin-gual frenulum (4). Chronic irritation can result in a traumatic fibroma on the frenulum (4).

Two possible, but rare, occurrences can be seen in the female recipient of oral–genital sex. One is a pneumoperitoneum. This can result after air is blown into the vagina, traverses the cervical canal and endometrial cavity, and enters the abdomen through the fallopian tubes (4). Cases have been reported in patients with their uterus in situ (4). Posthysterectomy cases have also been encountered, with the supposition that the air entered through a small dehiscence in the vaginal cuff (4,5). These patients generally have lower abdomi-nal pain, upper quadrant pain, or shoulder pain (4). Peritoneal signs tend to be absent, allowing for conservative management (5). The clinical course is benign, with the air being gradually absorbed spontaneously. Cuff defects should be repaired when encountered (4,5).

Air embolism is the second complication seen in the female recipient of oral–genital sex. It is uniformly fatal (4). Death occurs rapidly, and resuscita-tive measures are usually too late. This complication has been reported in

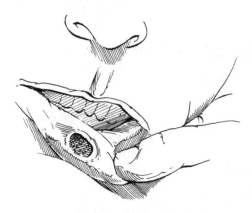

**FIGURE 27.1** Chancre behind lip.

seven gravid women, all at >20 weeks of gestation (4). Whether or not oral–genital–related air embolism can occur in nonpregnant women is not known.

Another possible, although rarely documented, complication of oral–genital sex is a vulvar hematoma from a human bite. One case report exists in the literature (11). Finally, oral–genital sex can lead to lesions of the oral cavity caused by sexually transmitted diseases. This should be kept in mind by the practitioner, so that information can be elicited from the patient (Fig. 27.1).

Trauma with coitus can range from hymenal tearing during initial intercourse to evisceration with hemorrhage. Small tears of the hymen are usually associated with minimal discomfort, but occasionally, profuse bleeding that requires repair can occur (4).

Vaginal lacerations and ruptures are rare, but when they are seen, it is usually in women of reproductive age who were having consensual intercourse (4,5,9). Metsala and Nieminen (9) found that approximately 88% of vaginal ruptures occurred during penile coital activity, with most of the remaining cases owing to other direct mechanical effects. The exact cause of the rupture often cannot be determined. Many predisposing factors have been suggested (4,7,9). In 1965, Purnell reported several cases of apparently spontaneous rupture of the vaginal vault (9). All of these cases were in postmenopausal women with vaginal atrophy. They occurred with sudden increases in intra-abdominal pressure during lifting, coughing, falling, or defecation. Purnell's theory was that the sudden intra-abdominal pressure acted through the pouch of Douglas on a weakened posterior fornix to bring about a rupture. Women in both these situations generally had vaginal bleeding as the presenting symptom. Exsanguination has been reported (4,6,7). Sometimes, a history of sharp vaginal pain during intercourse is obtained (6,7). Surrounding structures may also be injured, and evisceration of abdominal contents has been seen (Fig. 27.2) (4,8).

Management starts with controlling the bleeding and treating shock, if present. If the bleeding is heavy, a moist vaginal packing can be placed as a tamponade while the history and physical examination are completed, with particular emphasis on other signs of trauma. When the bleeding has slowed, the vagina can be examined to determine the extent of the laceration. Most lacerations are in the posterior and right lateral fornix (Fig. 27.3) (6,7,9). Often, the examination has to take place in the operating room under general anesthesia for patient comfort. If evisceration has occurred and the penetration is known to be by a penis, finger, or other blunt object, the physician may attempt to replace the

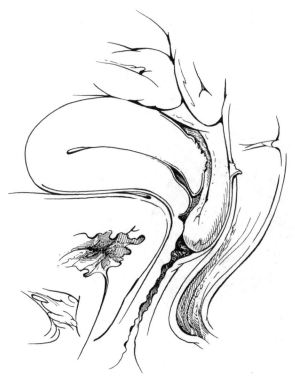

**FIGURE 27.2** Evisceration after vaginal laceration.

eviscerated organs, usually bowel, back into the abdomen using moist sponges and with the patient in the Trendelenburg position. If the bowel has passed beyond the introitus, it should be wrapped in moist towels until the patient can be taken to the operating room. Included in the evaluation should be a digital rectal examination to look for a rectal laceration. The bladder can be evaluated by instillation of indigo carmine and then observed for leakage. Cystourethrography may be necessary to look for intra-abdominal leakage (12). A flat plate of the abdomen is necessary to rule out an intraperitoneal foreign body.

Once the evaluation is complete and there are no other injuries besides the vaginal rupture known to be caused by a blunt object, simple vaginal repair with observation and intravenous antibiotics is indicated. Rarely does significant bowel injury occur in this situation (4). If further injury has been documented or evisceration outside the introitus is present, then abdominal repair becomes necessary. If bleeding persists even after closure and applied pressure to a vaginal nonpenetrating laceration, then laparotomy with hypogastric artery ligation is an option (13). A transverse incision has been advocated when an abdominal approach becomes necessary, because it is a stronger incision than those available when operating in a contaminated field. However, if bowel injury is even suspected, a vertical incision is necessary to evaluate the entire bowel fully. Upper abdominal bowel injuries have been reported after a history of blunt

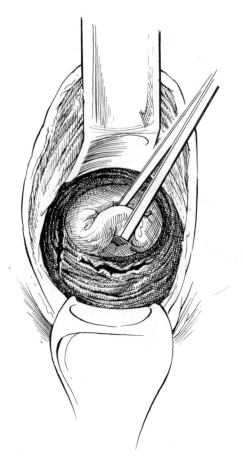

**FIGURE 27.3** Laceration of lateral and posterior vaginal fornices.

vaginal perforations (12). Repair of the vaginal laceration is performed after the abdominal part of the procedure is completed. Closed suction drains should be used routinely (12). Antibiotics are appropriate in all cases after cultures are obtained. Prophylaxis with tetanus toxoid should also be considered. Complications from penetrating vaginal wounds include pelvic abscesses, vaginal strictures, and vesicovaginal and rectovaginal fistulas (12).

Anal intercourse is a practice of the heterosexual as well as the homosexual communities. Various forms of trauma from this practice can present in women as well as men. Proctitis can occur and is generally the result of inflammation caused by trauma, but it may be due to chlamydia or herpes infection. Patients may have rectal bleeding from a rectal mucosal laceration. If a history of anal intercourse is obtained, then evaluation should include an upright abdominal film to rule out pneumoperitoneum and retained foreign body. Proctoscopy is then performed to determine the extent of the lesion. Most patients require no treatment, although transanal repair is occasionally necessary. Stool softeners and sitz baths are recommended. If disruption of the anal sphincter occurs from this form of sexual activity, repair should be done in the operating room. Occasionally, a patient is seen at the ED reporting loss of a sexual aid used in anal–rectal stimulation. Most foreign objects can be removed in the ED with appropriate instruments. Occasionally, general anesthesia is necessary to promote relaxation and patient comfort (10). If a vacuum has been created, passage of a Foley catheter around the object can break the seal (Fig. 27.4). The inflated bulb of the Foley can then help provide traction downward (4). If the object is beyond reach, the patient may be observed for 24 hours. The object will generally descend into the rectum within that time. Sigmoidoscopy should be performed after removal to rule out significant lacerations. If none are found and there are no signs of peritonitis, the patient can be discharged with close follow-up. Rectosigmoid colon perforations are rare but can be caused by foreign body manipulation. Peritonitis is generally the result. Attempts should be made to make the diagnosis without the use of barium enemas or Gastrografin enemas, because these enemas increase irritation and can increase bowel content spillage (4). A diversionary colostomy is necessary at the time of repair to allow the laceration to heal. Generous irrigation and broad-spectrum antimicrobial coverage are indicated. Perforations occurring below the peritoneal reflection do not cause peritonitis, thus possibly delaying their presentation and diagnosis (4). Treatment, however, is the same.

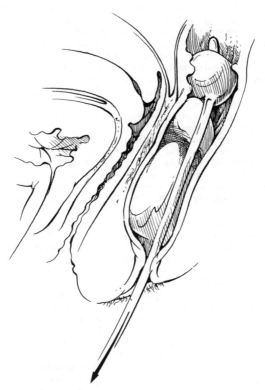

**FIGURE 27.4** Foley catheter removal of intrarectal foreign body.

## NONSEXUALLY RELATED TRAUMA

Many mechanical causes of vaginal lacerations have been reported, which are not always related to sexual stimulation. Tampons with plastic applicators have been incriminated (14). Patients can have acute bright-red bleeding or a several-week history of bleeding (14). Examination generally shows a linear lesion through the full thickness of the vaginal mucosa. Lesions tend to heal on their own with an extended absence of tampons in the vagina.

Pressurized water entering the vagina can also cause laceration or rupture. Multiple case reports exist involving water skiing, Jet-Skis, and water fountains (13,15–19). The typical fall taken while water skiing is backward with legs abducted. Thus, the speed at impact dictates the amount of pressurized water that enters potential spaces such as the vagina and rectum (20). The pressurized water has been documented to cause significant lacerations with significant blood loss (14,20). Previously published literature led to the conclusion that only the width and relaxation of the parous vagina allowed the forceful entry of water. But Perlman et al. (17) reported on a similar injury in a premenarcheal 9-year-old female. The "Jet-Ski douche" is much less common but has also been reported (18,19). The injuries occur when the rider falls backward off the Jet-Ski with legs abducted. The high-pressure water jet from the Jet-Ski is the offender. Both of these types of "water douches" can cause significant lacerations, usually deep in the vagina around the cervix. The blood loss can cause significant anemia. Often, exploration under anesthesia is required to visualize and repair the defect after the patient's condition has been stabilized. Because of the heavy bleeding, initial management in the field may include perineal pressure packs and antishock trousers. The use of antibiotics in these patients is unclear. There is the potential for infection from vaginal bacteria, as well as the flora from the water. If antibiotics are not used pro-phylactically, then observation for a fever seems prudent. The douche can also cause less visible injuries to the cervix, uterus, and fallopian tubes, such as salpingitis, tubo-ovarian abscesses, and precipitation of a miscarriage (16).

Laparoscopy or laparotomy should be considered when uncertainty as to intraperitoneal injury is present.

More serious gynecologic injuries are seen in automobile accident victims with pelvic fractures. Pelvic fractures in females can be associated with significant intra-abdominal gynecologic injury (21). Intra-abdominal soft tissue injuries are generally caused by tears and lacerations from sharp, bony fragments. Lacerations have been seen in the intestines and genitourinary tract, including the vagina and urethra (21,22). There have been reported cases of laceration to the uterus, tube, and ovary after a pelvic fracture as well as avulsion of the uterus (21,23). Retroperitoneal hematoma may result from such injuries (21). Avulsion of the uterus may result in hysterectomy (23). Infertility and obstetric complications are potential consequences of pelvic fractures as well as vaginal stricture, dyspareunia, osteomyelitis, and pelvic abscess (24). A gentle pelvic examination is warranted in women with pelvic fractures (21). The gentleness is emphasized, because the physician could create an open fracture through the vaginal wall. Delay in identifying lacerations could result in pelvic abscesses and higher rates of mortality. Once an abscess occurs, multiple operations are often necessary before complete cure is achieved (24). Future complications after the apparent resolution of abscesses include urethrovaginal fistula, vesi-covaginal fistula, and rectovaginal fistula (24). Sudden bladder rupture has been reported as a result of osteomyelitis (24).

Mechanisms by which pelvic fractures cause vaginal lacerations are multi-ple. Most obvious is penetration of a bone fragment through the vaginal wall (24). Diastasis of the symphysis pubis tends to result from straddle injuries (24).

The lateral tearing force of this injury lacerates deep pelvic soft tissues and sometimes extends to the vaginal wall. Bilateral ischiopubic rami fractures result in the anterior pelvic ring being freed from the weight-bearing portions of the pelvis. This can cause an avulsion of the vaginal vault or urethra (22). Finally, crushing injuries are capable of producing vaginal wall lacerations. Foreign bodies such as tampons and contraceptive devices can increase the chances of a vaginal laceration (24). Urethral and bladder neck injuries occur in about 6% of females with a pelvic fracture (25–32). These patients present with either blood at the introitus or gross hematuria. The physician should have a high suspicion of urethral or bladder neck injury in any female patient presenting with this combination of findings.

Niemi and Norton (24) recommend repair of vaginal lacerations as early as possible. A severely comminuted open pelvic fracture with associated rectal injuries and fecal contamination requires a diverting colostomy to allow the best chance of healing (24). Urethral avulsions have been reported to heal after primary end-to-end reanastomosis (22). Intravenous antibiotics are always indicated with an open fracture.

In one study of 102 major pelvic fractures, the mortality rate was 16%. The researchers suggested that the most significant determinant of mortality was the life-threatening injuries, along with the hemorrhage from lacerated pelvic vessels. Promptly recognizing and treating injuries to the bowel or bladder are also important (24).

Rarely, one finds gynecologic injury after blunt abdominal trauma unassociated with pelvic fracture. Stone et al. (25), in their study of 220 patients with blunt abdominal trauma, found that the most frequent gynecologic injury was a ruptured and bleeding corpus luteum. The ovarian laceration can be simply oversewn, thus preserving the ovary. Also, vaginal evisceration following a simple slip and fall has been reported (31). This particular case occurred in a patient with long-standing procidentia and hypoestrogenemia even without a history of surgery. Wide-spectrum antibiotics should be used and preservation of the bowel in a moist saline wrap should be done while awaiting arrival in the OR. A vaginal approach to repair is reasonable as long as there are no signs of intra-abdominal injury or bowel incarceration.

Vulvar injuries and hematomas are another major area of gynecologic trauma. Injuries to the vulva and perineum of young girls are fairly common. Often, these injuries consist of slight tears that heal on their own. However, more severe cases, including urinary retention from vulvar injury following straddling the bar on a boy's bike or other toy, have been reported (26). Even a small mucosal tear of the vulva or vestibule can cause intense pain or burning on urination so that the child inhibits voiding. This cause should be considered in young girls with urinary retention. They often will not volunteer information about the injury, so the diagnosis may not be made unless there is a high level of suspicion. Applying lidocaine gel to the tear with each urge to void, as well as voiding in a tub of warm water, is helpful and may prevent the need for catheterization.

Vulvar hematomas from trauma are seen in both young girls and women (Fig. 27.5). Naumann et al. reported two cases of vulvar hematoma that occurred while riding a "mechanical bull," although such injury can result from any blunt trauma (27–29). Both women experienced abrupt pain and bleeding. One woman had a small hematoma merely treated with ice packs as an outpatient. The second woman had a large vulvar hematoma, producing urethral obstruction that required a Foley catheter for 7 days. She initially had a significant decrease in her hematocrit, which stabilized after 24 hours of conservative management with ice packs and observation. The ice pack is the primary treatment, with surgical evacuation reserved for rapidly enlarging hematomas or drainage of large hematomas following clot lysis (27–29). It is important to make the correct diagnosis,

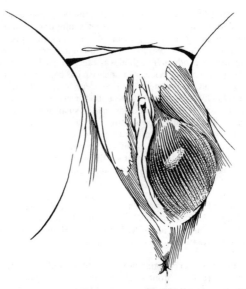

**FIGURE 27.5** Vulvar hematoma.

because evacuation in the first 24 hours could decompress the bleeding vessel, resulting in further blood loss. However, as discussed earlier, an infected vulvar hematoma must be incised, drained, and debrided as soon as possible. The bleeding site in this case must be localized quickly and ligated.

The final topic is iatrogenic gynecologic trauma. One reported case is of bilateral vaginal tears causing the loss of approximately 1,000 mL of blood from a routine speculum examination in a patient with vaginismus (30). No gross vaginal abnormality was apparent. The patient had to be taken to the operating room for repair and was transfused with 2 units of blood.

## SUMMARY

Genital trauma in women can have multiple etiologies. Accurate information obtained from a cooperative patient is imperative to guarantee proper management. Compassion and nonjudgmental manner are therefore all-important in ensuring that the appropriate management is rendered.

### *References*

1. Claytor RN, Bath KL, Shubin CI. Evaluating child sexual abuse, observations regarding ano-genital injury. *Clin Pediatr.* 1989;28:9.
2. Suram D. Child sexual abuse: relationship between sexual acts and genital findings. *Child Abuse Negl.* 1989;13:211.
3. Slaughter L, Brown CRY. Cervical findings in rape victims. *Am J Obstet Gynecol.* 1991;154:528.
4. Elam AL, Ray VG. Sexually related trauma: a review. *Ann Emerg Med.* 1986;15:576.
5. Christiansen WC, Danzl DF, McGee HJ. Pneumoperitoneum following vaginal insufflation and coitus. *Ann Emerg Med.* 1980;9:480.

6. Smith NC, Van Coeverden De Groot HA, Gunston DK. Coital injuries of the vagina in nonvirginal patients. *S Afr Med J*. 1983;64:746.

7. Parakevaides EC. Severe post-coital puerperal vaginal tear. *Br J Gun Pract*. 1990;44:777.

8. Cullins V, Anasti J, Huggins GR. Vaginal evisceration with pneumoperitoneum, a case report. *J Reprod Med*. 1989;34:426.

9. Metsala P, Nieminen U. Traumatic lesions of the vagina. *Acta Obstet Gynecol Scand*. 1986;47:482.

10. Cummings PH, Cummings SP. Foreign object-induced sexual trauma. *J Emerg Nurs*. 1981;7:24.

11. Mathelier AC. Vulvar hematoma secondary to a human bite: a case report. *J Reprod Med*. 1987;32:618.

12. Grindlinger GA, Vester SR. Transvaginal injury of the duodenum, diaphragm and lung. *J Trauma*. 1987;27:575.

13. Druzin ML, Gottesfeld SA. Management of serious vaginal injury: a case report. *J Reprod Med*. 1986;31:151.

14. Gray MJ, Norton P, Treadwell K. Tampon-induced injuries. *Obstet Gynecol*. 1981;58:667.

15. Gray HR. A risk of waterskiing for women: a letter to the editor. *West J Med*. 1982;136:169.

16. Kizer KW. Medical hazards of the water skiing douche, a case report. *Ann Emerg Med*. 1980;9:268.

17. Perlman S, Hertweck SP, Wolfe, WM. Water-ski douche injury in a premenarcheal female, a case report. *MD Consult*.1995;96:783.

18. Ramos JP, Cari-ison D, Phillips DL. Unusual vaginal laceration due to high-pressure water jet, a case report. *West J Med*. 1998;169:171.

19. Haefner IIK, Andersen HF, Johnson MP. Vaginal laceration following a jet ski accident. *Obstet Gynecol*. 1991;78:986.

20. Kalaichandran S. Vaginal laceration: a little-known hazard for women water skiers: a letter to the editor. *Can J Surg*. 1991;34:107.

21. Doman AN, Hoekstra DV. Pelvic fracture associated with severe intra-abdominal gynecologic injury. *J Trauma*. 1988;28:118.

22. Netto NR, Ikari O, Zuppo VP. Traumatic rupture of the female urethra, case reports. *Urology*. 1983;22:601.

23. Smith RJ. Avulsion of the nongravid uterus due to pelvic fracture, a case report. *South Med J*. 1989;82:70.

24. Niemi TA, Norton LW. Vaginal injuries in patient with pelvic fractures. *J Trauma*. 1985;25:547.

25. Stone NN, Ances IG, Brotman S. Gynecologic injury in the non-gravid female during blunt abdominal trauma. *J Trauma*. 1984;24:6226.

26. Manaker JS. Gynecologic trauma, non-obstetrical vulvar, urethral, and vaginal injuries. *J Kans Med Soc*. 1980;81:329.

27. Naumann RO, Droegmueller W. Unusual etiology of vulvar hematomas, a communications in brief. *Am J Obstet Gynecol*. 1982;142:357.

28. Shesser R, Shulinan D, Smith J. A nonpuerperal traumatic vulvar hematoma, a case report. *J Reprod Med*. 1987;32:618.

29. Vermesh M, Deppe G, Zbella E. Non-puerperal traumatic vulvar hematoma, a case report. *J Gynaecol Obstet*. 1984;22:217.

30. Rafla N. Vaginismus and vaginal tears, a case report. *Am J Obstet Gynecol*. 1988;158:1043.

31. Bozkurt N, Korucuoglu U, Bakirci Y, Yilmaz U, Sakrak O, Guner H. Vaginal eviseratio after trauma unrelated to previous pelvic surgery. *Arch Gynecol Obstet*. 2009 Apr; 279(4):595–597.

32. Black PC, Miller EA, Porter JR, Wessells H. Urethral and bladder neck injury associated with pelvic fracture in 25 female patients. *J Urol*. 2006;175(6):2140–2144.

# Imaging in Gynecologic Emergencies

**Marcia E. Murakami and Joseph G. Cernigliaro**

Ultrasound is the most useful imaging modality in the evaluation of gynecologic emergencies. Moreover, ultrasound does not pose the risk of ionizing radiation, which is a consideration when examining the potentially pregnant patient. Transvaginal imaging, in particular, permits exquisitely detailed examination of the uterus and ovaries, so that a specific diagnosis can often be made with great confidence. Plain radiographs are rarely useful as the initial screening study. Computed tomography (CT), in selected cases, can provide more global information for extensive disease, especially when the pathologic process extends out of the pelvis.

Although some authors think that transvaginal scanning (TVS) alone is sufficient for defining pelvic pathology (1,2), it is our view that transabdominal scanning (TAS) should be performed first. For patients who are suspected of having an emergent gynecologic problem, the sonographer quickly scans the upper abdomen to exclude free intraperitoneal fluid, which is highly suspicious for hemoperitoneum in this patient population. Scanning through the urinary bladder affords a wide field of view and a survey of the entire pelvis. Although the diagnosis often can be made using TAS alone (Fig. 28.1), TVS almost always follows to better characterize the transabdominal findings (Fig. 28.2). The transvaginal examination is therefore directed and performed with the confidence that pathology is not outside the limited field of view of the transvaginal probe. Other authors suggest that TVS may be performed first, with addition of TAS as needed (3–5).

## THE PREGNANT PATIENT

The development of an accurate and rapid pregnancy test has narrowed the differential diagnosis of otherwise nonspecific clinical findings. Still, the list of diagnostic possibilities in the early stages of pregnancy remains long and includes intrauterine pregnancy (IUP), ectopic pregnancy, embryonic or fetal demise with missed or incomplete abortion, completed abortion, and molar pregnancy. Ultrasound can make a specific diagnosis in a number of cases or at least aid in the clinical management of the patient. Establishing the presence of a normal IUP essentially excludes an ectopic pregnancy. Evaluation of the gestational sac and its contents can often confirm embryonic demise. Often, correlation of the ultrasound findings with the clinical history may strongly suggest incomplete or completed abortion.

### Normal Early IUP

At the time of implantation, between day 20 and day 23 (menstrual age), the conceptus is only about 0.1 mm in diameter (6), much too small to be detected by transabdominal or transvaginal probes. Focal echogenic thickening of the endometrium can be visualized at the implantation site between 25 and 29 days. The earliest that a sac may be seen within the uterus is at 3.5 weeks, as a tiny anechoic fluid collection within the thickened decidua, termed the

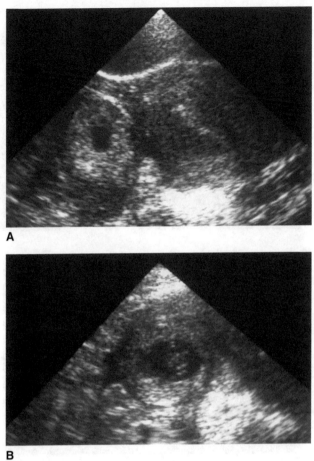

A

B

**FIGURE 28.1** Value of transabdominal technique. **A:** Transverse scan through the fundus of the uterus shows echogenic ring in the right adnexal region. Uterus empty. **B:** High-resolution image of the right adnexa shows embryonic pole. Cardiac activity was observed, diagnostic of a living pregnancy. TVS, even with knowledge of the transabdominal findings, could not visualize the ectopic pregnancy.

*intradecidual sign* (Fig. 28.3) (7). More commonly, an early gestational sac is reliably detected at approximately 4.5 weeks' menstrual age by TVS and at 5 weeks' menstrual age by TAS (8). Correlation with serum human chorionic gonadotropin (hCG) levels is extremely helpful. Sac detection discriminatory levels of 1,800 IU/L (Second International Standard [2nd IS]) or approximately 3,600 IU/L (International Reference Preparation [IRP]) TAS (9–11) and 1,000 IU/L (2nd IS) or about 2,000 IU/L (IRP) TVS (10,11) have been established. (The 2nd IS is approximately half the IRP value.) At these levels or higher, a definite intrauterine gestational sac should be visualized. Below

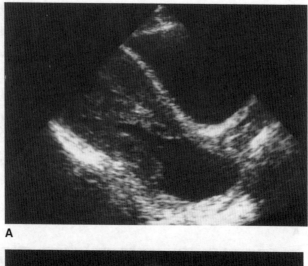

A

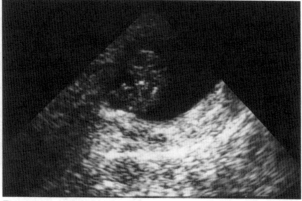

B

**FIGURE 28.2** Value of transvaginal technique. **A:** Large, irregular fluid collection expands the cervix and the lower endometrial cavity. **B:** Transvaginal imaging detected an embryo without cardiac activity within the fluid collection, indicating embryonic demise and abortion in progress.

these levels, a normal intrauterine gestation may be too small to detect. If the hCG level is disproportionately low relative to the gestational sac size, an abnormal pregnancy should be suspected (9). In general, the intrauterine findings of an early pregnancy are visualized on TVS approximately 1 week earlier than on TAS (12).

The *double decidual sac sign* (13) may be the earliest confirmatory sign of an IUP on TAS or TVS (Fig. 28.4) (14,15). Although a definite double decidual sac sign is not identified in all normal IUPs, when this sign is clearly present, it is a very useful indicator of IUP (16). It is based on the visualization of the chorionic cavity

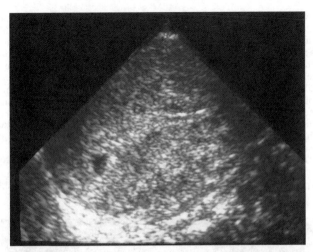

**FIGURE 28.3** Intradecidual sign. The very small eccentric fluid collection within the decidua represents a very early (<4-week) IUP.

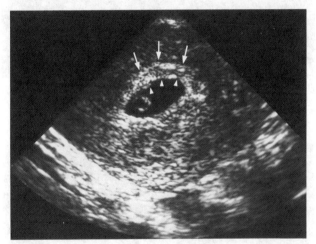

**FIGURE 28.4** Double decidual sac sign. Decidua capsularis and chorion (*arrowheads*) and decidua parietalis (*arrows*) form the two arcs of the double decidual sac in a 5.2-week gestation. The yolk sac is clearly visible.

surrounded by two layers of echoes, the inner echogenic ring representing the decidua capsularis and chorion and the outer echogenic ring, the decidua parietalis. The combination of the gestational sac plus the decidual layers forms a much larger complex than the chorionic cavity itself and may be more readily identified at an earlier stage.

Normally, the yolk sac is the first structure seen within the gestational sac (Fig. 28.5). It should always be visualized with a mean sac diameter (MSD) of 20-mm TAS (17) and 8-mm TVS (18). (The MSD is calculated by dividing the sum of the three orthogonal dimensions of the fluid sac by three.) Whereas the double decidual sac sign is not absolutely specific for an intrauterine gestation, the presence of a yolk sac is definitive (14). Between 5 and 10 menstrual weeks, a yolk sac should never exceed 5.6 mm in diameter (19). As early as 5.5 weeks, a second sac may be seen adjacent to the yolk sac. This second sac represents the amnion, and this, together with the yolk sac, forms the *double bleb sign* (20). The embryonic disc lies between the two sacs. The amnion continues to grow and eventually fills the chorionic cavity by weeks 14 to 16. Normally, the amnion may be seen as a separate membrane until this time (Fig. 28.6).

Once a yolk sac is visualized within the gestational sac, a search should be made for an embryo immediately adjacent to the yolk sac (Fig. 28.7). Transabdominally, pulsation of the embryonic heart may be identified at real time, establishing a

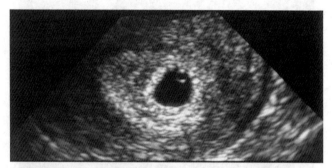

**FIGURE 28.5** Yolk sac. Perfectly spherical, thin-walled yolk sac is noted in the periphery of the gestational sac. The 10-mm MSD corresponds to a 5-week gestation. Note the double decidual sac sign.

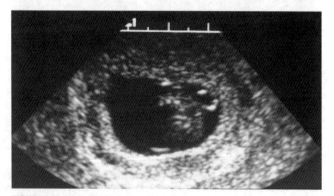

**FIGURE 28.6** Yolk sac and amnion. The delicate amniotic sac envelops an 8-week embryo. The amnion has not yet fused with the chorion. Note the yolk sac adjacent to the embryo.

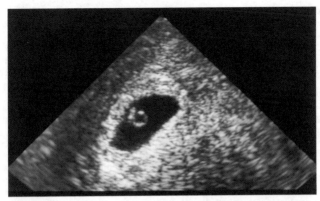

**FIGURE 28.7** Embryo. Gestation of 5.5 weeks (13-mm MSD) with yolk sac and adjacent embryo. Cardiac activity was present.

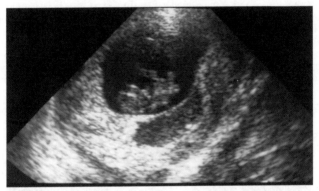

**FIGURE 28.8** Subchorionic hemorrhage. A 9.5-week living IUP in a patient who was first seen with acute vaginal bleeding. Hemorrhage is more echogenic than the fluid within the gestational sac.

live pregnancy, even though a distinct embryo is not visible (21). An embryo should always be visualized with an MSD of 25-mm TAS (9) and 16-mm TVS (10). An embryo is consistently detected transabdominally once it has reached a crown–rump length ≥5 mm. Cardiac activity is often visible transvaginally in embryos with a crown–rump length of 2 to 4 mm (about 6 weeks). However, TVS can identify normal embryos without cardiac activity when they are <5 mm (22). The absence of cardiac activity in these small embryos should not be construed as embryonic demise.

Subchorionic hemorrhage is a common finding late in the first trimester and may be associated with vaginal bleeding. The hemorrhage causes elevation of the chorionic membrane, appearing acutely as a fluid collection more echogenic than amniotic fluid (Fig. 28.8), becoming more hypoechoic in 1 to 2 weeks. The significance of these hematomas is somewhat controversial. Some researchers believe that the prognosis depends on the volume of the hemorrhage, with a better prognosis associated with the smaller hematomas. Others suggest that the vast majority of pregnancies with subchorionic hemorrhage detected before 20 menstrual weeks end in a normal term delivery (23).

Corpus luteum cysts are commonly detected in the first trimester. The cysts may be simple or hemorrhagic (Fig. 28.9). They are usually 3 to 6 cm in size but may be as large as 10 cm. These cysts usually resolve spontaneously by 16 weeks.

### Abnormal Early IUP

Ultrasound has proved to be extremely helpful in the evaluation of the failed pregnancy. With TVS, a single examination is often conclusive in establishing embryonic demise. A large gestation sac (MSD, >25-mm TAS [9] or >16-mm TVS [10] without an embryo; MSD, >20-mm TAS [9] or >8-mm TVS [10] without a yolk sac) is diagnostic of an anembryonic gestation or blighted ovum (Fig. 28.10). Distorted gestational sac shape is also highly specific for abnormal pregnancy, although it is a somewhat subjective feature and is relatively insensitive. Suggestive but less specific findings include a thin (<2 mm), weakly echogenic or irregular choriodecidual reaction, absent double decidual sac sign, and low position of the sac within the endometrial cavity (9).

The yolk sac itself should not measure >5.6 mm in diameter between 5 and 10 weeks or ≤2 mm between 8 and 12 weeks (19). If a normal embryo cannot be identified adjacent to an abnormally large yolk sac, the diagnosis of blighted ovum or anembryonic pregnancy is made (Fig. 28.11). Conversely, it is also abnormal if a yolk sac is not visualized in the presence of an embryo demonstrated by TVS (8). This is associated with embryonic demise either at the time of the scan or on follow-up examination. Calcification of the yolk sac is also seen with embryonic demise (Fig. 28.12) (24). Just as a gestational sac too large for its contents is abnormal, a gestational sac too small also carries a poor prognosis (Fig. 28.13). Despite the presence of cardiac activity within embryos between 6

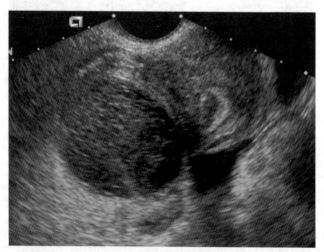

**FIGURE 28.9** Hemorrhagic corpus luteum cyst. Transvaginal image shows a 4-cm complex mass arising from the ovary compatible with a hemorrhagic cyst. Note adjacent uterus and small amount of simple free fluid.

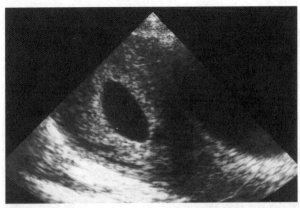

**FIGURE 28.10** Blighted ovum: empty gestational sac. No embryo is visualized and decidual reaction is weak.

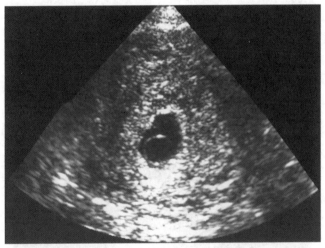

**FIGURE 28.11** Blighted ovum: abnormally large yolk sac. A 9-mm yolk sac occupies about one half the volume of the gestational sac. No embryonic pole could be detected.

and 9 weeks, those with a gestational sac size too small for the crown–rump length almost always end in miscarriage (25). Therefore, management of these pregnancies should be cautious.

Cardiac activity establishes embryonic life. In a high-quality TAS, once an embryo is visualized, cardiac activity should always be present (Fig. 28.14). Transvaginally, however, a normal embryo <5 mm in crown–rump length may or

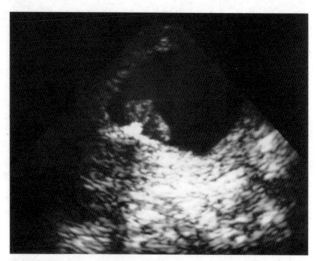

**FIGURE 28.12** Embryonic demise: calcification of the yolk sac. Densely echogenic structure with shadowing is presumed to be calcified yolk sac immediately adjacent to the embryo. No cardiac activity was visualized.

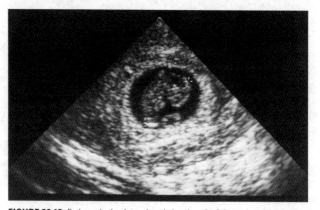

**FIGURE 28.13** Embryonic demise: missed abortion. An 8.2-week embryo is too large for the gestational sac size, which corresponds to a 6.7-week gestation. Cardiac activity was not present.

may not exhibit cardiac activity, and follow-up sonography may be of benefit to establish normal development (22).

Embryonic bradycardia is also a sign of impending fetal demise. The normal embryonic heart rate at 5 to 6 menstrual weeks is approximately 100 bpm. At 8 to 9 menstrual weeks, the rate is approximately 140 bpm. It has been demonstrated

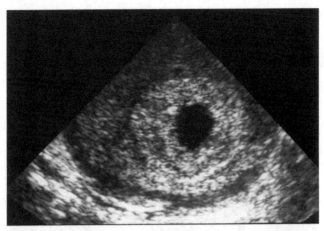

**FIGURE 28.14** Incomplete abortion. Intrauterine fluid and markedly thickened endometrium. No yolk sac or embryo is detected.

that embryos between 5 and 8 weeks of menstrual age with heart rates of <85 bpm end in fetal loss (26).

Retained products of conception from an incomplete abortion are quite variable in appearance and are often difficult to differentiate from a pseudoges-tational sac or decidual cast of an ectopic pregnancy. The endometrium may appear abnormally thick (>5 mm), with fluid and debris within the uterine cavity (Fig. 28.14). If the endometrial stripe is thin (<2 mm), there is little likelihood of retained products (27).

At times, an abortion in progress can be observed at real-time ultrasound. The uterine contents move lower in the uterus toward the cervix with active con-traction of the uterus, and the cervical canal may be fluid filled and dilated (Fig. 28.2). A completed abortion is often identical in ultrasound appearance to a normal empty uterus. In the presence of a positive pregnancy test, the differen-tial diagnosis must include very early IUP and nonvisualized ectopic pregnancy.

Early trophoblastic disease is usually indistinguishable from an incomplete abortion, demonstrating abnormal echogenicity within the uterine cavity. Hydropic villae may not develop vesicles until 12 weeks or more, making detec-tion by even TVS difficult until that time (28).

### Ectopic Pregnancy

The sine qua non for diagnosis of an ectopic pregnancy is the demonstration of an extrauterine embryo with cardiac activity (Fig. 28.15). TVS has increased the detection of live extrauterine embryos compared with TAS (29,30). Practically speaking, the presence of a normal intrauterine gestation excludes ectopic pregnancy. The likelihood of coexistent intrauterine and ectopic pregnancy, also known as heterotopic pregnancy, is variably estimated as 1 in 30,000 to 1 in 7,000 (16).

A *pseudogestational sac* or decidual cast must be differentiated from a very early IUP (13). The pseudogestational sac represents an intrauterine fluid collec-tion surrounded by a single decidual layer rather than the concentric arcs of the

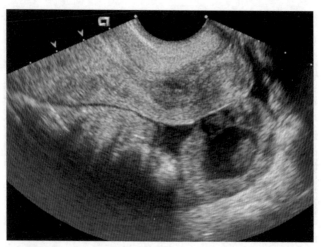

**FIGURE 28.15** Ectopic pregnancy. An 8-week living ectopic pregnancy in the cul-de-sac. Note the empty uterus and free fluid. Cardiac activity was present.

double decidual sac sign (Fig. 28.16). It may be impossible to distinguish a decidual cast from a spontaneous incomplete abortion (Fig. 28.17).

If an IUP is not identified in the patient who is suspected of having an ectopic pregnancy, the adnexal regions should be carefully examined. An adnexal mass is highly suspicious for ectopic pregnancy in this setting. The appearance of the mass is variable but is usually complex (Fig. 28.18). An ectopic *tubal ring* may be seen separate from the ovaries, a finding strongly associated with an unruptured tubal pregnancy (Fig. 28.19) (31,32). The ring is an echogenic structure created by the trophoblast of the ectopic pregnancy. If this ring is carefully examined, a yolk sac or embryo may be identified within it. Increased flow surrounding a tubal pregnancy on color Doppler or *ring of fire* is a nonspecific finding as a corpus luteum cyst may also have this appearance. This sign is probably most helpful when an ectopic pregnancy is not visualized but suspected and color Doppler is used as an adjunct to gray scale imaging to detect the extrauterine pregnancy separate from the ovary (33).

A search for free fluid should be made in the cul-de-sac, over the fundus of the uterus (34), in both paracolic gutters, in the hepatorenal space, and about the spleen (Fig. 28.20). The fluid of hemoperitoneum is often echogenic. The presence of even relatively small amounts of echogenic fluid should alert the examiner to the strong possibility of an ectopic pregnancy, despite the absence of other abnormal findings (35). Small amounts of free, simple, nonechogenic fluid can be normal and do not necessarily indicate hemoperitoneum.

Interstitial or cornual pregnancies are suggested by the eccentric location of the gestational sac within the fundal region of the uterine cavity (Fig. 28.21). The myometrium surrounding the sac may be thin or incomplete, with the gestational sac within 5 mm of the uterine serosa (31,36). The *interstitial line sign*, a thin echogenic line from the endometrial canal to the cornual sac, is a more sensitive and specific finding (37). A high degree of clinical suspicion should be maintained because these pregnancies tend to rupture later than other tubal gestations, often with massive intraperitoneal hemorrhage.

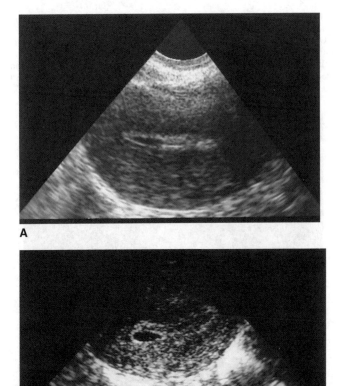

**FIGURE 28.16** Pseudogestational sac versus early IUP. **A:** Small fluid collection within the uterus surrounded by a single echogenic layer in a patient with proven ectopic pregnancy. **B:** For comparison, a <5-week IUP with the double decidual sac sign.

Cervical pregnancies are extremely rare but must be distinguished from an abortion in progress. The gestational sac of a cervical implantation is expected to be round or oval, fixed in the cervical canal and may contain a yolk sac or embryo; a mobile, collapsed or crenated sac would suggest spontaneously aborting products of conception (38).

## PELVIC INFLAMMATORY DISEASE

Pelvic inflammatory disease (PID) is a multimicrobial ascending infection of the female upper genital tract and adjacent pelvic spaces. Prompt recognition and treatment are needed to decrease long-term sequelae of chronic pain and inflammation, infertility secondary to adhesions, and increased risk of future ectopic pregnancy as a result of tubal scarring.

Once the diagnosis of PID is suspected, ultrasound is the study of choice in the emergent setting. The combination of TAS and TVS is able to detect and evaluate the complications of PID. The ultrasound findings of PID will vary based on the degree, duration, and distribution of the disease. In mild cases, the ultrasound may be normal.

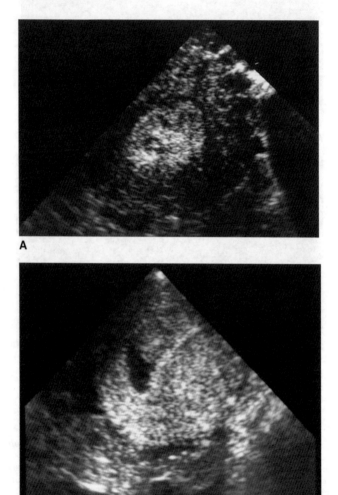

**FIGURE 28.17** Decidual cast of ectopic pregnancy versus spontaneous incomplete abortion. Four different patients. **A, B:** Decidual cast of ectopic pregnancy. *(continued)*

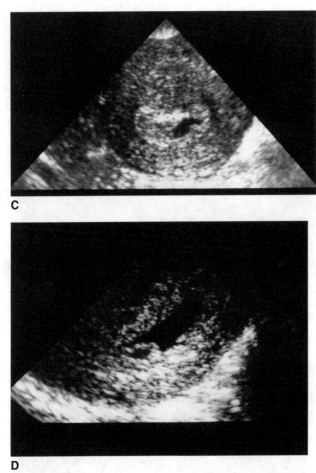

**FIGURE 28.17 (Continued) C, D:** Incomplete abortion. The nonspecificity of the intrauterine findings is quite evident.

### Endometritis

Cases of endometritis are more common after iatrogenic intervention (e.g., cesarean section and dilatation and curettage). Ultrasound findings include endometrial thickening of >12 mm, increased or decreased echotexture of the endometrium with poor definition of its interface with the myometrium, fluid in the endometrial canal, and a poorly defined uterine margin resulting from pelvic exudate or adhesions (39).

### Salpingitis and Tubo-ovarian Abscess

It is uncommon to identify thin, tortuous, normal-sized fallopian tubes. Tubes can be seen when they are filled with or surrounded by fluid. In acute PID, the tubes can be filled with purulent material or blood (pyosalpinx [Fig. 28.22] or

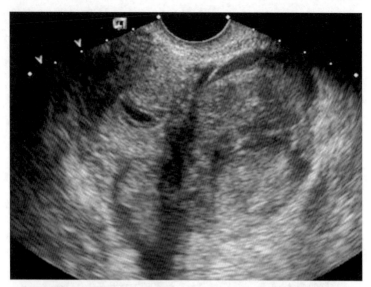

**FIGURE 28.18** Ectopic pregnancy: nonspecific adnexal mass. Transverse image shows a large, complex, predominantly solid mass in the left adnexa. The uterus contains a small amount of fluid. Left ectopic pregnancy was found at surgery.

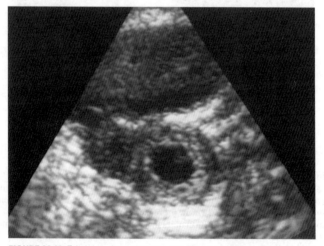

**FIGURE 28.19** Tubal ring of ectopic pregnancy. Transvaginal image shows an echogenic ring <2 cm in diameter found to be a tubal pregnancy at surgery.

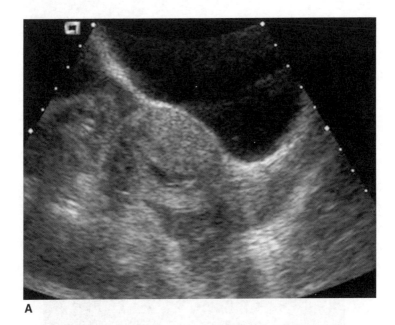

A

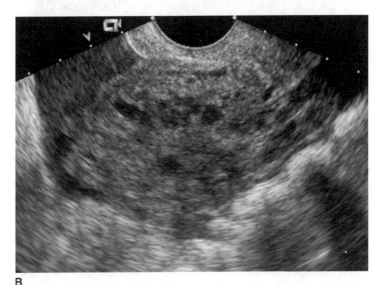

B

**FIGURE 28.20** Hemoperitoneum. **A:** Sagittal scan shows echogenic fluid in the cul-de-sac and between the uterine fundus and the bladder. **B:** Echogenic fluid adjacent to adnexal mass in patient with proven ectopic pregnancy. *(continued)*

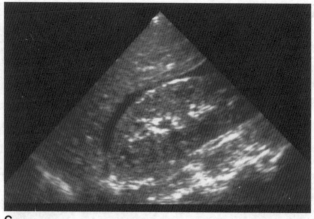

C

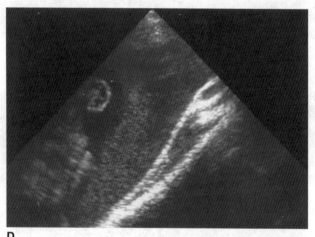

D

**FIGURE 28.20 (Continued) C:** Free fluid between the liver and the right kidney in Morison's pouch. **D:** Image of right iliac fossa shows bowel loops floating in echogenic fluid.

hematosalpinx). On ultrasound, one can recognize the enlarged tube as a serpiginous dilated continuous tubular structure with diffuse internal echoes, which sometimes layer. The process is often bilateral. On occasion, nodular excrescences representing salpingeal fold remnants can be seen (40). After treatment, and with time and proteolysis, the pyosalpinx/hematosalpinx can completely resolve or convert to a hydrosalpinx (Fig. 28.23), which is a dilated, water-filled tube. On ultrasound, this appears as a dilated anechoic tube with a well-defined wall. Color Doppler and real-time observation help to differentiate dilated tubes from dilated pelvic veins or peristalsing bowel.

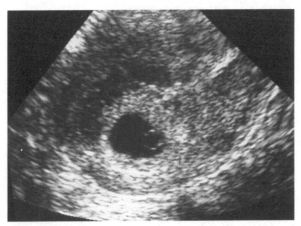

**FIGURE 28.21** Interstitial ectopic pregnancy. A highly echogenic ring surrounding the gestational sac eccentrically located in the periphery of the fundal portion of the uterus. Myometrium extends incompletely about the ring and the endometrial echo points directly to the ring (interstitial line sign). Note the yolk sac within the gestational sac. (Courtesy of Maribel U. Lockwood)

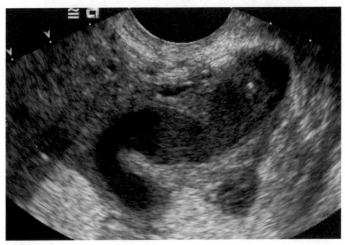

**FIGURE 28.22** Pyosalpinx. Tubular adnexal structure containing low-level echoes immediately adjacent to the ovary.

Although the ovaries are relatively resistant to infection, oophoritis and tubo-ovarian abscesses (TOAs) do occur. Oophoritis is characterized on ultrasound as enlarged globular and multicystic ovaries. Leakage of purulent material results in pelvic inflammation and adhesions. Eventually, if the process is untreated or inadequately treated, the dilated tubes and enlarged cystic

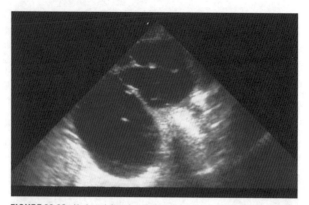

**FIGURE 28.23.** Hydrosalpinx. Anechoic tubular and tortuous structure in the adnexal region. Good through transmission of sound is indicative of its fluid content.

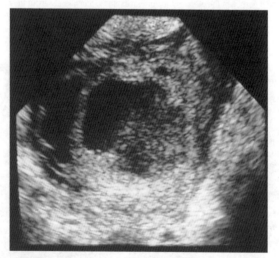

**FIGURE 28.24** Tubo-ovarian abscess. Complex adnexal mass with solid and cystic components. The cystic components contain internal echoes consistent with pus. (Courtesy of Maribel U. Lockwood)

ovaries become a large indistinguishable mass known as a TOA (Fig. 28.24). These masses can have a variable ultrasound appearance ranging from nearly solid to unilocular or multilocular cystic lesions with or without thick walls or fluid–fluid levels. An echogenic focus with "dirty" posterior acoustical shadowing in the TOA represents gas. A TOA cannot be differentiated from a pelvic abscess of nongynecologic origin. Without clinical history, ovarian neoplasm, ectopic pregnancy, and endometriomas can also be confused with a TOA.

CT, although rarely used in initial evaluation, may be useful if there is a concern about an abscess of another source or a TOA poorly responsive to antibiotic therapy. These abscesses may require percutaneous or surgical drainage.

## OVARIAN TORSION

Torsion of the ovary is seen most commonly in young women and girls with ovarian cysts, tumors, and other masses (41), but it may also be seen in patients with normal ovaries (42,43). Sonographic findings are nonspecific, but usually, an adnexal mass, either complex or predominantly cystic, can be demonstrated (Fig. 28.25). If the ovary is identified, it is enlarged and may have multiple

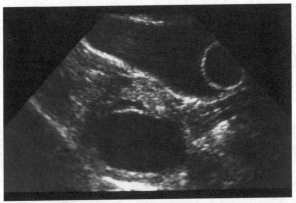

**A**

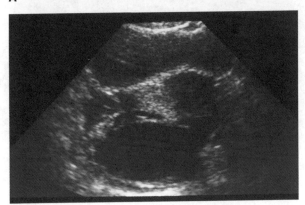

**B**

**FIGURE 28.25** Ovarian torsion in a 15-year-old female. **A:** Longitudinal transabdominal scan. **B:** Transverse transabdominal scans. Complex, predominantly cystic mass within the cul-de-sac and slightly to the right. Note balloon of Foley catheter within the urinary bladder. At surgery, a 6-cm blue necrotic mass compatible with torsion was found in the cul-de-sac originating from the left adnexa.

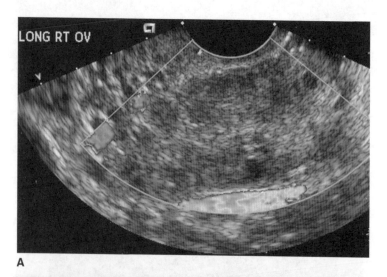

A

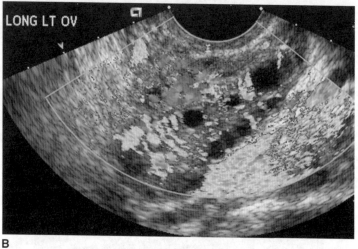

B

**FIGURE 28.26** Right ovarian torsion. **A:** Color Doppler shows no flow within the right ovary. **B:** Compare color flow in normal left ovary. (Courtesy of Douglas L. Brown)

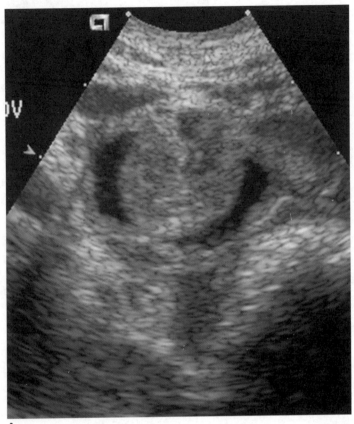

**A**

**FIGURE 28.27** Whirlpool sign of ovarian torsion. **A:** Adnexal mass. *(continued)*

prominent peripheral follicles, presumably from transudation of fluid from vascular congestion (44). Color Doppler may be useful if no flow is detected within the torsed ovary (Fig. 28.26) or if the *whirlpool sign*, a swirl of vessels in the adnexal region, is present (Fig. 28.27) (45). However, vascular flow, both arterial and venous, can be detected in ovarian torsion due to the dual arterial blood supply to the ovary. This must be kept in mind when considering this diagnosis (46).

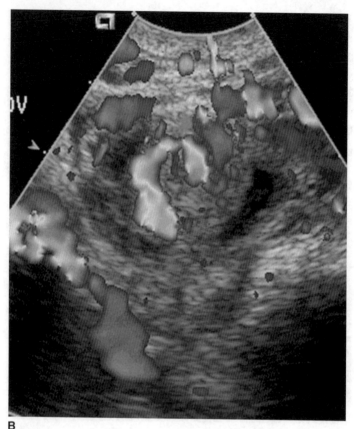

**B**

**FIGURE 28.27 (Continued) B:** Color Doppler reveals swirling configuration of blood vessels in the mass. At surgery, ovarian pedicle was twisted 10 to 12 times.

## RUPTURED OVARIAN CYST

A patient with a ruptured cyst may have extreme pain, clinically similar to torsion. The collapsed cyst may or may not be visualized on ultrasound examination. Hemoperitoneum, identical in appearance to that from a ruptured ectopic pregnancy, can be present (47).

## REFERENCES

1. Dashefsky SM, Lyons EA, Levi CS, Lindsay DJ. Suspected ectopic pregnancy: endovaginal and transvesical. *Radiology.* 1988;169:181–184.
2. Tessler FN, Schiller VL, Perrella RR, Sutherland ML, Grant EG. Transabdominal versus endovaginal pelvic sonography: prospective study. *Radiology.* 1989;170:553–556.
3. Mendelson EB, Bohm-Velez M, Joseph N, Neiman HL. Gynecologic imaging: comparison of transabdominal and transvaginal sonography. *Radiology.* 1988;166:321–324.

4. Lande IM, Hill MC, Cosco FE, Kator NN. Adnexal cul-de-sac abnormalities: transvaginal sonography. *Radiology*. 1988;166:325–332.

5. Coleman BG, Arger PH, Grumback K, et al. Transvaginal and transabdominal sonography: prospective comparison. *Radiology*. 1988;168:639–643.

6. Moore KL. The beginning of development: the first week. In: Moore KL, ed. *The Developing Human: Clinically Oriented Embryology*. 4th Ed. Philadelphia, PA: WB Saunders; 1988:13–37.

7. Yeh H-C, Goodman JD, Carr L, et al. Intradecidual sign: a ultrasound criterion of early intrauterine pregnancy. *Radiology*. 1986;161:463–467.

8. Levi CS, Lyons EA. The first trimester. In: Rumack CM, Wilson SR, Charboneau JW, eds. *Diagnostic Ultrasound*. St. Louis, MO: Elsevier Mosby; 2005:1076–1077.

9. Nyberg DA, Filly RA, Filho DLD, Laing FC, Mahony BS. Abnormal pregnancy: early diagnosis by US and serum chorionic gonadotropin levels. *Radiology*. 1986;158:393–396.

10. Nyberg DA, Mack LA, Laing FC, Jeffrey RB. Early pregnancy complications: endovaginal sonographic findings correlated with human chorionic gonadotropin levels. *Radiology*. 1988;167:619–622.

11. Levine D. Ectopic pregnancy. In: Callen PW, ed. *Ultrasonography in Obstetrics and Gynecology*. 5th Ed. Philadelphia, PA: Saunders Elsevier; 2008:1022–1024.

12. Bree RL, Edwards M, Bohm-Velez M, Beyler S, Robert J, Mendelson EB. Transvaginal sonography in the evaluation of normal early pregnancy: correlation with HCG level. *Am J Roentgenol*. 1989;153:75–79.

13. Nyberg DA, Laing FC, Filly RA, et al. Ultrasonographic differentiation of the gestational sac of early intrauterine pregnancy from the pseudogestational sac of ectopic pregnancy. *Radiology*. 1983;146:755–759.

14. Nyberg DA, Mack LA, Harvey D, Wang K. Value of the yolk sac in evaluating early pregnancies. *J Ultrasound Med*. 1988;7:129–135.

15. Jain KA, Hamper UM, Sanders RC. Comparison of transvaginal and transabdominal sonography in the detection of early pregnancy and its complications. *Am J Roentgenol*. 1988;151:1139–1143.

16. Filly RA. Ectopic pregnancy: the role of sonography. *Radiology*. 1987;162:661–668.

17. Nyberg DA, Laing FC, Filly RA. Threatened abortion: sonographic distinction of normal and abnormal gestation sacs. *Radiology*. 1986;158:397–400.

18. Levi CS, Lyons EA, Lindsay DJ. Early diagnosis of nonviable pregnancy with endovaginal US. *Radiology*. 1988;167:383–385.

19. Levi CS, Lyons EA, Lindsay DJ. Ultrasound in the first trimester of pregnancy. *Radiol Clin North Am*. 1990;28:19–38.

20. Yeh H-C, Rabinowitz JG. Amniotic sac development: ultrasound features of early pregnancy—the double bleb sign. *Radiology*. 1988;166:97–103.

21. Chadkin AV, McAlpin J. Detection of fetal cardiac activity between 41 and 43 days of gestation. *J Ultrasound Med*. 1984;3(11):499–503.

22. Levi CS, Lyons EA, Zheng XH, Lindsay DJ, Holt SC. Endovaginal US: demonstration of cardiac activity in embryos of less than 5.0 mm in crown-rump length. *Radiology*. 1990;176:71–74.

23. Laing FC, Frates MC, Benson CB. Ultrasound evaluation during the first trimester of pregnancy. In: Callen PW, ed. *Ultrasonography in Obstetrics and Gynecology*. 5th Ed. Philadelphia, PA: Saunders Elsevier; 2008:205–206.

24. Laing FC, Frates MC, Benson CB. Ultrasound evaluation during the first trimester of pregnancy. In: Callen PW, ed. *Ultrasonography in Obstetrics and Gynecology*. 5th Ed. Philadelphia, PA: Saunders Elsevier; 2008:208–209.

25. Bromley B, Harlow BL, Laboda LA, Benacerraf BR. Small sac size in the first trimester: a predictor of poor fetal outcome. *Radiology*. 1991;178:375–377.

26. Laboda LA, Estroff JA, Benacerraf BR. First trimester bradycardia: a sign of impending fetal loss. *J Ultrasound Med*. 1989;8:561–563.

27. Kurtz AB, Shlansky-Goldbert RD, Choi HY, Needleman L, Wapner RJ, Boldberg BB. Detection of retained products of conception following spontaneous abortion in the first trimester. *J Ultrasound Med*. 1991;10:387–395.

28. Woodward RM, Filly RA, Callen PW. First trimester molar pregnancy: non-specific ultrasonographic appearance. *Obstet Gynecol*. 1988;55:315.

29. Pennell RG, Baltarowich OH, Kurtz AB, et al. Complicated first-trimester pregnancies: evaluation with endovaginal US versus transabdominal technique. *Radiology*. 1987;165:79–83.

30. Thorsen MK, Lawson TL, Aiman EJ, et al. Diagnosis of ectopic pregnancy: endovaginal vs transabdominal sonography. *Am J Roentgenol.* 1990;155:307–310.

31. Fleischer AC, Pennell RG, McKee MS, et al. Ectopic pregnancy: features at transvaginal sonography. *Radiology.* 1990;174:375–378.

32. Cacciatore B. Can the status of tubal pregnancy be predicted with transvaginal sonography? A prospective comparison of sonographic, surgical, and serum HCG findings. *Radiology.* 1990;177:481–484.

33. Levine D. Ectopic pregnancy. *Radiology.* 2007;245(2):385–397.

34. Nyberg DA, Laing FC, Jeffrey RN. Sonographic detection of subtle pelvic fluid collections. *Am J Roentgenol.* 1984;143:261–263.

35. Nyberg DA, Hughes MP, Mack LA, Wang KY. Extrauterine findings of ectopic pregnancy at transvaginal US: importance of echogenic fluid. *Radiology.* 1991;178: 823–826.

36. Jafri SZH, Loginsky SJ, Bouffard JA, Selis JE. Sonographic detection of interstitial pregnancy. *J Clin Ultrasound.* 1987;15:253–257.

37. Ackerman TE, Levis CS, Dashefsky SM, et al. Interstitial line: sonographic finding in interstitial (cornual) ectopic pregnancy. *Radiology.* 1993;189:83–87.

38. Paspulati RM, Turgut AT, Bhatt S, Ergun E, Dogra V. Ultrasound assessment of premenopausal bleeding. *Ultrasound Clin.* 2008; 345–368.

39. Bowie JD. Ultrasound of gynecological pelvic masses: the indefinite uterus and other patterns associated with diagnostic errors. *J Clin Ultrasound.* 1977;5:323.

40. Abbitt HP. *Ultrasound: A Pattern Approach.* New York, NY: McGraw–Hill; 1995: 379–387.

41. Helvie MA, Silver TM. Ovarian torsion: sonographic evaluation. *J Clin Ultrasound.* 1989;17:327–332.

42. Han BK, Babcock DS. Ultrasonography of torsion of normal uterine adnexa. *J Ultrasound Med.* 1983;2:321–323.

43. Graif M, Itzchak Y. Sonographic evaluation of ovarian torsion in childhood and adolescence. *Am J Roentgenol.* 1988;150:647–649.

44. Graif M, Shalve J, Strauss S, Engelberg S, Mashiach S, Itzchak Y. Torsion of the ovary: sonographic features. *Am J Roentgenol.* 1984;143:1331–1334.

45. Vijayaraghavan SB. Sonographic whirlpool sign in ovarian torsion. *J Ultrasound Med.* 2004;23:1643–1649.

46. Stein MW, Ricci ZJ, Novak L, Roberts JH, Koenigsberg M. Sonographic comparison of the tubal ring of ectopic pregnancy with the corpus luteum. *J Ultrasound Med.* 2004;23:57–62.

47. Salem S, Wilson SR. Gynecologic ultrasound. In: Rumack CM, Wilson SR, Charboneau JW, eds. *Diagnostic Ultrasound.* St. Louis, MO: Elsevier Mosby; 2005:557–558.

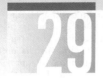# Urogynecologic Emergencies

### Bela I. Kudish and Cheryl B. Iglesia

While urologic emergencies related to gynecology are relatively rare and most are not life threatening, their management should be done in a logical and timely fashion.

## URINARY TRACT INJURY FOLLOWING PELVIC SURGERY

Lower urinary tract injuries (bladder and ureter) accompany <2% of hysterectomies, with bladder injuries outnumbering ureteral injuries five to one (1). Ureteral injuries can result from devascularization, crushing, ligation, or transection and, most commonly, occur at the time of abdominal or laparoscopic hysterectomy (2). Although ureteral injury is a rare occurrence, many injuries are not recognized at the time of initial surgery and present as delayed complications with infection, hydronephrosis, urinoma with subsequent ileus, ureterovaginal fistulas, or silent kidney death. In cases of unilateral ureteral obstruction, patients may present with abdominal and flank pain, fever, and leukocytosis. An ultrasound or intravenous pyelogram showing a dilated renal collecting system will suggest the diagnosis, while cystoscopy with retrograde dye studies will confirm it. If the ureter has been transected, the patient can present with abdominal distention, nausea, vomiting, ileus, or clear vaginal discharge suggestive of a ureterovaginal fistula. Cystoscopy with retrograde ureteral stent placement, ureteroscopy, or percutaneous nephrostomy with antegrade stent placement aided by a fluoroscopic dye study will help localize the site of transection (3). Computed tomography with intravenous contrast material is helpful in assessing an intra-abdominal or retroperitoneal process that may be involved in extrinsic ureteral obstruction or compression. After localization of the ureteral leak or site of obstruction, placement of a percutaneous nephrostomy drainage or transvesical ureteral stenting allows for nonoperative diversion and salvage of the remaining renal function. Complete transections of the ureter require definitive repair (ureteroneocystostomy or bladder reimplantation of the ureter, ureteroureterostomy or end-to-end anastomosis, and bladder mobilization and extension). The choice of method is based on the location of the injured ureteral segment.

In cases when a urinary tract fistula is suspected, the emergency room (ER) provider can utilize the "tampon test" to aid in the diagnosis. This test can also help differentiate between a ureterovaginal and a vesicovaginal fistula. The bladder is filled with 250 mL of indigo carmine-dyed water or saline, and the vagina is inspected for leakage. If no leakage is visualized but the suspicion of a fistula remains high, a tampon can be placed into the vagina, and the patient is then instructed to ambulate for a minimum of 15 to 30 minutes. Observation of the blue dye on the tampon suggests vesicovaginal fistula which can be confirmed with cystoscopy. The presence of nondyed urine in the vagina suggests ureterovaginal fistula. The appearance of a ureterovaginal fistula is usually preceded by a pyelitis, including history of fever spikes and unilateral costovertebral angle tenderness. Intravenous pyelogram and ureteroscopy are diagnostic.

Only physicians with expertise should repair complex ureterovaginal or ureterovesicovaginal fistulas. Vesicovaginal fistulas are amenable to transvaginal repair, while ureterovesicovaginal fistulas require transabdominal or endoscopic surgery with ureteral reimplantation and omental graft superimposition (4). The role of the ER physician is to recognize the possible symptoms of ureteral injury in a patient who has undergone pelvic surgery which may include abdominal distention with ileus and urine ascites; fever, chills, and flank pain; oliguria, pyuria, or hematuria; pyelonephritis or a urinary tract infection not responding to appropriate antibiotics; and a ureterovaginal fistula with continuous vaginal discharge. Treatment for an underlying infection as well as appropriate and prompt urologic consultation is necessary to avoid further loss of kidney function.

## URINARY RETENTION FOLLOWING UROGYNECOLOGIC PROCEDURES

While many pelvic surgeries can lead to acute or subacute urinary retention, urogynecologic procedures, in particular anti-incontinence operations, have the highest incidence of this complication. Patients with urinary retention typically present to the ER with complaints of incomplete bladder emptying, poor urinary stream, dribbling or lower abdominal pain, and bladder distention. These symptoms usually occur in the first few days after the surgery, even though the patient may have documented normal voiding trials and post-void residual volumes. The ER provider must recognize this condition and should attempt to decompress the bladder with a transurethral catheter. An expeditious bladder decompression is necessary to prevent over-distention injury to the bladder. Urinalysis and cultures should be obtained when indicated. In rare instances, such as in the case of an overcorrected repair, a transurethral catheter cannot be passed, and the urologic service should be consulted for cystourethroscopic evaluation and possible suprapubic catheter placement. Transurethral catheters should be placed with caution especially with those who have undergone primary urethral surgery. Medications such as $\alpha$-agonists and anticholinergics can aggravate urinary retention and should be discontinued when possible. In cases of mechanical obstruction, further surgical intervention to include urethrolysis or revision of a suburethral sling may be indicated. Patients with incomplete bladder emptying following urogynecologic surgery should be taught intermittent self-catheterization to avoid complications such as recurrent urinary tract infections and upper urinary tract damage.

## URETHRAL CARUNCLES AND PROLAPSE

Urethral caruncles, small polyps of urethral mucosa protruding through the meatus, are seen almost exclusively in postmenopausal females, whereas urethral prolapse, defined as an eversion of the urethral mucosa through the external meatus, can be found in both postmenopausal women as well as young girls. The two urethral pathologies may be difficult to distinguish from one another. They commonly present with irritative voiding symptoms. Furthermore, it is not uncommon for urethral prolapse to present with vaginal bleeding. Classically, urethral prolapse is described as a fleshy erythematous mass of tissue surrounding the meatus. It occurs in the setting of vaginal atrophy and may be related to repeated straining, trauma, the placement of periurethral bulking agents, or, rarely, urethral tumors (5). Urethral caruncles, in contrast, are focal and not circumferential. The primary treatment for both is topical estrogen cream. The ER provider must ensure that the patient is not obstructed, in which case a transurethral catheter needs to be placed. If the urethral mucosa appears ischemic due to strangulation or thrombosis is noted, then resection of exposed urethral mucosa may be indicated and urologic consultation is recommended.

## BOWEL EVISCERATION FOLLOWING VAGINAL SURGERY

Vaginal evisceration is a rare but serious condition. It has been reported to occur following trauma from intercourse, obstetrical tears, foreign bodies, and vaginal surgery. Most commonly, evisceration will occur following hysterectomy in patients with prolapse, enteroceles, urogenital atrophy, and history of radiation therapy (6). Other predisposing factors include a vaginal cuff left open at the time of hysterectomy and cuff cellulitis or hematoma (7). The distal ileum is most commonly involved in vaginal evisceration (8).

When the patient presents with vaginal evisceration in the ER, the bowel should be wrapped in sterile gauze soaked in saline, and an immediate surgical consultation should be made. Prompt and appropriate surgical intervention is necessary to prevent mortality, which can occur in 6% to 10% of cases due to septicemia and thromboembolism. In general, emergent laparotomy with inspection of the bowel and resection of any compromised areas with reanastomosis is recommended (9). Resection of necrotic tissue at the vaginal cuff and closure of the cuff with interrupted absorbable sutures should be followed by copious irrigation and placement of an appropriate suction drain. Nasogastric drainage may be required for treatment of a prolonged ileus associated with the small bowel resection (10).

## FOURNIER'S GANGRENE

Although rare, Fournier's gangrene is one of the most capricious and deadly urogynecologic emergencies seen in the ER. Fournier's gangrene is an aggressive form of necrotizing fasciitis of the perineum that, even if aggressively treated, can result in death in 22% to 40% of cases (11). It can present subacutely and with nonspecific symptoms before progressing to its fulminant form associated with extensive tissue destruction and systemic toxicity. The diagnosing physician therefore requires a high index of suspicion.

Fournier's gangrene is a mixed infection caused by both aerobic and anaerobic bacteria and occurs most commonly after surgical procedures, after vaginal delivery, or associated with primary perirectal infections. This disease can complicate minor vaginal surgical procedures, such as tension-free vaginal tape placement, or newer larger reconstructive vaginal surgeries utilizing mesh (12,13). Patients with diabetes and peripheral vascular disease are at increased risk. The predominant isolates found in patients with necrotizing fasciitis are *Staphylococcus aureus, Escherichia coli*, group A strepococcus, *Peptostreptococcus* species, *Bacteroides fragilis*, and *Clostridium* species (14).

This infectious process starts in the perineal area or within the vagina with penetration of the gastrointestinal or urethral mucosa by enteric organisms. It is a deep-seated infection of the subcutaneous tissue that results in the destruction of fascia and fat but may spare the skin. These infections begin abruptly, usually with pain over the affected site. In many patients, this initial presentation is overlooked because in postoperative or postpartum patients these symptoms are part of the normal convalescence. Diabetics may present late owing to absence of pain secondary to peripheral neuropathy. Erythema may be present diffusely or locally, but in some patients, excruciating pain in the absence of any cutaneous findings is the only clue of infection. Within 24 to 48 hours, erythema may develop or darken and turn to a reddish-purple color, frequently with associated blisters and bullae. Once the bulla stage is reached, there is already extensive deep soft-tissue destruction, and such patients usually exhibit fever and systemic toxicity including malaise, myalgias, diarrhea, anorexia, and possibly septic shock (15).

The diagnosis is often difficult to appreciate in the early stages. Pain is usually out of proportion to physical findings, and laboratory findings are non-specific. Blood tests may demonstrate leukocytosis with marked left shift and elevations in serum creatinine or creatinine kinase (16). Imaging studies such as soft-tissue x-rays, computed tomography scans, and magnetic resonance imaging are most helpful but may only show soft-tissue swelling and cannot distinguish necrotizing fasciitis from cellulitis or inflammation (17). Gram stain or cultures via punch biopsies at the site are also ineffective in clarifying the diagnosis rapidly, and therefore, aggressive surgical exploration should proceed immediately once the diagnosis is suspected. Any delay increases mortality. The ER personnel should begin broad-spectrum intravenous antibiotic coverage empirically and aggressively treat any evidence of shock with fluid resuscitation. A surgical team should be organized quickly including general surgery, urology, and gynecology to manage these patients appropriately.

## INCARCERATED UTEROVAGINAL PROLAPSE

Stage III or IV uterovaginal prolapse is visible prolapse that protrudes outside the hymenal ring. The term "procidentia" refers to stage IV uterovaginal prolapse or prolapse of the uterus and the cervix with a completely inverted vagina. In rare instances, the prolapse may become impossible to reduce back into the vagina. Women presenting with irreducible or incarcerated prolapse to an office or ER are often older and might have neglected routine gynecologic visits. Additionally, an examining physician may find ulcers or areas of erosion of the exposed vaginal mucosa or cervix. Biopsies of any suspicious ulcerations should be performed to rule out any underlying malignancy.

When evaluating a patient with a prolapse that is difficult to reduce, a full history and an examination should be performed to determine the cause for incarceration—a large palpable bladder stone, fibroid uterus, pelvic mass, or cul-de-sac abscess. The bladder should be emptied initially with a straight catheter which will allow for evacuation of any elevated residual bladder volumes which are frequently found in patients with incomplete bladder emptying because of urethral kinking from the prolapse. Once the bladder has been emptied and no mass has been palpated in the cul-de-sac through a transrectal examination, the prolapse can be gently squeezed to try to decrease the tissue edema. Alternatively, the uterus can be wrapped in bandages soaked in hypertonic saline, and gentle but steady pressure can be applied on the prolapse with the patient in the lithotomy or Trendelenburg position. Knee–chest positioning has also been recommended to reduce intra-abdominal pressure (18). Once reduced, the vagina will need to be packed until an adequately sized pessary is available for placement.

The donut, Gehrung, Gellhorn, ring-with-support, cube, or Inflato-ball type of pessary is typically used for procidentia. A patient with a widened genital hiatus may be unable to retain the pessary and will therefore need either definitive surgical correction or a pessary with concomitant perineoplasty to reduce the size of the hiatus. Alternatively, local anesthesia can be used to place bilateral labial stitches to hold the pessary in place until surgery. Definitive surgical correction, a partial or complete colpectomy or vaginal hysterectomy with subsequent colpocleisis or reconstructive surgery, should be delayed until the tissues have healed and the surrounding infection and edema have resolved. Bladder calculi if found will need to be treated via cystoscopy or cystotomy.

Emergency requiring ICU admission for stabilization and reduction of prolapse to allow for appropriate urine flow may result from acute renal failure secondary to bilateral ureteral obstruction in rare cases of procidentia (19). This obstruction is secondary to distal kinking of the ureters. Unless there is preceding chronic renal disease, these patients generally recover once the obstruction has been alleviated.

## THE NEGLECTED PESSARY

Women using pessaries should have adequately estrogenized vaginas and ideally should remove the pessary nightly. For patients who lack the necessary manual dexterity, a caregiver can remove and clean the pessary two to three times per week, or a health care provider can remove and clean the pessary and inspect the vagina every 8 to 12 weeks. Patients with neglected pessaries will present to the ER with foul-smelling vaginal discharge or vaginal bleeding and, in rare cases, urosepsis (20). The neglected pessary can lead to superficial and full-thickness vaginal erosions from pressure necrosis. These can progress to form vesicovaginal or rectovaginal fistulas. The ER provider must remove the pessary and closely inspect the vagina for evidence of erosion or fistulae. If no lesions are found, the vagina can be cleaned and treated with Trimosan® or other antibacterial creams. The pessary can be replaced once the infection has resolved. Any necrotic tissue should be debrided. Superficial erosions can be treated effectively with topical estrogen cream which should be applied topically for several weeks. If a vesicovaginal fistula is suspected, an indwelling Foley catheter should be placed until surgical correction can be performed. Patients with suspected rectovaginal fistula should also be referred urgently to the appropriate surgical service.

## FECAL IMPACTION

Fecal impaction is one of the most common urogynecologic presentations to the ER and is defined as the inability to pass a hard collection of stool. The risk factors include a history of constipation with decreased colonic motility, poor eating habits, severe rectocele leading to trapping of stool in the rectal vault, and patient immobility. The pathophysiology involves a combination of these factors, which result in stasis of stool and reabsorption of water, leading to hardening of the stool. This is aggravated by continuous colonic motility, which packs the stool in the rectum. Because of the decreased sensation, the rectoanal reflex becomes dysfunctional, leading to an inability to coordinate defecation. The result is a large bolus of hard stool in the rectal vault, leading to obstruction (21).

The patients are generally elderly, institutionalized, and poor historians but often present acutely with symptoms of obstipation including nausea, vomiting, severe abdominal or rectal pain, paradoxical diarrhea, and fecal incontinence. With severe posterior compartment distension, the urinary tract may also be affected and patients may present with chronic urinary tract infections or irritative voiding. A patient history including bowel habits, systemic disease (i.e., diabetes, multiple sclerosis, hypercalcemia, hypothyroidism), dyschezia, or a history of fecal evacuation disorders should be obtained. The need for the patient to use perineal splinting, digital disimpaction, or unusual positions during defecation suggests pelvic outlet dysfunction. If a sensation of rectal fullness predominates, this could indicate rectal prolapse, internal intussusception, or rectocele (22). Physical examination may reveal a distended abdomen and large hard stool in the vault. Occasionally, impaction may be proximal to the reach of a digital examination. If diagnosis is apparent on history and physical examination, and there is no suspicion of an acute intra-abdominal process, and electrolyte abnormalities have been ruled out, these patients can be treated in the ER. Otherwise, a more extensive workup including radiographic evaluation is warranted.

Acute treatment for fecal impaction generally involves digital disimpaction. Using lidocaine gel for local anesthesia, one or, ideally, two fingers are gradually inserted into the rectum and the stool is extracted. This technique may be aided using transvaginal pressure with the opposite hand. Stool may be softened using glycerin suppositories or mineral oil transrectally. Other options include saline and Fleet enemas. If these are ineffective, a rectal tube or Foley catheter can be carefully passed beyond the presenting fecal bolus, and normal saline solution can be injected promixal to the obstruction. Alternatively, oral treatments including magnesium citrate, oral Fleet's, polyethylene glycol, and other nonabsorbable sugars such as lactulose and sorbitol can be used. These agents should be used with caution, in particular, oral Fleet's, which has been reported to cause severe electrolyte disturbances and even death in some patients. Stimulant laxatives such as docusate salts are not as effective for fecal impaction and should not be used in combination with mineral oil on a chronic basis because of the damage this can cause to the myenteric plexus (23).

If fecal impaction can be resolved in the ER, these patients and their caregivers need to be given instruction on prevention. A high-fiber diet with fluids is needed to bulk up stool. The patient should be on a bowel regimen to promote bowel movements at a minimum of every 3 to 4 days. These patients will require close follow-up by their primary care providers, and if fecal impaction persists, further evaluation should be undertaken.

## References

1. Ibeanu OA, Chesson RR, Echols KT, Nieves M, Busangu F, Nolan TE. Urinary tract injury during hysterectomy based on universal cystoscopy. *Obstet Gynecol.* 2009; 223(1):6–10.
2. Jelovsek JE, Chiung C, Chen G, Roberts SL, Paraiso MF, Falcone T. Incidence of lower urinary tract injury at the time of total laparoscopic hysterectomy. *JSLS.* 2007;11(4): 422–427.
3. Liatsikos EN, Karnabatidis D, Katsanos K, et al. Ureteral injuries during gynecologic surgery: treatment with a minimally invasive approach. *J Endourol.* 2006;20(12):1062–1067.
4. Blaivas JG, Heritz DM, Romanzi LJ. Early versus late repair of vesico-vaginal fistulas: vaginal and abdominal approaches. *J Urol.* 1995;153:1112.
5. Harris RL, Cundiff GW, Coates KW, et al. Urethral prolapse after collagen injection. *Am J Obstet Gynecol.* 1998;178(3):614–615.
6. Ramirez PT, Klemer DP. Vaginal evisceration after hysterectomy: a literature review. *Obstet Gynecol Surv.* 2002;57(7):462–467.
7. Cardosi RJ, Hoffman MS, Spellacy WN. Vaginal evisceration after hysterectomy in premenopausal women. *Obstet Gynecol.* 1999;94:859.
8. Kambouris AA, Drukker BH, Barron J. Vaginal evisceration. *Arch Surg.* 1981;116: 949–951.
9. Kowalski LD, Seski JC, Timmins PF, et al. Vaginal evisceration: presentation and management in postmenopausal women. *J Am Coll Surg.* 1996;183(3):225–229.
10. Nichols DH. Evisceration one year after vaginal hysterectomy without colporrhaphy. In: Nichols DH, DeLancey JOL, eds. *Clinical Problems, Injuries and Complications of Gynecologic and Obstetric Surgery.* 3rd Ed. Baltimore, MD: Williams & Wilkins; 1995: 179–181.
11. Lauks SS. Fournier's gangrene. *Surg Clin North Am.* 1994;74:1339–1352.
12. Riedler I, Primus G, Trummer H, et al. Fournier's gangrene after tension-free vaginal tape procedure. *Int Urogynecol J.* 2004;15:145–146.
13. Diwadkar GB, Barber MD, Feiner B, Maher C, Jelovsek JE. Complication and reoperation rates after apical vaginal prolapse surgical repair: a systematic review. *Obstet Gynecol.* 2009;113(2):367–373.
14. Brook I, Frazier EH. Clinical and microbiological features of necrotizing fascitis. *J Clin Microbiol.* 1995;33:2382–2391.
15. Stevens DL. Necrotizing infections of the skin and fascia. UpToDate Version 12.1.

16. Simonart T, Simonart JM, Derdelinckx I, et al. Value of standard laboratory tests for the early recognition of group A beta-hemolytic streptococcal necrotizing fasciitis. *Clin Infect Dis.* 2001;32:E9.

17. Schmid MR, Kossmann T, Duewell S. Differentiation of necrotizing fascitis and cellulites using MR imaging. *Am J Roentgenol.* 1998;170:615.

18. Delancey JOL. Uterovaginal prolapse that is difficult or impossible to reduce. In: Nichols DH, DeLancey JOL, eds. *Clinical Problems, Injuries and Complications of Gynecologic and Obstetric Surgery.* 3rd Ed. Baltimore, MD: Williams & Wilkins; 1995: 147–151.

19. Sudhakar AS, Reddi VG, Shei M, et al. Bilateral hydroureter and hydronephrosis causing renal failure due to a procidentia uteri: a case report. *Int Surg.* 2001;86(3): 173–175.

20. Roberge RJ, McClandish MM, Dorfsman ML. Urosepsis associated with vaginal pessary use. *Ann Emerg Med.* 1999;33:581–583.

21. Wald A. Approach to patient with constipation. In Yamada T, Alpers D, Kaplowitz N, et al., eds. *Textbook of Gastroenterology.* 4th Ed. Philadelphia, PA: Lipincott Williams & Wilkins; 2003.

22. Prather CM, Ortiz-Camacho CP. Evaluation and treatment of constipation and fecal impaction in adults. *Mayo Clin Proc.* 1998;73:881–887.

23. Sloan S. Medical management of constipation In: Brubaker LT, Sclarides S, eds. *The Female Pelvic Floor: Disorders of Function and Support.* Philadelphia, PA: F. A. Davis; 1996.

# Emergency Room Communication Issues: Dealing with Crisis

## Marghani M. Reever and Deborah S. Lyon

The emergency department (ED) is a fast-paced environment dealing primarily with short-term interventions. Because of this setting and the nature of this type of care, the importance of good communication is often overlooked. For female patients, this is a particular concern, especially for women with obstetric or gynecologic health problems. A large body of literature discusses the different communication styles of men and women (1–6). Because of these differences, discussing obstetrics or gynecologic health problems, particularly with a male provider, is likely to be a problematic area. This issue takes on even more importance when one considers that communicating sensitive information in an emergency situation is often limited by the very nature of the setting in terms of continuity, engagement, and educational opportunities. Formal medical education provides limited opportunities to acquire or improve basic communication skills (7–14). Consequently, communicating sensitive medical issues to women in an emergency situation is a skill that is often obtained by experience, sometimes very negative experience.

Even though the problems of gender gap and setting are real, they are not insurmountable. Some thought given to this subject will be amply rewarded with improved personal comfort as well as patient satisfaction and compliance.

## COMMON EMERGENCY SITUATIONS REQUIRING SENSITIVE COMMUNICATION SKILLS

The ED provider will inevitably encounter situations in which sensitive communication skills are important. These situations include such events as fetal death, sexually transmitted diseases, domestic violence, rape, and potentially serious diseases (10,13,15,16). These issues are discussed herein. First, however, thought should be given to the more general aspects of provider–patient communication: process, content, and personality.

## PROCESS ISSUES

Men and women communicate differently. Men tend to be more focused on factual issues and tend to be action oriented. (What are the facts, and what needs to be done?) Women tend to focus more on emotional issues and work out solutions through dealing with the emotional aspects (2). Although these statements are generalizations and there is certainly a significant overlap in communication styles between the genders, the stereotypes are, nonetheless, well supported by research (1–6). To optimize communication with female patients, it may be helpful to consciously identify a communication style that is more emotionally oriented than one might embrace with male patients.

The process by which sensitive information is communicated is important and goes more smoothly if the physician considers some basic issues to be addressed (7,8,11–13,15,17–19). The first important issue to decide is who does the telling. Oftentimes in the ED, the physician does not have an ongoing relationship with the patient and, in fact, may have never seen her before. However, if sensitive information has to be communicated, it is usually better that it originally come from the physician rather than a nurse or a technician. This demonstrates respect for the patient, and for the seriousness of the situation, and bypasses the "I want to speak to the doctor" scenario. Many physicians consciously or unconsciously opt out of difficult or sensitive communication scenarios because they may be time-consuming or because the providers recognize their own inadequacies as communicators. Ultimately, both the provider and the patient are better served by the provider's making a deliberate effort to learn satisfactory communication skills than simply abdicating communication responsibilities.

It is also helpful, if possible, to have some support personnel in the room with the physician. One study indicates that team-based/family communication is preferable to physician–patient dyad communication (20). A social worker or nurse may be the one to provide support once the physician has left, and it may be helpful to make the connection while the unwanted news is being given. It also helps the patient understand that the support personnel have a relationship with the physician. This person may also be able to give the provider helpful insight that will allow further communication skills refinement. At times, it is impossible or impractical for the physician to be the communicator of sensitive news, but this should be the ideal.

After deciding who does the telling, attention needs to be paid to the setting (21). Standing in the middle of the hallway to inform a woman that she has a sexually transmitted disease is not optimal. The preferred setting would be a room (not a curtained cubicle) that is not a high-traffic area and where there is a place to sit. The physician needs to be at eye level with the patient, preferably sitting. Eye contact is important when talking with a patient. (This is a skill that can be formally rehearsed to improve performance.) The physician also needs to communicate to the staff that he or she needs uninterrupted time with the patient or family. Attempting to discuss sensitive information while being interrupted by staff or by a pager going off may increase the patient's anxiety, as well as inspire anger. Uninterrupted time in an appropriate setting is more likely to transmit a sense of care and concern on the part of the physician (22,23). The physician also needs to be conscious of his or her own communication style, including such issues as speed of delivery. Speaking at a slower speed and in a lower tone helps to reduce anxiety. Even though the physician may be feeling enormous pressure to complete the conversation and move on to other tasks, very little time is lost by techniques such as sitting down, pacing the delivery of news, and maintaining appropriate tone and speed of speech. Indeed, time may be saved if patients comprehend information more clearly on the first transmission.

Timing is also important. There is never a good time to present bad news. However, there are bad times to present bad news, such as when the patient or family members have been up all night with no sleep and are fatigued or when a large family group has just arrived and emotions are intense. One cannot always wait for the optimal time, but it is important that this issue be considered. Less urgent tasks such as acquiring consent for autopsy may be deferred until the family has had a chance to recover from the initial emotional blow.

Providing the patient with an opportunity for follow-up questions and clarification of issues is also important. If the physician cannot provide this opportunity, it is imperative that the patient or family members have contact with someone who can answer their questions. This allows closure to the current event and allows the patient or family members to know that someone will be there to help when they have dealt with some of the emotional issues of the situation. Many support groups exist to provide patients with information and assistance beyond what the ED can provide. Contact information for national

**TABLE 30.1** National Agency Support Services

| Agency | Phone Number |
|---|---|
| American Cancer Society | 1 (800) ACS (227)-2345 |
| National Child Abuse Hotline | 1 (800) 422-4453 |
| Sudden Infant Death Support | |
| Compassionate Friends | 1 (877) 969-0010 |
| First Candle | 1 (800) 221-7437 |
| AIDS Hotline | 1 (800) 448-0440 |
| AIDS (SIDA) Hotline (Spanish) | 1 (800) 232-4636 |
| National STD Hotline | 1 (919) 361-8488<br>1 (800) 344-7432 (Spanish) |
| National Sexual Assault Hotline | 1 (800) 656-4673 |
| Rape Abuse and Incest National Network | 1 (800) 810-7440 |
| National Mental Health Association | 1 (800) 273-8255 |
| National Domestic Violence Hotline | 1 (800) 799-7233 |
| National Stroke Association | 1 (800) 787-6537 |
| Endometriosis Association | 1 (414) 355-2200 |

agencies are listed in Table 30.1. It is helpful to have a similar list of local resources available (preferably in a pocket-card format) to all ED physicians.

## CONTENT ISSUES

Content issues might seem more straightforward than process issues, but they may, in fact, be equally difficult when communicating sensitive news. It is important to use terminology that the patient can understand. The patient receiving unwanted news may hear only a small portion of what is being said and may not understand the implications of certain medical terms (15,24). There is also a tendency for patients to nod as though in understanding, thus leading the provider to believe that communication has been successful. The words used by the provider need to be simple and basic to increase the understanding. Do not give too much information too soon. If the patient or family members do not appear to be comprehending the situation, back up, break it down to even smaller portions, and tell it again. The physician may need to repeat the same news a number of times or in several different ways. Open-ended questions ("What do you know about herpes?") are time-consuming but can provide great insight into what information needs repeating or reframing.

The literature indicates that one of the most important issues in receiving unwanted news is that the physician be honest and direct. More times than not, the patient or family members have some idea that there is a potential for bad news and they need to begin to deal with it on an emotional level. It is important to give hope but not false hope (23,25). Sometimes physicians can be vague when communicating sensitive news. This may be due to their own discomfort and is generally not what the patient wants or needs. One way to compromise between withholding information and overwhelming the patient is to let her guide the conversation by asking her questions such as "What would you like to be told about this problem?" or "Do you have concerns about how this might affect you?" (26).

Many physicians are uncomfortable with their own emotions (7,17,24,27–29). When discussing a sensitive medical issue with a patient or family, the physician often attempts to remain emotionally detached. A number of studies indicate that patients and families are more comforted by a physician who demonstrates some emotion. This allows the family members to feel that the physician is engaged in their situation and cares about them. Even having the physician express sorrow can be very helpful to the patient or family, and it may move the statement "We did everything we could" from the realm of defensiveness to one of shared loss and frustration. The physician's showing emotion is not seen as a sign of weakness by the patient or family.

Some physicians are very uncomfortable when the patient or family members have intense emotions. They may attempt either to squelch the expression of the emotions or to remove themselves from the emotional environment. But it is important to allow the patient or family members to express themselves. Becoming comfortable with the emotions of others takes practice but allows providers a much broader scope of healing than would otherwise be possible.

The most important skill that a physician can acquire in dealing with sensitive news is the ability to listen. By listening, the physician communicates respect, caring, and empathy. In addition, it provides the physician with direction as to where the conversation needs to go. Most people complain more about not being listened to than any other facet of their medical care.

## PERSONALITY ISSUES

All individuals involved in a communication situation bring aspects of their personalities to the interaction. Physicians need to be aware of their own personality type, as well as the type of personality they are dealing with, when communicating sensitive information. The physician, like any other person, has a way of looking at things such as death, the role of the doctor in the treatment process, and appropriate ways of expressing and coping with intense emotion (30). The physician's perspective affects the communication interaction (7). For example, a physician who believes that he or she represents health and wellness may feel a sense of failure when communicating serious illness or death. For a physician who believes that he or she is a facilitator working with the patient to obtain optimal health, the view of illness or death may differ.

In addition to physicians being aware of their own personality issues and belief systems, it is important to understand that each patient's personality affects communication. Not all women express their emotions in the same manner, and if a physician waits until the patient expresses her emotion in the manner that is expected, there may be discomfort and misunderstanding for all parties involved. Some patients are prone to anxiety, which may be expressed in several ways such as crying, anger, and pacing. Although it is not possible for an ED provider to know patients the way a primary care provider does, some attempts to identify the patient's personality type and needs will be rewarded with greatly enhanced communication patterns.

Another factor that needs to be considered is the patient's social/cultural environment. Having some information about what is going on in the patient's life may facilitate the communication that will take place. For example, if a woman has been attempting to have children for several years and has experienced a fetal death, her reaction may be much different from that of a woman who was not aware of being pregnant and has experienced a spontaneous abortion.

If a woman is going through a conflictual divorce, her reaction to any bad news may be compounded by her already fragile emotional state. The level of support that an individual receives from other sources such as family, clergy, and friends will also greatly impact her ability to receive sensitive communication. Even though the ED physician cannot know all these things, it is helpful simply to remember that there is a social/cultural context affecting the transmission and interpretation of information (25).

Furthermore, patients may have mental health issues in addition to their presenting complaints, and the mental health issues can sometimes overshadow the physical ones. Two categories of mental illness are of particular concern to the ED physician caring for women. The first is schizophrenia. Patients with this diagnosis often have difficulty establishing ongoing relationships and thus may receive most or all of their health care in the emergency setting. These patients' noncompliance with prescribed care regimens and their disordered and often disruptive thought processes can be extremely frustrating. Obviously, every effort should be made to establish a connection with a mental health professional. It may also be of some help to have the consultant to whom the patient will be referred for ongoing care of the problem actually come to the ED and begin establishing a relationship with the patient. This may make it easier for her to muster the trust necessary to continue her care regimen in a conventional fashion.

The second mental health disorder of particular significance to women's caregivers is borderline personality disorder. This Axis II disorder is three times more common in women than in men (31) and often goes undiagnosed. It is not amenable to treatment, but the highly disruptive effects of a borderline "acting out" can be contained if the provider is alert to the possibility of the diagnosis. Women with borderline personality disorder are extremely seductive, although this may not be enacted as sexual behavior. They may be victims, ceaseless caregivers, lost newcomers, or any other role calculated to win sympathy and special treatment. They are often excessively flattering regarding their current care situation, while being vituperative in their denunciation of the previous caregiver who somehow failed them. Underlying all actions of patients with borderline personality disorder is the insatiable need for attention. Even though initially interactions may be gratifying to providers who are being told that they are marvelous, borderline patients inevitably become disillusioned when interactions fail to escalate to what their fantasies lead them to expect. At this point, they may become angry, vengeful, and abusive. And at this stage, the special efforts that physicians may have exerted on these patients' behalf will inevitably be used against them.

The point of mentioning borderline personality disorder is not to discourage genuine care on the part of ED providers. Certainly, there are patients with extraordinary problems worthy of extraordinary care measures. Providers should be alert, however, to patients dressed seductively, those who describe outrageously inappropriate behavior on the part of previous caregivers, or those who actively campaign to elicit sympathy. Providers are particularly cautioned to pay attention to their own interaction style and how that may change from patient to patient. If one finds oneself taking extraordinary measures on behalf of a patient whose needs at face value do not merit such effort, it is best to disengage quickly. Such a patient is best managed by a team approach with the active involvement of a mental health professional, and the physician should never allow the patient to manipulate him or her into being alone with the patient for any portion of a physical examination. Once a borderline patient has been identified, it is best to have chaperonage even for interviews to help contain inappropriate self-disclosures or solicitations.

Unfortunately, the seductive behavior patterns of borderline patients, along with their explosive interaction patterns, tend to make them frequent victims of rape, domestic violence, and battery. Awareness of the patient's underlying personality disorder in no way lessens the tragic nature of these situations or diminishes the need for provider concern and compassionate care. It is vital, however, that providers protect their own interests as well as those of the patient.

## SKILLS FOR SPECIFIC SITUATIONS

### Fetal Death

Emotional response to a fetal death may be influenced by several factors. Gestational age of the fetus is highly likely to play a role. Generally, the more advanced the pregnancy, the more intense the grief reaction. This is true not only because of the expectancy of a live birth but also because of the amount of planning the mother and family have done to welcome a new baby. The more preparation that has been made, the more difficult it is to move on emotionally. Life experiences of the parents may also play a part. Young parents who have experienced very little grief in their lives are likely to respond with greater difficulty to a fetal death than older parents who have had other grief experiences. On the other hand, a woman who has undergone an extensive infertility workup to become pregnant is more apt to experience an intense grief response than a woman whose pregnancy was unintended. Social support is important in helping a mother deal with a fetal loss. Women who have a high degree of social support are more likely to be able to handle the situation better than women who are socially isolated.

The most difficult area to evaluate with regard to grief experience is the importance of the pregnancy to the mother. The issue of planned versus unplanned pregnancy may have an effect on the emotional response. If the pregnancy was unplanned and consideration was given to terminating the pregnancy, feelings of intense guilt may result. Even if the mother felt somewhat ambivalent toward the baby, guilt may result. If the pregnancy was planned and anticipated, the emotional response to the loss is likely to be significant. Each woman is different, and her grief will be acknowledged, felt, and expressed in a unique way. Providers should be aware that a broad spectrum of emotional responses may occur and that many full-blown grief reactions occur after the patient is sent home from the ED. Every effort should be made to ensure both adequate medical follow-up and availability of appropriate emotional support. Most communities have fetal loss support groups, and every patient should be given this information for possible further reference.

### Sexually Transmitted Disease

Communicating the presence of a sexually transmitted disease should be straightforward and matter-of-fact, without expression of judgment. Most patients accept this information without significant emotional reaction, particularly in an urban medical environment. However, for some patients, notification of a sexually transmitted disease such as herpes is devastating. All patients should be approached with the consideration that they may have an intense emotional reaction to the news. Additionally, there has been a dramatic increase in the diagnosis of pelvic inflammatory disease (PID) (10). Women with PID are often not told that it is the consequence of an untreated sexually transmitted disease. This leads to social embarrassment as well as a high likelihood of reinfection if sexual partners or behaviors are not modified. Because of its social and medical consequences, the diagnosis should not be made without careful consideration of a differential diagnosis, and the patient should be informed of the etiology of PID, so that she can make informed decisions regarding her lifestyle habits.

## Domestic Violence

Domestic violence is more prevalent than many would like to acknowledge. The most likely medical arena in which domestic violence will be discovered is the ED. It is very important when discussing the possibility of domestic violence with a woman that the spouse or partner not be in the room. Most victims of domestic violence are unlikely to acknowledge the problem without some probing. One of the barriers to communication between a physician and a victim of domestic violence is the failure of the physician to ask directly about possible abuse (32). Additionally, providing messages to patients that they are worth caring about has been found to be an intervention that is effective in overcoming barriers to women receiving much-needed help (33). This is a situation in which the ability to communicate sensitively is very important.

One of the convenient ways many providers find to have a private conversation with a woman is to establish a standing policy that there will be no family members present in the examination room when a pelvic examination is being conducted on an adult. This allows for an opportunity to talk with the woman without making her partner suspicious. If the partner is reluctant to leave the room, this may be a warning sign.

Questions regarding abuse should be frank and explicit. Many abused women do not consider being slapped or punched by a partner to be abnormal, so specific questions should be asked about the etiology of injuries. Many women also collude to hide abuse, either because of fear of retaliation or because of a genuine desire not to see the partner harmed. If there is a high index of suspicion that domestic violence is occurring but the patient refuses to acknowledge it, information regarding shelters and victims services should be provided in such a way that the woman can secure it for future use. Consideration should be given to making this information available in the waiting room or in the women's bathrooms. Some women will use this information at a later date even if they are not prepared to do so at the time of presentation. Additionally, each state has specific laws regarding suspicion or knowledge of domestic violence. All providers should be aware of the law in their state.

## Rape

Rape or attempted rape is one of the most difficult situations that a woman may experience. The reaction is often far more severe than even that to aggravated assault, in part because rape threatens the deepest sense of self and personal control that most women possess. Research shows that about 12.4% of the estimated 12 million American women who have experienced a completed rape will develop chronic posttraumatic stress disorder (PTSD) (34). Upon the arrival of law enforcement officials, the patient is often drawn into what feels very much like a second assault: first, by having to repeat her story in detail and, then, by being subjected to the most meticulous and invasive medical examination imaginable. The ability to communicate with a rape victim in an empathic and sensitive manner is of vital importance in this situation.

In some cases, it is believed that litigation is absolutely not under consideration and the patient just wants a medical evaluation that is briefer and much easier on the patient and the staff. However, some patients subsequently change their minds and the best time to collect evidence is immediately after the assault, so if there is any potential for litigation, evidence should be collected immediately and following the standard protocol. The patient may be very poorly suited to make this decision immediately following an assault. It is the job of the provider, in this case, to be the patient's advocate in assessing the opportunity for improving litigation outcome versus the immediate cost to the patient.

Careful communication with the victim is vital. As with any severe emotional trauma, patients who are victims of rape may not be able to hear or understand information or instructions. It is important that all information be presented often and in many different ways, so that the patient can absorb it. The patient should be informed of what is to happen next at each phase of the examination, and whenever possible, she should be given choices about her examination and treatment. This begins to restore some sense of control for her. Particularly if the protocol involves plucking hair or scraping nails, the patient should be allowed to do this herself rather than have medical providers virtually reenact her assault. Psychomotor retardation is common in sexual assault victims and can be maddening to busy providers, but the patient must be allowed to move at her own pace.

Law enforcement officials often have their own agendas regarding reporting of sexual assault. They may push for access to the patient before she has been fully evaluated or before she is emotionally able to communicate with them. Again, the provider may need to serve as the patient's advocate in controlling access to her.

### Potentially Serious Diseases

Patients do not often receive first notification of a serious or life-threatening disease in the ED. However, they do sometimes come to the ED shortly after receiving the news. Kubler-Ross, in her book *On Death and Dying* (35), discusses the five stages of grief (anger, denial, depression, bargaining, and acceptance) and notes that patients may move often and at varying speeds back and forth through each of these. It is expected that patients given the news that they have a serious disease will begin to traverse these stages almost immediately. The ED physician is unlikely to know where a particular patient is in her grief process. It is therefore in the best interest of the patient and the provider to consider consulting the treating physician early in the patient's ED assessment, regardless of her presenting complaint.

If the ED physician is the first person to share the news of a serious or life-threatening disease, the following process should be considered. Never lie. Acknowledge that a limited knowledge base about the problem exists and provide enough information to get the patient to the next level of care. It is important for the ED physician not to overstep his or her knowledge base, although the patient or family may press for such information. For example, if a patient says she has been told that she has pancreatic cancer, she should not be told that she has only 6 months to live. The information may or may not be true and will not be helpful regardless. As much optimism as should be expressed as the situation will allow, along with the repeated emphasis that prompt treatment by the best qualified specialist is vital to the patient's emotional as well as physical well-being. If possible, the patient should be associated with the next level of care before leaving the ED. This connection is potentially the most important thing that the ED physician can do for the patient.

### Other Communication Issues

When a patient receives serious news, there is almost always some follow-up needed. If there is follow-up medical treatment, an appointment should be made before the physician ends the communication, if possible. If there has been a death, the patient or family will need to know what to do next. Many times, the patient or family is in emotional shock and can only understand the most basic of instructions. Some people have never dealt with death before and have no idea as to the process of dealing with funeral arrangements, hospice care, do-not-resuscitate orders, or other complex instructions. It should be the ethical commitment of the medical staff to ensure connection to someone who can direct the patient or family through whatever process is necessary. The worst thing that can happen to a patient is to feel that she has been abandoned.

Patients also benefit from having access to support opportunities (36). If a social worker is assigned to the ED, he or she should be involved as soon as possible. There are many groups that have been developed to help with specific traumatic situations. They include such organizations as support groups for those who have lost a spouse or a child, cancer support groups, and support for victims of domestic violence. These support groups also help the patient get answers to all her questions regarding her situation. If possible, all ED personnel should have a laminated information card with basic information regarding available support services. The ED staff can then be prepared to make prompt, appropriate referrals.

Another aspect of communicating sensitive information is dealing with support persons and family members. Much of the literature regarding communicating bad news revolves around how much should be told and to whom. When possible, ask the patient. She not only has the right to know what is going on with her health but also has the right to decide who else has access to that information (37). Extended families may improve a patient's support structure, but there is also a higher potential for conflict and chaos. A clear understanding of the patient's desires can allow safety in the minefield of such conflicts. On the other hand, the litigation fears inherent in modern medicine often inhibit warm communication with needy family members. The physician is well advised to temper confidentiality concerns with good judgment in deciding who is informed of difficult news. If the patient has no support system, the physician may do well to inquire if he or she can contact the hospital social worker or a member of the clergy to be involved in the situation.

## SUMMARY

The ED is a particularly difficult environment for learning or maintaining good communication skills. It is also, however, a place where those skills are most highly valued. Attention to the more global aspects of patient care is essential to ensure compliance, continuity, and patient satisfaction. The skills necessary may not be intuitive, and almost certainly were not taught or emphasized in medical school, but can be learned if they are valued by the caregiver. Many sources are available from which to learn these skills, including textbooks, references cited here, and good mentoring from a clinician respected for his or her ability to communicate. Such effort will be amply rewarded by generally shorter, less conflictual patient interactions and by better patient compliance with prescribed therapy. Resources are available for patient support and should be liberally used.

## References

1. Griffin EM. *A First Look at Communication Theory.* New York, NY: McGraw-Hill; 1994.
2. Gray J. *Men Are from Mars, Women Are from Venus.* New York, NY: Harpercollins; 1992.
3. Hickson ML, Stacks DW. *Nonverbal Communication: Studies and Applications.* Madison, WI: Brown & Benchmark; 1985.
4. Horn S. *Tongue Fu! How to Deflect, Disarm and Defuse Any Verbal Conflict.* New York, NY: St. Martin's Press; 1996.
5. Mulac A, Bradac JJ, Gibbons P. Empirical support for the gender-as-culture hypothesis: an intercultural analysis of male/female language differences. *Hum Commun Res.* 27:121–152.
6. Tannen D. *You Just Don't Understand: Women and Men in Conversation.* New York, NY: Morrow; 1990.
7. Chisolm CA, Pappas DJ, Sharp MC. Communicating bad news. *Obstet Gynecol.* 1997;90:637–639.

8. Fallowfield L. Giving sad and bad news. *Lancet.* 1993;341:476–478.

9. Gallup DG, Labudovich M, Zambito PR. The gynecologist and the dying cancer patient. *Am J Obstet Gynecol.* 1982;144:154–161.

10. Lichter ED. Obstetrics and gynecology in the emergency room: a teaching opportunity. *Obstet Gynecol.* 1987;70:936–937.

11. Miranda J, Brody RV. Communicating bad news. *West J Med.* 1992;156:83–85.

12. Travaline JM. Communication in the ICU: an essential component of patient care; strategies for communicating with patients and their families. *J Crit Illn.* 2002;17(11): 451–456.

13. Vandekieft GK. Breaking bad news (discussion of preparation and techniques). *Am Fam Phys.* 2001;64(12):1975–1978.

14. Rappaport W, Witzke D. Education about death and dying during the clinical years of medical school. *Surgery.* 1993;113:163–165.

15. Girgis A, Sanson-Fisher RW. Breaking bad news 1: current best advice for clinicians. *Behav Med.* 1998;24(2):61–72.

16. Heggar A. Emergency room: individuals, families and groups in trauma. *Soc Work Health Care.* 1993;18:161–168.

17. Krahn GL, Hallum A, Kime C. Are there good ways to give bad news? *Pediatrics.* 1993;91(3):578–582.

18. Michaels E. Doctors can improve on the way they deliver bad news, MD maintains. *Can Med Assoc J.* 1992;146:564–566.

19. Sharp MC, Strauss RP, Lorch SC. Communicating medical bad news: parents' experiences and preferences. *J Pediatr.* 1992;121:539–546.

20. Wittenberg-Lyles EM, Goldsmith J, Sanchez-Reilly S. Communicating a terminal prognosis in a palliative care setting: deficiencies in current communication training protocols. *Soc Sci Med.* 2008;66(11):2356–2365.

21. Ptacek JT, Ptacek JJ. Patients' perceptions of receiving bad news about cancer. *J Clin Oncol.* 2001;19(21):4160–4164.

22. Ambuel B, Mazzone MF. Breaking bad news and discussing death. *Prim Care.* 2001; 28(2):249–267.

23. Meert KL, Eggly S, Pollack M, et al. National Institute of Child Health and Human Development Collaborative Pediatric Critical Research Network. Parents' perspectives on physician-parent communication near the time of a child's death in the pediatric intensive care unit. *Pediatr Crit Care Med.* 2008;9(1):2–7.

24. Creagan ET. How to break bad news and not devastate the patient. *Mayo Clin Proc.* 1994;60:1015–1017.

25. Metzger-Ngo Q, August KJ, Srinivasan M, Liao S, Meyskens FL Jr. End-of-life care: guidelines for patient-centered communication. *Am Fam Physician.* 2008:77(2): 167–174.

26. Lyon DS, Lyon D, Benrubi G, Reever M. The gynecologist and the dying patient. *Glob Libr Women's Med.* 2008; doi: 10.3843/GLOWM.10426.

27. Charlton R. Breaking bad news. *Med J Aust.* 1992;157:615–621.

28. Dosanjh S, Barnes J, Bhandari M. Barriers to breaking bad news among medical and surgical residents. *Med Educ.* 2001;35(3):197–205.

29. Ptacek JT, Fries EA, Eberhardt TL, Ptacek JJ. Breaking bad news to patients: physicians' perceptions of the process. *Support Care Cancer.* 1999;7(3):113–120.

30. Moyer T. Code of denial. *Discover Science, Technology and the Future.* Published online 1 October 1999.

31. American Psychiatric Association. *Diagnostic and Statistical Manual of Mental Disorders.* 4th Ed. Washington, DC: American Psychiatric Association; 1994.

32. Rodriguez MA, Sheldon WR, Bauer HM, Perez-Stable EJ. The factors associated with disclosure of intimate partner abuse to clinicians. *J Fam Pract.* 2001;50:338–344.

33. Gerbert B, Caspers N, Milliken N, Berlin M, Bronstone A, Moe J. Interventions that help victims of domestic violence. *J Fam Pract.* 2000;49:889–895.

34. Resnick HS, Kilpatrick DG, Dansky BS, Saunder BE, Best CL. Prevalence of civilian trauma and posttraumatic stress disorder in a representative national sample of women. *J Consult Clin Psychol.* 1993;61(6):984–991.

35. Kubler-Ross E. *On Death and Dying.* New York, NY: Macmillan; 1973.

36. Ptacek JT, Eberhardt TL. Breaking bad news: a review of the literature. *JAMA.* 1996;276:496–502.

37. Asai A. Should physicians tell patients the truth? *West J Med.* 1995;163:36–39.

*Note:* Page numbers followed by *f* indicate figure; those followed by *t* indicate table.